Caring for Older Adults Holistically

SIXTH EDITION

Tamara R. Dahlkemper, MSN, CNE
Associate Professor
School of Nursing
Weber State University
Ogden, Utah

F.A. Davis Company • Philadelphia

F. A. Davis Company
1915 Arch Street
Philadelphia, PA 19103
www.fadavis.com

Printed in the United States of America

Last digit indicates print number: 10 9 8 7 6 5 4 3 2 1

Publisher: Terri Wood Allen
Content Project Manager II: Amy M. Romano
Illustration and Design Manager: Carolyn O'Brien
Electronic Project Manager: Sandra Glennie

As new scientific information becomes available through basic and clinical research, recommended treatments and drug therapies undergo changes. The author(s) and publisher have done everything possible to make this book accurate, up to date, and in accord with accepted standards at the time of publication. The author(s), editors, and publisher are not responsible for errors or omissions or for consequences from application of the book, and make no warranty, expressed or implied, in regard to the contents of the book. Any practice described in this book should be applied by the reader in accordance with professional standards of care used in regard to the unique circumstances that may apply in each situation. The reader is advised always to check product information (package inserts) for changes and new information regarding dose and contraindications before administering any drug. Caution is especially urged when using new or infrequently ordered drugs.

Library of Congress Cataloging-in-Publication Data

Caring for older adults holistically / [edited by] Tamara R. Dahlkemper. — Sixth edition.
    p. ; cm.
  Includes bibliographical references and index.
  ISBN 978-0-8036-4549-3
  I. Dahlkemper, Tamara R., editor.
  [DNLM: 1. Geriatric Nursing—methods. 2. Aging—physiology. 3. Geriatric Assessment—methods. 4. Holistic Nursing—methods. WY 152]
  RC954
  618.97'0231—dc23
                                          2015032631

This book is dedicated to
Dr. Mary Ann Anderson the
original author of this book.
She was my mentor
and my friend.

Preface

The book is a postmodern book, with content designed to assist students to enter the postmodern era of nursing. Students will study Dr. Jean Watson's Theory of Human Caring, Maslow's Hierarchy of Needs, and other current or well-established theories that will enhance their practice. Unique to this book is information on Gerotranscendence, transitions and caring theories designed for gerontological practice.

The foundation of this book is that of critical thinking. It is full of compelling questions that illustrate what it is to be a nurse. The critical thinking assignments draw the reader into the realm of wondering, "what if . . . ?" rather than thinking "this is . . ." It is designed to be reader friendly in that it conveys a feeling of conversation with a group of wise nurses who care deeply about nursing and its participants. This book also conveys a deep respect for every person who provides the most valuable kind of care, that art of caring for those who have gone before us and made the world a better place because of their effort; the elderly.

New to this edition is information focused on QSEN and Evidence-based practice. This edition also includes a new chapter on Safety. Each chapter has a presentation on what should be the priority focus of the chapter and assignments that can be done in or out of class, if the teacher chooses to use them. Chapter Concepts are now identified at the beginning of every chapter, to support use of this text in programs with concept-based curricula.

There is ample opportunity for students to use the case studies, critical thinking activities, review questions and other web-based interactive media to enhance their learning. For the faculty there are PowerPoint presentations and a well-developed test bank located on DavisPlus.

Registered nurses, who maintain a clinical practice and value the role of the licensed practical/vocational nurse (LPN/LVN), wrote this book. The purpose of this book is to assist the future nurse to give informed and holistic care to the growing population of elderly persons who have the courage to live.

Contributors

Vickie Anderson, RN, CIC
Infection Control Coordinator
Intermountain Health Care
Salt Lake City, Utah

Kathleen Paco Cadman, MSN, RN, RAC-CT, CNE
Assistant Professor
School of Nursing
Weber State University
Ogden, Utah

Kathleen R. Culliton, APRN, MS, GNP
Associate Professor
School of Nursing
Weber State University
Ogden, Utah

Richard Dahlkemper, PhD
Associate Professor
Health Administrative Services
Weber State University
Ogden, Utah

Deborah M. Judd, DNP, APRN, FNP-C
Associate Professor
School of Nursing
Weber State University
Ogden, Utah

Diane Leggett-Fife, PhD, RN
Associate Professor
School of Nursing
Weber State University
Ogden, Utah

Susan B. Thornock, EdD, RN
Professor and Department Chair
School of Nursing
Weber State University
Ogden, Utah

Kristiann T. Williams, DNP, APRN, FNP-C
Assistant Professor
School of Nursing
Weber State University
Ogden, Utah

PRIOR CONTRIBUTORS

The following people contributed material to prior editions that was used in this edition.

Judith Pratt, MSN, RN
Associate Professor
School of Nursing
Weber State University
Ogden, Utah

Emily Ravsten, MSW
Thornton, Colorado

Alicebelle Maxson Rubotzky, PhD, RN
Associate Professor
Department of Nursing
Rhode Island College
Providence, Rhode Island

Reviewers

Acknowledgments

I want to recognize the gerontological nurses, in professional practice, who exhibit their caring skills to those who have grown older. The job you do is challenging and requires your very best. Thank you for being willing to do it! I also want to acknowledge the nursing faculty who incorporate concepts related to caring for older adults in their courses. You are teaching the future generation the importance of caring for the older adults in our lives.

I wish to acknowledge F. A. Davis editors Lisa Houck, and Elizabeth Hart and Amy Romano for their patient assistance.

Table of Contents

UNIT ONE | **Foundations of Care for the Older Adult** | 1

Chapter 1 | **Holistic Caring** | 3

Chapter 2 | **The Aging Experience** | 19

Chapter 3 | **Supporting Life Transitions and Spirituality in the Elderly** | 37
Diane Leggett-Fife

Chapter 4 | **The Use of the Nursing Process and Nursing Diagnosis in the Care of Older Adults** | 57
Kathleen R. Culliton

Chapter 5 | **Legal, Ethical, and Financial Considerations Regarding Older Adults** | 89

Chapter 6 | **Promoting Wellness** | 105
Diane Leggett-Fife

Chapter 7 | **Safety** | 125
Kathleen Paco Cadman

Chapter 8 | **Nutrition for Older Adults** | 145

Chapter 9 | **Culturally Specific Care** | 161
Diane Leggett-Fife

Chapter 10 | **Activity, Rest, and Sleep as Criteria for Health** | 181

Chapter 11 | **End-of-Life Issues in Older Adults** | 197

Chapter 12 | **Environments of Care** | 211
Kathleen R. Culliton

Chapter 13 | **Management and Leadership Role of the Licensed Practical/Vocational Nurse** | 225
Susan Thornock

UNIT TWO | **Clinical Practice** | 253

Chapter 14 | **Infection** | 255
Vickie Anderson

Chapter 15 | **Common Medical Diagnoses** | 269

Chapter 16   **Physiological Assessment**   291
             Kathleen R. Culliton

Chapter 17   **Common Clinical Problems: Physiological**   313

Chapter 18   **Psychological Assessment**   333

Chapter 19   **Common Clinical Problems: Psychological**   349

Chapter 20   **Rehabilitation and Restorative Care**   371
             Kathleen R. Culliton

Chapter 21   **Pharmacology and Its Significance
             for Older Adults**   389
             Kathleen R. Culliton

Chapter 22   **Laboratory Values and Older Adults**   409
             Deborah M. Judd

Appendices

Appendix A: **Sample Advance Directives: Living Will and Power
            of Attorney for Health Care**   439

Appendix B: **Answers to Review Questions**   455

Index   457

unit ONE

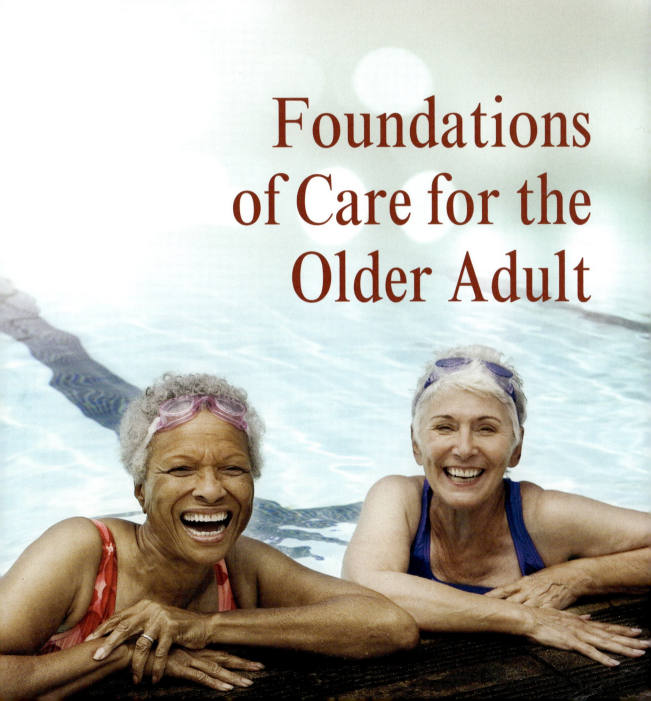

Foundations of Care for the Older Adult

Holistic Caring

TAMARA DAHLKEMPER

CONCEPTS

Advocacy

Caring

LEARNING OUTCOMES

1. Define gerontological nursing.

2. Discuss the current demographics of people older than age 65 years.

3. Write a one-sentence nursing philosophy.

4. Define the word *holism* as it relates to gerontological nursing.

5. Discuss the theory "The Science of Human Caring" by Dr. Jean Watson as it relates to clinical practice.

6. Describe five examples of how you, as a novice nurse, can use Watson's theory as you give nursing care to older adults.

7. Define the concept of "gerotranscendence."

CASE STUDY

You have been out of school for 1 year, and although you have learned a great deal as you have been working, you are aware there still is much to learn. You enjoy your job at the Country Meadows Nursing facility, where you work full-time on the day shift. It is a bright, open place that actually is surrounded by country meadows.

You work on the locked Alzheimer's disease (AD) unit and have learned to love the residents there. Even though there is a great deal of agitated behavior, you understand the phrase, "There is a reason for every behavior." This is because you take the time to observe and listen to residents carefully to understand what is going on inside their minds. Then you act on what you have seen and understood. You seem to do this naturally, based on your knowledge of holistic and caring nursing care, and have received compliments from your nurse manager on your skills.

The nurse manager has hired John, a new certified nursing assistant (CNA), and she has asked you to orient him to your philosophy of care for persons with AD. You have worked with John for two shifts and are concerned about some of his behaviors. You have noticed the following:

1. He consistently calls the residents "honey," "dearie," and "sweetie."

2. He is impatient when the residents are slow in walking, eating, or asking for things.

3. He refuses to learn their names.

4. You noticed one resident who did not have her glasses on or dentures in, and it was 10:00 a.m.

5. He got into an argument with an older man who was confused and wanted to leave the building.

6. He does not listen to you or treat you with respect.

Make a narrative summary of your thinking regarding the following questions. Be prepared to submit your answers to your faculty person. Add more ideas and comments to your paper than what is listed in the solution. Apply the principles you read in this chapter. Expound on the list noted in the solution. Use it as a foundation of thinking only.

■ How does the CNA's behavior conflict with your holistic and caring philosophy?

■ What are you going to do about the problem?

Welcome to gerontology! This is where you will learn information and skills that will assist you in being successful in all areas of nursing. "How can one class touch all segments of health care?" you may ask. "How" is by the simple growing numbers of persons older than age 65 who are living instead of dying. Caring for them is what gerontology is by definition. The growing number of older adults in the United States need, and will continue to need, health care because of the normal consequences of aging as well as the acute and chronic diseases that occur in all age groups. Older adults connect with all age groups, and because of their increasing numbers, we as nurses will be seeing them in more roles than ever before in our history.

 ## GERONTOLOGICAL NURSING

It is important to understand the vocabulary that goes with the speciality of gerontological nursing. The word *gerontological* comes from the Greek words *gero,* meaning "related to old age," and *ology,* meaning "the study of." The word *gerontology* refers to the study of the complex world of human aging. It includes physical, emotional, social, spiritual, and economic considerations. It is an aspect of nursing that impacts all areas of society, including health care resources, politics, housing, education, business, and law making. Another commonly used word is *geriatrics*. The Greek word *geras* means "old age," and the word *iatro* means "relating to medical treatment." The word *geriatrics* refers to the medical speciality that deals with the diagnosis and treatment of elderly adults. The word *geriatrics* is very specific; it refers to medical treatment only. *Gerontology* covers several aspects of need for older adults. This definition is appropriate because of the holistic nature of nursing practice.

If you are a gerontological nurse, you are guaranteed a future in nursing because older adults are the fastest growing segment of the population in the United States. There are elderly people in home health settings, hospitals, homeless shelters, assisted living centers, and nursing homes. People older than age 65 occupy approximately 65% of the beds in acute hospital settings. The percentage of people older than the age of 65 increases in

Priority Setting

As you enter your new profession of licensed practical/vocational nursing, you will be expected to determine priorities that relate to the person receiving care, the environment, and the health-care team, among other things. In each chapter of this book, there will be a box titled "Priority Setting." It will focus on your development as a professional and the management of the priorities of care for the elderly people for whom you are responsible as a nurse. Setting priorities is a challenge. When you are licensed as a practical nurse, you will realize that others expect you to identify and meet the demands of patient-care priorities.

Thoughtfully read the Priority Setting boxes and work to incorporate the priorities identified into your nursing practice. Some may seem simple; others may seem a bit daunting. I want to assure you, though, that all of them are important in your role as an LPN.

Here is your first Priority Setting challenge.

The priority for this chapter is to incorporate within yourself holistic caring because this puts you on the cutting edge of health-care delivery and transforms you into a professional nurse.

As a nurse in the 21st century, you are expected to practice the skills of this profession on the cutting edge. Holistic approaches to care that are guided by what the literature refers to as a *caring ontology* (caring philosophy) are on that cutting edge. Historically, nurses have been very task-oriented. Such nurses carried the notorious list I referred to in the chapter. When everything was checked off the list, the nurse considered his or her work completed. There is more expected in this era of nursing. Everything on the list has to be done, as "the list" contains the critical interventions that will improve the health of the person receiving care—yet it needs to be done within the framework of holistic caring.

You will need to reread this chapter if you finish it and are unsure what the characteristics of holistic caring are.

Why? Because you need to start now and work to incorporate them into your philosophy of nursing and daily practice.

- You must learn to listen to people both verbally and nonverbally.
- You probably need to slow down. Don't rush people or even seem to be in a hurry when with a patient or family. This is especially true of older adults, who may need to do things more slowly because of the process of aging.
- Consider family members and significant others as critical to the care you administer. They need to be involved with every stage of treatment and are a valuable source of information.
- Give your *full* attention to the individual to whom you are giving care at the moment. Consider that person's feelings, personal needs, and strong individuality while you are with him or her. Learn from the individual as you teach him or her, and respect the person for the life that he or she has lived.

These are some of the components of transpersonal caring. Learn to live this concept as you practice your art of nursing.

home health and hospice settings. They are also more frequently present in pediatric and neonatal intensive care units as custodial grandparents for children whose parents are unable to provide appropriate care. You will be relating to and caring for older people throughout your career wherever you work.

Gerontology is a relatively new nursing specialty and has within it certified nurses, clinical specialists, and geriatric nurse practitioners who give care only to people older than age 65 years. There are nurses in the specialty who have a great deal of experience and novice (or new) nurses just like you. Together, all of us, experienced and novice nurses, make a valuable team for the frail and vulnerable older adults in need of nursing care and for the well elderly persons who are focused on health promotion. Gerontological nursing is exciting and varied, and I compliment you for being interested in this area of health care.

Early in my more than 30 years of experience as a registered nurse, I chose to be a gerontological nurse. I made this choice at a time when gerontological nurses were thought to be lesser skilled nurses. "If they were any good, they would be working in the intensive care units (ICUs), wouldn't they?" was a common comment. Fortunately, things have changed.

Gerontological nurses have a specific body of knowledge that they must master (similar to the ICU nurse) to be effective in their practice. For example, did you know that most elderly persons who have heart attacks are less likely to have chest pain? In addition, medication doses for a middle-aged person may overwhelm the systems of an elderly person with devastating results. Aging brings with it stages of life development that are different from any previous stage; gerontological nurses need to know and understand these stages. The knowledge required to give gerontological care needs to be learned, understood, and implemented for the elders in this society to have the best quality of life possible.

In the current health-care environment, people respect gerontological nurses for their multiple skills and abilities. If they don't, those persons may be ageists, or prejudiced against older adults. Ageism has long been a social construct of the United States and is something every gerontological nurse should be willing to work toward eliminating. Who but a nursing-home nurse can pass medications to 42 residents twice in one shift without

This elegant woman represents the growing number of older women in the United States who are living longer than older men.

making a mistake? Who has the skill and knowledge to calm a pacing, agitated older person with dementia by using validation therapy, a communication technique specifically for demented elderly persons? I am proud to be a gerontological nurse and willingly talk to others about how wonderful my career has been because of that choice made long ago to work with older adults.

DEMOGRAPHICS OF AGING

Old age is new. I find that simple statement to be true because of my age. I actually feel the consequences of aging. I am sure many of you reading this book do not notice from week to week or month to month that you are aging. I am 64 years old, have some chronic diseases, and feel them. Growing older is new for every person who experiences it, and it is new for our society as well. In the history of the United States, there never have been so many people older than age 65. The composition of the American population is different today from that of any previous generation.

The numbers of old people previously were small compared with the number of older adults who are age 65 and older today. In the 2002 U.S. census, there were 35.6 million older adults, and they constituted 12.3% of the population. Based on the most recent U.S. census completed in 2010, individuals 65 and older now make up 13% of the population. It is predicted that 19% of the population will be age 65 and older by 2030. In 2002, there were 20.8 million women older than age 65 but only 14.8 million men. In 2010, there were almost 23 million women and 17 million men in that age group. The U.S. Census Bureau also projects that the number of people who are 85 years and older will increase from 4.6 million to 9.6 million by 2030.

What is the makeup of this growing number of older adults? The increase in number is attributed to the group referred to as the "baby boomers," who are people born between 1946 and 1965 after World War II. Baby boomers constitute 30% of the U.S. population. In 2011, the first individuals who turned 65 began applying for Social Security and Medicare. This places federal financial concerns over paying for baby boomer retirement at the forefront.

Besides the sheer number of the aging baby boomers, other reasons for the increased number of older persons in our society include better nutrition, sanitation, and overall living conditions; lower infant mortality rates; and more effective medical management of acute and chronic diseases. There are specific trends, however, related to gender and race. Because more women reach 65 years of age than men, there are more older women than men in the older-than-85 category. This also means there are more single older women than single older men. The U.S. Department of Commerce (2010) states

---

Point of Interest

The increased numbers of elderly people in the United States have resulted in new definitions of aging. The term *young-old* is used for people 65 to 74 years old; *middle-old* is used for people 75 to 84 years old; *old-old* is used for people 85 to 100 years old; and *elite-old* is used for people older than 100 years. It is necessary to define the differences for each age group because of the health needs, medication dosages, and frailty that relate specifically to each age category.

Compare the previous numbers with the fact that, in 1776, when the Declaration of Independence was signed, a child born in the United States had a life expectancy of 35 years. In 1930, life expectancy was 59.7 years; in 1965, it was 70.2 years. Today, the average life expectancy is 81.1 years for women and 76.3 years for men (National Vital Statistics Report, 2012). An older adult who reaches age 65 can expect to live for another 18.1 years, or to reach 82.9 years of age.

Point of Interest

The Bureau of National Health Statistics (2008) lists the following 10 diseases as the leading chronic conditions affecting people older than age 65 years:

1. Arthritis
2. Hypertension
3. Problems hearing
4. Heart conditions
5. Visual impairment
6. Deformities or orthopedic disability
7. Diabetes
8. Chronic sinusitis
9. Hay fever and allergic rhinitis
10. Varicose veins

that there are fewer than 7 men to 10 women in the older-than-65 age group. The current trends show, however, that the ratio of men to women is slowly increasing. Unfortunately, even with the increase in life expectancy, it varies by race. Since the 1980s to the present, the gap in life expectancy between white and black elders has widened because the elderly black population has declined. This decline is attributed to death by homicide and acquired immunodeficiency syndrome (Eliopolis, 2014).

Older adults today have more education and financial resources than ever before in U.S. history. Because they initiated the fitness movement, they are more likely to have regular exercise programs. They also have fewer children to assist in their care.

Less than 5% of older adults live in nursing homes, assisted living centers, and other institutions. That leaves 95% living in homes either alone or with their aging spouses or family members.

 ## NURSING PHILOSOPHY

I love working with older adults because doing so allows me to practice within the framework of my nursing philosophy. My first job was at a Catholic hospital, and I was taught to "Serve the Sick as Though They Were Christ in Person." I embraced that philosophy and still practice it today. When I care for elderly persons in all settings, I am able to give them excellent physical and emotional care as well as to be caring. When I add holism to my caring approach, I have a successful format for delivering quality nursing care within the framework of my nursing philosophy. This book is based on the two concepts of holism and caring, and the purpose of this chapter is to share these critical concepts with you.

Critically Examine the Following

Think about the elderly people (older than age 65) in your family or among your other acquaintances. Identify three people and think about them. Use their name for the heading and list the characteristics of older people, just discussed, that apply to them. What are their race, gender, age, living conditions, general health, source of income, and other factors that contribute to their quality or lack of quality of life? The purpose of this exercise is to assist you in really seeing older adults. If you don't know the answers, go visit the people you chose and ask them just what it is like to be 65+ in the 21st century.

Understanding the diversity and uniqueness of older adults is important to giving them excellent health care. One professional aspect of yourself that will assist you in meeting the objective of excellence is a nursing philosophy.

Have you considered what your nursing philosophy might be? As a beginning nurse, you may not know what a nursing philosophy is, let alone have defined one for yourself. This is a personal concept that has to come from within you. At this point in your career, you may find a philosophical statement that you like, and as you obtain more education and clinical experience, it is something you may change.

I have shared my philosophy with you. It is (1) simple and (2) specific and (3) has great meaning

 ## Point of Interest

Important definitions follow:

1. Medicare: Federal regulations that provide health care for individuals older than age 65 or who are permanently disabled.
2. Medicaid: Federal and state-supported health care for individuals who are financially disadvantaged.
3. Social Security: Federal benefit check paid to retired workers of a specific age, disabled workers of any age, and spouses and minor children of deceased workers.
4. Supplemental Social Security (SSI): Federal benefit check paid to persons older than age 65 or with disabilities that do not allow employment.

for me. These are three characteristics of a valuable nursing philosophy. Let me repeat it: "To serve the sick as though they were Christ in person." Obviously, I am a Christian; this philosophy would not work for someone of a different religion. I suggest you develop your own nursing philosophy to use as a guide and measurement for the work you do in nursing.

Holistic Nursing

The word *holism* or *wholism* is derived from the Anglo-Saxon root *hal,* which means "whole" or "to heal" (Random House College Dictionary, 2008). Its very definition makes the word and its concepts important to the profession of nursing. Holistic care refers to care of the body, mind, socialization, and spirit of the person for whom you are responsible. Holistic care occurs when you, the caregiver, make healing the whole person (all of the person's "parts") your priority. It goes beyond healing a surgical incision and includes all aspects of the individual that need attention so there is a wholeness of the person.

When you examine the career of Florence Nightingale in your nursing history class, it will be apparent to you that she was able to integrate holistic concepts into her personal nursing practice. She considered touch, light, empathetic listening, music, and quiet reflection essential components of good nursing care Dossey & Keegan (2013). If she were not holistic, she would have considered just the soldier's wound and nothing else. You will learn that Nightingale is known as the "Lady with the Lamp." This is because when the other nurses had gone to bed, she would walk through the wards at Scutari with her lamp to check on the wounded; she wrote letters for them; and she spent her own money to buy them fruit and vegetables so they would have better nutrition. These are examples of holistic care.

Holistic nursing is something Florence Nightingale practiced without a textbook or a teacher to explain it to her. How did she, the Mother of Modern Nursing, capture the essence of holism with her patients in Scutari? More importantly, how do we, as modern nurses, accomplish that vision today?

Basic Concepts of Holistic Care

Understanding the concepts of holistic nursing is important for the practice of 21st-century nursing. It is a philosophy that weaves the demanding technical skills of nursing with the social science skills that

enhance the humanity of the nurse and the person receiving care.

The philosophy of holism, which was first formulated in the 1930s, emphasizes the importance of understanding a person's whole being rather than treating only specific parts. When a patient is recovering from a total hip replacement, the patient definitely wants the hip fixed and fixed properly! There may be other needs, however, such as loneliness, fear about being able to live alone again, or a misunderstanding about medications. The person needs more than treatment for the hip.

The philosophy of holistic care should put an end to comments such as "the gallbladder down the hall," which ignores the person and focuses on the illness alone. A holistic identification of the "gallbladder down the hall" should be the person's name or something pleasantly descriptive, such as "the grandmother who knits all of the time."

If you are a holistic nurse, you will take an active role in developing a healing relationship with the patient. This relationship focuses on the

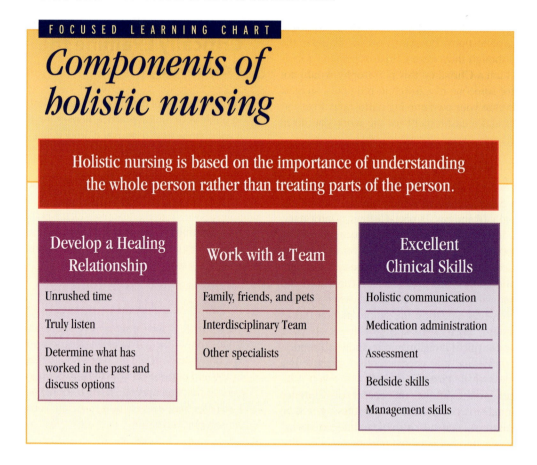

FOCUSED LEARNING CHART

Components of holistic nursing

Holistic nursing is based on the importance of understanding the whole person rather than treating parts of the person.

Develop a Healing Relationship

Unrushed time

Truly listen

Determine what has worked in the past and discuss options

Work with a Team

Family, friends, and pets

Interdisciplinary Team

Other specialists

Excellent Clinical Skills

Holistic communication

Medication administration

Assessment

Bedside skills

Management skills

---

multiple needs of persons who are ill and how they can best be resolved. The critical activity to promote holistic care is listening. This approach encourages people who are sick to be more involved in their care. The nurse should listen to what has worked in the past for patients and discuss their ideas as to what would be best for them in the current situation. The nurse needs to provide an environment in which the patient is able to make decisions that are honored by the health-care team.

Holistic nursing practice can be imple-mented in many ways. Following are four basic concepts:

Rule #1: Always follow the physician's orders. If the patient refuses the treatment or medication ordered, call the physician. That is an excellent way to validate that you are listening to the patient. Be sure to share the patient's concerns with the physician.

Rule #2: You will develop clinical expertise; use it.

Rule #3: Draw on the personal intuition and creativity patients have to resolve their own health problems. You will need to consider the patients' values and life experiences when devising treatments. Remember, all of the older adults you will be giving care to are the survivors; they are the people who did not die, and they are strong and smart and have lived with their body long enough to know what it needs. Can you imagine telling a man who endured imprisonment and torture as a prisoner of war how to manage his postoperative pain? I wouldn't do it. Instead, I would listen to what he had to say about it.

Rule #4: Take every opportunity to develop a closer relationship with family members or significant others. This is your true entry into getting support and assistance for the older person who is ill. You also will learn many things about the patient in your care.

Holistic Care Is Based on Teamwork

The holistic approach to nursing is effective when dealing with most populations, and it is an excellent way to deliver care to older adults. One of the principles of holistic care is that neither you nor the older person is alone. There always is a team of people working for the best outcome for the person needing care.

These teams look very different for each person. Most holistic teams have family members, although that is not always true. Some have a treasured family pet—a very valuable member. Others have an entire health-care team, such as an older adult in a nursing home who has the advantage of an interdisciplinary team. This is a team of professionals, such as a dietitian, physical therapist, nurse, pharmacist, social worker, and others, who work toward the best condition for the resident. They meet at least monthly to discuss each resident, and the resident and family members are invited to attend this meeting.

The premise is that you, the nurse, will work closely with the team members who are most important to the older adult. The focus of the teamwork should be to provide care, health promotion, and, if possible, cure. This means that you will advocate for the 15-year companion, Suzie the dog, to make regular visits to the nursing home. If you have a home health patient who needs

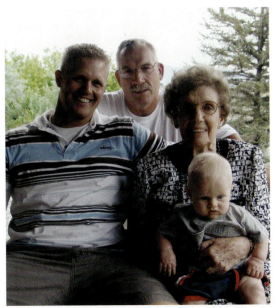

This elderly woman fell and broke her hip 10 days after this picture was taken. Her son and grandson were instrumental in her recovery. Her great-grandson brought her great joy when his parents brought him to see her at the hospital and nursing home.

assistance with getting into bed at night, you need to work to make arrangements with family, neighbors, or friends for the necessary assistance. If the person to whom you give care has six adult children and you get calls from each one each week, you need to be grateful that there are children who are willing to be involved.

A holistic nurse does not wait for the varied team members to come to the nurse. Instead, it is essential to be on the lookout for any sign or mention of the people who will make a difference in the life of the older person. I remember a blind woman who was brought to the hospital for terminal care. She was brought in an ambulance, and consequently none of her personal things accompanied her. She had no children, and her spouse was deceased, but she did have a dear older friend and neighbor. One morning I entered this woman's room and found her crying. With a bit of encouragement, she told me that she missed having her pictures with her. She had several treasured photos of herself and her husband, and she liked to hold them and think about the wonderful life she and her husband had shared. She was blind, right? But she still wanted those pictures! I located her neighbor, who brought her pictures to the hospital. I know that being able to hold her pictures assisted this woman in having a better quality of life before her death. It simply made her happier.

Some nurses would dismiss the need to be concerned about pictures for a blind woman, and others would not take the time to locate her friend. A holistic nurse would do both things because of the reality of caring about *every* aspect of *every* person in his or her care. Holistic care is a powerful concept and works best when complemented by the nursing theory of human caring.

HUMAN CARING

The Science of Human Caring is a nursing philosophy that was developed by Dr. Jean Watson, former Dean and Distinguished Professor at the School of Nursing, University of Colorado. Dr. Watson's theory is taught worldwide and serves as the basis of teaching and caregiving for many of the world's nurses. Watson (2013) proclaims that a theory assists us, as nurses, to "see" what it is we do more clearly. It is her hope that the individuals studying and using her theory of nursing will see the world of health care in a "new and different lens." She wants us to be open to new ideas that are based on caring, and she wants us to put them into our practice as nurses.

Watson focuses on looking at the person to whom a nurse gives care as a whole human being, with attention needed for the body, mind, and spirit. This theory calls on you, as a nurse-to-be, to use your imagination and creativity to solve problems in ways that are personal for the people to whom you give care.

There is much more to Dr. Watson's nursing theory, but for the moment, concentrate on these three concepts. In summary, they are:

1. All human beings are valuable, and as a nurse, you have the responsibility to assist, nurture, and provide care for them.

2. It is essential to focus on the human relationship you have with all persons in your care and their relationship with the environment.

3. Developing a human-to-human relationship is critical to being a caring nurse.

Why Study Caring?

Many nurses and other health-care providers tell me they are caring already and ask why they need to study it. I understand the question they are asking. Yet I often see acts of uncaring behavior, as demonstrated by the absence of the human-to-human connection. The following is just one example:

One thing I often see are nurses with lists in their hands as they move quickly from room to room to reassure themselves of the safety of their patients or residents. Many times I have seen a nurse go into a room and say "good morning" without looking at the person and acknowledging him or her personally. Then, with list in hand, the rushed nurse checks the intravenous solution, the bladder catheter, and any dressing or wound completes the electronic charting, says "good-bye," and leaves the room. Everything the nurse did should have been done, but something very serious was missing. There was no human connection, no transpersonal caring; the nurse was not at all holistic in his or her approach.

How could the same things (checking critical items) be done in a caring mode? First, on the same list with the IV and dressing information should be the person's name. Note it as you go into the room and use it. My personal rule of thumb is to use Mr. or Mrs. the first time I meet an older person. Then, if individuals ask me to use their first names, I do, but only if invited to do so. This is a respectful way to communicate. Look the person in the eye as you say "good morning." Really look at the person's face and see if it has good color, if there are grimaces from pain, or if the person seems sad or depressed. When you get close enough to the person, reach out to touch an arm or a hand if it seems appropriate. This action demonstrates an effort to use transpersonal caring, and it gives you the opportunity to feel if the skin is dry and hot or cold and clammy. Some of these things can be done while you are walking into the room, and none of them take any extra time. After you have connected with the person (human-to-human connection), you can check the IV, the wound, and the

---

QSEN

COMPETENCY: Patient-Centered Care

Human Caring

You are working in a nursing home that takes care of a variety of older adults. After a thorough orientation to the facility, which includes their philosophy of human caring, you are assigned to work on the admissions unit. This is where all new admissions go for the first 3 days to evaluate where they should be placed to receive care specifically suited for their physical and emotional needs. The police bring in a 76-year-old intoxicated man to be admitted. The police tell you he is homeless and an alcoholic. He is dirty, smelly, and uncooperative. His hair is matted, and his beard is overgrown and crusted with food. He has been incontinent, his eyes are bloodshot, and he is drooling. The police remove his handcuffs and quickly leave the area.

Patient-centered care means providing holistic care to *every* patient.

- What is the reaction many people would have about being assigned to admit this man?
- What is your reaction as a nurse who is practicing "The Science of Human Caring"?
- How can you put the relationship you have with this man as the highest priority?
- What can you do to make the environment more conducive to the needs of this person?

FOCUSED LEARNING CHART

Climate of caring: environmental management

Privacy	Personal Space	Safety	Stimulation/ Personalization
Knock on door before entering	Respect personal items	No clutter or throw rugs	Multiple opportunities for individual choice
Privacy with family members	Respect personal space	Proper shoes	Encourage independent function
Respect time to be alone	Use touch only if it is acceptable to the other person	Sometimes pets	
Pull cubicle curtains		No frayed cords or broken furniture	Cherished furniture and decorations
			Meaningful pictures

Notice how this LPN is touching the resident and looking directly into her eyes. She is down to the resident's level so the resident can see and hear as the LPN talks to her. What else does the LPN's nonverbal communication tell you?

catheter. Then lean close so that the older person can see you and hear you, and tell him or her "everything is all right," or "I need to check with the registered nurse (RN)," or whatever is appropriate. Be honest and pleasant in all of your communications. Let the person know approximately when you will return.

Consider John, the CNA, who is the case study at the beginning of the chapter. After reading the first part of this chapter, do you have a better idea as to how you will help John provide holistic care to the residents assigned to him? What key concepts of Dr. Watson's theory does John need to learn in order to provide humanistic care to the residents in his care?

 Point of Interest

Remember the list of 10 chronic conditions most common for people older than 65? Visual and hearing problems were on that list. With that information, can you understand why it is so important to move in close so that an older adult can see you and hear you?

Point of Interest

When speaking to older adults, some people address them as "honey," "dearie," or "sweetie." This is an example of the caregiver treating the patient or resident as a child. It is called *paternalism*. Think for whom those comments are generally reserved; it is children. You may hear others use such terms, but you should talk to gerontological patients as the older adults they are rather than as children. It is a matter of respect.

Expanding the Concept of the Science of Human Caring

To truly be a caring person, as defined by Watson, you need to use her principles in all aspects of your life. I do not know your personal or family environment, but I do know that you can choose to behave in any way you wish. I have been screamed at by family members of older adults, but I never scream back. I simply let them "get it out." While they are screaming, I observe them and really listen to their words so I can understand the problem. When the screaming is done, the person generally is crying with sorrow or fear. I keep in mind that there is a reason for every behavior, and I consider it my responsibility to learn the reason for the behavior before I react.

This one application of caring theory in your personal life will improve your ability to relate well to the people you care for the most. Other examples are to listen to people when they are talking and respond thoughtfully. Caring people "get into it" and help others when they need it. This could mean cooking a meal for a sick neighbor, working with the community to make a vacant lot a safe play area, or telling your mom that you love her. (Being a mom, I really like that idea!) I am simply saying that to be a caring nurse, you need to be a caring person, too.

Critically Examine the Following

Take 5 minutes to think about nothing except how you feel about people with lesser resources for health care. What I mean by that term is people without insurance, people who live at or below the poverty level, people who do not speak English, homeless people, and people with disabilities. These groups of people are often referred to as marginalized people. That means they are on the "margin" of society and not really in it. Can you honestly value each person to whom you give care? Are you willing to use transpersonal caring in your health-care delivery to everyone? Are you willing to make the human-to-human connection with every individual who counts on you for safety and care?

After you have thoughtfully considered how you feel about these questions and any others that come to you, discuss your thoughts with others. They could be classmates, friends, or family. It is an intriguing topic of conversation if you approach it earnestly.

 GEROTRANSCENDENCE

Eric Erickson spent his life studying the psychological developmental tasks of people. His concept was that people would have good psychological health if they fulfilled the developmental tasks associated with each age group. Developmental tasks are the skills and knowledge learned through life experiences that allow us to meet the challenges that occur as we age. Erickson identified eight life stages with specific tasks that need to be accomplished. They are the following:

• Infancy: Trust vs. Mistrust
• Toddler: Autonomy vs. Shame
• Early childhood: Initiative vs. Guilt
• Middle childhood: Industry vs. Inferiority
• Adolescence: Identity vs. Identity diffusion
• Adulthood: Intimacy vs. Isolation
• Middle age: Generativity vs. Self-absorption
• Old age: Integrity vs. Despair

Point of Interest

How do elderly people you know work at achieving gerotranscendence? It is very challenging to develop more connections to others when their normal physical changes do not allow for convenient socialization (i.e., diminished vision and hearing, perhaps the inability to drive). Make some observations and discuss what you learn with someone who is older than you are. See what insight you can develop.

If older adults have accomplished integrity, they have likely experienced *gerotranscedence,* which is one of the critical tasks of old age.

Tornstam (2005) identified the concept of gerotranscendence. He states that older adults desire a life with more connections to other people, a life that is significant to self and others. This concept indicates that aging involves a transition to a lesser concern with material possessions, meaningless relationships, and self-interest. With gerotranscendence, older people are satisfied with the lives they have led and look forward to living a full life for the rest of their days; without gerotranscendence,

older people are more likely to feel despair with their lives—past, present, and future. These ideas and other insights into gerotranscendence will be integrated throughout this book in an effort to provide you with information that will assist you to help older adults achieve satisfaction with the lives they have lived.

CONCLUSION

I am confident that you can see how holism and caring complement each other. If you are caring, you look at the body, mind, and spirit of the person. If you are holistic, you also look at the entire person. Both approaches look at how the environment affects the person, and they work with the individual to make the environment more healing. Family members and other loved ones also are essential to delivering both types of nursing care, and understanding gerotranscendence is key to helping older adults feel more satisfied with the lives they have lived so far. There is much more to these concepts. My goal is for you to have an understanding of the basic principles of each approach to nursing care. Then it makes sense for you to discuss, think about, and put into practice the things you have learned. If you can gradually incorporate the material in this chapter into your daily caregiving, you will be the type of nurse you would want to take care of the people you love most. Best wishes for the journey!

Evidence-Based Practice

Dossey, B.M. (2010). Holistic nursing from Florence Nightingale's historical legacy to 21st-century global nursing. Alternative Therapies in Health and Medicine, 16(5), 14-16.

This article discusses Florence Nightingale's approach to holistic nursing during the 20th century and how many of her thoughts and ideas translate to the 21st century.

Question

As a 21st-century nurse, how will you incorporate the concept of holistic care into your nursing practice?

CASE STUDY SOLUTIONS

■ How does the CNA's behavior conflict with your holistic and caring philosophy?

It seems that he has not embraced either concept into his caregiving, even after you have role-modeled and discussed appropriate behaviors for him.

1. He is not respectful. Examples are the "cutsie" names he uses rather than learning the residents' names and his disrespect toward you.

2. He does not listen. An example is the argument he got into with a demented resident. If he would have listened to the resident, he would have understood the "reason behind the man's behavior."

3. He is not caring. An example is his impatience with the slowness of older persons.

4. He does not give good technical care. This CNA not only is *not* caring or at all holistic, but he doesn't give good physical care. We know this because of the glasses and teeth that were not in place by mid-morning.

■ What are you going to do?

It is only day 2 and there already are many problems with this employee. You are a relatively new LPN, but you know how nursing care should be delivered. His care is dangerous. What if he got into another argument with a resident and hit the person? It is a serious point of concern.

You have role-modeled for him and tried to explain things to him, yet he hasn't changed. This indicates that he doesn't want to change and probably won't. His lack of respect for you also is a point of concern in terms of how decisions are made on the unit. There will be many times when he will need to do what you tell him to do. You must question if he actually will do what you ask. This puts residents at risk.

You should carefully document his actual behaviors, both positive and negative. Then make an appointment with the nurse manager *before* he comes to another day of work. Carefully and objectively explain everything to her and leave the decision as to what to do with her. If she asks you to assist in continuing to evaluate or teach him, do as you are asked in a caring manner. If the CNA is terminated, that is the responsibility of the nurse manager and not your responsibility.

REVIEW QUESTIONS

1. Gerontological nursing refers to the nursing care of:
   1. the "old-old" population.
   2. people who are older and in need of assistance.
   3. people age 65 and older.
   4. a specialized body of knowledge regarding holistic and caring principles of nursing.

2. Older adults constitute:
   1. 12.3% of the U.S. population.
   2. 8.4% of the U.S. population.
   3. 25% of the U.S. population.
   4. 10% of the U.S. population.

3. The underlying concept of holism is:
   1. to include family and pets in the care plan.
   2. to recognize persons as individuals and to see them as an entire or whole person
   3. to identify team members who will make the nursing care easier.
   4. to look at the patient's face and note how he or she looks.

4. The purpose of a nursing philosophy is to be able to:
   1. think like a philosopher.
   2. have something positive to write on a job application.
   3. talk to other nurses about philosophy.
   4. have a personal conviction of the type of nursing care you will give to others.

5. "The Science of Human Caring" is:
   1. a nationally accepted philosophy of nursing.
   2. authored by Dr. John Wadsworth, former Dean and Distinguished Professor at the University of Colorado.
   3. a philosophy that addresses the body, mind, and physicality of all human beings.
   4. a philosophy of nursing that calls for the practice of individual caring.

6. Gerotranscendence is:
   1. one of the critical tasks of old age.
   2. based on Dr. Watson's developmental task of integrity vs. despair.
   3. a concept that refers to an elderly person's transition to a more materialistic mindset.
   4. a task that, when accomplished, makes older people despair the lives they have led.

REFERENCES

Bureau of National Health Statistics (2008). http://www.cdc.gov

Dossey, B.M., Keegan, L., & Guzzetta, C.E. (2013). *Holistic nursing* (6th ed.). Gaithersburg, MD: Aspen Publication.

Eliopolous, C. (2014). *Gerontological nursing* (8th ed.). Philadelphia, PA: J.B. Lippincott. National Vital Statistics Report (2012)

Random House College Dictionary (2008). http://www.randomhouse.com

Tornstam, L. (2005). *Gerotranscendence: A developmental theory of positive aging.* New York, NY: Springer Publishing.

U.S. Census Bureau. ACS Data Base (2010). http://factfinder2.census.gov/faces/nav/jsf/pages/index.xhtml

U.S. Department of Commerce (2010). http://www.commerce.gov/

Watson, J. (2013). Caring Science. http://watsoncaringscience.org/about-us/caring-science-definitions-processes-theory/

WEB RESOURCES

Watson Caring Science Institute and International Caritas Consortium: http://watsoncaringscience.org/

American Holistic Nurses Association: http://www.ahna.org/

The Aging Experience

2

TAMARA DAHLKEMPER

LEARNING OUTCOMES

1. Define the term *ageism*.

2. Discuss six common theories of aging.

3. Identify age-related changes in the following body systems:
   Cardiovascular   Gastrointestinal
   Respiratory   Genitourinary
   Musculoskeletal   Neurological
   Integumentary   Special senses

CONCEPTS

Assessment

Health, Wellness, and Illness

Professional Behaviors

Self

CASE STUDY

Ms. B. is 76 years old and lives in a duplex with her 83-year-old sister. Last year, the sister had a mild stroke, leaving her with left-sided weakness. Ms. B. manages the household and coordinates her sister's care, including home health aides, physical and occupational therapy, and visits to the doctor's office.

Ms. B. describes herself as healthy. She also comments, "Okay, I had cancer of the colon 2 years ago, but I had surgery and some chemotherapy too, and now I'm okay. Oh, I sometimes get constipated, but that has nothing to do with the cancer."

She states that she tires more easily these days and tries to rest every afternoon. Still, she maintains a full schedule of grocery shopping, visiting friends, cooking and cleaning, and caring for her sister's needs. She has no breathing problems, and her appetite is excellent. "I can't eat as much as I used to at each meal, but my sister and I have a snack in the afternoon and at bedtime."

She does complain about nocturnal voiding two or three times a night and has had two urinary infections this year. "Sometimes I dribble urine, and I use those pads."

Both sisters are always cold; their home is kept very warm, and they always seem to be wearing sweaters and heavy stockings. Every Sunday is beauty day at the B.'s residence, when they apply face and hand cream to dry skin, style their thinning hair, and care for their nails, which are getting thick and brittle. Both claim that they have become shorter in the past few years; Ms. B. often feels weary at night because of joint pain. She has learned to adjust her daily schedule to changes in endurance. She says, "No matter where I go, I take my time, sit down, and pace myself. I know where every bench and restaurant is in South Philadelphia."

Ms. B. has noticed that she needs to wear her glasses all the time when reading or paying bills; she invested in 100-watt light bulbs for every lamp "because we both need stronger light to read by these days." She is never without her sunglasses to avoid glare; every shade is always lowered at their house during the day. Ms. B. claims, "I don't think as clearly lately as I used to; it takes me longer to figure things out and make decisions." But she continues to manage the household and lead an active life.

"I have my friends, my neighborhood, my home, and, of course, my sister. We have been together all of our lives. We care about each other, and we do pretty well, taking each day as it comes, each day expecting another good day."

Discussion

1. What age-related changes has Ms. B. experienced?

2. Would you consider Ms. B. to be a healthy older adult? Explain.

 INTRODUCTION

The aging experience is a significant part of personal and societal living. Sometimes called "the graying of America," this dramatic change in our population has many ramifications in politics, economics, health care, recreation, and entertainment. All facets of life, not just health care, are affected by the fact that many more older adults are living today than lived in the past.

People 65 years old and older constitute 13% of the population in the United States—that is more than one in every eight Americans.

Here are two important pieces of demographic information that will impact your practice as a licensed practical nurse (LPN):

1. The older white population will grow more slowly than before, and in the next 40 years, it will begin to decline compared with African American and other

ethnic minority groups. Current minority populations are projected to represent 42% of the elderly population in 2050.

2. The fastest-growing segment of the population in the United States is people who are older than 85 years of age. Projections indicate that the size of this age group will almost double between 2010 and 2050. At present, there are more people having their 85th birthday every day in the United States than babies being born.

 ## IMPACT OF AGING ON NURSING

The great increase in the number of older people means that nursing practice must be different from what it has been in the past. Current national statistics state that 65% of all patients in acute-care hospitals are age 65 or older, as are 83% of people in home care and 92% of residents in nursing homes. In 2000, Tim Porter O'Grady, a nursing futurist, said that if a nurse was not preparing for a job in gerontology, that nurse was not preparing for the nursing jobs of the future. The graying of America calls for gerontologically qualified nurses who can work in diverse health-care settings. The purpose of this book is to assist you to meet that objective.

Health care has changed in various ways because of the number of people who are aging. As a group, older citizens are a very powerful political force; they have influenced the actions of Congress and the President on health-related issues and will continue to do so.

Older adults want and expect to have a say in the kind of health care they receive, where they receive it, and from whom. They are better educated than any other generation of older adults and have the knowledge to make more sophisticated demands on the health-care system. For instance, demand is growing for home-care services from older people who need assistance and nursing care but prefer to be cared for at home.

This population of new clients in the health-care system requires you, the nurse, to consider them in a new way. Never before have nurses had to care for such a large number of older adults who

Critically Examine the Following

Before reading the next section, take the time necessary to complete this critical thinking exercise. Critical thinking is an essential component of nursing. These exercises are a positive way to begin to develop that all-important skill.

How Will It Impact Your Nursing Practice to Have:
1. Increasing numbers of old-old people as your patients?
2. Increasing numbers of nonwhite older adults as your patients?

I am going to answer the questions as though I were a student. It is hoped that this will assist you in considering how you will answer the questions. Your faculty person may request this assignment to be turned in at the next class session, or it may be used as a point for class discussion. However it is used, it is an opportunity for you to think critically and compare your thinking with your classmates. Here are my responses:

1. When I planned on going to nursing school, I wanted to be a maternal-child nurse. I was excited to think about working in labor and delivery, and I cannot imagine anything nicer than working in the newborn nursery. However, if the population of older people, especially the very old, is growing, I need to consider working in gerontology. If that is where I am going to be because of the need for nurses, I am going to become very good at taking care of fragile old-old or elite-old people. They sound like my type of challenge!
2. I live in Utah, where 95% of the population is white. I will have an adjustment to make when my patients are not mostly white and of the same working-class, emigrant society. I need to learn about the cultures of other ethnic groups so that I can be an effective nurse and meet their needs on a high level.

have survived the Great Depression, two world wars, the Holocaust, the Korean and Vietnam Wars, and rock and roll! Because the survival experiences and life skills of these elderly people are new to health care, they require society to address them in a new way.

 ## ATTITUDES TOWARD AGING

The study of aging is a very important part of nursing. Many myths, stereotypes, and prejudices about old age exist in our culture, and nurses need to be able to separate myths and prejudices from fact. Modern researchers are intently studying the aging experience (another indication of the importance of this topic in today's world). This chapter draws from their findings to represent a realistic picture of the processes and effects of aging.

Myths and prejudices about old age are pervasive in our society. Browsing through a greeting card display reveals some very good examples of the stereotypes and fables of aging:

"I won't say you're old," reads one greeting card, "but in horse years, you'd be glue on this envelope."

"Happy birthday, Hot Stuff! Who says people our age can't still live in the fast lane?" reads another. The inside message: "Voila! Adult diapers with racing stripes."

As the contents of many of the cards imply, old age conjures up images of rocking chairs, dentures, memory loss, and incontinence. People laugh at the humor in the birthday cards, but a

Home health care is one of the health-care changes that elderly people have demanded as part of their health-care options. People want to stay at home and be near family, friends, and the things that are familiar to them.

 # Point of Interest

The word *geriatrics* is the term that describes the medical study of older adults, and the word *gerontology* describes the nursing study of older adults. You need to know the definitions of both words to discuss gerontological issues knowledgeably.

 # Evidence-Based Practice

Flood, M.T., & Clark, R.B. (2009). Exploring knowledge and attitudes toward aging among nursing and non-nursing students. *Educational Gerontology, 35,* 587-595.

This study evaluated and compared the knowledge and attitudes of non-nursing and nursing students toward elderly persons. Research has shown if nurses have negative stereotypes of older adult patients, it has an impact on the patient's physical and psychological well-being. Literature also shows that if nurses are knowledgeable about how to provide the needed level of care for older adults, they are better able to meet the challenges related to caring for their older patients.

This study showed that nursing students who had prior experience working with older adults or had some geriatric content as part of their nursing education felt better prepared to care for their older patients. The authors of the study also suggest that nursing programs must continue to offer geriatric content and opportunities for students to interact with older adults. These experiences will promote a better understanding of the older adult population that will decrease negative attitudes toward older patients.

Questions

1. What can you do to increase your knowledge about caring for older adults?
2. While in a clinical setting, how can you apply your new knowledge?

serious societal danger lurks in such negative and prejudicial images. Stereotypes, myths, and distortions concerning aging and old people lead to actions that discriminate against the aged. American culture glorifies youth. Print and television advertising, clothing fashions, and other expressions of the desirable norm all push the image of zestful youth. Because today's adults have grown up in this culture, they pick up its values and prejudices without realizing it.

 ## AGEISM

The term *ageism* was coined in 1968 by Robert Butler (1969) to describe negative attitudes and practices that were directed toward old people. He defined ageism as a systematic stereotyping of and discrimination against people simply because they are old. Ageism is very similar to racism and sexism, which discriminate against people because of skin color and gender. We as a society are outraged by acts of racism and sexism, but we seem to accept ageism as a norm for behavior. Old people are categorized as confused, rigid in thought and manner, and old-fashioned in morality and skills. Yet older adults are as individual and unique as people of all other age groups. It simply seems easier to place them in a negative category and ignore them. Ageism allows the younger generation to see older people as different; they subtly cease to identify with their elders as human beings.

In the decades since Dr. Butler first wrote about ageism, a steady improvement in attitudes toward the aged has been seen. This change partly resulted from general public education, increased attention in the media, and broadening of education about gerontology in colleges and universities. Seriously negative attitudes toward the aged still exist. They appear subtly, covertly, and even unconsciously. Similar to racism and sexism, ageism is still persistent.

 # Priority Setting

The priority you need to take from this chapter is that of recognizing and combating ageism. Why is that the priority I chose? Ageism is a powerful, negative form of discrimination.

Because you are going to be giving care to older adults, you need to be their champion and assist them in combating this negative influence in their lives.

How can you meet this priority of recognizing and fighting ageism?

- Start with becoming acutely aware of what ageist behavior is. It could be something as simple as not laughing at the discriminatory cards that mock older people and the aging process. They simply are not funny. Look for age-based discrimination. Once you can recognize it, you can begin to change within yourself if that is needed.
- Look at older adults as "wise and wonderful." They really do have the wisdom of the ages. Just think of all the problems they have solved by living in a war-torn and tumultuous world (world wars, the Great Depression). They deserve to be heard, so listen!
- Be patient with older people. Their bodies are wearing out because of the *normal* process of aging. Don't hold that against them.
- Along with patience, speak up, move in close so you can be seen, touch if it seems appropriate, smile, and learn to enjoy your time with someone older. You may need to start with enjoying your grandparents or older aunts and uncles. Both generations have so much to offer each other. Don't be too busy to take advantage of this opportunity.
- Be brave! Speak up when someone says or suggests doing something that is ageist. You don't need to be aggressive, but you should state your opinion. You don't need to defend what you say because the statement should speak for itself.
- Read about ageism, ponder what you read, talk to others about it, consider how you would like to be thought about and treated when you are older. If you don't like what you foresee, how can you change it?

An example is the cosmetic industry, which thrives on the sale of products that eliminate age spots, smooth away wrinkles, conceal gray hairs, and make one look younger than one's actual age. Growing old is represented as a calamity, and being old as having a dreaded disease. The last years of life are pictured as time spent in death's waiting room.

In reality, elderly people do not offer a panorama of doom and death. Many senior citizens live well into their 80s and 90s with "youthful vigor," in relative physical comfort and safety, and in good health. Many others do have chronic health problems, but because the problems are well managed and well controlled, such people consider themselves healthy and lead active, fulfilling lives. Still others have significant limitations that affect their independence and activity, but they are able to enjoy a rich and varied existence because they live with family members or in other protected environments.

Negative images of nursing homes envisioned by some people are in part an expression of ageism. Most nursing homes give excellent care to a frail and vulnerable population that cannot be cared for elsewhere. Another point of information, unknown by many people, is that only 5% of people older than 65 years are in nursing homes at any one time Administration on Aging (2011). Today's nursing home is characterized by a concept of *rehabilitative,* not *custodial,* care, a perspective that calls for nursing interventions intended to support the highest possible level of independence despite physical and cognitive limitations.

It is easy for society to judge, criticize, and ignore an older person. Do an internal examination to determine if you are ageist. Do you get impatient when an older person is in front of you driving on the freeway? I tell my gerontology students that they will not pass the class until they have conquered that type of impatience. I give them assignments to sit down and unhurriedly talk to a well elderly person. I suggest they go to lunch or shopping, even to the grocery store. The students are encouraged to ask the person about living with ration cards, going to war, or being left a widow or widower after 50 to 60 years of marriage. The ageism in our society has kept most of us from knowing about the aging process and respecting those who survive it. It is time for this situation to change (King, Roberts, & Bowers, 2013).

An important concept to remember is the uniqueness of the individual. Just as every child and every middle-aged adult is unique in some way, so is every older adult. The mistaken belief that one old person is just like another is an expression of ageism, and this perception can lead to potentially harmful treatment. Physicians and nurses sometimes treat older patients as they might treat a child, calling them by their first names without asking how they wish to be addressed or, worse yet, calling them "honey" or "dearie." Caregivers often are guilty of "infantilizing" the elderly. It is easy to see how such treatment increases dependence and frailty, rather than fostering independence, even for a person with limitations. Not all old people are cranky and gloomy, although a man or woman who was cranky and gloomy at age 40 is probably more so at age 80. People tend to become more and more like themselves as they age. All individuals who work in the health-care field need to examine their own attitudes and biases about older adults in general and about frail or ill older adults in particular to battle ageism successfully.

 ## THEORIES OF AGING

Theories of aging are a scientific effort to assist people to understand what contributes to aging in a positive or negative manner. As a nurse, you need to understand the basic theories to assist and support your older adult patients and residents to live healthier lives. There are physiological and psychological theories to assist you in understanding aging. There are many theories available for study; the following are three from each category that will assist you in giving effective nursing care.

Physiological Theories of Aging

Genetic Factors

The theory of genetic factors is easy to understand if you critically examine yourself and your family members. You already know that you may have inherited your hair and eye color, height, and body size from your ancestors. There are many other things you also may have inherited, such as musical or athletic ability. Have you considered that the aging of your body also is inherited? This theory says that it is. Interview your grandparents or older aunts and uncles. Are their siblings still alive? How long did their parents and grandparents live? I know of a family in which all of the men died before the age of 50 with heart disease, but the women lived to be in their 70s. I know a family of

QSEN

COMPETENCY: Patient-Centered Care (Attitudes)

Attitudes Toward Older Adults

If you were to ask other students where they plan to work when they graduate, very few will say they plan to work in assisted living or a nursing home. Yet, most nurses working in acute-care facilities will work with older adults as their primary patient population. It is important for all nurses to have the necessary knowledge to provide quality care for their older patients.

Because of earlier experiences with older adults, some nurses may have a negative attitude toward their elderly patients. Beyond the ability to know how to provide needed care, a nurse must also value the individual for whom they are providing care.

- What is your attitude toward older adults?
- Do you have any biases toward taking care of older adults?
- What are some things you can do to overcome your personal ageism?

Spend time pondering the issue of ageism. Really grasp what it means for you on a personal level. This can be done by talking to your colleagues and peers and, more importantly, by talking to older people.

six sisters who all went through menopause at age 52. I have a friend whose mother had 11 brothers and sisters; they all lived to be in their 80s. Consider Ms. B. in the chapter case study. Can any of her aging issues be related to genetics?

This theory claims that animals and humans are born with a genetic program that predetermines their life span. This may seem discouraging to people who are working hard to obtain or maintain optimum health. A healthy diet, exercise, and stress control, among other things, will certainly support a higher quality of life, however, if not add to one's longevity.

Just as nurses interview people about their family history regarding diseases, it would be appropriate use of this theory to ask about their parents and siblings and their aging process. This information may assist you in working with the patient or resident. The most important aspect of this theory is for you to recognize that it is one way to accept aging as the inevitable process it is. With that acceptance, you should develop an additional acceptance of the normal and abnormal aspects of aging and the eventual death of each of us. According to this theory, it is predetermined and inevitable.

Wear and Tear

If you were to go to a senior citizen center or a nursing home dayroom, you would easily identify the basis for the wear and tear theory. As people age, their body parts show the effects of the complex and sophisticated work the body does through the years. People will be walking with canes or walkers; some will be on oxygen; others will simply moan when they get up from a chair. Similar to all fine-tuned machinery, body parts wear out or become less effective. Knees need to be replaced because of the lack of cartilage that comes with aging, joints develop arthritis, and hips break because of decreased bone mass or lack of balance leading to a fall.

Think of all the running and jumping you did as a child. Perhaps you were an athlete during high school. Think of how you use your body now that you are in school. The body is well used and sometimes abused, and its parts simply wear out.

Understanding this theory should assist you in accepting that older adults walk slower, hear less effectively, and need to stop and rest and overall do things at a slower and safer pace. If you understand and accept this theory, you will accept the changes that require your attention in giving care to specialized, older people.

Critically Examine the Following

Spend time with your parents or older relatives and discuss the genetic factor theory with them. Ask questions about your ancestors, and identify traits that you may have inherited from them. Inquire about the longevity of your ancestors as well as their major diseases. When you have enough information, predict how long you will live and the predominate diseases you will have. Justify what you predict from your family history. Prepare the information into one paragraph that could be read in class.

Nutrients

Chapter 8 in this book is devoted to nutrition. The focus is on nutrition for older persons. When considering the nutrient theory, however, you should focus on your own nutritional intake. This theory states that aging and the quality of aging depend on a person's nutrition intake over the span of his or her life. This is easy to understand because, as a health-care worker, you recognize the negative effects of obesity, lack of exercise, and high cholesterol, all of which may be attributed to food consumption. The quart of chocolate ice cream, mountain of french fries, and large steak are not ways to promote a successful aging process. The nutrient theory states that good nutritional intake at any age assists in improved health as one ages. The longer you eat healthy foods, the longer you will live with a better quality of life. Now is a good time to start.

Whenever you are giving care to an older person, you should examine the individual's eating habits and determine if you can teach him or her something new that will improve health. Ask the nurse manager about having a dietitian visit the person or arrange for fresh fruits to be available for snacks if that would help. You need to take care of yourself and share your knowledge with those you love. Teach them the things you will learn in the nutrition chapter and apply the principles to yourself as well. There is little in life that is better than a healthy old age!

Psychological Theories

Developmental Tasks

Eric Erikson (1963) is famous for his eight stages of personal development of individuals. He begins with infancy and progresses through old age. His focus is on ego development, which gives people the strength to manage their lives. The task for old age, according to Erikson, is Integrity vs. Despair. If older people can find meaning in the life lived, then they will have the ego integrity to adjust and manage the process of aging. If they do not have integrity, they will be angry, depressed, and feel inadequate; in other words, they will feel despair.

You may encounter older persons who are feeling despair. They complain constantly and keep saying they wish "this" or "that" had happened in their life. Also frequently heard is the phrase "if only . . . ." Such people need your time and acceptance of them and their lives. Ask them to talk about their life experiences and reinforce the valuable things they have done. Help them to see what they have contributed to the world. Your efforts should focus on identifying the actions in their life that will assist in building the feeling of ego integrity. Similarly, you may also find older adults who are happy in their lives and have been able to adjust to the process of aging. An example is Ms. B., the woman introduced in the chapter case study. Although she is dealing with issues related to the normal aging process, Ms. B. states "she has her friends, her home, and her sister and that she takes each day as it comes and expects more good days." I would say Ms. B. has reached Erickson's eighth stage and has developed ego integrity.

Subculture Theory

This theory defines older people as a subculture. In anthropological terms, this theory indicates that older people have their own cultural norms and standards. This includes attitudes that cross over to multiple members of the group and beliefs, expectations, and behaviors that make them different from others.

You will study the cultural and ethnic differences in people throughout your education. It is important to understand people, their differences, and their needs. This theory indicates that elderly people are another group worthy of your study. You need to observe older people and note their similarities. They will not be the same because, similar to all people, they are strongly individualized, but they will exhibit similarities. In reference to this theory, you need to note their similarities.

Continuity Theory

In simple terms, the continuity theory states that as people change, their basic personality and behavioral patterns do not change. If you are an angry person at age 20, then you will be even better at being angry at age 70. The same is true of a teacher, who will find a way to keep teaching as he or she ages. A loving mother will find a way to continue to mother people (perhaps her grandchildren or children in the neighborhood), musicians will keep playing, and athletes will still keep trying to win.

The continuity theory recognizes the unique and individualized characteristics of people and their ways of adapting to aging. This theory is easy to apply to your practice. You simply need to talk to the older person and the family members about what type of person your patient was in his or her youth or adulthood. Then you will know what type

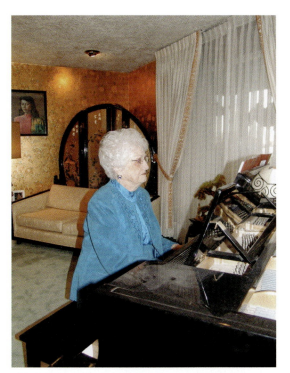

This 82-year-old woman has always played the piano. Now that she is older, she is better at it than ever before in her life. Which psychological theory does this demonstrate?

of behavior to expect now that he or she is an older adult. Don't try to change older people; rather, respect them for who they are.

NORMAL AGING PROCESS

Since the early 1950s, much research has been done in Europe and the United States on identifying and classifying common physiological and psychosocial changes that occur as people grow older. These changes have been termed *normal* because they represent alterations in body structure and function that occur gradually throughout life (Hyman, Oden, & Wagner, 2010). In this context, aging is seen as a natural process, and the changes associated with it are considered to be expected and continuous. If you are curious about your potential normal aging changes, you need to look at your grandparents. What acute and chronic diseases do they have? At what age do people in your family die? Do the men go bald; do the women develop osteoporosis? We all will age until we die. To me, that comment makes aging the desirable choice between the two. I would sooner grow old than die young.

To understand the normal aging process fully, nurses must realize that aging is a normal

---

FOCUSED LEARNING CHART

Theories of aging

Physiological Theories

Genetic Factors
Born with a genetic program that predetermines life span.

Wear and Tear
All life is a fine-tuned machine. Body parts wear out as they age.

Nutrients
Aging and the quality of life depend on the person's nutritional intake over his or her life span.

Psychological Theories

Developmental Tasks
Eric Erickson defined eight developmental tasks from infancy to old age. The task for old age is integrity versus despair.

Subculture Theory
Defines old people as their own subculture with cultural norms and standards.

Continuity Theory
People change physiologically as they age, but their basic personality and behavioral patterns do not change.

developmental event and that patterns of aging vary dramatically among older adults. Although the profession studies normal age changes that are universal, every person ages in a particular, individualized way. No two individuals are alike; the number of ways in which people age may be seen as equal to the number of people who have lived into old age. As individuals age, they become more diverse, not more alike. The range of "normal" aging characteristics is wide, and each individual exhibits a unique interplay of physical, social, and environmental influences that define the personal aging experience.

Older adults often have a chronic or acute illness superimposed on age-related changes, but development of disease is not a normal part of aging. It is essential for you, the LPN, to understand this perspective and develop a positive approach to normal aging. It also is important to remember that most older adults live actively and independently in the community and cope successfully with age-related changes and chronic illnesses (remember that only 5% of them are in nursing homes). Health for older adults might be defined as the ability to function at an individual's highest potential despite the presence of age-related changes and risk factors.

ESSENTIAL FACTS ABOUT THE NORMAL AGING PROCESS

- As individuals age, they become more diverse, not more alike.
- Age-related changes develop in each individual in a unique way.
- Normal aging and disease are separate entities.
- Normal aging includes gains and losses and does not indicate decline.
- Successful adaptation to the aging process is accomplished by most older adults.

NORMAL PHYSIOLOGICAL CHANGES ACCORDING TO BODY SYSTEMS

Specific age-related changes are described in terms of the body systems with which they are associated. Common functional changes experienced by older adults as a result of physiological alterations also are discussed. The term *function* refers to an older adult's ability to perform activities of daily living (ADLs) and independent activities of daily living (IADLs) and takes into consideration the quality of life of the individual. As the older adult experiences an increase in the number and intensity of age-related changes, functional independence is often jeopardized. Nursing approaches to prevent losses and promote self-care in light of age-related changes also are considered in this section.

Cardiovascular System

The cardiovascular system loses its efficiency with age, but because older adults require less oxygen at rest and during exercise, many people effectively compensate for changes in circulatory function. The high incidence of cardiovascular disease in the older population often makes it difficult, however, to distinguish normal age-related changes from changes related to sickness. One of the "good news" facts about cardiovascular disease and elderly people is that it is no longer the number one cause of death as it has been for decades. Older adults now know more about taking care of themselves, which improves their cardiovascular system. Cancer is now the leading cause of death in older adults.

Age-Related Changes
HEART
- Cardiac muscle strength is diminished.
- Heart valves become thickened and more rigid.
- The sinoatrial node, which is responsible for conduction, is less efficient, and impulses are slowed.
- Heart contractions may be weaker, blood volume decreases, and cardiac output declines.

BLOOD VESSELS
- Arteries become less elastic.
- Capillary walls thicken and slow the exchange of nutrients and waste products between blood and tissues.
- The greater rigidity of the vascular walls increases systolic and diastolic pressures.

BLOOD
- Blood volume is reduced owing to an age-related decline in total body water.
- Bone marrow activity is reduced, which leads to a slight decrease in levels of red blood cells, hematocrit, and hemoglobin.

Point of Interest

Function is the ability to take care of one's ADLs—basic personal needs, such as eating, dressing, washing, toileting, and moving. Function also refers to the ability to live independently in one's community, performing IADLs including cooking, shopping, taking medications properly, cleaning, traveling locally, and managing finances. This information will be addressed in more detail in Chapter 16.

Functional Changes

In summary, with normal aging, some atherosclerosis is expected as well as decreased cardiac output, but cardiovascular response remains adequate if cardiac disease is not present. Older adults usually adjust to cardiac changes but find they may need to pace their physical activity.

Respiratory System

Respiratory functioning shows minimal age-related decline in healthy older adults. The age-related changes that affect the respiratory system are so gradual that most older adults compensate well for these changes.

Age-Related Changes

SKELETAL CHANGES
- The rib cage becomes rigid as cartilage calcifies.
- The thoracic spine may shorten, and osteoporosis may cause a stooped posture, decreasing active lung space and limiting thoracic movement.

ACCESSORY MUSCLES
- Abdominal muscles weaken, decreasing inspiratory and expiratory effort.
- The diaphragm does not seem to lose mass.

Intrapulmonary Changes
- Lung elastic recoil is progressively lost with advancing age.
- Alveoli enlarge and become thin, and although their number remains constant, the number of functioning alveoli decreases overall.
- The alveolus-capillary membrane thickens, reducing the surface area for gas exchange.

Functional Changes

Structural changes in the respiratory system affect the rate of airflow into and out of the lungs as well as the rate of gas exchange at the alveolar level. Because of limited elastic recoil, residual volume increases; less ventilation occurs at the bases of the lungs, and more air and secretions remain in the lungs. In addition, the shallow breathing patterns of older adults—secondary to postural changes—contribute to this reduced airflow. Decreased chest muscle strength contributes to a less effective cough response and places an older adult at greater risk of pulmonary infection. The shallow breathing pattern also affects gas exchange. Oxygen saturation is diminished. For example, the partial pressure of oxygen in alveoli (P_{AO_2}) is about 90 mm Hg for a healthy young adult, whereas a value of 75 mm Hg at age 70 years would be acceptable. This decline may result in a decreased tolerance for exercise and the need for short rest periods during activity.

Musculoskeletal System

Most older adults experience alterations in posture, changes in range of motion, and slowed movement. These changes account for many of the characteristics normally associated with old age.

Age-Related Changes
BONE STRUCTURE
- Loss of bone mass results in brittle, weak bones.
- The vertebral column may compress, leading to reduction in height.

MUSCLE STRENGTH
- Muscle wasting occurs, and regeneration of muscle tissue slows.
- Muscles of the arms and legs become thin and flabby.
- Muscles lose flexibility and endurance with inactivity.

JOINTS
- Range of motion may be limited.
- Cartilage thins, so that joints may be painful, inflamed, or stiff.

Functional Changes

Loss of muscle mass is a gradual process, and most older adults compensate for it well. Regular exercise has been shown to reduce bone loss, promote increased muscle strength, and improve flexibility and muscle coordination. Conversely, immobility and sedentary lifestyles lead to loss of muscle size and strength.

Loss of bone mass and bone density results in osteoporosis and porous, brittle bones that are at greater risk of fracture. This problem can be due to estrogen deficiencies and low serum calcium levels; calcium supplements and estrogens are often prescribed. More recent research has raised some questions, however, about the use of estrogen therapy. This should be discussed with the older person's physician.

In summary, changes caused by osteoporosis, lack of joint motion, and decreased muscle strength and endurance may affect the functional ability of the older adult. An effective exercise program, together with adequate diet and a healthy outlook that includes independence and an active lifestyle, can reverse or slow down musculoskeletal changes. The phrase "Use it or lose it!" directly applies to an older adult's musculoskeletal functional ability.

Integumentary System

Changes involving the skin and hair probably are symbolic of the aging process more than those of any other system. The formation of wrinkles, the development of "age spots," graying of the hair, and baldness are constant reminders of growing old. In addition, no other system is so highly influenced by previous life patterns and environmental conditions, particularly exposure to the sun.

Age-Related Changes

SKIN
- The skin loses elasticity, leading to wrinkles, folds, and dryness.
- The skin thins, giving less protection to underlying blood vessels.
- Subcutaneous fat diminishes.
- Melanocytes cluster, producing the skin pigmentation known as age spots.

HAIR
- Decreased activity of hair follicles results in thinning of the hair on all areas of the body.
- Decreased rate of melanin production results in loss of original color and graying.
- Women may develop hair on the chin and upper lip.
- Men may develop an increase in ear, nose, and eyebrow hair.

NAILS
- Decreased blood flow to the nailbed may cause nails to become thick, dull, hard, and brittle, with longitudinal lines.

SWEAT GLANDS
- Decreases in size and number occur.

Functional Changes

Intact skin is the first line of defense against bacterial invasion and minor physical trauma. Age-related skin dryness and decreased elasticity increase the risk of skin breakdown and skin tears, leading to increased potential for injury and infection. Body temperature regulation is impaired by decreased sweat production. Because of this, older adults may not exhibit diaphoresis with elevated body temperatures.

Conversely, the loss of insulation in the form of a fat layer may make older adults feel cold. They often ask for extra sweaters when younger adults are comfortable with the ambient temperature. Nurses need to be aware of temperature discomforts when bathing, dressing, or examining an older adult and respond appropriately to the older adult's concern.

Age-related changes in the integumentary system affect the essential mechanisms of body protection and temperature regulation and greatly influence one's perception of aging. Earlier health practices related to nutrition, grooming, bathing,

This grandmother and granddaughter team go swimming together twice a week. It provides a special time for them to be together and a great opportunity for meaningful exercise.

and physical activity as well as genetic, biochemical, and environmental factors are powerful determinants of integumentary status.

Gastrointestinal System

Changes in the gastrointestinal (GI) system, although not life-threatening, often cause the greatest concern to the older adult. Indigestion, constipation, and anorexia are common GI problems that greatly affect functional status.

Age-Related Changes
ORAL CAVITY
- Reabsorption of bone in the jaw may loosen teeth or cause a loss of teeth, reducing the ability to chew.
- Saliva production decreases.

ESOPHAGUS
- The gag reflex weakens, causing an increased risk of food aspiration.
- Smooth muscle weakness delays emptying time.

STOMACH
- Decreased gastric acid secretions may impair absorption of iron, vitamin B_{12}, and protein.

INTESTINES
- Peristalsis decreases.
- Weakening of the sphincter muscles leads to incompetent emptying of the bowel.

Functional Changes
The slowing of peristalsis and the loss of smooth muscle tone delay gastric emptying so that a feeling of "fullness" is present after eating only small amounts of food. In addition, delayed gastric emptying time and reduced gastric acid secretions may lead to indigestion, discomfort, and reduced appetite. Frequent small meals, rather than three large ones, may be better tolerated. Decreased peristalsis also contributes to slower transit time in the large intestine and allows more time for water reabsorption and hardening of the stool. Because of this factor, the nurse must recommend a diet adequate in fiber and fluids.

Fatigue, discomfort, activity intolerance, and sensory losses may make food preparation difficult for an older adult living at home. This problem could result in a nutritionally inadequate diet. In summary, effective GI functioning creates peace of mind for the older adult and greatly influences well-being.

Urinary System

Changes in the genitourinary system affect the basic bodily functions of voiding. This issue is often difficult for an older adult to discuss. A commonly held belief is that having genitourinary problems such as incontinence is a normal result of aging. It is not, but the belief that it is often causes an older adult to delay seeking treatment. Helping the older adult to maintain optimal genitourinary function is often a challenge for the nurse.

Age-Related Functions
RENAL FUNCTION
- Renal blood flow decreases because of decreased cardiac output and reduced glomerular filtration rate.
- Ability to concentrate urine may be impaired.

BLADDER
- Loss of muscle tone and incomplete emptying may occur.
- Capacity decreases.

MICTURITION
- In men, increased frequency owing to enlargement of the prostate is possible.
- In women, increased frequency may be caused by relaxation of the perineal muscle.

Functional Changes
Despite decreased renal blood flow and the loss of kidney mass, the genitourinary system continues to function normally in the absence of disease. Functional impairments result from decreased bladder capacity and include urinary frequency, nocturia, and retention of urine. These changes may eventually cause dysfunction, leading to infection, urgency, and incontinence. Although urinary incontinence is not a normal outcome of the aging process, loss of perineal muscle mass may contribute to one of the most common forms of incontinence in women—stress incontinence. This condition involves leakage of urine that occurs with coughing, sneezing, laughing, or lifting. Pelvic floor exercises are an effective strategy to strengthen muscle tone and prevent involuntary leakage.

Enlargement of the prostate, which occurs in most elderly men, is most often benign. It can cause, however, urinary retention, frequency, overflow incontinence, and, eventually, renal damage. Older men should have regular examinations of the prostate.

Changes in voiding, particularly incontinence, may contribute to embarrassment and general discomfort for an older adult. By showing sensitivity and acceptance, the nurse can intervene effectively to improve genitourinary functional response.

Reproductive System

Age-Related Functions
FEMALE REPRODUCTION
- The vulva may atrophy.
- Pubic hair may fall out.
- Vaginal secretions diminish, and vaginal walls thin and become less elastic.
- Breast tissue atrophies.

MALE REPRODUCTION
- Testes atrophy.
- The prostate may enlarge.

Functional Changes
Because of the aging process, female genitalia exhibit many changes. As a result of a decrease in vaginal secretions and changes to the tissue, women may experience painful sexual intercourse. To alleviate these symptoms, some women choose to take low doses of estrogen, which can lead to postmenopausal bleeding resulting from the endometrium's response to hormonal stimulation. Any postmenopausal vaginal bleeding is considered abnormal and should be checked by a health-care provider.

The structural changes in male genitalia can cause a reduction in sperm count, but these changes do not affect the physical ability of men to achieve erection or ejaculation.

Despite the changes in the male and female reproductive system, many older adults are still able to enjoy intercourse and other forms of sexual pleasure. For many older adults, discussing reproductive issues can be embarrassing, but these issues need to be assessed by the nurse.

Nervous System

Age-related changes in the nervous system affect all body systems and involve vascular response, mobility, coordination, visual activity, and cognitive ability. Most misconceptions about normal age-related changes involve the nervous system. For example, there is a misconception that mental decline or "senility" is inevitable with aging or that intellectual capacity diminishes with age. The nurse needs to teach older adults that general decline of neurological function is not an automatic response to aging and that, in the absence of disease, the older adult's neurological system functions adequately.

Age-Related Changes
NEURONS
- Neurons are steadily lost in the brain and spinal cord.
- Synthesis and metabolism of neurotransmitters are diminished.
- Brain mass is lost progressively.

MOVEMENT
- The kinesthetic sense is less efficient.
- Balance may be impaired.
- Reaction time decreases.

SLEEP
- Insomnia and increased night wakening may occur.
- Deep sleep (stage IV) and rapid eye movement sleep decrease.

Functional Changes
As motor neurons work less efficiently, reaction time slows, and the ability to respond quickly to stimuli decreases. Research studies indicate that although response time may be prolonged, older adults are willing to give up speed for accuracy and tend to respond more slowly but with greater precision. There seems to be little correlation between brain atrophy and cognitive loss. Older adults are generally well oriented to time, place, and person, with minimal changes in memory performance despite decreased synthesis of neurotransmitters and diminished brain size.

Older people are particularly at risk for falls, owing to a slower reaction time in maintaining balance and the potential for hypotensive reactions secondary to decreased blood volume. Resulting symptoms of dizziness, light-headedness, and vertigo contribute to impaired balance. Nurses should allow older adults adequate time for position change; dangling at the bedside and standing briefly before ambulation may be indicated.

Older adults generally sleep less at night but take naps during the day, so that cumulative sleep time is usually adequate. The frequent awakenings may cause restless sleep and abrupt wakefulness that are often troubling to an older adult. Thorough sleep assessment is necessary to determine actual sleep time. Additionally, the nurse may suggest afternoon exercise and a decrease in stimulants at bedtime.

Environmental changes, such as noise control and regulation of room temperature, may be helpful.

Common age-related changes of the nervous system, particularly slowed reaction time, affect movement, sleep, and cognition, the functions of which are vital to optimal performance of ADLs.

Special Sense Organs

The sensory organs of sight, hearing, taste, touch, and smell facilitate communication with the environment. Loss of sensory function, particularly vision and hearing, severely alters an older adult's self-care abilities and quality of life. Age-related changes that result in loss of sensory function may be the most difficult for a person of any age to accept and cope with effectively. The nurse must be extremely sensitive to sensory changes and their impact on each person.

Age-Related Changes
VISION
- Ability to focus on close objects is diminished.
- Increased density of the lens occurs, and lipid accumulates around the iris, causing a grayish yellow ring.
- The production of tears decreases.
- The pupils decrease in size and become less responsive to light.
- Night vision decreases, and the iris loses pigment so that eye color usually becomes light blue or gray.

HEARING
- The ability to hear high-frequency tones decreases.
- The cerumen contains a greater amount of keratin so that it hardens and becomes more likely to become impacted.

TASTE
- Ability to perceive bitter, salt, and sour tastes diminishes.

TOUCH
- Ability to feel light touch, pain, or different temperatures may decrease.

Functional Changes
Despite normal age-related changes in vision, most older adults have adequate visual function using corrective lenses for self-care activities. Because dark and light adaptation takes longer, simple activities, such as entering or leaving a theater or going to the bathroom at night, put older people at risk for falls and injury. Yellowing of the lens makes vision for low-tone colors (violet, blue, green) difficult; use of yellow, orange, or red colors on signs or on bedroom walls increases the older adult's ability to read. Decreased production of tears by the eye may contribute to irritation and infection; artificial tears are often prescribed.

Functional hearing changes result initially in an inability to hear high-pitched tones. The nurse should speak in a normal tone of voice without shouting and without increasing pitch.

Because it takes more sensory stimulation to trigger the taste experience, older adults may use more salt to produce a salt taste on their food effectively. Sensory changes have a profound impact on the functional ability of older adults. The nurse must always determine whether the patient uses corrective lenses or a hearing aid and ensure that the older person has these assistive devices available at all times.

Later in this book, the reader will be able to compare abnormal physiological changes of older adults with the normal changes explained here. As a future gerontological nurse, you should have a thorough understanding of both aspects of physiological aging.

CONCLUSION

This chapter has pointed out the importance of understanding the older adult in today's society. As the number of aged individuals increases, and as more and more older adults require nursing care, you need to develop a strong knowledge base in gerontological nursing content. It is equally important to explore the myths, stereotypes, and prejudices about old age to begin the process of seeing older adults as unique individuals who have special histories and life experiences. Understanding the various theories of aging can promote a more positive attitude toward the process. Normal aging changes each person in a unique way. As you acquire the specific knowledge and skills to be an effective caregiver of older adults, it is hoped that you will embrace the attitude that all older adults are unique and should be encouraged to function at their full potential. With this critical understanding, you are the generation of nurses who will define the application of gerontological nursing. Best wishes with the task!

CASE STUDY SOLUTIONS

1. Ms. B. has experienced age-related changes in all the following areas:

Cardiovascular

Decreased activity tolerance

Fatigue with increased activity

Musculoskeletal

Loss of muscle strength

Height loss

Joint pain

Integumentary

Dry skin

Brittle, thickened nails

Thinning hair

Gastrointestinal

Delayed gastric emptying leading to fullness

Reduced GI motility

Genitourinary

Urinary retention, which may contribute to infection

Urgency and stress incontinence

Nervous

Delayed reaction time

Special Senses

Diminished ability to focus on close objects

Inability to tolerate glare

Poor vision in reduced light

2. Ms. B. is a healthy older adult because she functions at an optimal level despite the presence of age-related changes. She feels good about her life and about her coping skills. She expects continued "good days."

REVIEW QUESTIONS

1. Your client is 84 years old. What normal change in vital signs would you expect to assess?
    1. A higher than normal temperature
    2. A slower pulse
    3. A shallower breathing pattern
    4. A lower blood pressure

2. Immobility or sedentary lifestyles have what effect on the older adult?
    1. Loss of muscle size and strength
    2. Decreased serum sodium levels
    3. Loss of skin elasticity
    4. Thinning of cartilage in joints

3. Mrs. Jones, aged 86 years, complains of fullness after eating only small amounts of food. This is primarily due to which GI change?
    1. Delayed gastric emptying time
    2. Increased gastric acid secretions
    3. Hypertonicity of gastric muscles
    4. Loss of ability to chew

4. Mrs. Smith, aged 79 years, is admitted to the hospital. Based on your understanding of normal age changes in the nervous system, what behavior might you expect Mrs. Smith to exhibit?
    1. Decreased intellectual function
    2. Forgetfulness and confusion
    3. Lack of orientation to time and place
    4. Longer response time to questions

5. Which of the following statements most accurately describes normal aging changes in an older adult?
    1. As individuals age, they become more diverse.
    2. Most older adults experience chronic illness and functional impairment.
    3. Age-related changes are similar in each older adult.
    4. Normal age changes most commonly describe decline and loss of function.

REFERENCES

Butler, R.M. (1969). Ageism: another form of bigotry. *Gerontologist,* 9, 243-246.

Erikson, E.H. (1963). *Childhood and society* (2nd ed.). New York, NY: Norton.

Hyman, B., Oden, G., & Wagner, M. (2010). The aging process: physiological changes and implications for educators and practitioners. *Activities, Adaptation, & Aging,* 34(2), 148-153.

King, B.J., Roberts, T.J., & Bowers, B.J. (2013). Nursing student attitudes toward and preferences for working with older adults. *Gerontology & Geriatrics Education,* 34 (3), 272-291.

WEB RESOURCES

Age Related Changes in Health. ConsultGeri.org: http://consultgerirn.org/topics/normal_aging_changes/want_to_know_more

Supporting Life Transitions and Spirituality in the Elderly

3

DIANE LEGGETT-FIFE

LEARNING OUTCOMES

1. Discuss the significance of transitions and spirituality in the lives of elderly people.

2. Describe what a transition is and the impact it has on people.

3. List four to six activities the nurse can perform that will facilitate a successful transitional outcome.

4. Define how the "progressively lowered stress threshold" concept can assist in the management of negative behaviors in older adults.

5. Recommend three transitions common to older adults.

6. Compare and contrast spirituality and religion.

CONCEPTS

Communication

Caring
  Interventions

Teaching and
  Learning

Collaboration

Advocacy

Ethics

Stress and Coping

Grief and Loss

Family

CASE STUDY

Mrs. Goldstein, age 82, was living at the local Hebrew Nursing Home after the death of her husband 8 months ago. She was admitted because she confused her heart medication with her arthritis medication and became dehydrated and fell. The fall resulted in a broken left humerus. She adjusted well to the nursing home and was allowed to bring in two of her favorite pieces of furniture, pictures of her husband and son, and artwork for the walls. Mrs. Goldstein is an Orthodox Jew who continued to practice her religion while in the home.

Mrs. Goldstein became confused during the night and fell while trying to get out of bed. She fractured her femur and bumped her forehead. After assessing her, the nursing home sent her by ambulance to St. Mary's hospital. You are Mrs. Goldstein's nurse postoperatively.

As Mrs. Goldstein is being wheeled down the hall to her room, from surgery, you hear her crying out and repeatedly saying, "My head, what have you done to my head?" She is grabbing at her head while she repeats her question. When she is recovered enough to eat something other than clear liquids, you bring her a light supper. On the tray are cheese, crackers, Jell-O, and a small slice of turkey. She immediately demands to know who fixed the food and where it was prepared. She pushes the tray away, and by doing so, knocks it onto the floor. The next day is Saturday, and Mrs. Goldstein refuses to go to physical therapy. This is very serious because the therapy department is closed on Sunday.

Discussion

1. Why is Mrs. Goldstein asking about her head? How will you approach her to discuss her concern?

2. Why is Mrs. Goldstein refusing her food? Determine what has caused this behavior and how you can assist her with what seems to be a problem.

3. Why is Mrs. Goldstein refusing to go to physical therapy? How will you resolve this problem?

4. Consider all three problems and determine what you can do to help Mrs. Goldstein.

 ## INTRODUCTION

With today's harried workloads in health-care environments, you, the licensed practical nurse (LPN), may think that there is not time to deal with the issues of transition and spirituality. There are too many medications, too many treatments, and definitely too much paperwork! In addition, there are not enough licensed nurses and too many budget cuts. It is challenging and difficult for this generation of nurses to be able to deliver humanistic (vs. mechanistic) care. Transitions are a consistent part of life, however. Think of Mrs. Goldstein, who had faced several transitions and was expressing frustration from not having her needs met. Even the choice to be a more humanistic, holistic nurse requires a transitional period, during which time the nurse needs to work out the details of how to treat elderly people in a more caring and holistic manner, while still fulfilling all of his or her responsibilities on time. This chapter will assist you in understanding transitions and spirituality so that you can learn to incorporate holistic care into your daily practice.

 ## SIGNIFICANCE OF TRANSITIONS AND SPIRITUALITY

Whatever your age, you have experienced a lifetime of *transitions,* which are the moments between what was old and what is new. One author describes transition as the moment when you let go of a trapeze bar (the old life) and are soaring through the unknown until you reach the second trapeze bar (the new life). That time between the bars, when you are hurtling through space, is frightening, unpredictable, and lacks familiar reference points. The time of the unknown, which is usually marked by the stress provoked by the change, is the *transitional* moment (Schulweis, 2003).

You experienced transitions after you chose to attend school. The need to pay for school, arrange child care, the need to complete house work and/or school work, and the need to maintain a part-time job are some possible challenges that you faced during the transition. Do you remember the stressful feelings you had until you worked out the details successfully? That period of stress and the unknown was the transitional period. You eventually resolved the stress of the changes and are now a successful student.

Youth is a period of constant growth and learning. A child learns to ambulate by first crawling, then standing up, and then walking; the child may then learn to ride a tricycle and then a bicycle. All of these instances involve periods of uncertainty as the child learns the new skill. Adults, too, experience transitions as they commit to an education and career, a spouse, and possibly children.

As people reach older adulthood, there is still much to learn and many new skills to master; however, it is also a time when more of life's changes include loss. I am referring to children leaving their parents' home for work, school, or adventure, among other choices. One's parents may die and siblings or friends may move or succumb to accident or disease. Retirement is a big change for most people, resulting in a loss of work friends, income, and often social position. As people age, some develop the chronic diseases of normal aging and other diseases such as heart disease, diabetes mellitus, or a debilitating stroke that results in physical and emotional losses.

Many of the life occurrences that accompany aging are challenging experiences, and all of them require older adults to make a life transition. No one experiences only one transition in a lifetime, and sometimes there is more than one transition at a time. Each loss or change requires transitional effort from the person experiencing it. Think of Mrs. Goldstein and the transitions she has faced: the loss of her husband, moving to a new location unexpectedly, and the loss of independence and some mobility. All of these required transitional effort on her part.

Another example is a young-old friend who lives out of state, who called me recently. She had fallen while attempting to do yard work; although she lives alone, a neighbor noticed that she was lying in her front yard crying with pain. She was found to have a broken wrist and a sprained rotator cuff (shoulder). Her wrist was put into a brace, her arm was placed in a sling, and she was instructed to see an orthopedic surgeon that upcoming Monday. Yet on Sunday, she had so much pain in one of her teeth that she had an emergency root canal (I am not making this up!). She is a strong woman who has lived her life well. When I talked to her this morning, however, she was feeling despair. The changes she was dealing with were major and painful, and she was managing them alone. She needed assistance to move through the changes: someone kind who would keep her informed, provide honest hope regarding her situation, and care for her as the total person she is rather than the crying older woman she appeared to be. Humanistic health-care providers can assist her and people like her through this transition.

Now let us consider how spirituality fits into the concept of transition. *Spirituality* is often part of the process of transition for older people. Most people have a belief in God, the Divine, or a greater power. With this belief, there is a connection with something more powerful than oneself. When individuals have this connection, it links them to others with a similar belief. It also can be a link to nature or to familiar rituals and behaviors. Spirituality is comforting and can provide for many people a method for understanding the losses that are being experienced.

Spirituality can also provide the purpose for moving forward, for accepting and adapting to the losses that are occurring, and for finding the strength to deal with one's life changes. This ability to "move on" results in an improved quality of life and death. Let us return to my friend who had fallen in her yard. She is a very religious person, and I know that she would want to see a clergyman and would appreciate someone to pray with her. I realize that you may not believe in God and may not pray. If that is the case, as her nurse you could offer to sit with her while she prays, and you could offer to call the clergyman. Because her religious beliefs have helped her through previous transitions in her life, she will benefit from them again. Accepting and accommodating a person's spirituality to the

Think Like a Nurse

You have been assigned care of a patient recently admitted for repair of a fractured ulna on the right side. She was given pain medication in the emergency department before being transferred to your care. She does not have family with her at this time and reports that all her family lives out of the state. She has voiced concern about being able to care for herself because she is right handed. What would be some physical and transitional priorities for this patient?

Responses

- The developmental stage for this patient is to maintain integrity (see Eric Erickson's stages of development in Chapter 2). Communication with and for the patient is key to identifying and meeting the needs of the patient.
- Physical priorities should include pain management to prevent feelings of hopelessness, physical therapy consultation to address changes in mobility and use of the right arm, and occupational therapy consultation to assist in the transition to home from the facility.
- Transitional care priorities would include communication with all health-care providers involved in the care and any family members or significant others (neighbors or friends) who will be assisting in the care. This communication should address available services to be accessed, should provide consistent information to those involved in the care across the continuum, and should be leveled according to the educational level of the patient. The patient needs to feel that needs are and will be met throughout the time of recovery.

best of one's ability is one of the many ways a holistic nurse can help a person through a transition. Think of Mrs. Goldstein and the solutions offered for her care relating to her spirituality. The nurse recognized that she was in a Catholic hospital but was a practicing Orthodox Jew. With this information, the nurse offered her a cover for her head, arranged for kosher food, and took time to listen to her as a caring nurse.

UNDERSTANDING TRANSITIONS

Ralph Waldo Emerson, a poet, essayist, and philosopher who is described as belonging to the tradition of "wisdom literature," commented,

"Not in all his goals, but in his transitions a man is great." (ThinkExist, n. d.). Emerson understood change and its powerful impact on the life quest for individuals. Transitions are significant, universal human experiences. Because transitions are interconnected with the growth of the person and, consequently, the world, understanding transitions has rich significance for your personal and professional life and for your practice of human caring.

As a holistic nurse, your objective is to assist the older person in your care to be successful in making the transition and managing the stress. Doing so alleviates despair and promotes integrity for the individual, and it achieves your objective of excellent caregiving. Most people have experienced a critical transition; if you assist people in remembering the behaviors that were helpful to them in the past, they can use those behaviors again to help them through the transition that they are currently facing.

Common Transitions

High school graduation, sudden loss of a job, marriage, significant illness, death of a loved one, pregnancy, divorce, and relocation to a new home are some of the life events you may have experienced. These events are marked by beginnings and endings and a new phase of life change (the time between the trapeze bars). Joy and celebration at a transition are common, although some transitional events result in a deep sense of loss and sadness. Whether pleasant, painful, anticipated, unexpected, temporary, or permanent, all transitions, by their nature, evoke some degree of stress.

Patients often face health-illness transitions, which occur when changes in health status result in a change in role relations, expectations, and abilities. Multiple transitions occurring simultaneously are common and particularly challenging. For example, a health-illness transition precipitated by a severe stroke can require a person to relocate to a hospital, which could be followed by a second or even third relocation to a nursing home or rehabilitation center. In addition, there are the physical losses from the stroke: perhaps the loss of one's job and social role as the breadwinner. Dependence on others often is a difficult transition for most people to make.

The time span of a complex transition, such as having a stroke, extends from the first anticipation of transition until a sense of stability in the new

Priority Setting

The priority for this chapter is to help you understand your own personal transitions. It is only through personal experience that a person can successfully and sincerely apply transitional theory. Examine your own life and critically consider what has happened to you in terms of transitions, and then learn to identify your personal strengths. How did you manage your last three transitions? Were they effective coping skills? What would assist you in the future? When you understand this concept on a personal level, you will be able to apply it to elderly people. Remember, you also want to achieve gerotranscendence, so now is a good time to begin working toward it.

situation has been achieved. A transitional period can last weeks or months, which indicates the critical need for nursing staff to know and understand the concept of transition. Only by understanding can the nurse be therapeutic.

Four Common Features of Transitions

Transitions are serious, life-altering experiences. They are processes of change that are lasting in their effects; they force one to give up how they view the world, and they necessitate the development of new thinking and skills. Transitions generally cause great emotion and require the person experiencing the transition to work hard to survive the change. Transitions warrant the attention of health-care professionals.

Critically Examine the Following

Think back to your most difficult transition. How did you feel? What assisted you to manage the transition? Take the time to make a list of the people, activities, or thoughts that assisted you to "hang on" during the space between the trapeze bars.

According to researchers (Davies, 2005; Jungers, 2010), there are four common features to transition:

1. A phase of turmoil
2. Disturbances in bodily function
3. Mood and cognition changes
4. An altered time perspective

These four characteristics are commonly seen in older adults in health-care facilities. Have you had experience with an older person who was in a state of turmoil, was unable to control bowel or bladder, seemed confused, and did not know the time or date? I realize that this could be a person with mental illness or any form of dementia, that a loss in bodily function is expected when someone has a stroke, and that time confusion is something that happens to people who are no longer tied to work schedules or routines.

So are these characteristics being exhibited because of illness or because of transition? All of these behaviors demonstrate a change for the person experiencing them, and so they are due to transitions. As a nurse, you can play a strong role in assisting a person to make sense of the change and to manage it with minimal symptoms. The objective is integrity vs. despair. With your thoughtful application of transition theory, you can assist the older people in your care to achieve integrity and improve their quality of life and death.

HOW TO INFLUENCE A TRANSITIONAL OUTCOME

You can influence the outcome of transitions for elderly people. The following factors have been identified as having a strong influence on transitional outcomes:

1. Degree of choice in the transitional process
2. Extent or degree of change
3. Preparation for the change
4. Characteristics of the individual experiencing the transition
5. The individual's perception of the change
6. The characteristics of the prechange and postchange environment, including support systems (Anthony & Hudson-Barr, 2004; Davies, 2005; Jungers, 2010; Ryan & Deci, 2000).

The moments of our lives combine to make a lifetime of transitions. This picture of a grandmother, mother, and daughter is symbolic of that concept.

Let's examine these influences and see how nurses can use these influences to help ease older people into necessary transitions.

Give People a Degree of Choice and Respect Their Decisions

People who think they have freely chosen the transition are more likely to embrace it or own it. Think of the differences between your decision to come to LPN school and the fact that you "had" to go to high school. Choice is an essential part of being human, and it should be honored and respected.

I spent some time as a consultant at a large (700-bed) nursing home on the East Coast. While I was there, I learned some valuable lessons. The most profound lesson that I learned occurred on the very large Alzheimer's Unit. Everyone, and I mean *everyone,* included the residents in the decision making. For example, a resident refused his medication, and the polite and caring nurse agreed with the decision and came back within 10 minutes and tried again (successfully). She understood that the resident had the right to refuse any treatment, had the need to have some control over his life, and that—within just a few minutes—may forget that he refused the medication and might be amenable to taking it later. When the housekeeper asked to clean a resident's room and was told no, the decision-making authority to the resident was respected and the housekeeper did not go in, but returned when the resident was not in the room. The housekeeper accepted the negative answer, but did not neglect professional responsibility. Everything was done, just at a slightly later time.

Evidence-Based Practice

Schoenborn, N.L., Arbaje, A.I., Eubank, K.J., Maynor, K., & Carrese, J.A. (2013). Clinician roles and responsibilities during care transitions of older adults. *Journal of the American Geriatric Society, 61,* 231–236.

This qualitative study explored what constituted successful care transitions for older adults when transitioning to a variety of care settings. Despite literature outlining challenges to optimal care for the older adult, the role of clinicians in the resolution of these challenges remains poorly documented. This study examined the perspectives of health-care professional regarding processes, roles and responsibilities, and barriers during the transition of care for the older adult. The researchers found that little information is available for clinicians to define roles during transition of care, and this lack of information may result in placing the older adult at greater risk of readmission.

Questions

Which of the following inferences can you make? State whether the study summary provides extensive, limited, or no evidence to support each inference.

1. Clinicians are anxious to transition the older adult to other care facilities.
2. Roles and responsibilities for clinicians during care transition are not clearly outlined or defined.
3. Older adults transitioning to other care facilities will benefit from more organized processes.
4. Health-care professionals do not always understand or know their roles during transitions of care of the older adult.
5. Readmission to a health-care facility is not the concern of health-care professionals.

Mrs. Goldstein was unable to participate in many of the decisions regarding her because of the situation. As a nurse, if you realize the importance of the desire to have some degree of choice in decision, you would have been able to offer her something as simple as choosing her meal. When she was included in the physical therapy participation appointment decision, she was more calm and willing to negotiate.

Make the Extent or Degree of Change More Manageable

Transitions can be made smoother if the apparent obstacles are removed and the changes are manageable. A family asking their aging mother to relocate from a rural farmhouse to a city apartment to be closer to health-care services would require their mother to make a huge change, which would be very disruptive for the older woman. To ease their mother into the transition, a family member who lives in the city could invite her to stay for either a long weekend or a 2-week period so that she could get a feel for city life. Additionally, when the family members find an apartment that meets the physical requirements necessary for their mother, they could verify that there are people near their mother's age who live in or around the complex. Is there a senior citizen's center nearby where she can crochet with newly made friends? Is there a grocery store that is within walking distance? All of these are thoughtful considerations of a loving family that would make their mother's transition easier. They represent humanistic caring rather than mechanistic caring. The mechanistic solution would be to find an apartment that meets the location and safety needs of the mother, while doing nothing to make the transition less stressful. Which approach would you like someone to use with you?

Another example of humanistic caring is the nurse's willingness to negotiate care with Mrs. Goldstein. The nurse also brought some personal items to the facility to help in the adjustment of the change.

Help Prepare People for the Transition

Although preparation for a transition is something logical to do, reflect on how often people fail to prepare for a transition even though it is expected. Consider a person diagnosed with a chronic disease like diabetes. This individual needs to know what to expect and how this disease will impact his or her life in order for them to start the transition process. Death is something we all will experience, and yet it seems difficult for people in our society to discuss it and plan for it. Psychologists often say that the closer a family is, the easier it is

to discuss the topic. When transitions are identified as part of one's future, preparation is a key factor in being able to manage them.

Talk to your patients and residents about changes that are anticipated. Give them all appropriate information and be willing to repeat it as often as necessary. You should involve the family members as well. Use your creative thinking and do all you can for each individual to prepare him or her for changes that are coming.

Consider the Characteristics of the Individual

Transitions can be very threatening to persons who are cognitively impaired or who require a high degree of structure and predictability in their environments. Research has shown that relocating people who are mentally ill or confused is associated with higher death rates compared with people with similar impairments who are not moved. Some people who are cognitively intact don't deal well with change, either. It is common for people to fear or avoid change.

A person's personality, past experiences, and coping skills are important factors to consider when helping that person through a transition. Generally, being in good health increases resiliency during stressful times (Sapolsky, 2004). Adequate sleep, nutrition, exercise, and satisfying social relationships are also important to transitional outcomes.

When considering past experiences and coping skills, think back to Mrs. Goldstein. She had lost her husband only 8 months earlier, she had been moved to a nursing home and now was facing another major transition. The nurse took the time to talk to her in an effort to discover what coping skills she had used previously.

Learn How the Person Perceives the Transition

All of us create meaning and give our experiences labels. Different individuals can view the same transition as an opportunity, blessing, crisis, challenge, or disaster. Use your communication skills to listen to how a person perceives a transition and gain insight into the unique meanings that are attached to it for the person. It is dangerous to assume that you know what someone is thinking. It is better to invite their reflection on the transition and accept that there are differences in the way people think.

Critically Examine the Following

Think back to your decision to go to school. What fears did you experience? Were there changes that you tried to avoid? Now think of an older adult in your life, either someone to whom you have given care or someone who is a friend or family member who has recently experienced a transition. Did you recognize their fears or resistance at the time? Do you see them now? They are there even if you did not recognize them.

Remember the example of the woman who needed to move to the city from her farm? It is possible that she would love to be closer to her grandchildren, that she is excited about being near a wider variety of stores for shopping, and that she recognizes that she needs to be closer to healthcare services.

Taking time to talk to individuals, as the nurse did with Mrs. Goldstein, provides valuable information to assist both you as the nurse and the individual with the transition. It is important to listen and, as mentioned, not assume you know what is going to be said. Listening is how you will learn about the individual.

Help Improve Environmental Characteristics

We all live in an environment with its variable aspects. When you walk onto a unit in a hospital or nursing home, can you sense what the environment really is like? I am not talking about cleanliness or colorful or drab decoration schemes, although they are important for a healing environment. I am referring to aspects of the environment such as cheerfulness, relaxation, nurturance, and respectfulness. These environmental components are the opposite of harsh, demanding, restrictive, and joyless environments. In caregiving situations, nurses have the power to cocreate, with the older adults, healing environments that are loving, empowering, and respectful. Remember the personal items the nurse brought to the hospital for Mrs. Goldstein? Seeing the picture of her husband gave her renewed hope to work on recovery.

 ## PROGRESSIVELY LOWERED STRESS THRESHOLD

The "progressively lowered stress threshold" (PLST) is a care concept (Hall & Buckwalter, 1987) designed to be used when planning personalized, holistic care for elderly individuals. The concept of PLST originates from the importance of personal freedom and control. According to the PLST theory, dysfunctional or negative behaviors of humans often occur because of increased anxiety. If people perceive that they have lost their personal freedom or their control over a situation because of an increasing amount of outside stressors, they can become anxious and stressed, which leads to frustration and anger.

A classic example with which most people are familiar is getting children to eat their vegetables. Imagine a scene at the family dinner table when parents tell their children to eat their vegetables. By telling the children to do something, the children's personal freedom and control are taken away. Generally, this situation results in a power struggle (*note: no one* wins in a power struggle) and in the children not eating their vegetables.

An elderly person's freedom is restricted during the time he or she resides in a health-care facility. In hospitals and nursing homes, meals are generally served at set times, and baths are given at the convenience of the staff rather than of the patient or resident. No one is encouraged to stay up late and watch or read a good mystery! There are rules in health-care facilities, and they usually are enforced.

When people have limited control over their life, there is a higher likelihood that stress will occur. With unresolved stress comes frustration, and unresolved frustration leads to anger (Sapolsky, 2004). That is a normal human reaction. What does anger look like? It is different for every person because of individual personality traits, but it can include raising one's voice, screaming, hitting, or a high level of criticism of the environment and the people in it. If you perceive that the reason behind the anger is stress because of lack of control, you can apply your understanding of PLST to your practice and work at giving the people in your care as much personal control over their lives as is safe for them.

Critically Examine the Following

Take some time and think back to any recent experience when you were told what to do. How did you feel? Did it make you feel like a child? That is the feeling that comes to me. I like suggestions, interesting information, even metaphors, but I do not like being told what to do. I have learned over the years how to handle this feeling so that a situation does not degenerate into a power struggle, but I still have to take time to consider my reaction.

Write a brief paragraph regarding how you feel when someone imposes on your personal freedom. Note how you handle being told what to do and what your thought processes are regarding it. Then consider how your feelings compare with those of any elderly person with whom you have had experience. Does the older adult like being told what to do? How does he or she handle the situation? Be prepared to share your ideas in class either verbally or by handing in the paragraph.

Common Stressors

Five common stressors that tend to result in the highest levels of stress for older persons are:

1. Fatigue.
2. Change in environment, routine, or caregiver.
3. Misleading or inappropriate stimuli (sounds or noise are examples).
4. Internal or external demands to achieve that exceed one's functional ability.
5. Physical stressors such as pain, discomfort, infection, acute illness, or depression (Hall & Buckwalter, 1987).

I am sure that you can immediately see the relationship between transition and these five stressors. It is like "the perfect storm." Changing living environments is tiring (stressor 1), and it is a dramatic change in environment, routine, and caregiver (stressor 2). The person going through the transition may have great expectations from self to "do well" so as not to worry "my daughter/son" or to assure a return to one's home (stressor 4). Deteriorating health or a new illness (stressor 5) may be the very reason the elderly person was moved.

With this basic information on PLST, do you see how transitions and most other stressors will, in all likelihood, result in the older person showing signs of stress? Even under ideal circumstances most of us would feel the effects of stress; thus this is something that needs to be recognized as a reality in giving care to susceptible older people.

Application of Progressively Lowered Stress Threshold

Your objective, each day you go to work, needs to be to decrease the stress of the persons in your care. This often includes the certified nursing assistants (CNAs) and other people in your work environment. Settle disputes among the staff, keep noise levels low, provide places of rest for elderly people in the facility to avoid fatigue, and expect stress-related behavior to occur.

When such behavior does occur, don't be upset and get involved in the problem. Instead, use your knowledge, and work to eliminate the stress. Perhaps taking an elderly man who is angry and combative off the unit for a "special walk" with you will remove him from what is upsetting him. Try to find out what is the stressor for any person who is acting stressed, and involve the other members of the health-care team in correcting the problem.

Remember the initial premise of the PLST model. It is to give as much control as possible to the individuals in your care. After all, they are adults who are accustomed to making their own decisions, and, in most situations, they should be allowed to continue. This premise requires the entire health-care team to understand and agree to provide such an environment.

Transition is challenging, and being older can be difficult. The role of the LPN is to do everything possible to make these realities less stressful and enhance the quality of daily life for older adults.

Read the following poem. It is charming and meaningful. Read the poem to enjoy it, and then read it again to look for the impact of transition and PLST on human life.

Point of Interest

I remember a cold and snowy winter afternoon in Utah. My daughter, one of her friends, and I were traveling in the car. The girls were laughing and playing noisy games in the backseat, the radio was blaring something I didn't recognize, and, unknown to me, the temperature was falling. I recognized the fall in temperature the moment my tires started to slide on the newly formed ice into a monstrous snowdrift on the side of the road. If I corrected the slide, I would head into the oncoming traffic. I was stressed!

Within a brief second my entire personality changed. I turned off both the heater and the radio, I literally yelled at the girls to be quiet, and then miraculously (or so it seemed to me) I was able to stop the car with minor damage caused by the snowdrift. When the initial stress was over, I spoke with great concern and tenderness to the girls, turned the heater back on, and got out my cell phone to get the help I needed.

Why did my behavior change so abruptly? It was because of the stress. Without thinking, I turned off the radio and heater because they were stressors to me. Much to my chagrin, I yelled at the girls because their noise was a stressor as well. Then, with less external stress, I could handle the immediate situation.

Have you seen exasperated mothers of young children raise their voice at them in a store? A man swearing out loud because of a flat tire? Two children or two adults hitting each other? I observe that they usually are exhibiting such behavior because they are stressed. Relate the concept of stress and the resulting behavior to yourself. Once you understand how it affects you, you will have a better understanding of how and why it makes a big impact on elderly people, who often have fewer physiological resources.

Sunshine Acres Living Center
Marilyn Krysl, RN

The first thing you see up ahead is
Mr. Polanski,
wedged in the arched doorway,
like he means absolutely
to stay there; he shouldn't
be there in the first place, put here
by mistake, courtesy of that grandson
who thinks he's a hotshot, and too busy
raking in the dough to take time
for an old man.

If he had anyplace to go, you know he'd
be out instantly, if he had any money.
So he intends to stay in that doorway,
not missing a thing, and waiting for trouble.
Which of course will come.
And that could be you—you're handy, you
  look
likely, you have the authority. And you're
new here, another young whippersnapper,
doesn't know ankle from elbow, but has
been given the keys.

Well, he's ready, Mr. Polanski. So you go right
to him. "Mr. Polanski, good morning." You

say it in Polish, which you learned a little of
when you were little, and your grandmother
taught you a little song about lambs, frisking
in a pen, and you danced a silly dance with
your grandmother while the two of you sang.

So you sing it for him in the dim, institutional
light of the hallway, light which even you find
insupportable, because at that moment
it reminds you of the light in the hallway
in the rest home where, when your
grandmother died, you weren't there.
So you're also singing to console yourself.
And at the moment you pay her this silly
little tribute.

Mr. Polanski steps out of the doorway. He
who had set himself to resist you, he who
made himself a first, Mr. Polanski,
  contentious
  often combative
  and always inconsolable
hears that you know the song. And he steps
  out
from the fortress of the doorway, begins to
  shuffle
and sing along.

This poem captures many aspects of human relationships and struggles. You may want to discuss your insights about the poem's message with fellow students or family members. As an LPN, you will have many opportunities to meet people like Mr. Polanski.

Understanding the mediating factors of control and decision making, preparation, support, meaning and perception, and maintaining optimal health will assist you in your own transitions as well as in supporting and caring for older people.

COMMON TRANSITIONS FOR OLDER ADULTS

As I have stated, transitions occur at every stage of life. It is important to examine the transitions that commonly occur in the lives of older adults to anticipate them and develop the knowledge base to be supportive when they occur. As you know, not all transitions happen for everyone, but some can be anticipated because of their frequency in the aging process. Job changes and retirement, family role changes, and health changes are common impetuses for transitions that occur with older people.

Job Changes and Retirement

Job changes and retirement can have a dramatic impact on the aging population. Common changes include the following:

1. *Role change.* When an older person retires, the role change can be a very difficult transition. The person retiring has to adjust to the loss of what was their purpose and position for 8 or more hours a day.
2. *Lower income.* A retiree's income often is decreased. This can be the cause of several other changes. Health care can be reduced because of the financial need to maintain the house or replace a furnace. Good nutrition may be impacted because of the expense of essential medication. Plans of traveling or other leisure activities may have to be cancelled.
3. *Dissatisfaction with employment status.* Older adults generally were raised with a strong work ethic and believe that unemployment is an unacceptable situation whatever the cause.

4. *Unpreparedness for the future.* Many people do not prepare for their eventual retirement. They have not developed interests outside of work, prepared financially for a decreased income, or nurtured their dreams. Without preparation, retirement can be fraught with profound losses for the individual.
5. *Loss of identity.* For some people, the loss of their job, with retirement or other factors, threatens their identity. Most people derive their identity from the work they have done throughout their lifetime. Be it mother, physician, teacher, or nurse, part of who we are rests solidly on what we do. When that crucial role is gone, it is a struggle to redefine one's personal identity, and that struggle is not always successful.
6. *Lack of social interaction.* Someone who has been focused on their work setting often has many friends there. With retirement comes a separation from those people. This can be a serious transition unless the retiree has been wise enough to maintain relationships outside of work. Without friends to join in social activities, life can be very lonely.

Family Role Changes

Family roles and relationships change as each of us age. Common changes in old age are the following:

1. *Grandparenting.* Because of the aging of America, more people experience grandparenting, and many are able to enjoy this phase of life longer than ever before in U.S. history. There can be serious transitional concerns, however, with the various roles grandparenting can take.
2. *Distant family members.* Adult children move out of the house, and many are scattered throughout the United States or the world. Older people of today frequently were raised with the responsibility to build their adult lives in a location near their parents to promote family closeness and to care for their aging parents. Today's grandparents often have to adjust to not seeing children and grandchildren as frequently as they would like, and they may not be able to count on adult children

to assist them to remain in their homes as they age.

3. *Parenting for parents.* Some grandparents are assisting single parents by providing child care or are tending children while both parents work, while others may be grandparenting full time. For many older adults, this can be too much responsibility in the day-to-day activities of their children and grandchildren.

4. *Role crisis.* Parents eventually die. In some situations, the illness and death are lingering, which requires the caregiver to be part of what is known as the "sandwich generation." This role often goes to the woman. The sandwich generation caregiver is a person who is raising children while caring for aging parents. As this person ages, the children leave the home, and the parents die. This can cause a role crisis because there is no one left who needs the "sandwiched" person.

5. *Death of spouse.* The death of a spouse is more common as people age. It is an event that has a dramatic impact on all aspects of life for the surviving partner. When an older spouse dies, the survivor has lost the person with whom he or she has spent most of his or her life. The intimacy that was shared is gone as is the help, understanding, and often part of the income. Their experiences together can be the most significant happenings that have occurred during their lifetime. With the deceased person go dreams, plans for the future, and a lifelong companion. The loss can be intolerable.

6. *Insufficient income.* More women than men experience the death of a spouse. Because of their age, many older women have not worked outside of the home and are poorly prepared to supplement their income. Their life role generally has been focused on their spouse and children. These women end up alone, without the income they need, and with fewer friends because most of their previous friends were couples. If their children and grandchildren are living in other states, the situation is even more difficult because they are truly alone.

Health Changes

Health changes are complex concerns for older adults. They can affect every system in the body and cause a change in one's health that has a life-altering impact. Some common health changes are as follows:

1. *Illness and disability,* which are major reasons that older adults need assistance and support. It is estimated that at least 50% of the population in the United States over the age of 60 is living with at least two chronic diseases. These chronic diseases lead to disabilities that limit doing yard work or housework (Agency for Healthcare Research and Quality, 2002). This may extend to cooking as well. Along with the disappointment over what they are unable to do, older adults with disabilities often worry about being placed in an institution such as a nursing home or assisted living facility. The overall fear is the loss of independence.

2. *Acute diseases.* It could be the flu or pneumonia, a heart attack, or some type of infection. Regardless, older adults often do not have the strength to fight such acute illnesses as they did when they were younger. The immune system commonly is weaker because of aging (Mauk, 2014). Every winter, numerous older people die of pneumonia because their bodies are no longer strong enough to ward off the disease.

3. *Body image.* Adjusting to a new body image is another challenge of growing older. There may be crippling from arthritis that interferes with routine activities such as cooking or walking. The older body gains weight and becomes shorter, hair color changes, and vision and hearing diminish. There are also changes related to acute and chronic diseases. All of these conditions can cause an altered body image or lower one's self-esteem.

4. *Longer physiologic response time.* The aging body does not work as efficiently as it once did. Fatigue is often a daily occurrence along with decreased memory function and slower response time (Mauk, 2014).

It is important for you to keep these transitional situations in mind as you care for older people. For example, even if you have seen numerous people put into wheelchairs because of the pain and danger of arthritis, remember that it is each person's first time doing so. During the transition, there are fear and concern on the part of the older adult and the need for support and understanding from you. Preparing yourself to assist people through the transition is a critical aspect of giving holistic nursing care.

SIGNIFICANCE OF SPIRITUALITY

In the lifelong search for integrity vs. despair, spirituality has a significant role. Most people feel they are part of something very important when a spiritual bond connects them to others. There is a commonality in belief and understanding of the universe. The belief system often provides a social system as well. These aspects of spirituality are supportive to someone going through one or several transitions.

Religion and Spirituality

There is a difference between religion and spirituality. *Religion* is the organized practice of one's belief regarding God or a higher power. Most religions have a formal building for worship and prescribed actions (prayer) or practices (partaking of the sacrament). Some religions worship personages other than a God or simply believe in a Divine power. Religion is an organized practice, whereas *spirituality* is the feeling within that communicates to individuals there is a higher power at work in the universe. Many spiritual people do not belong to a religion but practice beliefs they feel strongly about regarding a higher power (Fontaine, 2011; Taylor, 2002).

Humans, by their nature, are spiritual. It is the part of being human that seeks meaningfulness through some type of connection such as with nature or with other humans (Taylor, 2002). This makes awareness of and concern for another's spiritual and religious needs a significant aspect of nursing care. Being supportive while sharing and participating in a person's spiritual beliefs is an important aspect of holistic care.

Realizing their connection to something greater than themselves assists all people to rise above their challenges. For older adults, this sense of connection to a greater being is very important because of the numerous losses and transitions they make as they age. Spirituality and the practice of formal religion can assist people to overcome their problems, manage their despair, and find the peace that will help them to accept the change that is occurring (Fontaine, 2011; Taylor, 2002). Spirituality and religion help provide the essential step toward integrity and gerotranscendence.

Assessing Spiritual Needs

Assessing people for their spiritual needs and identifying how you can assist in meeting them may be a new skill for you. Most health-care facilities list the religious preference of the person on the chart. That is the place to start. Use your observation skills to identify religious jewelry or other artifacts in the person's personal belongings. Are there religious books in the room such as the Koran, Book of Mormon, or Bible?

The facility where you work may have a spiritual assessment. If not, think about what it is you need to know to be helpful. The information you need should include the following:

1. Does the person belong to a formal religious group? If so, does he or she want the leader of the group or other members to be contacted? Are there special rituals the person would like to have performed, such as a blessing for health, a prayer circle, or something else?
2. You need to know the person's specific spiritual beliefs, so ask. Then inquire if there are any specific practices the person would like to see performed. This may include a Shaman from the Navajo Indian culture, being allowed out of bed to pray on the floor facing East for a Muslim, incense burning, or specific foods. You cannot meet an individual's spiritual needs unless you know what that person believes.
3. When a person in your care is found crying, exhibits depression, or simply does not seem interested in what is going on in the environment, these could be symptoms of spiritual distress. A person may continuously question, "Why is God

doing this to me?" or, "What have I done to deserve all of these problems?" Comments of this type often are expressions of an unmet spiritual need.

4. Some people exhibit anger at God or the Divine power because of the severity of

---

QSEN

COMPETENCY: Patient-Centered Care (Knowledge, Skills, Attitudes)

Respect for Patient Preferences, Values, and Needs

Alman Ahmini, a 72-year-old man who practices the Islamic faith, has been admitted to the hospital for pneumonia. He requires oxygen by nasal cannula and has been encouraged to increase his intake of fluids by mouth. He has brought with him a book that he refers to as the Qur'an and informed the admitting personnel that it was Ramadan for the next 3 days. You are the nurse assigned to his care for the evening.

At approximately 6 in the evening, you hear a commotion coming from his room. You enter to find him attempting to climb out of bed and tangled in his oxygen tubing. As you try to assist him back to bed, he begins protesting and pushing you away. You also notice that his evening meal tray remains untouched, and he refuses to have any fluids by mouth.

You request assistance to help him back in bed. The individual who comes in to assist has spoken with a family member and informs you of the desire for the patient to say his prayers and to honor Ramadan by not eating or drinking until after sundown. With this information, you and the assistant help the patient into position for prayers while making sure the oxygen is still in place. After helping him back to bed following prayers, you notify the primary health-care provider of the patient's desire to remain faithful by not eating or drinking during the daylight hours and make a note in the chart of the patient's requests.

- Should the nurse allow and/or assist the patient out of bed? Why or why not?
- How did the nurse and assistant show respect for the preferences of this patient?
- How would you describe the values and needs of this patient?

---

the transition that must be made. Loss of basic physical ability because of a severe stroke or unmanageable pain from cancer could be examples. An older adult may feel betrayed by God and express unusual anger. This symptom of unmet spiritual needs should be addressed with understanding and empathy.

Resolving Spiritual Needs

Research indicates that a meaningful spiritual or religious practice promotes health and healing in many people (Haber, 2003). Because of this fact alone, you need to strive to identify unmet spiritual needs. When you have identified such needs, determine interventions that will help the older adult in your care. You should do all you can to assist the person to meet the unmet needs. This may require quiet listening, meaningful discussions, and the involvement of outside people from the religious or spiritual groups of the person. Remember the nurse caring for Mrs. Goldstein and the time she took to work with her to resolve issues of attending physical therapy because of the conflict with religious beliefs. Lack of physical therapy could have impacted her recovery.

To learn what you need to be helpful, you need to *listen attentively*. Ask questions if you do not understand what has been said. Plan time so that you can stay with the person until he or she is through with what he or she wants to say. Then take this new understanding to your nurse manager and, together, identify a way to resolve the spiritual need.

It is essential that you *accept the beliefs* of the person in your care, even if you do not agree with them. Your support of another's belief system is as important as your support when you assist someone to walk. Work with the family and spiritual leaders to provide the spirituality that will assist with comfort and healing.

Provide the people in your care with time alone so that they can participate in religious activities. This time could be spent praying, reading religious or other meaningful books, or meditating in solitude. Solitude is a valuable asset for most spiritual people. Do all you can to provide it for your patients while still caring for their physical needs.

Remember the spiritual need that is expressed with anger toward God or a Divine power? It generally is based on the need to make sense of the transition that has occurred. *Do **not** be judgmental* when you hear this anger. Be empathetic, and do

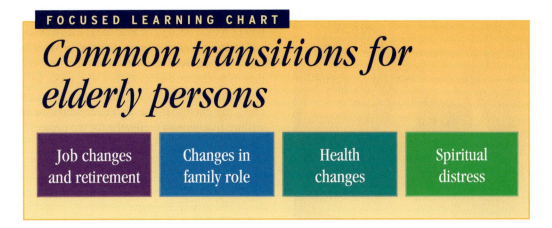

Common transitions for elderly persons

| Job changes and retirement | Changes in family role | Health changes | Spiritual distress |

all you can to understand the person's point of view. Look at the situation as if you were the person so that you can more readily understand the frustration being expressed. Let's be honest: Some things are not fair, but nevertheless they do happen. Do not join in the anger and do not criticize the anger; rather, listen and make nonjudgmental comments designed to be comforting.

Prayer is a common tool for spiritual people. I realize you may or may not pray; however, if a person in your care requests someone to pray with, please do what you can to assist the person. You might hold a hand or sit near and be reverent during the prayer. If you are uncomfortable with prayer, find a coworker who can assist the person. The objective is to support the person with unmet spiritual needs so that he or she can achieve management of the illness or problems being faced. You play a crucial role in that goal achievement.

RESOLVING TRANSITIONAL PROBLEMS

At this point, you understand the basics of transitional and spiritual care. I hope that you also understand the importance of meeting the needs that arise based on those concepts. Meeting such needs contributes greatly to improved health, the ability to manage distress, and the all-important objective of achieving integrity and eventually gerotranscendence. Gerotranscendence allows an older person to live life without regret and to die well, which is something we all would like to achieve. That makes finding a way to implement the resolutions to transitional situations a quality-of-life as well as a quality-of-health issue.

I realize that your workloads are heavy and that fulfilling the medical orders and personal care needs of the individuals to whom you give care is essential for you to do. If you believe in holistic care, however, assisting an older adult who is under the stress of seemingly insurmountable transitions is also essential and needs to be addressed. You may need to talk to your nurse manager and determine if family members or volunteers could be thoroughly oriented to the skills needed to take over that responsibility. If volunteers are used, ensure that there is an effective way for them to communicate with you regarding what they learned. Perhaps the patient or resident mentioned a spiritual person or ritual he or she would like to be with or experience, or perhaps there is a person the patient or resident wronged and wishes to apologize to before death. It is important you learn of the unmet needs so that these can be resolved, if possible.

One way to help older people resolve transitional problems and move toward integrity and gerotranscendence is life review. Staff members who value the lives of older people are also key to providing holistic care and guidance to aging residents and patients.

Life Review

The objective of this activity and the activities described subsequently is to assist older people to review their lives and appreciate them. If there are items the older adults feel need to be resolved, life review also gives them that opportunity.

I often hear families complain about having to listen to the same stories over and over again from their elderly parent or grandparent. This storytelling is not unhealthy behavior. Instead, it is exactly what the older adult should be doing to

This home health nurse is assisting her patient with reminiscence therapy. Notice how involved the older woman is in telling her story or memory after seeing pictures in her scrapbook.

achieve integrity. When health declines and the older person's social system gets smaller, it is healthy to reflect on the accomplishments of one's life. In that reflection, the older person can identify strengths that will assist with current transitions as well as feel the satisfaction of good deeds and good times.

This crucial behavior requires time from you or others assigned to do life reviews. Volunteers with maturity and a deep sense of responsibility can be taught to do effective reviews.

Sometimes there is an event in life about which the person feels shame and remorse. It may be difficult for you or the volunteer to listen to older persons reveal their mistakes and talk about the people they have hurt. Yet, this information should be shared. Talking about life errors to a kind and attentive listener is therapeutic and should be encouraged. Sometimes referrals to a counselor or therapist should be made. This is a strong reason for you to keep in close contact with volunteers who may do life reviews on the unit. In addition to verbal life reviews, written and visual life reviews can be created by the older adult and their caregivers and loved ones.

Writing One's Life Story

When writing a life story, many adults do not feel as if it is something they can do. It is especially difficult if they hand-write rather than use a computer. This is where a volunteer would be very effective. Initially, the volunteer needs to develop a relationship with the older person. It can be determined if a recording device or simply talking would be the best way to share the person's life story. The volunteer would need to be able to type on a computer while the older person is talking or, if using a recording device, interview the older person and then type the information that was recorded on a computer. There is a great satisfaction in recording one's life events. It is even better when there is a willing listener and facilitator for the project.

Imagine the satisfaction of having your life recorded or documented, even if it is just you who reads it. That is seldom the case, however. This type of life review meets the same needs as previously discussed. Perhaps the family could be involved and copies made for the children and grandchildren. A copy of a life story could be put on each chart or in a specific file so that staff members could read it and know the person better. Keep in mind that you would need permission from the person, whose story it is, to share it with the staff. You will also need to be aware of HIPAA regulations regarding the sharing of information.

Collecting and Organizing Photos

Many people I know have boxes of photos that are unlabeled and disorganized. When those boxes exist for an older adult, it could represent the disorganization they are feeling in their life. Suggesting to a family member or recruiting an effective volunteer to assist in the organization and labeling of, quite literally, one's life is a significant thing to do. This is another way to do a life review. It provides the opportunity for the older person to relive precious moments, note the voids in pictures because of a family argument, or simply enjoy the grandchildren's pictures when they were babies.

The final product, the photo album, often becomes a treasured item to be shared with others. The significance of one's life is then visually apparent. The scrapbook provides the opportunity to reassess one's life and experience a sense of accomplishment.

Staff Who Value the Lives of Older People

If you are working on a unit that has a large percentage of older adults, or if you work in a nursing home, I hope that people who value the lives of older people surround you. As you go through your daily workload, take the time to ask older adults about their life as a child or young adult. Hopefully you know about the person and his or her culture and can ask questions that have significance for the person. When you ask a question, take the time to listen. Be especially alert for coping mechanisms that worked in the past for that individual. Listen for accomplishments and success stories that can be shared with the staff, and hopefully someone will ask to have the story told again.

Think of your own transitional stress and what helped you, then provide the same support for your patient. Consciously strive to be a truly holistic nurse by embracing the body, mind, and spirit of the person to whom you give care. You do this by following the medical plan of care (body), addressing transitional stress needs and all that accompanies those needs (mind), and meeting spiritual needs (spirit).

 CONCLUSION

Transitions are an undeniable part of life. It is important to provide elderly patients and residents with holistic and humanistic care, assist them as they develop or hone the skills they need to manage their transitions, and support them in their religious beliefs and their spirituality. Accept the challenges, resolve the problems, and move the profession forward.

CASE STUDY SOLUTIONS

1. Quietly approach Mrs. Goldstein after she has been transferred to her bed. Be calm and do not react to her crying out. Instead, calmly ask her "what is wrong?" Gently touch her arm, if she is receptive. Maintain eye contact; do not move quickly.

   The problem is that this patient is an Orthodox Jew. It is part of her religion to keep her head covered as a statement of humility. When she awoke to find her head uncovered she was very upset. She explained to you that she would not have to worry about such things at the Hebrew Home. She requests to go back there immediately.

   You cannot return her to the nursing home as quickly as she wishes, but you can find her scarf or locate something suitable so that she can cover her head. She calms down and then you feel you can do her postoperative assessment.

   As you leave her room, you recognize that it may be a transitional stress for her to be at a Catholic hospital rather than a Hebrew nursing home. You plan to ask her about her spiritual needs as well.

2. You were thinking about Mrs. Goldstein and how to help her transition to an acute hospital when the certified nursing assistant (CNA) comes out into the hallway looking frantic. She announces that Mrs. Goldstein threw her dinner on the floor. You rush to the room, and once again ask, "what is wrong?" "This is not kosher food," she screams. "You are trying to kill me!"

   The CNA timidly followed you into the room, and you send her for a kosher tray for Mrs. Goldstein. Apologize to her for not recognizing that her diet should be kosher. Ensure that the hospital prepares kosher meals all of the time and that the mistake will not happen again. Stay with the patient because she is very upset. Sit and look relaxed; listen to what she has to say about her husband's death. Listen for clues to what helped her with that major transition, and determine if it would be helpful in the current situation. If it is possible, stay with her until her tray comes, and make sure it is satisfactory.

3. You are back on duty Saturday morning and Mrs. Goldstein refuses to go to physical therapy (PT). By this time, you had anticipated the problem. This woman is very serious about her religious rituals, and you and the staff were unaware of their importance to her. You go in and talk to her about PT. You discuss the significance of having PT the day after surgery, and you ask her if there is any type of compromise she can make. With some effort, the two of you work out a partial PT schedule for the day. Then you talk to the staff for Sunday, when PT is closed, and see if they will assist her with some basic exercises.

4. When you come back on Monday, you bring the picture of her husband and son from the nursing home. She cries when she sees it and states that she can do anything if Fred (her husband) is with her. She is wearing her head scarf, cheerfully eating a kosher breakfast, and is excited about working with the physical therapist. Her recovery will be challenging simply because of the seriousness of the fracture and her age, but you can see that you have made it easier for her.

REVIEW QUESTIONS

1. The overall objective of recognizing and assisting clients with transitions is to:
   1. Resolve shame vs. doubt
   2. Decrease complaints filed on your unit.
   3. Achieve Maslow's esteem level of need.
   4. Deliver humanistic and holistic care.

2. The importance of understanding PLST is to:
   1. Give firm directions to older adults so they won't feel insecure.
   2. Provide health-care environments where older people have complete freedom to make decisions.
   3. Lower the stress threshold of the environment where older adults are given care.
   4. Assist older adults in making the decision to make a transition or to perform PLST.

3. The difference between spirituality and religion is:
   1. One is done in a formal building; the other can't be.
   2. One is a feeling that comes from within.
   3. The age of the person determines the difference.
   4. Spirituality is a category of highly functioning religious people.

4. Research with spirituality and religion indicates that:
   1. It does not impact people who believe in a Divine power only.
   2. It does promote health and healing.
   3. It should not be considered when planning nursing care.
   4. It is too personal to discuss with patients and residents.

5. The value of life review is to:
   1. Find something useful for the volunteers to do.
   2. To keep older people busy while they are hospitalized.
   3. To publish a book of older adults' lives and sell it as a fundraiser project.
   4. To gain understanding into one's successes and mistakes.

6. When discharging (or transitioning) a patient from the hospital to a long-term care facility, it would be important for the nurse to include:
   1. A detailed description of the medications for the patient to review.
   2. Contact cards for the patient of various therapies involved in the care.
   3. All communication, contacts, medications, and therapies for the facility.
   4. Detailed information regarding family involvement in the patient's care.

REFERENCES

Agency for Healthcare Research and Quality (2002). Preventing disability in the elderly with chronic disease. *Research in Action, 3,* 1-7. U.S. Department of Health and Human Services: www.ahrq.gov

Anthony, M.K., & Hudson-Barr, D. (2004). A patient-centered model of care for hospital discharge. *Clinical Nursing Research, 13*(2), 117-136.

Davies, S. (2005). Nursing theory and concept development or analysis: Meleis's theory of nursing transitions and relatives experiences of nursing home entry. *Journal of Advanced Nursing, 52*(6), 658-671.

Fontaine, K.L. (2011). *Complementary & alternative therapies for nursing practice* (3rd ed.). Upper Saddle River, NJ: Pearson Education, Inc.

Haber, D. (2003). *Health promotion and aging: Practical applications for health professionals* (3rd ed.). New York, NY: Springer Publishing Inc.

Jungers, C.M. (2010). Leaving home: an examination of late-life relocation among older adults. *Journal of Counseling & Development, 88*(4), 416-423.

Mauk, K.L. (2014). *Gerontological nursing: Competencies for care.* Burlington, MA: Jones & Bartlett Learning.

Ryan, R.M., & Deci, E.L. (2000). Self-determination theory and the facilitation of intrinsic motivation, social development, and well-being. *American Psychologist, 55*(1), 68-78.

Sapolsky, R.M. (2004). *Why zebras don't get ulcers* (3rd ed.). New York, NY: Henry Holt and Company.

Schulweis, H.M. (2003). *In God's mirror.* Brooklyn, NY: KTAV Publishing, Inc.

Taylor, E.J. (2002). *Spiritual care: Nursing theory, research, and practice.* Upper Saddle River, NJ: Pearson Education, Inc.

ThinkExist.com Quotations (n. d.). Ralph Waldo Emerson quotes. http://en.thinkexist.com/quotes/ralph_waldo_emerson/

WEB RESOURCES

Elder Care Online: www.ec-online.net

Transitions and the Elderly: http://www.ec-online.net/knowledge/articles/brandttransitions.html

Spirituality and Aging: http://cas.umkc.edu/casww/sa/Spirituality.htm

4

The Use of the Nursing Process and Nursing Diagnosis in the Care of Older Adults

KATHLEEN R. CULLITON

LEARNING OUTCOMES

1. Describe the nursing process as a problem-solving technique in the context of assessment of the older adult, plan of care, nursing interventions, and nursing documentation.

2. Identify the use of the nursing process minimum data set (MDS) and Care Area Assessments (CAAs) in developing nursing care plans for residents in nursing facilities.

3. Use the nursing process to develop a care plan for the presented case study.

CONCEPTS

Clinical Decision Making

Managing Care

CASE STUDY

Resident Admission

December 1, 2015, 1 p.m.: Mr. B., 82-year-old white widowed man, is admitted to Room 112 of Quality Care Health Facility from Mercy Hospital via ambulance accompanied by daughter-in-law. Admitted with diagnosis of fractured left wrist, multiple hematomas and abrasions, Alzheimer's disease, diabetes mellitus, and a history of HF. Dr. Ben Johnston notified of admission and verified orders. Dietary notified of 2 g sodium/no concentrated sweets diet. Medication orders faxed to the pharmacy:

furosemide (Lasix) 40 mg qd for HF and COPD

Lisinopril 25 mg qd for HF

potassium chloride (K-tabs) 2 tabs qd for CHF

Metformin 800 mg q a.m. for diabetes

oxazepam (Serax) 20 mg qhs for insomnia

ducosate (Dulcolax) sodium suppository qd prn constipation

acetaminophen (Tylenol) 1,000 mg q4h prn pain

hydrocolloid gel (DuoDerm) to open area on coccyx change qod

mupirocin (Bactroban) to abrasions bid

nystatin (Mycostatin) ointment to perineal rash bid 3 to 10 days

Ace wrap and splint to left wrist at all times

Return to clinic in 2 weeks

Son has durable power of attorney for financial and health-care decisions and has signed the advanced directive form for "Do Not Resuscitate." Resident has a living will, and his wishes are known to his family.

Daughter-in-law reports that he has no known allergies, wears bifocals and reads large-print *Reader's Digest* occasionally, has upper and lower dentures, does not use a hearing aid, and has minimal difficulty hearing unless in a noisy room. Uses a cane to ambulate. Height, 5'9''; weight, 124 lb.

Mr. B. is alert and oriented to self and daughter-in-law but states that it is 1936, that the season is winter, that the month is September, and that he is in Denver. Since his wife died 6 months ago, he has been living with his son and his family. His daughter-in-law has been his principal caregiver. Caring for Mr. B. has been quite stressful at times. He does not strike out but repeatedly asks the same questions over and over, even when the question has been answered. His daughter-in-law took a leave of absence from her job because Mr. B. could no longer stay in the house alone without becoming very anxious. He would call friends on the phone repeatedly and ask for his deceased wife. He would often go for walks and get lost.

Mr. B. was admitted to Mercy Hospital after he had fallen on an uneven sidewalk four blocks from home and sustained a concussion, multiple facial hematomas, abrasions on his right arm and shoulder, a fractured left wrist, and a large hematoma on his left hip. His daughter-in-law had been in the basement folding laundry when Mr. B. left the house. The family is expressing much guilt over the decision to place Mr. B. in a long-term care facility, but they admit that he would be safer there.

Mr. B. is able to walk with his cane but favors the left hip when he stands and is very unsteady. He forgets where he is and cries out for help. He is able to dress himself but must have supervision to remind him of what he is doing. Mr. B. is able to feed himself but has not been eating and has lost a significant amount of weight in the past 3 months. Mr. B. has been generally continent of his bladder and bowel except while in the hospital, where he was incontinent of both.

CASE STUDY *continued*

Mr. B. was an accountant before he retired, and he would often spend hours with a paper and pencil "doing the books." He has always enjoyed classical music and was quite an accomplished pianist. He had season tickets to the ballet and the opera and would go often before his wife died 6 months ago.

Physical Assessment

General Appearance: Thin white man

Head and Neck:	White hair. Scalp dry with multiple areas of white dry flaking. Face symmetrical. Two 5-cm hematomas on left cheek and jaw; 2-cm hematoma on left forehead. Skin also is dry. Eyes are clear with no drainage, conjunctivae pink, pupils are equal at 5 mm and react briskly to light, consensual, and accommodative. No drainage from nose; patient is able to breathe through both nostrils. No drainage from ears. Did not appropriately respond when asked in a whisper to raise his arm. Oral mucous membranes are pink and dry. No denture irritation noted. No saliva pooling noted between gum and cheek. Tongue pink with no coating; remains at midline when extended from mouth. Throat dry with no pharyngeal drainage or redness noted; no cervical lymph nodes palpable; no thyroid nodules or enlargement palpated.
Chest:	Symmetrical chest movements. Breath sounds clear throughout except for expiratory crackle in base of left lower lobe that cleared with cough. Apical pulse: 78 and regular. No extra heart sounds noted. Back has multiple waxy, light brown to medium brown, 2- to 3-cm, flat, raised lesions. Moderate kyphosis of spine.
Abdomen and Buttocks:	Large (8 × 12 cm) hematoma over left hip and left lower abdominal area. Hard stool in rectum. Active bowel sounds in all quadrants. Abdomen soft. No masses palpable. Stage 2 pressure ulcer 2 × 1.5 cm over coccyx that is oozing serous drainage. Three small fluid-filled vesicles in gluteal fold of right buttocks.
Genitourinary:	Normal male genitalia. Urinary meatus reddened. Urine dark amber and foul-smelling. Fiery red rash noted on inner aspects of both upper thighs and scrotum.
Extremities:	Full range of motion (ROM) of shoulders, elbows, right wrist, and fingers. Left wrist is splinted with a rigid plastic splint and wrapped with an Ace bandage that he is constantly unwrapping. Radial and brachial pulses strong and equal bilaterally. Healing abrasions noted over lateral aspect of left upper arm and left shoulder. Limited ROM of both hips with complaints of pain with movement of left hip. Full ROM of both knees and ankles. Femoral and popliteal pulses strong and equal bilaterally. Left pedal pulse weak and 1+ pitting edema noted in left ankle. Right pedal pulse strong and right ankle edematous with no pitting noted. Homans' sign not present bilaterally, and

continued on page 60

CASE STUDY *continued*

no complaints of calf tenderness to palpation. Eschar 1 cm in size noted along medial nail of the left great toe. No drainage noted, but there is slight redness around the eschar.

July 10, 2:00 p.m.: Mr. B. was found in another resident's room, pulling clothes out of the closet. This is a daily occurrence. Mr. B. cannot explain why he is in the other resident's room and does not know the way back to his room. He yells at his roommate to get out and yells randomly at other residents in the facility. When he is in his room, he cries for help but does not have any requests or needs when the staff members answer. He went 3 days without having a bowel movement and was incontinent of stool in the hallway 30 minutes after being given a suppository. Mr. B. attends activities when asked to go, but he often leaves the activity early. He naps for 1 to 2 hours in the afternoon and is awake frequently at night, when he has to be reminded to stay in bed. He was found one night stuck between the side rails and incontinent of urine.

The MDS for Mr. B. is shown in Figure 4.3 at the end of the chapter.

Discussion

Use the following nursing diagnoses to organize your assessment data and develop a nursing care plan for Mr. B. Following each nursing diagnosis, you will find possible problems you can address.

1. Nursing Diagnosis: *Self-Care Deficit* related to confusion manifested by inability to perform ADLs independently secondary to Alzheimer's disease and fractured wrist.

   ADL Function/Rehabilitation Potential

   Visual Function

2. Nursing Diagnosis: *Injury, high risk* for related to altered mobility as manifested by unsteadiness and wandering, secondary to hip injury and Alzheimer's disease.

   Falls

   Behavior Problems

3. Nursing Diagnosis: *Nutrition, altered: less than body requirements* related to lack of appetite as manifested by significant weight loss in last 30 days secondary to Alzheimer's disease.

   Nutritional Status

   Dehydration/Fluid Maintenance

4. Nursing Diagnosis: *Urinary Elimination, altered and Incontinence* related to confusion mobility as manifested by not going to the bathroom to void secondary to Alzheimer's disease.

   Urinary Incontinence and Indwelling Catheter

5. Nursing Diagnosis: *Confusion* related to inaccurate interpretation of environment as manifested by inability to state season and date, inability to remember names of staff members, and inability to follow commands secondary to Alzheimer's disease and possible use of antipsychotic and sedative medication.

   Delirium

   Cognitive Loss/Dementia

   Communication

   Mood State

   Behavior Problem

   Psychotropic Drug Use

   Psychosocial Well-being

CASE STUDY *continued*

6. Nursing Diagnosis: *Skin Integrity, impaired* related to a fall and being restrained in bed during hospitalization manifested by hematomas, abrasions, blisters, and stage 2 coccyx pressure ulcer.

   Pressure Ulcer

7. Nursing Diagnosis: *Constipation* related to decreased fluid intake as manifested by bowel movements hard and difficult to pass and use of suppository secondary to Alzheimer's disease, altered nutrition intake, and dehydration.

   Dehydration and Fluid Maintenance

   Nutritional Status

 ## INTRODUCTION

Licensed practical nurses (LPNs) work in a variety of care settings. Each setting may require the LPN to function in a different capacity, yet each practice area expects the practical nurse to be involved with the assessment, planning, implementation, and evaluation of older adults and the care they receive.

 ## ENVIRONMENTS OF CARE

Home Care

LPNs in home care work under the direction of a registered nurse. They provide nursing care such as changing dressings, monitoring blood glucose levels, administering medications, and assessing the status of chronic disease processes in the older adult's home.

Hospital Care

LPNs work in various capacities with acutely ill older patients in the hospital. Often, the LPN is paired with a registered nurse to form a care team in providing nursing care. Other care delivery models may require the LPN to have specific tasks on the unit, such as treatments or passing medications for all of the patients on the unit.

Long-term Care Facilities

The LPN may be employed in many types of long-term care facilities. *Skilled nursing facilities* and nursing facilities were previously thought of as nursing homes. These facilities generally provide a high level of nursing intervention. *Assisted-living facilities* provide care to older persons who may

 ## Priority Setting

There is a great deal of information in this chapter, and all of it points you toward the behaviors and thought processes of a licensed nurse. One of the unwritten objectives for you in attending school is to learn to think like an LPN, and this chapter provides the foundation for that type of thinking. Your priority for this chapter is to learn and put into practice the nursing process.

Using the nursing process in your everyday life will assist you in learning to think like a nurse. Remember the five stages of the process:

• Assessment
• Nursing Diagnosis
• Planning
• Implementation
• Evaluation

I suggest that you purposefully think in those five stages. It would work in most everyday situations. For example, when fixing dinner, you need to assess the number of people who will be eating and their likes and dislikes as well as the food you have on hand. Your nursing diagnosis would be the selection of food you choose to serve to a specific number of people. Then you plan the actual meal, implement the plan by serving the meal, and then evaluate the meal by obtaining feedback from those who ate it.

I know this seems simplistic, but it is critical to learn to think like a nurse. By going through the steps several times a day, you soon will think that way automatically.

need assistance with activities of daily living (ADLs) but who do not require complex, skilled intervention (Eliopolous, 2010). *Continuing care retirement communities* have several levels of care, including skilled nursing, assisted living, and independent living apartments. Wellness clinics are frequently provided for residents living in independent apartments. LPNs could be employed in any one of these long-term care settings.

In the long-term care environment, the practical nurse works with the registered nurse to collect admission data, provide input to the plan of care, carry out the nursing interventions that are outlined in the plan of care, and assist with the evaluation of the effectiveness of these interventions in meeting the goals of the care plan for the older adult. The registered nurse and LPN confer with the interdisciplinary health-care team (IDT) to share observations and clarify the plan of care. The LPN in these settings very often is responsible for working with nursing assistants to ensure the plan of care is carried out. Practical nurses often call physicians to clarify orders and to report changes in the resident's health status. The practice of LPNs in nursing facilities is the practice model referred to in this chapter.

NURSING PROCESS

The nursing process is a problem-solving model that describes what nurses do. It identifies the way nurses approach patient care, and it recognizes the ongoing and changeable nature of the care that nurses provide, care that is based on the individual needs of the patient. Consider the following example.

An LPN in a long-term care facility walks into a resident's room and finds the resident with a supper tray in place. The resident is unable to talk and is turning blue. The nurse thinks that the resident is choking. Quickly, the nurse moves the meal tray out of the way and uses a two-handed thrust under the resident's diaphragm to attempt to dislodge the food that is obstructing the airway. After the nurse does the abdominal thrusts, the resident is assessed for respiratory movements. If the person is breathing again, the nurse takes a deep breath, cuts the resident's meat into smaller pieces, and observes the resident eating the rest of the meal. If the resident is not breathing, the nurse may attempt another abdominal thrust or reposition the resident so that another abdominal thrust can be done from behind.

This short scenario is an example of the nursing process (Fig. 4.1). When the LPN entered the room and saw the older person with hands clenched on the throat and turning blue, the nurse was collecting data. In a split second, the nurse identified the resident's problem as choking. The nurse's next thought was to set a goal for this resident's care: the resident will expel the food that is causing the choking. With the goal of expelling the lodged food, the nurse designs the plan from nursing knowledge and immediately implements abdominal thrusts. After the nursing intervention, the nurse evaluates the situation to determine whether the resident has expelled the food. If the resident has not, the nurse must rethink and redesign the plan and immediately implement the revised nursing actions.

Nurses are faced with many patient-care or resident-care problems every day (note that residents are people who have been admitted to long-term care facilities). The nursing process provides a structure for nurses to plan and give high-quality, individualized care.

This woman soon will be discharged from the nursing home where she has been for the past 2 weeks because of a fractured hip. While at home, she will receive nursing and physical therapy as home care. Because of the multiplicity of services available to her, she spent only 3 days in the hospital and will be home much quicker than she would have been a decade ago.

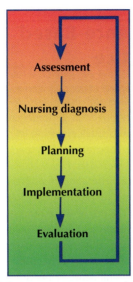

FIGURE 4.1. Nursing process model. The circular nature of this model demonstrates that the process is ongoing.

Assessment

The first step in the nursing process is to collect all of the information the nurse will need to identify clearly the older person's strengths and current and potential problems. Usually, the assessment starts with the call or written summary from the agency or department that is transferring the older adult to your nursing care area. Before the actual transfer takes place, your nursing care area should have the following information regarding the incoming patient or resident:

- Name, age, and insurance identification numbers
- Medical diagnoses, advanced directives, and disease prognosis
- Family support
- Need for equipment (Does the person need special equipment, such as a special bed, oxygen, intravenous [IV] setup, or feeding pump?)
- Functional ability (How does the person transfer, ambulate, move in bed, bathe, toilet, and eat?)
- Medications (Which prescription and over-the-counter medication does the person take?)
- Cognitive ability (Is the person oriented? How is the person's memory?)
- Special needs (Is the person depressed or at risk for skin breakdown or other health risks?)

This information is very important for the preparation of the older person's bed and room and makes the transfer to your care as smooth as possible.

After the older person is transferred, the nurse makes a focused assessment that culminates in a comprehensive assessment. The admission assessment includes a nursing history, observations, physical examination, review of laboratory values, and an interview with the older adult and his or her family.

In 1987, the federal government enacted legislation that set minimum standards for the assessment and care-planning processes in nursing facilities certified for Medicare reimbursement. This legislation is known as the Omnibus Budget Reconciliation Act of 1987 (OBRA 1987). This legislation was followed by OBRA 1990, which clarified some of the questioned areas of OBRA 1987. The minimum data set (MDS) and resident assessment protocols (RAPs) were a part of the legislation that had been implemented across the United States in nursing facilities that accept Medicare and Medicaid funding as reimbursement for the care they provide.

In 2010, the Resident Assessment Instrument (RAI) was updated to 3.0, and the RAI 3.0 includes the MDS 3.0. The RAPS have been replaced with Care Area Assessments (CAAs).

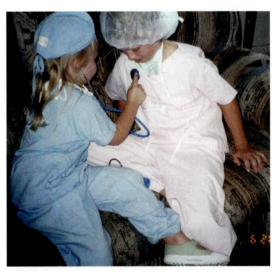

Although these children are only "playing nurse," they are illustrating what each reader of this book needs to do—practice, practice, and practice physical assessment skills until you have confidence in them.

Resident Assessment Instrument (RAI)

The RAI for long-term care includes the MDS, CAAs, and the RAI Utilization Guidelines. These forms detail a step-by-step process of completing the interdisciplinary assessment and designing a comprehensive plan of care for every resident in a long-term care nursing facility (Estabrooks, C.A. 2010).

Minimum Data Set (MDS)

The MDS is just that—the absolute smallest amount of information that must be collected on every resident. It is standardized so the information is collected on all residents. Nurses in long-term care facilities walk around asking each other "… have you done the MDS on Mrs. Hashamoto?" "… on Mr. Nay?" and others. The MDS contains information from all disciplines that work with the resident (i.e., nursing, social work, physical therapy, and dietary). The MDS must be completed within the first 7 days of admission. This allows the interdisciplinary team members some time to get to know the resident as they complete the MDS (Hutchinson, Milke, Maisey, Johnson, Squires, Teare & MDS 3.0 RAI Manual, 2014).

Care Area Assessment (CAA)

When the MDS is completed, it provides a comprehensive assessment as well as indicators of risk for the resident. These risk areas are the CAAs. The CAAs are the areas identified with MDS data.

Embedded within the MDS responses are Care Area Triggers (CATs). For example, if a resident has fallen within the last week, a fall risk would be triggered. When an area is triggered, the resident needs to be assessed further by using the CAA process to help decide if the area to be addressed in the resident's plan of care. This is the decision-making that is part of the nursing process.

The MDS is the assessment and the CATs trigger the decision-making process. Refer to Box 4.1 for a list of care areas.

Nursing Diagnosis

Developing the nursing diagnosis is a primary responsibility of the registered nurse. It involves the use of diagnostic reasoning to reflect the older person's strengths, problems, and potential problems. The registered nurse considers the assessment data MDS, and the triggered Care Areas to select the specific nursing diagnosis supported by the data. organize them and to decide whether they meet criteria for a specific nursing diagnosis. The North American Nursing Diagnosis Association (NANDA) has

Evidence-Based Practice

Wittenberg-Lyles, E.M., Oliver, D.P., Demiris, G., & Regehr, K. (2009). Exploring interpersonal communication in hospice team meetings. Journal of Gerontological Nursing, (35)7, 38-45.

Researchers examined the communication at 4 different hospice agency interdisciplinary team meetings. They reviewed 81 team discussions and 1,917 messages. Research assistants reviewed the transcripts and identified message control types and indirect messages in the conversations. The results were interesting. Forty percent of the messages were one-up messages. They included interruptions and topic changes. At times these messages did not even respect the flow of an opening report. Twenty percent of the messages were one-down messages aimed to stimulate discussion and obtain input. One-across messages almost equaled one-up messages. The one-across message is neutral in control and actually seeks to continue the conversation. The other area reviewed in the transcripts was the indirect messages sent and received. It revealed that some team members only received one-up or one-down messages from some team members, and some team members communicated differently with different team members. The authors pointed out that it was a small study but that the results suggest that members of the interdisciplinary team (IDT) should reflect on their behavior in IDT meetings. The authors also noted that every member should be encouraged to share. The authors discussed the need for an established or standardized process for how information is introduced.

Questions

1. The minimum data set 3.0 is an interdisciplinary form and process for completing. Do you think there may be disagreements over assessment coding on the form? How do you think these IDT disputes should be resolved?

2. As part of the Resident Assessment Instrument process, IDT meetings are scheduled with the resident and his or her family. What would you think would be a good agenda for that meeting? What would be the priorities? Who would chair or moderate the meeting?

FOCUSED LEARNING CHART

Resident Assessment Instrument (RAI)

Federal law requires all facilities that have Medicare or Medicaid residents to have a Resident Assessment Instrument (RAI) that has minimum data sets (MDSs).

Essential information that must be collected on residents	Care Area Assessments (CAAs)	Information is used for:
Nursing observations	Areas that require further assessments before designing care plans	Meeting federal requirements
Physical assessments		Referring IDT members to the list of problems to be addressed
Health history	Specialized assessments done by IDT members	
Interviews with older adult and family		

identified diagnoses that are widely accepted and understood by multiple disciplines and are viewed as the national standards for nursing diagnoses. The NANDA diagnoses are not specific to older people, but they are useful in providing consistent expression of nursing diagnoses for all disciplines and in all settings. An example of a NANDA diagnosis is the following: *Comfort altered, Pain, related to: degenerative joint disease.*

In the long-term care setting, nurses often prefer to use nursing diagnoses that incorporate the MDS language and format. An example of an MDS-related nursing diagnosis is the following: *Potential for joint pain due to degenerative joint disease.* Common nursing diagnoses for older adults include the following:

- Self-Care Deficit
- Physical Mobility, impaired
- Nutrition, altered: less than body requirements
- Injury, high risk for
- Urinary Elimination, altered

BOX 4.1   TWENTY PROBLEM AREAS IDENTIFIED FROM THE MINIMUM DATA SET

Delirium

Cognitive loss/dementia

Visual function

Communication

Activities of daily living: function/ rehabilitation potential

Urinary incontinence and indwelling catheter

Psychosocial well-being

Mood state

Behavior problem

Activities

continued

BOX 4.1   TWENTY PROBLEM AREAS IDENTIFIED FROM THE MINIMUM DATA SET—cont'd

Falls

Nutritional status

Feeding tubes

Dehydration/fluid maintenance

Dental care

Pressure ulcers

Psychotropic drug use

Physical restraints

Pain

Return to Community Referral

• Constipation
• Confusion
• Skin Integrity, impaired: high risk for

The registered nurse is responsible for ensuring that nursing diagnoses address the comprehensive assessment. The nursing diagnosis is an important part of the nursing process and addresses the potential and actual problems of the older adult.

Nursing Diagnosis and Medical Diagnosis

There are two basic ways to communicate the nature of an older adult's health problems. One way is by medical diagnoses, and the other is by nursing diagnoses. Medical diagnoses are made by a physician and describe a disease or a disease process. Diseases are diagnosed by identifying a specific group of signs and symptoms. For example, diabetes mellitus is diagnosed when a person has elevated fasting blood glucose levels, weight loss, thirst, and a large urine output. A person who has an area of dead brain tissue on magnetic resonance imaging (MRI) and computed tomography (CT) scans, along with speech and swallowing difficulty and left-sided paralysis, would be diagnosed with a cerebrovascular accident. Both of these medical diagnoses are common for older adults and communicate information to the nurse about what physical or psychological processes are happening to the person.

QSEN

COMPETENCY: Informatics (Skills)

Using Available Information to Plan Patient Care

At shift report the night nurse expressed frustration with Mr. R. because he did not sleep. He paced up and down the hall and in his room all night. She asked if you could call the doctor and get him a "sleeping pill" or something to "knock him out." Because Mr. R. is a new admit, the charge nurse pulled up his chart and his minimum data set (MDS) online. She noticed that he had a diagnosis of Alzheimer's disease and that confusion has been triggered as a problem on his care assessment. Going to the plan of care, she saw that one of the written goals in the plan is to decrease agitation, sun-downing, and relocation trauma. Suggestions included nonpharmacological approaches such as the following:

1. Keeping the room and hall well lit
2. Having a clock and other visual cues such as a calendar available in the resident's room
3. Having familiar items in the room such as a favorite chair and family pictures
4. Making sure resident is wearing his hearing aid and glasses
5. Giving appropriate care cues to bedtime: helping the resident with brushing his teeth and washing his face along with putting his pajamas on, making sure he empties his bladder and has a glass of water at his bedside, and offering a back rub and a foot or hand massage to help with relaxation
6. Putting on soft music and trying to eliminate bells, alarms, and other irritating noises
7. Introducing yourself with every encounter and reassuring the resident
8. Encouraging family and friends to visit and walk with resident around the facility to help familiarize him to surroundings

The MDS assessment and Care Assessment Triggers automatically will bring up problems to address in the plan of care. For a new resident, it is important to check the plan of care and to provide appropriate care to the resident.

1. Why didn't the night nurse attempt the approaches identified in the plan of care?
2. How would implementing the items in the plan of care actually save time for the night nurse?

The major problem with planning care based only on medical diagnoses is that they do not describe the individual problems of the older adult or the impact the disease has on the person's day-to-day life. Nursing diagnoses are specific to the individual older person's nursing care needs and frequently relate to the areas in which the older person has difficulty functioning. For example, an obese person who is newly diagnosed with diabetes mellitus may have the following nursing diagnoses:

- *Nutrition, altered: more than body requirements and knowledge deficit related to poor dietary practices*

A patient with long-term diabetes may be experiencing problems with a heel ulcer that will not heal. In this case, the nursing diagnosis would be as follows:

- *Skin Integrity, altered*

Both of these people have the same medical diagnoses but different health-care needs, as shown in their nursing diagnoses. When writing your care plan for Mr. B., you will want to include all of the nursing diagnoses that apply specifically to him.

Planning

After organizing the assessment data and noting the nursing diagnoses identified by the registered nurse, you, the LPN working with the older adult, the family, and the health-care team, begin the planning part of the nursing process. The planning portion of the nursing process includes setting priorities, identifying goals and outcomes of care, and designing and documenting interventions.

Setting Priorities

The nurse reviews the nursing diagnoses and places them in priority order. Remember the example at the beginning of this section? Removing the lodged food so that the resident could breathe would be a higher priority than putting on the resident's shoes!

One of the most popular models used to assist the nurse in setting priorities is Abraham Maslow's hierarchy of needs. This framework gives life-sustaining needs the highest priority. These needs are followed by safety and security needs, love and belonging needs, self-esteem needs, and self-actualization needs.

Because the nursing process is focused on the older person as an individual, it also is necessary to consider the priorities of the resident. Often, a resident will state that the highest priority is to go home. The resident may refuse treatments, medications, and activities that would maintain personal health because no one is assisting in the patient's discharge. Although discharge may not be realistic (at this time), you, as the nurse, will probably be more successful in providing nursing care if the plan of care addresses discharge to home as a high priority.

Following is an example of how the nutrition nursing diagnosis can be considered:

- *Nutrition, altered: less than body requirements*
  - Resident refuses to eat and drink.
  - Discuss with the resident what is usually eaten at home and how it is prepared.
  - Review how the resident's current health status would affect the ability to buy food, prepare it, and eat at home.
  - Discuss strategies and plans for ensuring that the resident is able to eat after returning home.
  - Include the resident's food preferences in meals.

Goal Setting or Identifying Outcomes

After identifying the priorities for the resident's care, the nurse identifies goals or outcomes for each of the nursing diagnoses. Setting goals is something that most of us do all of the time. Sometimes our personal goal may be to clock out on time or to survive a busy day. The goals that are part of the planning process describe the specific resident outcomes and identify the goals that direct nursing care. To direct care and describe outcomes, goals must be:

- *Measurable*—measurable outcomes need to be identified. "Eating 100% of a meal" can be measured, whereas it is difficult to measure "appetite will improve."

 Point of Interest

Did you notice how many times the term *resident* was used in the previous explanation on outcomes? In the 1987 OBRA Act, the federal government determined that persons living in a long-term care facility are to be referred to as residents. The reason is because they live there; they are residents of the facility.

- *Realistic*—the goal must fit in with the resident's abilities. "The resident will recall the correct date and time" is probably an unrealistic goal for a person with Alzheimer's disease.
- *Specific*—the goal should identify certain behaviors or conditions to aid in their attainment and evaluation. "The resident will feel better" is not specific. It could be better worded as, "The resident will state that he has less nausea."
- *Timely*—a time frame needs to be established for the attainment of each goal. "The resident will walk 100 feet" does not specify a time frame for achievement of this goal. Adding "by the end of December" provides a time frame.
- *Attainable*—the goal should be written in such a way as to communicate a motivating factor to the resident and the nursing care staff. For an older adult with left hemiplegia, a goal such as "The resident will be independent in self-care by the end of the year" may be a strong motivator to work harder at the occupational and physical therapy sessions.

In nursing facilities, the documentation regulations under OBRA 1987 and OBRA 1990 require that the status of goal attainment be systematically addressed. These documentation requirements are the monthly summaries (a comprehensive review of outcomes every 30 days) and the quarterly reviews (comprehensive interdisciplinary review of the resident's plan of care every 90 days) (Box 4.2). With new admissions or specific insurance carriers, the nurse may be required to conduct monthly comprehensive assessments of the outcome of care. This provides a 30- or 90-day time frame in which goals can be designed. It also helps the nurse think about what is realistic in that specific time frame. For a resident who is rehabilitating after having a hip replacement, "Ambulate independently" may be a realistic goal in 6 months. "Stand and walk 10 steps with a walker" may be a more realistic goal for 30 days. Following are examples of goals:

- The resident will eat more than 75% of each meal for the next 30 days.
- The resident will toilet independently when reminded to go to the bathroom for the next 90 days.
- The resident will attend one activity daily for the next 90 days.
- The resident will have no signs and symptoms of a urinary tract infection for the next 90 days.
- The resident's supplemental oxygen needs will be decreased to 1 L in the next 30 days.

Look back at these goals. What do you notice about them? Each goal identifies something that the resident will or will not do or will or will not experience. The resident's behavior is the major focus of goals as outcomes. Nursing care is not part of the goal. "Bathe the resident" is a nursing intervention, not an outcome or a goal. Nursing standards also are not part of the goal statements. "Administer all medications within 30 minutes of their ordered time" is a nursing standard, not a resident goal.

Designing and Documenting the Plan of Care

After the goals or outcomes of care are identified, the LPN, along with the other members of the IDT, begins to plan the activities that will help the older person reach the goals. The planning phase involves discussion and pen-and-paper activity. Discussing and documenting the plan of care allow input from all members of the team to be communicated to all staff members who are providing care for that resident. Standards of nursing practice and federal regulations require that each resident have a written, comprehensive, and interdisciplinary plan of care. The plan of care includes the problem or potential problem to be identified, the actions or interventions to be taken to address the problem, the person or discipline responsible for each action, and the goals

---

BOX 4.2   ASSESSMENTS NEEDED FOR EACH NURSING HOME RESIDENT

Comprehensive admission assessment including Resident Assessment Instrument (RAI):

1. Minimum data set (MDS)
2. Care Area Triggers (CATs) and Care Area Assessments (CAAs)
3. Ongoing nursing assessment

Annual reassessment including RAI

Significant change in status assessment including RAI

Quarterly assessment including part of MDS

to be achieved. Because of Mr. B.'s multiple medical concerns, his care plan may be lengthy, but all of the information pertinent to him must be included for a complete plan of care. An example of interventions in an interdisciplinary plan of care follows:

- Document percentage of food eaten at each meal—*nursing*
- Feed resident and assess swallowing ability—*speech therapy*
- Review dietary preferences—*dietary services*
- Promote feeding of self—*restorative nursing*

The focus of this chapter is on developing interdisciplinary plans of care using the nursing process. All disciplines caring for the resident need to be represented in an actual plan of care. This is an important criterion for planning interventions: planned interventions must complement the interventions of other therapies. For example, it would be confusing for the resident to be ambulated with a walker by physical therapy and encouraged to walk with two canes by the nursing staff.

It is crucial that members of all disciplines discuss and develop the components of the interdisciplinary plan of care so that confusion among the staff does not occur. Residents who are asked to perform one way in physical therapy and another way on the nursing unit can become confused as to how they should perform. A coordinated approach between physical therapy and nursing helps residents improve quickly and maintain function longer. A coordinated approach among all disciplines enhances the effectiveness of the care given to the resident and minimizes duplication of efforts.

Nursing interventions also must consider the safety of the resident. "Administering a diuretic and a sleeping pill at bedtime" is an unsafe nursing action. The resident may fall while going to the bathroom at night if still groggy from the sleeping pill. Transferring a resident who is able to stand only with the assistance of one staff member may place that resident at risk of falling.

Selected nursing interventions should help to attain the identified goal. If a resident's goal is to "lose 1 lb a week," then giving "dietary supplements between meals and at bedtime" would not assist in achieving this weight loss. When the resident's goal is "will ambulate 100 ft by the end of the month," a nursing intervention must state that the nursing staff will assist the resident to ambulate.

Critically Examine the Following

Identify the correctly stated resident-based outcomes or goals in the following list. When the outcomes or goals are not properly expressed, explain what is wrong.

1. The resident will walk more in the next 90 days.
2. The nurse will toilet the resident every 2 hours for the next 30 days.
3. The resident will have no areas of skin breakdown in the next 90 days.
4. The resident's nutrition will improve.
5. The resident will drink 1500 mL a day for the next 90 days.

Nursing interventions also must be realistic for the resident, staff, resources, and equipment. A reality in the workplace is that there often is not extra time for staff to talk to the residents. Providing 30 minutes of one-on-one time every shift to discuss pain with the resident is an unrealistic intervention. Stating that each staff member "will ask the resident about hip pain whenever he or she interacts with the resident" is a more realistic intervention.

To be successful and effective, nursing interventions must be developed with input from certified nursing assistants (CNAs). CNAs are important members of the interdisciplinary team. Nursing assistants spend more time with residents in nursing facilities, assisted living facilities, and retirement communities and sometimes in the older adult's home than any other member of the IDT. They can offer important specific information for the assessment of the older adult. Because CNAs are so familiar with the daily routine and functioning of the residents, they can offer pertinent, realistic suggestions for individualized interventions to deal with specific problems. They also are frequently the first people to notice subtle changes in clients' conditions that may indicate onset of a new problem or success or failure of an intervention. A care plan meeting, including representatives of all disciplines, is generally held to discuss assessment information and develop the interdisciplinary plan of care. The CNA who works with the resident to be discussed should be invited to this meeting, and arrangements should be made to facilitate the CNA's attendance. The time away from the unit for the CNA is minimal compared with the value of the CNA's input into the care-planning process.

Successful nursing interventions require the resident's input and should be important to the resident. A resident may not want to "lift weights to strengthen and increase flexibility of his arms" but may be very willing to "comb his hair and wash his face." "Encourage the resident to drink 1,000 mL of water" may not work as well as "encourage the resident to drink 1,000 mL of fruit juice and water."

Nursing interventions also must include continuing assessment and monitoring of disease processes and effects of medications and treatments. If a resident has an IV, the IV site must be "assessed every shift for signs of infiltration, irritation, and infection." If a resident is receiving therapy with digoxin (Lanoxin), the "apical pulse must be taken and recorded before each dose." Residents with heart failure (HF) should be "assessed for edema and dyspnea."

The plan of care is part of the resident's permanent record. It needs to be routinely reviewed and updated as the resident's health status improves or declines. The monthly and quarterly review times provide excellent opportunities to revise the care plan to ensure that the resident is receiving appropriate nursing care.

Implementation

Implementation is the part of the nursing process that nurses do best. Being at the bedside of the resident providing care is one of the most rewarding aspects of being a nurse. Implementation means putting the plan of care into action. Along with providing the nursing care that has been outlined in the resident's nursing care plan, the LPN continues to collect data that can be used to update and revise the plan of care.

Many interventions from the plan of care are assigned to CNAs; this is another strong reason to have CNAs attend the care plan development meeting. If CNAs have an opportunity to provide input into the plan of care and if they are present when it is discussed and developed, they will be more likely to carry out the interventions than if they are merely told what to do or handed a care plan to read.

Because nursing assistants on all shifts cannot attend the care plan meeting, a major challenge for the LPN is communicating the plan of care back to all CNAs. Various communication techniques can be used. Some facilities provide nursing assistants with written assignments that list all of the interventions for each resident. Many facilities place the plan of care in a book and make it available to the staff. Very often, however, the book is rarely consulted. Meeting regularly with nursing assistants to discuss the plan of care, giving each CNA written assignments with information on the plan of care, and using primary CNAs who care for the same residents each day ensure the implementation of the plan of care. These actions make it a working document rather than a useless piece of paper completed only to comply with regulations.

Another difficult aspect of implementation is that it must be documented. Charting is an important part of implementing the plan of care. Documentation of interventions requires recording not only that the intervention was done but also the resident's responses to the intervention. An entry such as the following provides no information about the resident's response to the treatment:

12/16/15 1420 Wet to dry saline packing to coccyx ulcer

A better picture is given in the following chart:

12/16/15 1420 Wet to dry saline packing to coccyx pressure ulcer. Ulcer is 3 × 2 cm and 1.5 cm deep. Ulcer margins are pink, and there is granulation tissue evident. Small amount of yellow serous drainage on old packing. Resident complained of pain when old packing was removed and new packing inserted. Two small (6-mm) scabs on left buttocks from tape irritation. No redness or drainage noted.

Every visit with the resident is an opportunity to reassess nursing diagnoses and their implementation.

Think Like a Nurse

You are a student nurse working on an acute care unit. You are writing a care plan for your patient. The staff nurse comments that she doesn't write care plans for her patients. How might you respond to this nurse?

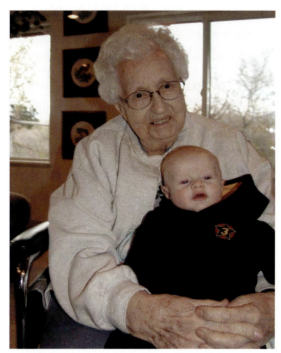

This woman was admitted to a nursing home with limited mobility, weakness, mild confusion, and heart failure. Her stated goal was to be strong enough to hold her great-grandchildren and to sit up and talk to her grandchildren, who ranged in age from 15 to 43. The MDS indicated several other goals to implement for her optimum health. As you can see, her priority goal as well as those identified through the MDS were met.

Following is a simple model that can be used to document the nursing process with nursing interventions and resident responses:

- *Assessment*—What the nurse observed and assessed. Includes:
  - Objective measurements (blood pressure, laboratory values)
  - What the resident did (response to nursing intervention)
  - What the resident said
- *Action*—What the nurse did (nursing interventions): treatments, turning the resident, giving a medication, increasing the oxygen flow rate, hanging a tube feeding, inserting a catheter
- *Plan*—What the nurse plans to do: call the physician, call the family, reassess with the next treatment, refer resident to social services

The assessment-action-plan charting format is simple, yet it sets up a framework for documenting the nursing process in a narrative format.

CNAs also may be involved in documentation and may provide information for the LPN's documentation. For example, nursing assistants can complete flow sheets, which include interventions from the plan of care and activities from the resident's day. Flow sheets can be used to document such interventions as ADLs, walking programs, bowel and bladder training programs, and dietary intake and feeding programs. Results and trends from the flow sheets can be incorporated into the LPN's regular progress charting.

Evaluation

Evaluation is the final step in the nursing process. The main purposes of evaluation are to decide if the resident has met the identified goals and to assess the outcomes of the nursing care provided. Remember how, in the discussion of implementation, the importance of assessing the resident and documenting the resident's responses to care was emphasized? The chart and resident assessments are reviewed as part of evaluation.

When goals have been stated in measurable terms, the LPN should be able to review all of the data and decide whether the goal has been met, has been partially met, or remains unmet. This is a straightforward look at the resident's response to the nursing interventions. The evaluation of goal achievement needs to be documented in a monthly summary, in a quarterly review, or in the nursing notes.

Evaluation also requires that the nurse review the nursing process. This review helps to keep the plan of care up-to-date and reflects changes in the resident's health status. It also is an opportunity to decide which nursing interventions were ineffective (Box 4.3).

BOX 4.3 SIGNIFICANT CHANGE IN RESIDENT'S STATUS

Decrease in level of functioning in two or more activities of daily living

Decrease or increase in the ability to walk or to use hands to grasp small objects

Decline in health status that is unresponsive to treatment

Changes in behavior or mood that cause daily problems in assisting the resident to achieve goals

The reassessment of the resident and the plan of care in evaluation really address the dynamic strength of the nursing process. Although the nursing process follows specific, organized steps, no step excludes collecting more data. Data collection is done by assessing the resident, updating goals and interventions, and conducting an ongoing evaluation of the outcome of the care that is provided. Nurses seem to use the nursing process even when they do not identify it as such. Consider the following example.

Mary Jones always was incontinent during the 1:00 a.m. rounds. The nursing staff decided to toilet her at 12:30 a.m.

In this example, the nursing staff assessed incontinence as a problem. Their unstated goal was, "the resident will not be incontinent at 1:00 a.m. rounds." Their intervention was to toilet the resident 30 minutes before she was usually incontinent. After toileting the resident at 12:30 a.m., the resident would be checked for urinary incontinence at 1 a.m. If she was not incontinent, the goal would be achieved, and the staff would continue to toilet the resident at 12:30 a.m. to maintain that outcome. If the resident was toileted at 12:30 a.m. and she still was incontinent at 1:00 a.m., the staff may decide to toilet the resident at midnight. The care plan and charting examples provided in Figure 4.2 demonstrate the use of evaluation.

As this example shows, evaluation is ongoing and occurs daily, not just at the mandatory reassessment intervals. Evaluation does not occur only when the quarterly assessment is due. Would you continue to carry out an intervention that was not working for 3 months until the quarterly review was due? Many people help you evaluate the plan of care each day. Residents give you information through their behavior and by telling you if an intervention is helping or not. Families tell you about changes they notice. Nursing assistants frequently note subtle changes in residents and may alter interventions to accommodate the change in the residents.

Making daily changes in the actual care given is common. Translating these changes into the written plan of care is less common. For the sake of communication and consistency among all staff, it is very important to ensure that the written plan of care is updated to reflect the actual care you want to be given.

COMPUTERS AND THE NURSING PROCESS

Computer and access to documentation supporting and submission networks have dramatically improved the RAI process. Imagine the difficulty interdisciplinary team members have if they all have to access the paper chart for a resident. Having the MDS, CAT, and CAA all available via a computer makes it easier to access the information for the entire team.

If you have never worked within a computerized documentation program before, you may be fearful of using it for your assessment and care plans. Completing the MDS and the care plan on the computer has many benefits. One of the most time-consuming portions of the process is computing the care areas triggered—that is, identifying the potential problem areas that need to be assessed further through the CAAs. Most MDS software packages compute the CATs and CAAs in a matter of seconds. Completing the interdisciplinary care plan on the computer saves the nurse from a great deal of handwriting and lends itself to regular updating without further lengthy handwriting. Some software packages print out nursing assistant forms that include all the interventions from the plan of care assigned to the nursing assistant. These forms can be used as assignment sheets that communicate the plan of care to the CNA.

CONCLUSION

As an LPN, you have major responsibilities for delivering meaningful nursing care to residents in long-term care facilities. Your responsibilities include the management of care given by nursing assistants, working with the IDT, completing documents required by the federal government, and delivering excellent care to the frail and vulnerable people in your care. It is essential that you understand and become highly skilled in the content of this chapter.

Nursing Diagnosis Problems Addressed	Goals Outcomes of Care	Nursing Interventions	Evaluation
Physical Mobility, impaired related to musculoskeletal impairment as manifested by inability to transfer and ambulate without assistance	Resident will increase ambulation with walker in PT to independent use with minimal supervision in 90 days	■ Assess and document: Orthostatic BPs (lying/sitting/ standing) ROM and strength of legs and arms Walking ability with walker and amount of assistance needed ■ Have walker in resident's reach at all times and use for all transfers and walking in room ■ Physical therapy for quad-strengthening exercises and ambulation with walker ■ Put on jogging pants for daily physical therapy	

DOCUMENTATION

October 11, 2015, 1:45 p.m.: Resident is transferred from bed to wheelchair with assistance of one. Uses walker to steady himself when standing. Ambulates with hold-on assistance from physical therapist using a walker. Ambulated two steps without hold-on assistance before becoming unsteady. Orthostatic BPs lying—138/82, sitting—110/80, standing—106/76, complained of being light-headed when he sat up. Dizziness passed in 5 minutes. Instructed to move slowly from lying–sitting–standing positions and not to move to another position until any dizziness or light-headedness passes. Will review medications and fluid intake for possible causes of orthostatic hypotension.

FIGURE 4.2 Sample care plan.

CASE STUDY SOLUTION

There is no specific format in which to write this care plan. Use the format you have been taught by your nursing instructors to develop and document the care plan for Mr. B.

REVIEW QUESTIONS

1. The nursing process is:
   1. A type of standardized care plan
   2. A framework for providing nursing care
   3. A procedure that registered nurses use to make care assignments
   4. An instinctive method of providing care

2. The steps in the nursing process are:
   1. Admission, inpatient care, and discharge
   2. Assessment, intervention, and documentation
   3. Assessment, nursing diagnosis, planning, intervention, and evaluation
   4. Admission, physical examination, interview, nursing history, and planning

3. Nursing diagnoses differ from medical diagnoses because they:
   1. Address the problems of the older person
   2. Are written in language that nurses understand
   3. Are standardized for any person who is receiving nursing care
   4. Are designed to address the medical treatment plan

4. When setting priorities during the planning stage of the nursing process, it is important to consider:
   1. The needs of the physician
   2. The needs of the family
   3. The needs of the nursing staff
   4. The needs of the resident

5. Evaluation of the nursing care plan is documented by means of:
   1. The nurse's notes
   2. The resident's care plan
   3. The physician's orders
   4. Revising the admission note

REFERENCES

Eliopoulos, C. (2010). *Gerontological nursing* (7th ed.). Philadelphia, PA: Wolters Kluwer Health/ Lippincott Williams & Wilkins.

Estabrooks, C.A. (2010). The Resident Assessment Instrument-Minimum Data Set 2.0 quality indicators: A systematic review. *BMC Health Services Research,* 10, 166-179.

Hutchinson, A.M., Milke, D.L., Maisey, S., Johnson, C., Squires, J.E., Teare, G., & MDS 3.0 RAI Manual (2014). http://www.cms.gov/Medicare/ Quality-Initiatives-Patient-Assessment-Instruments/ NursingHomeQualityInits/MDS30RAIManual.html

WEB RESOURCES

Comprehensive online resource for education and clinical care resources for care of older adults. Hartford Institute for Geriatric Nursing: http://hartfordign.org/practice

Centers for Medicare and Medicaid Services: http://www.cms.gov/

Geriatric assessment tools plus instructions how to use the tools. Hartford Institute for Geriatric Nursing: http://hartfordign.org/practice/try_this/

Nurses Improving Care for Healthsystem Elders: http://www.nicheprogram.org/

Resident **George T. Blair**   Identifier **784393**   Date **July 6, XXXX**

MINIMUM DATA SET (MDS) – Version 3.0
RESIDENT ASSESSMENT AND CARE SCREENING
Nursing Home Comprehensive (NC) Item Set

Section A	Identification Information

A0100. Facility Provider Numbers

A. National Provider Identifier (NPI):

1	2	3	4	5	6	7	8	9	0

B. CMS Certification Number (CCN):

9	8	7	6	5	4	3	2	1	0	9	8

C. State Provider Number:

5	6	7	8	9	0	1	2	3	4	5	6	7	8	9

A0200. Type of Provider

Enter Code **[1]**

Type of provider
1. **Nursing home (SNF/NF)**
2. **Swing Bed**

A0310. Type of Assessment

Enter Code **[0][1]**

A. Federal OBRA Reason for Assessment
01. **Admission** assessment (required by day 14)
02. **Quarterly** review assessment
03. **Annual** assessment
04. **Significant change in status** assessment
05. **Significant correction** to **prior comprehensive** assessment
06. **Significant correction** to **prior quarterly** assessment
99. **Not OBRA required** assessment

Enter Code **[9][9]**

B. PPS Assessment
PPS Scheduled Assessments for a Medicare Part A Stay
01. **5-day** scheduled assessment
02. **14-day** scheduled assessment
03. **30-day** scheduled assessment
04. **60-day** scheduled assessment
05. **90-day** scheduled assessment
06. **Readmission/return** assessment
PPS Unscheduled Assessments for a Medicare Part A Stay
07. **Unscheduled assessment used for PPS** (OMRA, significant or clinical change, or significant correction assessment)
Not PPS Assessment
99. **Not PPS** assessment

Enter Code **[0]**

C. PPS Other Medicare Required Assessment – OMRA
0. **No**
1. **Start of therapy** assessment
2. **End of therapy** assessment
3. **Both Start and End of therapy** assessment

Enter Code **[0]**

D. Is this a Swing Bed clinical change assessment? Complete only if A0200 = 2
0. **No**
1. **Yes**

Enter Code **[1]**

E. Is this assessment the first assessment (OBRA, PPS, or Discharge) **since the most recent admission?**
0. **No**
1. **Yes**

Enter Code **[0][1]**

F. Entry/discharge reporting
01. **Entry** record
10. **Discharge** assessment-**return not anticipated**
11. **Discharge** assessment-**return anticipated**
12. **Death in facility** record
99. **Not entry/discharge** record

MDS 3.0 Nursing Home Comprehensive (NC) Version 1.00.2 10/01/2010   Page 1 of 38

FIGURE 4.3 Sample minimum data set.

Resident **George T. Blair** Identifier **784393** Date **JULY 6, XXXX**

Section A	Identification Information

A0410. Submission Requirement

Enter Code **3**
1. **Neither federal nor state required submission**
2. **State but not federal required submission** (FOR NURSING HOMES ONLY)
3. **Federal required submission**

A0500. Legal Name of Resident

A. **First name:**

| G | e | o | r | g | e | | | | | |

B. **Middle initial:**

| T |

C. **Last name:**

| B | l | a | i | r | | | | | | | | | | | | |

D. **Suffix:**

| | | | |

A0600. Social Security and Medicare Numbers

A. **Social Security Number:**

| 0 | 0 | 5 | – | 0 | 6 | – | 7 | 8 | 0 | 0 |

B. **Medicare number** (or comparable railroad insurance number):

| 0 | 0 | 5 | 0 | 6 | 7 | 8 | 0 | 0 | A | |

A0700. Medicaid Number - Enter "+" if pending, "N" if not a Medicaid recipient

| N | | | | | | | | | | | | | | |

A0800. Gender

Enter Code **1**
1. **Male**
2. **Female**

A0900. Birth Date

| 1 | 0 | – | 1 | 5 | – | X | X | X | X |
| Month | | | Day | | | Year | | | |

A1000. Race/Ethnicity

↓ **Check all that apply**

☐	A. **American Indian or Alaska Native**
☐	B. **Asian**
☐	C. **Black or African American**
☐	D. **Hispanic or Latino**
☐	E. **Native Hawaiian or Other Pacific Islander**
☒	F. **White**

A1100. Language

Enter Code **0**
A. **Does the resident need or want an interpreter to communicate with a doctor or health care staff?**
0. **No**
1. **Yes** → Specify in A1100B, Preferred language
9. **Unable to determine**

B. **Preferred language:**

| E | n | g | l | i | s | h | | | | | |

FIGURE 4.3—cont'd

Resident **George T. Blair**   Identifier **784393**   Date **July 6, XXXX**

Section A	**Identification Information**

A1200. Marital Status

Enter Code [3]
1. **Never married**
2. **Married**
3. **Widowed**
4. **Separated**
5. **Divorced**

A1300. Optional Resident Items

A. **Medical record number:**

7	8	4	3	9	3				

B. **Room number:**

1	1	2						

C. **Name by which resident prefers to be addressed:**

G	e	o	r	g	e												

D. **Lifetime occupation(s) - put "/" between two occupations:**

A	c	c	o	u	n	t	a	n	t								

A1500. Preadmission Screening and Resident Review (PASRR)
Complete only if A0310A = 01

Enter Code [0]
Has the resident been evaluated by Level II PASRR and determined to have a serious mental illness and/or mental retardation or a related condition?
0. **No**
1. **Yes**
9. **Not a Medicaid certified unit**

A1550. Conditions Related to MR/DD Status
If the resident is 22 years of age or older, complete only if A0310A = 01
If the resident is 21 years of age or younger, complete only if A0310A = 01, 03, 04, or 05

↓ Check all conditions that are related to MR/DD status that were manifested before age 22, and are likely to continue indefinitely

	MR/DD With Organic Condition
☐	A. **Down syndrome**
☐	B. **Autism**
☐	C. **Epilepsy**
☐	D. **Other organic condition related to MR/DD**
	MR/DD Without Organic Condition
☐	E. **MR/DD with no organic condition**
	No MR/DD
☒	Z. **None of the above**

A1600. Entry Date (date of this admission/reentry into the facility)

0	7	–	0	6	–	X	X	X	X
Month			Day			Year			

A1700. Type of Entry

Enter Code [1]
1. **Admission**
2. **Reentry**

MDS 3.0 Nursing Home Comprehensive (NC) Version 1.00.2 10/01/2010   Page 3 of 38

FIGURE 4.3—cont'd

Resident **George T. Blair**   Identifier **784393**   Date **July 6, XXXX**

Section C   Cognitive Patterns

C0100. Should Brief Interview for Mental Status (C0200–C0500) be Conducted?
Attempt to conduct interview with all residents

Enter Code	
1	0. **No** (resident is rarely/never understood) ➝ Skip to and complete C0700–C1000, Staff Assessment for Mental Status
	1. **Yes** ➝ Continue to C0200, Repetition of Three Words

Brief Interview for Mental Status (BIMS)

C0200. Repetition of Three Words

Enter Code	
3	Ask resident: *"I am going to say three words for you to remember. Please repeat the words after I have said all three. The words are: **sock, blue, and bed.** Now tell me the three words."* **Number of words repeated after first attempt** 0. **None** 1. **One** 2. **Two** 3. **Three** After the resident's first attempt, repeat the words using cues ("sock, something to wear; blue, a color; bed, a piece of furniture"). You may repeat the words up to two more times.

C0300. Temporal Orientation (orientation to year, month, and day)

Enter Code	
0	Ask resident: *"Please tell me what year it is right now."* **A. Able to report correct year** 0. **Missed by > 5 years** or no answer 1. **Missed by 2–5 years** 2. **Missed by 1 year** 3. **Correct**
0	Ask resident: *"What month are we in right now?"* **B. Able to report correct month** 0. **Missed by > 1 month** or no answer 1. **Missed by 6 days to 1 month** 2. **Accurate within 5 days**
0	Ask resident: *"What day of the week is today?"* **C. Able to report correct day of the week** 0. **Incorrect** or no answer 1. **Correct**

C0400. Recall

Enter Code	
0	Ask resident: *"Let's go back to an earlier question. What were those three words that I asked you to repeat?"* If unable to remember a word, give cue (something to wear; a color; a piece of furniture) for that word. **A. Able to recall "sock"** 0. **No** - could not recall 1. **Yes, after cueing** ("something to wear") 2. **Yes, no cue required**
0	**B. Able to recall "blue"** 0. **No** - could not recall 1. **Yes, after cueing** ("a color") 2. **Yes, no cue required**
0	**C. Able to recall "bed"** 0. **No** - could not recall 1. **Yes, after cueing** ("a piece of furniture") 2. **Yes, no cue required**

C0500. Summary Score

Enter Score	
0 3	**Add scores** for questions C0200–C0400 and fill in total score (00–15) **Enter 99** if the resident was unable to complete the interview

FIGURE 4.3—cont'd

Resident **George T. Blair**   Identifier **784393**   Date **July 6, XXXX**

Section F	Preferences for Customary Routine and Activities

F0300. Should Interview for Daily and Activity Preferences be Conducted? - Attempt to interview all residents able to communicate. If resident is unable to complete, attempt to complete interview with family member or significant other

Enter Code **1**

   0. **No** (resident is rarely/never understood and family/significant other not available) → Skip to and complete F0800, Staff Assessment of Daily and Activity Preferences
   1. **Yes** → Continue to F0400, Interview for Daily Preferences

---

F0400. Interview for Daily Preferences

Show resident the response options and say: "*While you are in this facility...*"

↓ **Enter Codes in Boxes**

Coding:	Code	Question
1. **Very important** 2. **Somewhat important** 3. **Not very important** 4. **Not important at all** 5. **Important, but can't do or no choice** 9. **No response or non-responsive**	2	A. how important is it to you to **choose what clothes to wear?**
	3	B. how important is it to you to **take care of your personal belongings or things?**
	3	C. how important is it to you to **choose between a tub bath, shower, bed bath, or sponge bath?**
	3	D. how important is it to you to **have snacks available between meals?**
	2	E. how important is it to you to **choose your own bedtime?**
	1	F. how important is it to you to **have your family or a close friend involved in discussions about your care?**
	3	G. how important is it to you to **be able to use the phone in private?**
	3	H. how important is it to you to **have a place to lock your things to keep them safe?**

F0500. Interview for Activity Preferences

Show resident the response options and say: "*While you are in this facility...*"

↓ **Enter Codes in Boxes**

Coding:	Code	Question
1. **Very important** 2. **Somewhat important** 3. **Not very important** 4. **Not important at all** 5. **Important, but can't do or no choice** 9. **No response or non-responsive**	2	A. how important is it to you to **have books, newspapers, and magazines to read?**
	3	B. how important is it to you to **listen to music you like?**
	3	C. how important is it to you to **be around animals such as pets?**
	3	D. how important is it to you to **keep up with the news?**
	2	E. how important is it to you to **do things with groups of people?**
	2	F. how important is it to you to **do your favorite activities?**
	1	G. how important is it to you to **go outside to get fresh air when the weather is good?**
	3	H. how important is it to you to **participate in religious services or practices?**

F0600. Daily and Activity Preferences Primary Respondent

Enter Code **2**

Indicate primary respondent for Daily and Activity Preferences (F0400 and F0500)
   1. **Resident**
   2. **Family or significant other** (close friend or other representative)
   9. **Interview could not be completed** by resident or family/significant other ("No response" to 3 or more items)

MDS 3.0 Nursing Home Comprehensive (NC) Version 1.00.2 10/01/2010   Page 12 of 38

FIGURE 4.3—cont'd

Resident **George T. Blair**   Identifier **784393**   Date **July 6, XXXX**

Section G	**Functional Status**

G0110. Activities of Daily Living (ADL) Assistance
Refer to the ADL flow chart in the RAI manual to facilitate accurate coding

Instructions for Rule of 3
- When an activity occurs three times at any one given level, code that level.
- When an activity occurs three times at multiple levels, code the most dependent, exceptions are total dependence (4), activity must require full assist every time, and activity did not occur (8), activity must not have occurred at all. Example, three times extensive assistance (3) and three times limited assistance (2), code extensive assistance (3).
- When an activity occurs at various levels, but not three times at any given level, apply the following:
  - When there is a combination of full staff performance, and extensive assistance, code extensive assistance.
  - When there is a combination of full staff performance, weight bearing assistance and/or non-weight bearing assistance code limited assistance (2).

If none of the above are met, code supervision.

1. ADL Self-Performance
Code for **resident's performance** over all shifts - not including setup. If the ADL activity occurred 3 or more times at various levels of assistance, code the most dependent - except for total dependence, which requires full staff performance every time

Coding:

Activity Occurred 3 or More Times
0. **Independent** - no help or staff oversight at any time
1. **Supervision** - oversight, encouragement or cueing
2. **Limited assistance** - resident highly involved in activity; staff provide guided maneuvering of limbs or other non-weight-bearing assistance
3. **Extensive assistance** - resident involved in activity, staff provide weight-bearing support
4. **Total dependence** - full staff performance every time during entire 7-day period

Activity Occurred 2 or Fewer Times
7. **Activity occurred only once or twice** - activity did occur but only once or twice
8. **Activity did not occur** - activity (or any part of the ADL) was not performed by resident or staff at all over the entire 7-day period

2. ADL Support Provided
Code for **most support provided** over all shifts; code regardless of resident's self-performance classification

Coding:
0. **No** setup or physical help from staff
1. **Setup** help only
2. **One** person physical assist
3. **Two+** persons physical assist
8. ADL activity itself **did not occur** during entire period

	1. **Self-Performance**	**2.** **Support**
	↓ Enter Codes in Boxes ↓	
A. Bed mobility - how resident moves to and from lying position, turns side to side, and positions body while in bed or alternate sleep furniture	0	0
B. Transfer - how resident moves between surfaces including to or from: bed, chair, wheelchair, standing position (**excludes** to/from bath/toilet)	0	0
C. Walk in room - how resident walks between locations in his/her room	2	2
D. Walk in corridor - how resident walks in corridor on unit	2	2
E. Locomotion on unit - how resident moves between locations in his/her room and adjacent corridor on same floor. If in wheelchair, self-sufficiency once in chair	2	2
F. Locomotion off unit - how resident moves to and returns from off-unit locations (e.g., areas set aside for dining, activities or treatments). **If facility has only one floor**, how resident moves to and from distant areas on the floor. If in wheelchair, self-sufficiency once in chair	2	2
G. Dressing - how resident puts on, fastens and takes off all items of clothing, including donning/removing a prosthesis or TED hose. Dressing includes putting on and changing pajamas and housedresses	3	2
H. Eating - how resident eats and drinks, regardless of skill. Do not include eating/drinking during medication pass. Includes intake of nourishment by other means (e.g., tube feeding, total parenteral nutrition, IV fluids administered for nutrition or hydration)	1	1
I. Toilet use - how resident uses the toilet room, commode, bedpan, or urinal; transfers on/off toilet; cleanses self after elimination; changes pad; manages ostomy or catheter; and adjusts clothes. Do not include emptying of bedpan, urinal, bedside commode, catheter bag or ostomy bag	2	1
J. Personal hygiene - how resident maintains personal hygiene, including combing hair, brushing teeth, shaving, applying makeup, washing/drying face and hands (**excludes** baths and showers)	2	2

FIGURE 4.3—cont'd

Resident **George T. Blair**   Identifier **784393**   Date **July 6, XXXX**

Section G	**Functional Status**

G0120. Bathing

How resident takes full-body bath/shower, sponge bath, and transfers in/out of tub/shower (**excludes** washing of back and hair). Code for **most dependent** in self-performance and support

Enter Code	A. Self-performance
3	0. **Independent** - no help provided 1. **Supervision** - oversight help only 2. **Physical help limited to transfer only** 3. **Physical help in part of bathing activity** 4. **Total dependence** 8. **Activity itself did not occur** during the entire period

Enter Code	B. Support provided
2	(Bathing support codes are as defined in item **G0110 column 2, ADL Support Provided**, above)

G0300. Balance During Transitions and Walking

After observing the resident, **code the following walking and transition items for most dependent**

Coding:
0. **Steady at all times**
1. **Not steady, but _able_ to stabilize without human assistance**
2. **Not steady, _only able_ to stabilize with human assistance**
8. **Activity did not occur**

↓ **Enter Codes in Boxes**

1	A. **Moving from seated to standing position**
1	B. **Walking** (with assistive device if used)
1	C. **Turning around** and facing the opposite direction while walking
1	D. **Moving on and off toilet**
1	E. **Surface-to-surface transfer** (transfer between bed and chair or wheelchair)

G0400. Functional Limitation in Range of Motion

Code for **limitation** that interfered with daily functions or placed resident at risk of injury

Coding:
0. **No impairment**
1. **Impairment on one side**
2. **Impairment on both sides**

↓ **Enter Codes in Boxes**

1	A. **Upper extremity** (shoulder, elbow, wrist, hand)
2	B. **Lower extremity** (hip, knee, ankle, foot)

G0600. Mobility Devices

↓ **Check all that were normally used**

☒	A. **Cane/crutch**
☐	B. **Walker**
☐	C. **Wheelchair** (manual or electric)
☐	D. **Limb prosthesis**
☐	Z. **None of the above** were used

G0900. Functional Rehabilitation Potential
Complete only if A0310A = 01

Enter Code	A. **Resident believes he or she is capable of increased independence** in at least some ADLs
9	0. **No** 1. **Yes** 9. **Unable to determine**

Enter Code	B. **Direct care staff believe resident is capable of increased independence** in at least some ADLs
1	0. **No** 1. **Yes**

MDS 3.0 Nursing Home Comprehensive (NC) Version 1.00.2 10/01/2010   Page 15 of 38

FIGURE 4.3—cont'd

Resident **George T. Blair**	Identifier **784393**	Date **July 6, XXXX**

Section H — Bladder and Bowel

H0100. Appliances

↓ Check all that apply

☐	**A. Indwelling catheter** (including suprapubic catheter and nephrostomy tube)
☐	**B. External catheter**
☐	**C. Ostomy** (including urostomy, ileostomy, and colostomy)
☐	**D. Intermittent catheterization**
☒	**Z. None of the above**

H0200. Urinary Toileting Program

Enter Code [1]
A. Has a trial of a toileting program (e.g., **scheduled toileting, prompted voiding, or bladder training**) been attempted on admission/reentry or since urinary incontinence was noted in this facility?
0. **No** → Skip to H0300, Urinary Continence
1. **Yes** → Continue to H0200B, Response
9. **Unable to determine** → Skip to H0200C, Current toileting program or trial

Enter Code [1]
B. Response - What was the resident's response to the trial program?
0. **No improvement**
1. **Decreased wetness**
2. **Completely dry** (continent)
9. **Unable to determine** or trial in progress

Enter Code [1]
C. Current toileting program or trial - Is a toileting program (e.g., scheduled toileting, prompted voiding, or bladder training) currently being used to manage the resident's urinary continence?
0. **No**
1. **Yes**

H0300. Urinary Continence

Enter Code [2]
Urinary continence - Select the one category that best describes the resident
0. **Always continent**
1. **Occasionally incontinent** (less than 7 episodes of incontinence)
2. **Frequently incontinent** (7 or more episodes of urinary incontinence, but at least one episode of continent voiding)
3. **Always incontinent** (no episodes of continent voiding)
9. **Not rated,** resident had a catheter (indwelling, condom), urinary ostomy, or no urine output for the entire 7 days

H0400. Bowel Continence

Enter Code [2]
Bowel continence - Select the one category that best describes the resident
0. **Always continent**
1. **Occasionally incontinent** (one episode of bowel incontinence)
2. **Frequently incontinent** (2 or more episodes of bowel incontinence, but at least one continent bowel movement)
3. **Always incontinent** (no episodes of continent bowel movements)
9. **Not rated,** resident had an ostomy or did not have a bowel movement for the entire 7 days

H0500. Bowel Toileting Program

Enter Code [1]
Is a toileting program currently being used to manage the resident's bowel continence?
0. **No**
1. **Yes**

H0600. Bowel Patterns

Enter Code [1]
Constipation present?
0. **No**
1. **Yes**

MDS 3.0 Nursing Home Comprehensive (NC) Version 1.00.2 10/01/2010   Page 16 of 38

FIGURE 4.3—cont'd

Resident **George T. Blair** Identifier **784393** Date **July 6, XXXX**

Section M	Skin Conditions

Report based on highest stage of existing ulcer(s) at its worst; do not "reverse" stage

M0100. Determination of Pressure Ulcer Risk

↓ **Check all that apply**

- [X] **A.** Resident has a stage 1 or greater, a scar over bony prominence, or a non-removable dressing/device
- [X] **B.** Formal assessment instrument/tool (e.g., Braden, Norton, or other)
- [X] **C.** Clinical assessment
- [ ] **Z.** None of the above

M0150. Risk of Pressure Ulcers

Enter Code [1]

Is this resident at risk of developing pressure ulcers?
0. **No**
1. **Yes**

M0210. Unhealed Pressure Ulcer(s)

Enter Code [1]

Does this resident have one or more unhealed pressure ulcer(s) at Stage 1 or higher?
0. **No** → Skip to M0900, Healed Pressure Ulcers
1. **Yes** → Continue to M0300, Current Number of Unhealed (non-epithelialized) Pressure Ulcers at Each Stage

M0300. Current Number of Unhealed (non-epithelialized) **Pressure Ulcers at Each Stage**

A. Number of Stage 1 pressure ulcers

Enter Number [0]

Stage 1: Intact skin with non-blanchable redness of a localized area usually over a bony prominence. Darkly pigmented skin may not have a visible blanching; in dark skin tones only it may appear with persistent blue or purple hues

B. Stage 2: Partial thickness loss of dermis presenting as a shallow open ulcer with a red or pink wound bed, without slough. May also present as an intact or open/ruptured blister

Enter Number [1]

1. Number of Stage 2 pressure ulcers - If 0 → Skip to M0300C, Stage 3

Enter Number [4]

2. Number of these Stage 2 pressure ulcers that were present upon admission/reentry - enter how many were noted at the time of admission

3. Date of oldest Stage 2 pressure ulcer - Enter dashes if date is unknown:

☐☐ – ☐☐ – ☐☐☐☐
Month   Day   Year

C. Stage 3: Full thickness tissue loss. Subcutaneous fat may be visible but bone, tendon or muscle is not exposed. Slough may be present but does not obscure the depth of tissue loss. May include undermining and tunneling

Enter Number [0]

1. Number of Stage 3 pressure ulcers - If 0 → Skip to M0300D, Stage 4

Enter Number [0]

2. Number of these Stage 3 pressure ulcers that were present upon admission/reentry - enter how many were noted at the time of admission

D. Stage 4: Full thickness tissue loss with exposed bone, tendon or muscle. Slough or eschar may be present on some parts of the wound bed. Often includes undermining and tunneling

Enter Number [0]

1. Number of Stage 4 pressure ulcers - If 0 → Skip to M0300E, Unstageable: Non-removable dressing

Enter Number [0]

2. Number of these Stage 4 pressure ulcers that were present upon admission/reentry - enter how many were noted at the time of admission

M0300 continued on next page

MDS 3.0 Nursing Home Comprehensive (NC) Version 1.00.2 10/01/2010   Page 23 of 38

FIGURE 4.3—cont'd

Resident **George T. Blair**   Identifier **784393**   Date **July 6, XXXX**

Section M	Skin Conditions

M0300. Current Number of Unhealed (non-epithelialized) **Pressure Ulcers at Each Stage** - Continued

---

E. Unstageable - Non-removable dressing: Known but not stageable due to non-removable dressing/device

Enter Number: **0**
1. **Number of unstageable pressure ulcers due to non-removable dressing/device** - If 0 → Skip to M0300F, Unstageable: Slough and/or eschar

Enter Number: ☐
2. **Number of these unstageable pressure ulcers that were present upon admission/reentry** - enter how many were noted at the time of admission

---

F. Unstageable - Slough and/or eschar: Known but not stageable due to coverage of wound bed by slough and/or eschar

Enter Number: **1**
1. **Number of unstageable pressure ulcers due to coverage of wound bed by slough and/or eschar** - If 0 → Skip to M0300G, Unstageable: Deep tissue

Enter Number: **1**
2. **Number of these unstageable pressure ulcers that were present upon admission/reentry** - enter how many were noted at the time of admission

---

G. Unstageable - Deep tissue: Suspected deep tissue injury in evolution

Enter Number: **0**
1. **Number of unstageable pressure ulcers with suspected deep tissue injury in evolution** - If 0 → Skip to M0610, Dimension of Unhealed Stage 3 or 4 Pressure Ulcers or Eschar

Enter Number: ☐
2. **Number of these unstageable pressure ulcers that were present upon admission/reentry** - enter how many were noted at the time of admission

---

M0610. Dimensions of Unhealed Stage 3 or 4 Pressure Ulcers or Eschar
Complete only if M0300C1, M0300D1 or M0300F1 is greater than 0

If the resident has one or more unhealed (non-epithelialized) Stage 3 or 4 pressure ulcers or an unstageable pressure ulcer due to slough or eschar, identify the pressure ulcer with the largest surface area (length x width) and record in centimeters:

| 0 | 1 | . | 0 | cm | **A. Pressure ulcer length:** Longest length from head to toe |

| 0 | 1 | . | 0 | cm | **B. Pressure ulcer width:** Widest width of the same pressure ulcer, side-to-side perpendicular (90-degree angle) to length |

| - | - | . | - | cm | **C. Pressure ulcer depth:** Depth of the same pressure ulcer from the visible surface to the deepest area (if depth is unknown, enter a dash in each box) |

M0700. Most Severe Tissue Type for Any Pressure Ulcer

Enter Code: **4**

Select the best description of the most severe type of tissue present in any pressure ulcer bed
1. **Epithelial tissue** - new skin growing in superficial ulcer. It can be light pink and shiny, even in persons with darkly pigmented skin
2. **Granulation tissue** - pink or red tissue with shiny, moist, granular appearance
3. **Slough** - yellow or white tissue that adheres to the ulcer bed in strings or thick clumps, or is mucinous
4. **Necrotic tissue (Eschar)** - black, brown, or tan tissue that adheres firmly to the wound bed or ulcer edges, may be softer or harder than surrounding skin

---

M0800. Worsening in Pressure Ulcer Status Since Prior Assessment (OBRA, PPS, or Discharge)
Complete only if A0310E = 0

Indicate the number of current pressure ulcers that were **not present or were at a lesser stage** on prior assessment (OBRA, PPS, or Discharge). If no current pressure ulcer at a given stage, enter 0

Enter Number: ☐
A. Stage 2

Enter Number: ☐
B. Stage 3

Enter Number: ☐
C. Stage 4

FIGURE 4.3—cont'd

Resident **George T. Blair**   Identifier **78**   Date _____

Section V	**Care Area Assessment (CAA) Summary**

V0200. CAAs and Care Planning

1. Check column A if Care Area is triggered.
2. For each triggered Care Area, indicate whether a new care plan, care plan revision, or continuation of current care plan is necessary to address the problem(s) identified in your assessment of the care area. The <u>Addressed in Care Plan</u> column must be completed within 7 days of completing the RAI (MDS and CAAs)). Check column B if the triggered care area is addressed in the care plan.
3. Indicate in the <u>Location and Date of CAA Information</u> column where information related to the CAA can be found. CAA documentation should include information on the complicating factors, risks, and any referrals for this resident for this care area.

A. CAA Results

Care Area	A. Care Area Triggered	B. Addressed in Care Plan	Location and Date of CAA Information
	↓ Check all that apply ↓		
01. Delirium	☒	☒	Mood and behavior problems/Admit note NursesN
02. Cognitive Loss/Dementia	☒	☒	Poor short & Long term memory/admit note NurN
03. Visual Function	☒	☒	Wears glasses /Admit and Nurses note
04. Communication	☒	☒	Difficulty making needs known/admit Nurses Note
05. ADL Functional/Rehabilitation Potential	☒	☒	Assist with ADLs/ Nurses notes
06. Urinary Incontinence and Indwelling Catheter	☒	☒	Incontinent of Urine/ Admit note/ Nurses notes
07. Psychosocial Well-Being	☒	☒	Verbally abusinve/ Nurses Note
08. Mood State	☒	☒	Expressive of Distress/ Nurses Note
09. Behavioral Symptoms	☒	☒	Wandering/ Inappropriate Behavior/ Nurses Note
10. Activities	☐	☐	
11. Falls	☒	☒	Fell in last 2 weeks/ Admit note
12. Nutritional Status	☒	☒	Wt Loss Special diet/ Admit /Nurses Note
13. Feeding Tube	☐	☐	
14. Dehydration/Fluid Maintenance	☒	☒	Constipation\Nurses Note
15. Dental Care	☐	☐	
16. Pressure Ulcer	☒	☒	Coccyx pressure Ulcer Admit
17. Psychotropic Drug Use	☒	☒	Oxazepam HS/ Nurses Notes
18. Physical Restraints	☐	☐	
19. Pain	☒	☒	Had a fall/ Medicated at Hospital/acetaminophen
20. Return to Community Referral	☐	☐	

B. Signature of RN Coordinator for CAA Process and Date Signed

1. Signature *Alice Jones*

2. Date | 0 | 7 | – | 1 | 3 | – | X | X | X | X |
          Month   Day   Year

C. Signature of Person Completing Care Plan and Date Signed

1. Signature *Alice Jones*

2. Date | 0 | 7 | – | 1 | 3 | – | X | X | X | X |
          Month   Day   Year

FIGURE 4.3—cont'd

Resident **George T. Blair**   Identifier **784393**   Date **July 6, XXXX**

Section Z			Assessment Administration				

Z0400. Signature of Persons Completing the Assessment or Entry/Death Reporting

I certify that the accompanying information accurately reflects resident assessment information for this resident and that I collected or coordinated collection of this information on the dates specified. To the best of my knowledge, this information was collected in accordance with applicable Medicare and Medicaid requirements. I understand that this information is used as a basis for ensuring that residents receive appropriate and quality care, and as a basis for payment from federal funds. I further understand that payment of such federal funds and continued participation in the government-funded health care programs is conditioned on the accuracy and truthfulness of this information, and that I may be personally subject to or may subject my organization to substantial criminal, civil, and/or administrative penalties for submitting false information. I also certify that I am authorized to submit this information by this facility on its behalf.

Signature	Title	Sections	Date Section Completed
A. *Brenda Miller*	RN	M	07/013/XXXX
B. *Marcie Moeller*	LPN	All	07/08/XXXX
C. *Anna Schmidt*	LCSW	D, E, F	07/09/XXXX
D. *Grant Payne*	PT	O	07/13/XXXX
E. *Katie Charm*	OT	O	07/13/XXXX
F. *Alice Jones*	RN	All	07/13/XXXX
G. *Lisa de Bois*	Rec. Terapist	E,F	07/13/XXXX
H. *Cal Washington*	Pharmacist	J, N	07/13/XXXX
I. *Jennifer Jarvis*	Dietician	G,K	07/13/XXXX
J.			
K.			
L.			

Z0500. Signature of RN Assessment Coordinator Verifying Assessment Completion

A. **Signature:** *Alice Jones*

B. **Date RN Assessment Coordinator signed assessment as complete:**

0	7	–	1	3	–	X	X	X	X
Month			Day			Year			

FIGURE 4.3—cont'd

Legal, Ethical, and Financial Considerations Regarding Older Adults

5

TAMARA DAHLKEMPER

LEARNING OUTCOMES

1. Compare and contrast the terms *legal* and *ethical*.

2. Define the term *liability* and discuss the impact it can have on your career.

3. Define the guiding principles of a restraint-free environment.

4. Outline the role of the licensed practical nurse (LPN) in using advanced directives and informed consent.

5. Express an understanding of the ethical responsibility of working with older adults in meeting their sexual needs.

6. Explain the HIPAA law and the significance it has for your nursing practice.

7. Compare and contrast Medicare and Medicaid.

CONCEPTS

Legal Issues

Ethics

Advocacy

Violence

CASE STUDY

As the 7–7 charge nurse on a 20-bed unit at Cherry Dale Nursing Home, you have had concerns over the staffing on your shift. Often, you have found the nursing assistants restraining residents for their own good without telling you. You have discussed the problem with the nursing assistants and have taught them about the restraint-free environment at Cherry Dale. Despite your efforts, there still is one "old-time" nursing assistant who does not follow the facility's rules and regulations and ignores your instructions.

This is your first charge nurse position as an LPN. You recognize that the nursing assistants see you as an inexperienced nurse. This is especially true of the older nursing assistant. During your first 6 weeks on the job, you believe you have made progress in earning the trust you need from the nursing assistants. One or two are still restraining residents at night without telling you, however.

You discussed this problem with your nurse manager, and she simply told you that you were a charge nurse now, and it was your responsibility to follow the policies of the facility. The policy indicates that restraints are not used unless there is a documentable situation that risks the life of the older adult, such as displacement of a nasogastric tube or intravenous needle.

What are the ethical and legal ramifications regarding your current dilemma? How will you resolve the problem?

Discussion

Because you are the licensed nurse responsible for what occurs on your shift, you are legally and ethically accountable for the behavior of the nursing assistants who work with you. Because they are violating facility policy, it is as if you were actually performing the act.

It is unethical and illegal to restrain people without following the criteria discussed in this chapter. When the restraint of older adults occurs, and it breaks the rules and regulations of the facility, your legal accountability is compounded. It is important that you realize that the law is being broken every time the residents are restrained. It does not matter if you know about it or not. The point is that, as the charge nurse, you should know about it. Reporting the situation to your supervisor does not release you from responsibility either. She gave you clear instructions as to what to do; you are to follow the facility's policy regarding restraints. The ethical problems of restraining residents are as serious as the legal ones.

INTRODUCTION

Health-care decisions that are made daily across the United States are based on the legal and ethical definitions of health care. Advances in technology, increased resources, newer drug therapies, and other modalities of treatment continue to bring with them ethical and legal problems and solutions to the health-care system that are unprecedented. While the legislators and ethics committees of the United States debate the merits of treatment approaches, health-care providers deliberate every day regarding their own direct care role and often wonder if it is one of help or hindrance.

As a licensed practical nurse (LPN), you will be involved in making ethical and legal decisions that potentially are very complex. This chapter will assist you in understanding ethical and legal issues that relate specifically to the challenges facing older adults and their care.

ETHICS

Ethics is the study of moral actions and values. It is based on the principles of conduct that govern individuals and groups. Many people envision ethics as dealing with principles and moral concepts that determine what is good or bad behavior. The problem with this concept is determining who decides what is good and what is bad. Always ask yourself, "Is this decision one for the older adult, the nurse, the family, or an outside group like an ethics committee?"

A broader definition of ethics considers the value system of a person and the relationship of those values in determining what is good for an individual or group. It is important for LPNs to understand their own value systems and the ethical framework underlying the work performance that springs from them. The personal values of all the people involved in making health-care decisions for older adults form the most important aspect of the nurse's delivery of ethical health care (Burkhardt & Nathaniel, 2013).

Patient Care Partnership

The Patient's Bill of Rights was a document adopted by the American Hospital Association (AHA) in 1973. It was a single-page document that listed the ethical behavior that was seen as appropriate and proper for care of patients in a hospital. The AHA has updated and added content to the original Patient's Bill of Rights and refers to the new document as the Patient Care Partnership. By federal law, each nursing home must have available a similar document that discusses the rights of residents. Other organizations, such as the American Nurses' Association, have ethical codes that guide

the practice of each professional and are consistent with the Patient Care Partnership. Professional organizations publish standards of care that identify an ethical and legal model of practice. These models are often used in legal cases to determine the acceptable level of care.

The Patient Care Partnership is based on every individual's right to make decisions regarding health-care treatment. It is designed to serve as a model that defines acceptable behavior toward individuals in your care. All work done with persons of every age and condition should be based on the principles in the Patient Care Partnership. The new document stresses access to health care and coverage. It is clear in not allowing racial or ethnic disparities. It covers billing and collection policies, and it defines the right of every person to be a partner in health-care decisions and delivery. The vision statement of the AHA is as follows:

"Our vision is of a society of healthy communities where all individuals reach their highest potential for health."

Please read and review the Patient Care Partnership. The Patient Care Partnership should be the foundation for the work you do with elderly people. It has special significance when dealing with the older adults who may be struggling with the stress of a new situation, limited short-term memory, or chronic disease.

Critically Examine the Following

What do you value in life? Your values create the foundation for your ethical behavior. Make a list of the three things you value most in life in the left column. In the right column, put an example of a nursing situation in which that value would be either tested or proved. Be prepared to discuss your ideas in class. This is an example of how your submission should look.

My Values	Nursing Application
1.	1.
2.	2.
3.	3.

 Point of Interest

You can access the Patient Care Partnership document at http://www.aha.org/advocacy -issues/communicatingpts/pt-care-partnership .shtml. The document is currently available in seven different languages.

The Law

The legal system is based on rules and regulations that guide society in a formal and binding manner. These regulations are human-made rules capable of being changed by the legislative and judiciary systems of the United States, whose officials are elected and appointed as representatives of the public. The law gives you, as a health-care provider, a general foundation for guiding your work; it may or may not complement your personal value system.

Ideally, the care you give is ethical and legal. It is possible, however, for a legal approach to care to seem unethical to you because it conflicts with your value system. This is when ethical-legal dilemmas occur. For example, the law recognizes the right of a competent person to refuse therapy. All individuals have that right regardless of the agreement or disagreement of the health-care system with the decision. An older adult has the right to refuse to have a pacemaker replaced. Such replacement is essentially a benign procedure with minimal risk, and not to have it done may cause death. It is the person's right to accept or refuse the therapy, however. The values of the health-care provider do not change the principles of the law.

Another example is provided by Dr. Jean Watson in her theory the "science of human caring" and is explained in detail in her book *Human Caring Science: A Theory of Nursing* (Watson, 2012). In her book, Watson emphasizes the importance of valuing persons as individuals and avoiding objectifying them. She explains that a nurse gives legal care when going into a person's room to perform a complicated dressing change. The nurse assesses the wound site, plans what will be done, removes the old dressing, and replaces it with a new dressing. The dressing is then evaluated for effectiveness. (I hope you recognize the use of the nursing process here.) The law does not indicate that the nurse needs to talk to the person or to explain the procedure or the healing process. For that care to be ethical, the nurse must take the time to talk to the person, however, and treat the person as a human being rather than an object with a wound to dress. Another simple example is that of bathing persons with dementia. Federal law requires that persons in nursing homes be kept clean. It is possible for a nursing assistant to give a resident a bath that is abusive by allowing no protection of modesty, by not waiting for the water to warm, or by being verbally abusive. This situation could be described as a legal, but unethical, bath.

In the midst of the time pressures of the complex world of health care, one must be careful to define legal and ethical care. Nurses experience legal and ethical issues in their work every day. It is important to be able to distinguish between ethics and the law.

Laws can be developed and passed on national, state, and local levels. Nurses are influenced

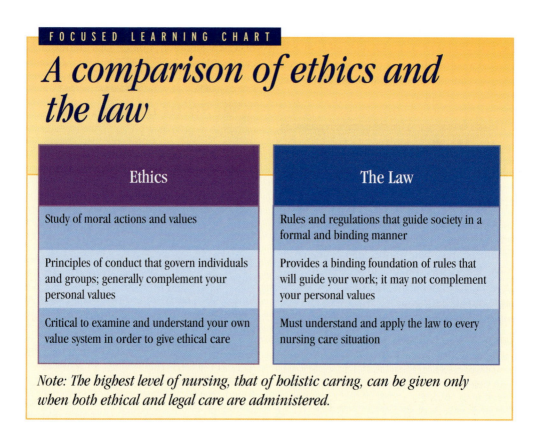

FOCUSED LEARNING CHART

A comparison of ethics and the law

Ethics	The Law
Study of moral actions and values	Rules and regulations that guide society in a formal and binding manner
Principles of conduct that govern individuals and groups; generally complement your personal values	Provides a binding foundation of rules that will guide your work; it may not complement your personal values
Critical to examine and understand your own value system in order to give ethical care	Must understand and apply the law to every nursing care situation

Note: The highest level of nursing, that of holistic caring, can be given only when both ethical and legal care are administered.

mostly by national (federal) laws and state laws. Examples of federal laws include the Patient Self-Determination Act of 1990, which requires asking people if they have living wills, durable power of attorney, or advance directives. There also is the Health Insurance Portability and Accountability Act (HIPAA), which includes regulations about patient privacy. This law was enacted in April 2003.

Nurse practice acts are state laws that tell the requirements for licensure and the limits of nursing practice. Every nurse needs to be familiar with the nurse practice act in the state where he or she is practicing. Nurse practice acts differ from state to state, so if you practice in more than one state, you need to know the differences.

Each hospital, home care agency, and nursing home has its own policies and procedures that must be in compliance with the state and federal laws. An employee of each health-care organization is a representative of that agency and is expected to follow all of the rules and regulations. Failure to do that is a reason for being terminated from a job. If an employee believes that laws are being broken by the agency's rules and regulations, there is a citizen's duty to report this to the agency authorities, such as a supervisor, or the legal authorities, such as the Department of Health, or both. This type of situation can lead to a serious legal and ethical dilemma. It is best to be certain of your facts before you take on such a serious risk. Consult a person who knows more about the law than you do.

LEGAL LIABILITY

Nurses do not commit wrongful acts deliberately, yet they are at risk every day for making a mistake for which they are liable. The term *liability* means that you are legally and morally responsible for an action taken. There are risky behaviors that can increase the possibility of making an error, increasing your risk of liability. These risks are apparent when the following occur:

1. Working when you are physically or emotionally exhausted
2. Working with inadequate staff
3. Not having the necessary equipment available to meet patient or resident needs
4. Not following the policies and procedures of the institution
5. Practicing beyond the scope of the nurse practice act
6. Allowing an impaired health-care provider to work without reporting him or her

The responsibility of the mistakes that can occur during any of the above-listed situations is a serious one and requires your best effort at all times to avoid it. Not only are you liable for your own actions, but you also are liable for any personnel working under your supervision. It is important to delegate only those tasks that an individual has the license or certification and knowledge to perform. For more information on delegation, refer to Chapter 13.

If there is a situation that puts anyone in your work environment at risk, do something to improve that situation. You are the licensed person, and not only do you want the situation to be changed, but also you could be liable for the situation itself. If any situation is present that could cause a medical or nursing error—including, but not limited to, the six previously listed risky behaviors and negligence, malpractice, and omission, which are discussed next—you need to work through the chain of command until the problem is solved. Working through the chain of command means going to your charge nurse, your nurse manager, and, if there is no resolution, the administrator. Because you are a new nurse, I understand that the very thought of going to a hospital or nursing home administrator might be intimidating. It would be nice if you and your charge nurse and nurse manager went to the administrator together, but in a risky situation, you must do whatever it takes, and I strongly suggest doing it before a patient injury occurs.

It is difficult to confront a serious problem, but your ethics will guide you, and I predict you would not be the only nurse troubled by the problem. Gather your resources and, in a patient and professional way, work with your nurse manager, the

 Priority Setting

The priority for this chapter is for you always to identify the nurse practice act for the state where you are practicing nursing as well as the rules and regulations at your place of employment. You are responsible for knowing the law and the policies that determine your practice. No one else can assume that responsibility for you.

unlicensed staff, and any others who can support you in making the work environment a safe and risk-free place to practice nursing.

ACTS OF NEGLIGENCE, MALPRACTICE, AND OMISSION

Two legal terms that are important to nurses are *negligence* and *malpractice*. Negligence is the failure of anyone to use care and caution to prevent harm to other people. Malpractice is the negligence on the part of a professional person in providing care to another person. Negligence and malpractice can occur if a medical professional fails to be cautious in doing something or fails to do something that needed to be done; the latter situation is called *omission*.

Every person is ethically and legally responsible and accountable for his or her own actions. Professional people who are licensed to care for others because they have special education, knowledge, and experience are held to a higher standard than other people. For example, as a nurse, you have a duty to protect and advocate for the people in your care as well as provide physical and emotional care for them.

Negligence is failure to exercise adequate care. The determination of negligence is based on the level of performance that is expected of an LPN as determined by the state nurse practice act, the policies and procedures for the facility where the LPN works, and what is considered safe and prudent care by other LPNs. For example, if you start an intravenous (IV) procedure, even in an emergency situation, and you are not IV-certified, you have broken the law as outlined in the nurse practice act, and you are liable for your behavior even if there is a good outcome from your actions. Why? Because you broke the law. Even if the outcome is good, you could be sued.

As a licensed nurse, you are liable for any acts of negligence and malpractice that you perform. If you are working on a team with CNAs, you are responsible or liable for their actions as well.

I remember being the charge nurse on a hospital-based nursing home unit when a patient was transferred from the medical/surgical unit. He was an elderly man who had fallen out of bed and had a bruise and gash on his forehead. I asked an experienced and trusted CNA to get him settled into his bed and to let me know when he was settled so that I could come in and do his admission assessment. The unit was full, and I had blood running. Although there were two LPNs working with me, neither of them could legally work with the blood except to observe it. I checked on the blood and the resident receiving the blood. Then I headed to the room with the new admit. Before I got to the room, someone met me and said to come quickly. The new admit was being walked to the restroom, lost consciousness, and fell, hitting his head again. I was horrified that the CNA had not used the wheelchair to move him! Although this case did not go to court, I was liable for the negligence of the CNA. The physician was called, and when he got to the floor, he asked for " … the stupid person who had let his patient fall!" The CNA walked up to him, but I got there in time to say, "I am responsible." It was the truth; I was legally liable for the CNA's actions.

The situation with the CNA was one of negligent care. If a nurse is accused of malpractice and is being investigated and tried in a court of law, how do judges and juries know the difference between good care, malpractice, and negligent care?

The legal system looks at what is the action that is expected from a reasonable and prudent person under the same circumstances. A prudent, responsible nurse is someone who is careful, thoughtful, and wise about his or her actions. This person also is a professional who renews nursing knowledge by reading, attending workshops and conferences, and simply "keeping up" with the profession. This is something I strongly recommend that you do.

Sometimes there is a small group of nurses who work together, cut corners, and neglect to follow rules unless someone in authority is watching. Such nurses are not prudent and responsible. A court would not use their behavior as a standard of care. Instead, the court would use expert witnesses, laws, agency rules, current textbooks, and standards of care published by professional organizations to show what a reasonable, prudent nurse would do under the circumstances.

Four conditions are needed to have malpractice or negligence:

1. A duty to the client
2. A failure to meet that duty or a breach of duty
3. An injury or negative outcome caused by not meeting that duty (causation)
4. Actual harm or damages suffered by the person who is receiving care

When these four criteria are met, the nurse is legally liable, or responsible, for the action in a court of law.

Many other nursing issues are closely related to meeting the criteria of the law. One additional issue is the concept of omission. Omission occurs when you omit something that is either ordered or expected as a normal part of treatment for a person. Classic examples of omission involve treatment or medication. Omission also could involve failure to notify a supervisor or primary care provider of a situation with a patient. Many lawsuits are based on omissions of care. Even though the act is something you did not do rather than something you did do, you are liable for your behavior.

Many issues within the realm of nursing are profoundly affected by ethical and legal concepts. The purpose of this section of the chapter is to discuss issues closely associated with nursing care of older adults, such as the use of restraints, advanced directives, informed consent, and elder abuse.

 ## USE OF RESTRAINTS

The long-practiced tradition of using restraints was an accepted aspect of nursing care of elderly adults until the 1980s. Nursing leaders joined other health-care professionals in drafting legislation and working with legislators to introduce and pass federal laws for reforming care of elderly adults in the United States. In 1987, the nursing home reform legislation was added to the Omnibus Reconciliation Act (OBRA) and became the law that was instrumental in dramatically changing and improving care of elderly residents in long-term care facilities. Gradually, states wrote and passed their own laws that reinforced the federal law and added improvements for the states. One very dramatic change was the reduction of the use of restraints and the gradual implementation of a restraint-free environment in the care of elderly residents.

Nurses who continue to use restraints often believe they are a means of preventing falls and wandering episodes. Evidence never did support that falls are prevented by restraints. Older adults who were restrained to prevent wandering often were seriously injured because of the restraint. Frequently, their injuries were worse than if they had been wandering and fallen. When restraints were used in large numbers, the injuries and deaths caused by the restraints outnumbered the injuries and deaths caused by wandering, even though the restraints were applied carefully and correctly. Most restraint deaths were from asphyxiation from crushing the trachea on a side rail or vest restraint or from obstruction of breathing owing to being pressed against the mattress between the bed and the side rail.

The legal system considers the use of restraints as well as the threat of using restraints as unlawful imprisonment. Anything that restricts a person's movement is considered a restraint. These items include side rails, protective vests, wheelchairs with trays, safety belts, and geriatric chairs. People fight and strongly resist being tied and shackled, which can cause death, severe injuries, skin excoriation, bruising, and pressure ulcers. These hard lessons were the reasons nurses took such strong political action in the late 20th century to "untie the elderly."

In the remote and rare situation when a restraint seems essential, the decision should be made with the interdisciplinary team (IDT) and by law must include informing the family. In hospitals, it

This woman is 82 years old and is proficient at using Facebook and e-mail. She gets a great deal of enjoyment out of them both. Also, she is an example of someone who is breaking one of the stereotypes of the elderly. The stereotype is that older persons do not like or know how to use technology. Do not let any negative stereotypes determine the degree of legal or ethical rights for older persons.

> ## *Think Like a Nurse*
>
> Mrs. Reed has been in bed for about 2 hours but is now awake and very agitated. Your facility is a restraints-free facility. What can you do instead of restraining Mrs. Reed to ensure her safety?

Evidence-Based Practice

Cotter, V.T., & Evans, L.K. (2010). Avoiding restraints in older adults with dementia. MEDSURG Nursing, 19(3), 197-198.

This article addresses best practices to avoid using restraints for older adults with dementia. The use of restraints is related to poor outcomes such as functional decline, agitation, serious injuries, and possibly death. The article provides several interventions nurses can use to address patient behaviors that may lead to the use of restraints.

Questions

1. What are some of the methods you can use to avoid the use of restraints on your patients with dementia?
2. What information is important for CNAs to know about the avoidance of restraint use?

sometimes is necessary to restrain a patient to maintain lifesaving procedures such as a tracheostomy, urinary catheter, or intravenous tubing. A physician's order for application of a short-term restraint requires the nurse to make careful observation and to perform periodic removal, skin care, and range-of-motion exercises. In an emergency, when it is necessary to protect the older adult or others from danger, a nurse may apply restraints without a physician's order or the IDT assessment and decision making. The circumstances and the observation and care given need to be documented carefully. In all instances, the least-confining restraint should be used (Said & Kautz, 2013).

Other Considerations

The staff in either a hospital or a nursing home should have some common strategies for managing confused older people. There may need to be a policy of placing mattresses on the floor or of lowering the bed near the floor to keep a night wanderer from falling out of bed. If wandering occurs more frequently at night or in the late afternoon, these are the times the staff should be increased so that residents can be closely monitored. At present in most facilities, evening and night shifts are times of minimal staffing, however. There are numerous

devices available to assist with this problem, including alarmed doors, wristband alarms, and bed alarm pads. With these devices, the older adult has freedom of movement, but the staff is immediately alerted when the older person is moving.

Implementing a restraint-free environment requires the education of everyone on staff, including ancillary people, to the principles of working there. Along with the education program, it is important to assist staff to focus on their personal values regarding care for the elderly person. This should help in establishing desirable approaches to care. A restraint-free environment is an innovative care strategy that also requires thought by bright and creative people who feel a commitment to the rights of all people, especially older adults.

INFORMED CONSENT AND ADVANCE DIRECTIVES

Informed Consent

Another very similar legal and ethical concern is the concept of *informed consent*. The Patient Care Partnership clearly outlines a person's right to information before giving consent to treatment. The law says that there needs to be a signature on the consent form. The ethical aspect of this situation is that the older adult and others have the right to all the information available on the treatment or procedure for which consent is being given.

As the nurse, you will assume the role of patient advocate. The physician is responsible for obtaining the consent by clearly informing the patient of all possible outcomes of the procedure and any alternatives to treatment that are available. A complete explanation of the procedure is essential. Would you stop a patient from going to surgery if, as you were assisting him or her onto the cart, the patient asked, "Tell me again, what is it the doctor is going to do?" Legal and ethical knowledge says that you should.

Think Like a Nurse

You are working with a patient who has a terminal illness and is refusing the placement of a feeding tube, but her daughter is insisting that a feeding tube be placed. You know this patient has an advanced directive that clearly states a feeding tube is not to be used. How do you handle this situation?

There are better ways to manage this type of situation than to postpone the scheduled surgery. One is simply to be sure ahead of time that the patient has the information needed to make decisions about the health and treatment plan. This situation can become challenging when the patient is a frail elderly person who is experiencing behavior that ranges from forgetfulness to dementia. Is it enough just to get the signature when you know the person will not remember the instructions? The answer to that is no, it is not enough.

You would need to ask yourself if you value the patient and his or her rights as outlined in the Patient Care Partnership. Do you value the principle behind the informed consent rule? It is hoped that you do. The work may involve reporting the forgetfulness or dementia to the nursing manager. In a nursing home environment, it would be important to share that information at the IDT meeting. Talking to the family may be something you do or that is delegated to the social worker. The priority is to ensure that the elderly person has complete information when asked to make a decision regarding health care.

Some older adults have a medical power of attorney entrusted to a family member or friend. If so, that is the person who should understand the procedure and sign the consent form. The elderly person also should be well informed even though the person may not remember the information. When elderly people do not have family members to assume this responsibility, the court appoints a legal guardian. The guardian is responsible for all legal documents.

Advance Directives

There are several legal and moral concerns with the issue of advanced directives. An advance directive is a legal document made and signed by a competent adult regarding life-sustaining issues and other concerns related to terminal care. Advance directives came into use when legal cases such as those involving Karen Ann Quinlan and Nancy Cruzan surfaced in the judicial system. In both of these legal cases, a young woman was kept alive on life support equipment but had no quality of life at the time and no possibility of improvement in the future. In both cases, the family members decided to remove the life support equipment and allow their daughters to die. In both cases, the health-care facility refused to remove the equipment, and the parents sued.

In 1989, the U.S. Supreme Court ruled that not even the family should make decisions for an incompetent patient without "clear and convincing evidence" that indicated the person's desire was to die if incompetent. In a five-to-four decision by the U.S. Supreme Court, the following rights were listed for states (Cruzan v. Director, 1990):

- The state has a right to assert an unqualified interest in the preservation of human life.
- A choice between life and death is a very personal matter.
- Abuse can occur when incompetent patients do not have loved ones available to serve as surrogate decision makers.

In 1990, Congress passed the Patient Self-Determination Act that requires all health-care institutions that receive federal funding (Medicare and Medicaid) to ask patients, on admission, if they have an advance directive. This could be a living will or a durable power of attorney, which gives another person the legal responsibility to make terminal care decisions (Box 5.1). If there is an advance directive, it is to be noted in the medical record. When the directive is noted, the patient's wishes should be followed. As an LPN, you need to determine what the law is in your state regarding advance directives. If they are required on admission, you need to know where they are

---

BOX 5.1 ADVANCE DIRECTIVES

Living will: A written document prepared by a competent person describing the type of medical care that he or she wants or does not want in a particular situation. The document needs to be prepared while the person is still able to make his or her own decisions.

Durable power of attorney or health-care proxy: A written document prepared by a competent person giving permission for someone to make health decisions on his or her behalf under certain conditions. This document should include clear instructions about the patient's wishes regarding feeding tubes, medications, resuscitation, and mechanical ventilation.

and what they say regarding your clients. It is the role of the nurse to be an advocate for the people to whom care is given. Knowledge about the advance directive and the state laws that govern its use is very important to you. When one is working with advance directives, there is more involved than just knowing the law.

The law represents legal responsibilities. These are serious responsibilities and should not be ignored; however, as with every issue, there is also an ethical component. It is the ethical responsibility of every nurse to ensure that the person signing the advance directive is not coerced and has full understanding of what is being signed. In most states, the nurse is not allowed to witness this document. It is important that outsiders who would not wield undue influence act as witnesses. Whenever you are giving care to a patient who is in a terminal condition, it is important that you listen as the person talks and provide honest answers to questions. If someone feels concern over what was written in the advance directive, you should bring that to the attention of the nurse manager. The instructions for completing an advance directive are provided in Appendix A of this book. In all situations, it is necessary to keep in mind the primary objective of the advance directive: to follow the wishes of the person who wrote it.

States have various laws regarding the use of a living will, and family members may have different ideas as to what the patient's terminal care should be. The best advice you can have for this complicated issue is to know the policies for the facility where you work and the laws of your state. You also may want to discuss this issue with a more experienced nurse before you have to deal with it. Dying is such a personal and permanent issue for each person. It is important for you to know what to do and how to manage the multiple situations that can occur by being prepared.

 ## ELDER ABUSE

Occurrences of elder abuse are increasing in the United States. It is estimated that about 500,000 older adults are abused each year, most often by a close family member. This is an underestimate of the amount of abuse because of individuals unwilling or unable to report their abuse to the authorities or family members (CDC, 2013). Abuse exists in family homes, nursing homes, and hospitals. It is done by

Whenever there is a question about elder abuse, immediately contact the social worker or ombudsman at the facility where you work. This social worker specializes in elder abuse investigation.

family members, paid caregivers, and strangers. It seems to be a consequence of life in Western society, which moves faster and faster, with more and more demands. Into this scenario comes an increasing number of older people who, as a natural consequence of aging, move more slowly and experience mental changes that require patience from caregivers. The United States has never had so many older citizens, and society does not seem adequately prepared to adapt to them and their needs.

Because of this lack of emphasis on understanding and meeting the needs of elderly adults, caregivers tend to experience burnout. Accompanying this phenomenon is the tendency to abuse the elder for causing the feelings of burnout and frustration. Elder abuse is the most extreme and destructive form of ageism that can be demonstrated.

Elder abuse is also against the law, and every state in the United States has laws that say that is true. As a licensed nurse, it is your responsibility to determine what the law is in your state and the policies and procedures for handling abuse in the organization where you work. Whatever the particulars of the law are, it will state that you are responsible, under the law, to report all suspected cases of elder abuse. For more information about elder abuse, refer to Chapter 7.

 ## PROVIDING FOR INTIMACY NEEDS

Another ageist concept in our society is that old people are asexual. Biologically, this is simply not true. Sexual needs are as basic as eating and so-cializing. The aging process does not remove that need from the physiological schema of older adults. The question is, how do you provide for the fulfillment or manage the needs of older adults for whom you are responsible?

Older people need love, too. I recall attending a conference many years ago in which the presenter, a music therapist, made the statement that every person needs 14 hugs a day. I do not believe that she had any scientific data to validate her point, but when she said it, I believed her! She continued to say that most of society finds old people very unlovable and unhuggable. I immediately began a lifelong quest to provide as many hugs to older people as I could give in a lifetime. Older people in our society are touch starved; often people do not readily touch or hug them. Does this flash of unscientific insight bring to your awareness that you can do something positive about meeting this need for older adults in your care? It would be very exciting to see a care plan that said: 14 hugs a day evenly distributed over 24 hours.

A myth that needs to be dispelled is that "dirty old men" are reaching and grabbing inappropriate parts of the female body. This unkind stereotyping is generally directed at an older, confused man. Instead of restraining or isolating that individual, you should assess him from a professional level.

An example of an intervention with an older man whose wife recently died could be sitting with him and asking, "You miss your wife, don't you?" to provoke a discussion of his sexual feelings. After your discussion with this man, you may learn strategies that will help him manage his sex-ual feelings in a more appropriate manner. Perhaps he needs a picture of his deceased wife that he can keep with him at all times, for instance, in the din-ing room or when he is in the hallway in his wheel-chair. It may take something as simple as teaching the nursing assistants to point to the picture of his wife and ask him to tell them about her to ward off his confused attempts at meeting his sexual needs. Perhaps the solution is more complex, and the nursing assistants need to be taught how to stop his inappropriate behavior in a respectful manner that recognizes sexual needs as normal and confu-sion as a reality. It is your responsibility, in an ethical framework, to determine the approaches and strategies that would provide for effective management of the sexual needs of the older people in your care.

Another problem that occurs sometimes is mas-turbation. Masturbation is a normal sexual outlet for people. Teenagers generally masturbate as part of their sexual experimentation. Adults often mas-turbate as part of their sexual relationships with other individuals. It is not abnormal for older peo-ple to masturbate. It is something they have either done intermittently or worked hard at suppressing throughout their lives. It is not wrong for an older adult to masturbate; however, because of different levels of cognitive ability, an older person may be participating in this activity in an inappropriate place. Masturbating in the dayroom or in any environment in front of others is inappropriate behavior. If this should occur, it is your responsi-bility gently and kindly to stop the activity and take the person to his or her room. It is appropriate to leave the person alone there to do as he or she wishes. This approach is an effective one to use if the person is acting out for attention or is forgetful or confused. If you walk into an older adult's room

---

QSEN

COMPETENCY: Patient-Centered Care (Attitudes)

Meeting Your Patients' Individual Needs

You have just admitted Mr. and Mrs. Bennett to your long-term care facility. Although they have a very close relationship, Mrs. Bennett has several health-care needs, so the decision was made by the primary care provider and the family to place them in separate rooms. On several occasions during the day, Mr. Bennett visits his wife in her room. The staff notices that Mr. Bennett sits very close to his wife's bed and rubs her arms and legs. Mrs. Bennett seems very responsive to his touch. On one occasion, one of the nursing assistants suggested that Mr. Bennett crawl into his wife's bed so he could be closer to her. The nursing assistant helped position both of them so they would be comfortable in the bed together. On leaving the room, she placed a "do not disturb" sign on the door.

Patient-centered care means providing for the individual needs of your patients.

■ Did the nursing assistant do the right thing?
■ Would you have done the same thing?
■ Are there any concerns that should be addressed in this situation?

and the person is masturbating, just excuse yourself and close the door.

Often in nursing home settings, there is controversy about allowing married couples to room together or to have time for conjugal visits. Sometimes it is unwise to have couples room together because one may need more care than the other, and the stronger person becomes worn out trying to administer to every need of the ill or degenerating spouse. Abusive behavior brought on because of dementia could be another reason. Only reasons that would jeopardize the health of one or both of the people involved are valid, however, for keeping a married couple separated. It is normal for married people to live together, and it is normal for married people to want to continue intimacy in their relationship.

Another situation that can occur is unmarried, consenting adults having an intimate relationship. You have the ethical and legal responsibility of protecting individuals with dementia and developmentally disabled or mentally ill persons from the sexual advances of others. If that person does not have the ability to make day-to-day decisions, the person doesn't have the ability to make the normal, everyday decision to have an intimate relationship. As a licensed nurse, you are responsible for protecting such a person from what could be defined as sexual abuse.

What about elderly residents who are not cognitively impaired? Counselors do not go around the halls of high schools or universities to keep teenagers and young adults from holding hands or kissing. Why does society think it is necessary to do that for older adults? Sexual feelings and

expressions are a normal part of living, even if one is old, disabled, or confused. Every dependent human being has the right to expect protection from sexual abuse, but every human being also has the right to express sexual feelings and have their intimacy needs met, within the framework of society's norms.

CONFIDENTIALITY

An underlying rule of professional health care is confidentially. Every individual in the health-care system deserves perfect confidentiality regarding his or her personal information. That includes age, weight, diagnosis, family matters, and any other item of personal living for the individual. No patient has only one caregiver, however. That means information has to be communicated verbally and in written format to others on the health-care team for effective care to be delivered to the person who is ill. That type of professional sharing is critical and needs to happen in an efficient manner. There is always the possibility, however, of a discussion at lunch or break with a colleague regarding someone or a procedure that is interesting. When you engage in such conversations, you are breaking the law.

The U.S. government developed the Health Insurance Portability and Accountability Act (HIPAA) as a strong effort to protect individuals' personal medical information. Confidentiality always has been an aspect of professional nursing; however, the HIPAA law brings the requirement of confidentiality in professional behavior to the forefront of practice. The law allows patients access to their medical records, provides a method for making formal complaints to the government when patients believe their confidentiality has been abused, and gives patients control over how their personal information may be used.

Maintaining confidentiality of information for every patient in your care is an essential moral behavior. It also is a legal responsibility.

It is your responsibility as a licensed nurse to learn the laws in the state where you practice. The excuse of "I didn't know" is unacceptable in any situation when you have broken the law or violated the nurse practice act.

FINANCIAL CONSIDERATIONS

In the United States, almost all citizens who have reached the age of 65 have health insurance coverage through the federal Medicare program. Many, if they have few assets and very low income, also qualify for Medicaid. Some seniors are still working and may have coverage through a plan offered by their employer.

Medicare

Medicare is a federal program managed by the United States government since 1966. It provides health insurance coverage to all people 65 years old and older who have been employed during their lifetime and have become eligible for Social Security benefits. Medicare provides coverage for hospital services, physician and outpatient care, home care, hospice services, and prescription drugs through various parts of the law as described in this section. Coverage is not 100%. There are deductibles that must be met and coinsurance that must be paid by the patient. Some services are not covered at all, most notably long-term care.

Medicare Part A primarily covers hospitalization. It is funded by payroll taxes on all workers that are then matched by their employers. There are no premiums for Part A, and coverage is automatic for anyone 65 years old or older who is eligible for Social Security retirement benefits. Part B primarily covers physicians' fees and outpatient services. Seniors may choose to join part B and must pay monthly premiums to be enrolled. Part D was added in 2006 to cover outpatient prescription drugs. Just as for Part B, those who wish to enroll in Part D must pay monthly premiums. Part C offers seniors a choice. If they wish, they can join a private health maintenance organization (HMO) or other managed care plan (called a Medicare Advantage plan) that replaces the other three parts. Many seniors have chosen to do this because they feel the Advantage plans offer better coverage at lower premiums.

One of the most important things for seniors and their care providers to know is that Medicare does not pay for long-term care. Under specific circumstances, Medicare will pay for some nursing and rehabilitation services but only for a limited period of time. Medicare members who have been hospitalized and on discharge need continuing skilled nursing and rehabilitation services can have those covered for a maximum of 100 days if the need is certified by Medicare and is periodically recertified as care progresses.

Medicaid

Medicaid was enacted by the federal government at the same time as Medicare in 1966. Each state is required to set up and manage its own Medicaid program that meets at least the minimum specifications of the federal law and regulations. To qualify for Medicaid coverage, people must have very few financial assets and very low income. Once a person does qualify, however, coverage is very broad, including both acute care and long-term care. There are no premiums to be paid for Medicaid coverage, and copayments are very minimal. Some seniors qualify for both Medicare and Medicaid.

Medicaid is the largest payer for skilled nursing facilities. Even if a resident does not initially qualify for Medicaid, that resident may qualify later after he or she has spent most of his or her assets to pay for care. At that point, Medicaid would take over payment to the skilled nursing facility. If a senior qualifies for Medicaid, it may also pay for portions of acute care, home care, and prescriptions not paid for by Medicare.

Private Health Insurance and Long-Term Care Insurance

A person who continues to work beyond age 65 may be covered through a private insurance plan offered by his or her employer. Such as person is still eligible for Medicare and can enroll if he or she wishes, but by law the employer's plan will be primary. That is, the employer's insurance will pay for services first as covered by that plan, and then Medicare may help fund some of the costs not covered by the private plan.

Neither Medicare nor employer-sponsored health insurance will cover long-term care. Because of this, some people choose to purchase long-term care insurance. These long-term care plans usually pay a fixed amount per day to help cover the cost of care provided in a nursing home, other certified facility, or even home care, as long as the needs can be documented as specified in the policy.

The Patient Protection and Affordable Care Act of 2010

The primary goal of the Patient Protection and Affordable Care Act (ACA) was to increase the number of people who have health insurance, and most of its provisions are aimed in that direction. However, there were some changes affecting seniors, even though nearly all seniors were already covered by Medicare. The reform law made some changes to Medicare Part D that will reduce out-of-pocket costs to members for outpatient prescription drugs. It also expanded Medicare coverage to include more preventive services. States were also allowed to expand Medicaid to include more people, which could make some seniors eligible sooner. Beyond those changes, most seniors will not see direct impacts of the ACA, but there are changes in the way doctors and hospitals are paid for services to Medicare patients that are intended to improve the coordination.

 ## CONCLUSION

This chapter covers several diverse topics that have legal, ethical, and financial ramifications for providing care to older adults. Every topic is important and needs to be addressed by you as a gerontological nurse. Older people have rights, and when these people come into the health-care system, you, the licensed nurse, are the unofficial advocate for them. Their legal and ethical rights are your responsibility. Understanding how health care is funded for the older adult is also important. The concepts explained in this chapter should help to provide you with a strong foundation for fulfilling that role.

CASE STUDY SOLUTIONS

There is more than one approach that could resolve this problem. The truth is that you may have to use them all before you find an appropriate solution.

Make it clear to all the nursing assistants that the law is being broken and the act of restraining residents on your shift is a criminal offense. Next,

- Use the experience and wisdom of the nursing assistants to process different solutions to the problem of residents wandering or potentially falling at night. The nursing assistants will appreciate being asked to assist in solving the problem rather than being told what to do. Try all ideas that do not go against the policy of the institution, the law, or your ethical standards.

- Share your creative solutions with the nurse manager. Let her know how prudent and safe the care is on your shift. (Remember that prudent and safe care is the care that most LPNs would give in the same situation.) You also should build a case for additional staffing on your shift, if that is the problem.

- Document the unique approaches of care you use on your shift, and share them with the other shifts by means of verbal report and the nursing care plan.

REVIEW QUESTIONS

1. Ethics is the study of moral actions and values. One of the dilemmas within ethical thinking is concern over:
   1. Who decides what is right and what is wrong
   2. Whoever pays the bill deciding what is ethical
   3. Ethical and legal behavior being the same
   4. The rules of ethical behavior changing daily

2. Because of Mrs. E.'s failing health and inability to live on her own, she has been admitted to a long-term care facility. Which method of financing cannot be used to cover her care in the facility?
   1. Medicaid
   2. Medicare
   3. Long-term care insurance
   4. Private pay

3. The legal concept of omission in care applies when:
   1. The physician has missed a diagnosis, and you have omitted treatment for it because nothing was ordered.
   2. You have intentionally or unintentionally missed an antibiotic dose.
   3. Residents are given baths only every other day.
   4. The RN does not work the weekend.

4. A restraint-free environment consists of an environment in which:
   1. Many of the residents fall or wander, but they do not sue the facility because they want to be without restraint.
   2. Mattresses are placed on the floor so that residents will not fall out of bed.
   3. The least-restrictive device is used on each resident.
   4. Restrictive devices are not used for any reason.

5. Elder abuse is a growing concern in modern society. Which of the following statements is correct?
   1. It is against the law to threaten abuse as well as to perform abusive acts.
   2. Elder abuse includes inflicting pain or injury but not confining an older person.
   3. Elder abuse is likely to happen to a male client, older than age 85, who lives with a relative.
   4. It is the legal responsibility of the RN to report all suspected cases of elder abuse; this is not the responsibility of the LPN.

REFERENCES

Burkhardt, M.A., & Nathaniel, A.K. (2013). *Ethics and issues in contemporary nursing.* Clifton Park, NY: Thomson.

Centers for Disease Control and Prevention. (2013). Elder abuse prevention. http://www.cdc.gov /Features/ElderAbuse/

Watson, J. (2012). *Human caring science: A theory of nursing.* (2nd ed.). Sudbury, MA: Jones and Bartlett Learning.

WEB RESOURCES

National Center on Elder Abuse: http://www.ncea. aoa.gov/index.aspx

Promoting Wellness

DIANE LEGGETT-FIFE

LEARNING OUTCOMES

1. Recognize aging as a normal process of living rather than a disease process.

2. Describe the role nurses play in health-promotion and disease-prevention activities for older people.

3. Recommend key health-promotion and disease-prevention activities appropriate for older people.

4. Examine the importance motivation plays in an older person's ability to participate in health-promotion and disease-prevention activities.

CONCEPTS

Teaching and Learning

Managing Care

Collaboration

Advocacy

Comfort

Mobility

Self

CASE STUDY

Mrs. C. is a 65-year-old widow who has lived alone since the death of her husband 2 years ago. She retired 1 year ago from her job of 25 years as a secretary. After retirement, she participated in a health-promotion and screening clinic at the senior center. After completing a lifestyle inventory and screening, the following problems were noted in the categories of health promotion:

Nutrition: 10 lb overweight

Exercise: Does no regular exercise

Stress: Cries easily, often unable to sleep at night, complains of fatigue and generally low energy

Relationships: Misses people at work, talks about missing deceased husband

Substance use or abuse: Takes an OTC sleeping pill and one glass of wine before bed

Self-care: Has not seen a physician since she had a hysterectomy 10 years ago; never had a mammogram and does not perform breast self-examination; cannot recall immunization history but is sure she has not had any in the past 10 years; has never had a flu shot or pneumococcal vaccine; recently had blood pressure taken at a drug store machine, which measured 150/92 mm Hg.

Discussion

1. List additional assessment data that should be known in each of the categories of health promotion.

2. How might you determine Mrs. C.'s greatest concern?

3. What part does Mrs. C.'s motivation play in developing a wellness plan?

4. What conditions or disease states might develop if Mrs. C. continues with no changes in her life?

5. What might be the first priority for Mrs. C.?

INTRODUCTION

One of the positive aspects of being a gerontological nurse is the variety of ways you are able to work with older people. The role of the licensed practical nurse (LPN) is crucial in the care of elderly persons. You are the person who gives direct care to most older people who seek out health-care services. Many nurses think only of care given in a nursing home when they consider gerontological nursing, yet you have learned that only 5% of people older than age 65 are nursing home residents. Where do the others live, and what type of nursing care do they need?

Many older adults need your knowledge and support to stay healthy. To help these individuals, you need skills and knowledge in holistic health promotion and wellness. Health has many definitions, one of which is the absence of disease. Most elderly persons have multiple chronic illnesses, however, for which there is only management, not cure. Can they ever be well? Yes, if you consider the concept of holistic wellness. When considered holistically, health implies " . . . a wholeness and harmony of body, mind and spirit" (Eliopolous, 2014). That will be the focus of wellness used in this chapter.

The search for eternal youth has a long history. People have died in their search for the Fountain of Youth, and others have killed for what they thought would prevent them from aging. The legends surrounding the "forever young" concept are taking on a new reality and meaning for the aging society in the United States because people are living to be older than ever before (remember the older-than-85-years age group and the elite-old?). The modern version of the legend of the Fountain of Youth is embodied in the concept of health promotion. The focus is on living longer and healthier, an opportunity offered to today's society that has not existed previously.

The older people of the United States are generally healthier than those of previous generations. This change is due to improved nutrition, sanitation, immunizations, and overall safety in work environments and everyday life. Today's older people have benefited from improved health care as well. People older than age 65 constitute 13% of the population (Werner, 2011), yet they use more than one-third of U.S. expenditures for health care (Stanton and Rutherford, 2005). The remarkable advances in surgery, pharmacology, and the technology available for diagnosis and treatment have made tremendous contributions to the prolonging of life for older people.

Some elderly people complain about getting old. They have not found the Fountain of Youth and are upset about it! It is important to acknowledge that normal processes of aging include some decrease in vision, hearing, and joint mobility from arthritis. There may also be some weight gain. Aging is associated with losses of friends and family because of death or nursing home placement; the loss of income is also a problem for some older people, as are the acute and chronic diseases that tend to accompany the aging process. Yet, the objective of wellness defined by harmony between the body, mind, and spirit can occur if individuals strive for gerotranscendence as they age. When aging individuals achieve this developmental stage, they are able to accept the naturally occurring losses of the aging experience. They also have plans for their future and have strong relationships with supportive and caring people.

Can you see how important these characteristics are to health and wellness? It can make the difference between good to excellent or poor quality of life. *Remember:* the objective is not to run a marathon or never to experience illness. Rather, the objective is harmony among the body, mind, and spirit.

Our society emphasizes age-related changes and common health problems as diseases experienced by older people, when actually they are normal consequences of aging. Not enough attention has been given to the positive side of aging and the beneficial effects of health-promotion activities to prevent disease and to slow the effects of chronic disease. Do you think that this lack of attention is another form of ageism? If so, what can you do about it as a nurse?

Current health-care concepts emphasize vitality and independence for older people as a primary concern. Regardless of age, as people laugh more, walk more, eat better, relax more, and think better of themselves and their relationships, they move beyond the neutral point of good health. Many of the complaints associated with the aging process, such as joint stiffness, weight gain, fatigue, loss of bone mass, and loneliness, can be prevented or managed by basic health-promotion activities. One does not have to be free of disease to experience the benefits of health and wellness.

Priority Setting

Do you remember Chapter 2, where your priority was to combat ageism? This chapter is a continuation of that idea.

Most older adults do not have the availability of health-promotion facilities, personnel, or financial support that other age groups have. Yet, if the health of older persons could be maintained, the medical bills in the United States would decrease immensely. That is secondary to the improvement in life quality that can happen for the wellness-focused older person.

Your priority for this chapter is to become well informed about wellness facilities and organizations that are specific for older adults. This information will be valuable for you as you render care to older people. You could visit the local senior citizens' center and become familiar with what they offer. The center can refer you to other organizations that assist elderly people to be healthy. Gather as much information as you can. As a licensed nurse, you need to have a broad spectrum of information available for use as you go about your daily work of caring for others. Assist older adults in recognizing the importance of holistic wellness. Encourage them to be involved in the organizations and activities you find. Teach them about the concepts in this chapter that will assist them in their personal wellness program. Become knowledgeable regarding wellness for older persons, and you will enhance the lives of those in your care and become a valuable resource to the health-care team.

Most health-promotion activities focus on exercise, stress management, nutrition, and dealing with substance abuse. In addition, it is important that wellness activities for older adults include relationships and self-care.

ILLNESS/WELLNESS AS A CONTINUUM

If you think of health as a continuum with illness on one end and health on the other, you can understand better the importance of health promotion. By using a holistic approach to examine the continuum, you focus your attention on the person's previous experience with life, existing support systems (e.g., family, church), and personal strengths. The point is that everyone wants health, and holistic health-promotion activities are the way to achieve that goal.

Primary care providers and nurses traditionally focus on working with patients who are on the illness end of the continuum or who have symptoms of disease or disability. As a person's health improves, traditional medicine becomes less involved in helping the person reach optimal well-being. In contrast, health-promotion efforts primarily are focused on the opposite, or wellness, side of the continuum. Think of Mrs. C. and how she participated in a health-promotion and screening clinic following her retirement. The information obtained at the clinic will assist her in to continue on the wellness path.

In more recent years, nurses have begun to use health-promotion efforts even when dealing with people on the illness side of the continuum. Special exercise and nutrition programs have been designed for cardiac rehabilitation, exercise and weight-lifting programs for chair-bound persons, and weight management programs for older persons. The remainder of this chapter focuses on health-promotion activities on the illness and the wellness sides of the health continuum.

Motivation

If you, as a nurse, want to be successful in promoting healthy choices in older people, you need to understand the importance of individual motivation. Desire must be present on the part of an older adult to make a change. It is critical to explore what motivates an older person to eat right, exercise, and avoid unhealthy behaviors on an individual basis. This is true for all people, even yourself.

Critically Examine the Following:

Motivation is an important concept to understand. You will understand it best if you comprehend what motivates you. Answer the following questions and be prepared to share your answers in class or submit them to your faculty person.

1. What are you wearing today? There is a reason for wearing it; do you know what that reason is? Whatever the reason, it is your motivation to wear it. It could be as simple as the outfit being your favorite color or being the last clean outfit in the closet.
2. What foods have you eaten today? Why did you choose those foods? Your choice of foods could be healthy or unhealthy, but you were motivated to choose them. What were your reasons for those choices?
3. Why are you in a nursing program? What is your motivation for being here? Spend time pondering this question. Understanding your personal motivation for such an all-important decision is critical.

As a part of human behavior, motivation is the incentive or drive that causes a person to act. Incentive to take action is based on needs and desires that are internal and external to the person. An older person may have an incentive to exercise three times a week if it helps the individual experience less discomfort or immobility from arthritis. For some people, the incentive may need to be more than physical wellness. A need also may exist for a mental wellness experience, such as that derived from socialization with others while exercising, such as in a water aerobic class, playing tennis, or with a group doing mall walking.

The nursing challenge is to assist older adults in identifying their own incentives for participation in health-promotion and disease-prevention activities. This information allows the nurse to have greater insight into ways to promote health and lessens the frustration experienced from what are often incorrectly referred to as *noncompliant patients*. Compliance occurs only if the individual can personally identify a need or desire to exercise, eat correctly, reduce stress, or make other changes necessary for improved wellness. This is motivation experienced by people in an individual way. Often, assisting to identify the motivation is one way that you, the LPN, can help an older adult. Think about Mrs. C's motivation to participate in the health-promotion and screening clinic. Will this same motivation keep her interested in addressing some of the issues listed? What could you do to increase her motivation?

Incentives

Studies have disclosed some of the reasons (incentives) for older people to participate in health-promotion behaviors, such as the following:

- A belief that activities improve fitness and health
- The enjoyment of socialization
- A belief that activities help maintain independence
- A desire to feel good and have fun (Marcus et al., 2006)

Knowledge about why a person participates in health promotion (or the incentives for doing so) can be determined through a caring and focused interview. After personal incentives have been identified, you can reinforce them in health-promotion activities. In addition to understanding individual motivation, you need to help individuals plan their short-term and long-term goals for making health changes. The secret to success in health behavior is to help the older adult choose personal goals with care and then learn to enjoy achieving them. Following an interview with Mrs. C., you may discover several areas that would increase her interest in obtaining the goals. Review her statements regarding missing people at work and her husband. Could socialization with group activities be a stimulus to keep her active?

Health-Promotion Activities

When older adults have identified an area of health promotion that is desirable, they have an incentive to maintain or improve their health. The challenge is to locate a properly designed activity. Many current health-promotion activities can be geared toward younger age groups and may exclude older adults by design. Four reasons underscore why the current focus on health-promotion activities is often inappropriate for older people:

1. The focus frequently is on life extension or on reducing the risks of premature death. If a person stops smoking, reduces fat intake, and exercises, the risk of a heart attack at an early age is reduced. For elderly people who have already lived beyond the average life expectancy, life extension may not be as important as quality of life. Stopping smoking, reducing fat intake, and exercising are important at any age, but for different reasons. The focus must be on health-promotion benefits specific to an older person.

2. Emphasis is often placed on advancing "youthfulness" and preventing aging. Older people recognize that they do not fit the image of youth and have already experienced some results of aging. This does not mean self-image and appearance are not important to older people, but that the image needs to match the older person's self-perception.

3. Health-promotion programs focus on preventing chronic disease. Remember that more than 50% of those age 65 or greater already have two or more chronic diseases. When these programs focus on management of the symptoms of the disease rather than on its prevention, more older adults have a reason to participate.

4. A focus on self-responsibility for health fails to consider the limitations imposed by personal circumstances. An individual who has a need and desire to walk daily for exercise may live in an unsafe neighborhood. An older adult may have a desire to eat a healthy diet but because of limited income may be unable to afford the proper food. The external environment may pose barriers to older people that are difficult to overcome. These problems need careful attention.

As you, the LPN, look at the key areas of health promotion for older people, your goals must be to design, plan, and provide activities that are sensitive to individual needs and responsibility.

Properly designed health-promotion activities should be:

- Accessible (transportation, time of day, location)
- Enjoyable and social (mental and physical wellness)
- Reasonable (focus on the right activity for the right reason)
- Sensitive to needs of older people (hearing, vision, functional level)

Health-promotion strategies must be based on the belief that the individual is the only one who can choose a path to a healthy life. Consequently, you, the nurse, must be sure that health-promotion activities are individually designed so that the pathways exist.

 ## REGULAR EXAMINATIONS

Before excellent health-promotion activities can be designed for an individual, physical examinations of most body systems need to be completed. An annual physical examination is important in terms of maintaining health and promoting wellness. Many older adults need to be seen more often for the management of the chronic diseases that may accompany aging. Some older people avoid making such appointments because they have limited funds to pay the co-pay, they lack convenient transportation, or they do not recognize that there is something that can be treated. Some people think that being ill is part of being old, so they accept their condition and do not seek treatment. Some people may be like Mrs. C. and with no health complaints do not feel the need to have regular examinations.

Regular visits to the physician can help prevent acute conditions and are an asset for managing chronic diseases. Regular blood work as an indicator of overall health is critical, as are examinations for colon, breast, cervical, and prostate cancers. The physician's visit is the time to obtain immunizations such as annual flu shots, tetanus immunizations (every 10 years), shingles immunization, and pneumonia immunization. ("Recommended Adult . . . ," 2014)

Medications should be monitored for effectiveness and drug interactions. Encourage your elderly patients to bring a list of all medications, including over-the-counter (OTC) drugs and supplements, with them when visiting the physician. The physician needs to know every medication, herb, or supplement taken, to avoid problems.

Feet often are a problem and may necessitate regular visits to a podiatrist to manage care of aging thickened toenails, bunions, corns, and calluses. Vision should be checked annually to monitor for glaucoma, cataracts, and other eye problems. Dental visits ideally should be twice a year and annually for people who wear dentures. Denture wearers still need to see a dentist because everyone should have an annual oral examination to check for denture fit, mouth soreness, or mouth cancer. Audiology examinations do not need to be done unless there is a hearing problem. The benefits of regular examinations of the body are to prevent, treat, and monitor physical conditions. Yet problems do occur even with careful attention to health-promoting activities. Chronic diseases are a common problem.

 ## CHRONIC DISEASE

As an LPN giving care to older adults, you need to understand the promotion of wellness in the holistic sense. This concept needs to go beyond the vision of physically well, older people living in their own homes independently. Remember that greater than 50% of individuals over the age of 60 are living with two or more chronic diseases (Agency for Healthcare Research and Quality, 2002). People older than 85 years experience increased difficulty with home management activities and are more likely to depend on assistance in their living situations. Regardless of age, living arrangement, or health condition, the goal for health promotion should be to assist older adults in reaching a state of optimal health—the legendary Fountain of Youth.

The most common health problems of older adults are associated with chronic diseases. The most frequent chronic conditions include arthritis, hypertension, heart conditions, hearing impairments, and dementia. Because of these conditions, older people visit physicians more often, are hospitalized more frequently, take more prescription and OTC drugs, and experience more functional problems than younger people. The focus of many medical treatment interventions in the United States is on *curing* acute conditions. Chronic illnesses, which are the predominate illnesses of older adults, cannot be cured, but instead require management with a focus on caring. It is important to understand that chronic diseases do not have a cure; instead, they can and do need to be managed.

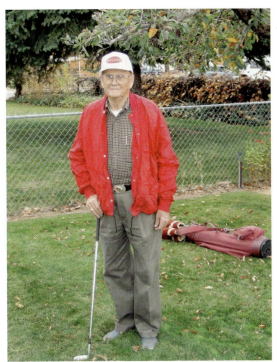

Although coronary artery disease generally is not considered a chronic disease, for this 72-year-old man, it is. He still goes golfing but rides a cart and sometimes elects to skip a difficult hole. This man has adapted to what has become, for him, a chronic disease.

Treatment Strategies

Management of chronic conditions involves treating symptoms and maximizing the strengths of an older person. You need to understand the aging process and older adults in general and advocate and lobby for what they need. For an older adult who has arthritis and who is in severe pain, it is important to treat the symptom of pain. If pain is minimized, the person is better able to stay active and prevent the further disabling effects of immobility. Nurses are the key people to recognize the symptom (pain) and administer the prescribed treatment (medication). As a gerontological nurse, you must go one step further and consider the impact of the disease and its treatment on the older person's ability to perform activities of daily living (ADLs), which include personal care, dressing, and eating. In addition, instrumental activities of daily living (IADLs), which are often more difficult, need to be considered. IADLs are activities such as shopping, doing the laundry, and cleaning the house. So consider:

What could be done to prevent the onset of pain?
What would be the side effects of the pain
  medication?
How has the older person coped with pain in
  the past? Would the same approach be
  effective now?

An LPN must recognize the importance of good health and its correlation with functional independence among older people. Understanding does not always make it clear, however, what kind of activities would promote health and prevent development of further secondary conditions that result in dependency.

Critically Examine the Following:

Reread the last paragraph of the introduction. Your health would improve if you paid more attention to the management of your personal exercise, stress, nutrition, substance use, relationships, and self-care. As a student in a very demanding program, you may need to examine your own health promotion critically. Make comments regarding how you can improve your health in the following areas. Be prepared to discuss them in class and relate how what you do for yourself may also assist an older adult.

1. Exercise
2. Stress management
3. Nutrition
4. Substance use and/or abuse
5. Relationships
6. Self-care

 Point of Interest

To meet the needs of older adults, nurses often seek interventions that come from external sources rather than empowering older people to use their inner sources. Most older people have lived a lifetime of taking care of themselves and their families; they have given service to the community, and many have managed devastating challenges. Be sure to use them as a resource by involving them in the planning stage of the nursing process.

NUTRITION

With advancing age, a person's general health is determined to a great extent by the effects of dietary patterns over the years. Staying physically and mentally active is important to all older adults, but it can be affected by dietary intake. They need to understand the role proper nutrition plays in their lives, even in later years.

As bodies age, four changes occur that affect what a person needs to have optimal nutrition:

1. The body's rate of metabolism slows and no longer needs the same amount of energy and food to do the same amount of work. Older adults often comment that they have not changed how they are eating and exercising, but they are now gaining weight. As people age, lean body mass decreases, and body fat increases. This may result in weight gain and can lead to obesity.
2. The senses of taste and smell may be less keen. Some or all of an elderly person's teeth may need to be replaced by dental appliances. As a result, older people may find themselves eating different foods and drinking less fluid.
3. Social aspects of eating are important. As people age, they retire, their families grow up and move, and their spouses and friends move away or die. This results in changes in the socialization of eating. One of the most difficult adjustments seems to be cooking for one and eating alone.
4. Environmental factors greatly influence nutritional habits of older adults. Lack of transportation to food stores and restaurants, inability to manage reading labels and shopping, and insufficient money to buy healthy food can be major barriers to eating properly.

Poor dietary habits contribute to many diseases that occur in older persons. Chronic diseases, such as heart disease and cancer, can be slowed—and for some people, prevented—by avoiding obesity and decreasing the amount of fat in one's diet. Studies from the American Heart Association (2013) indicate that high cholesterol levels increase the risk for atherosclerosis, which increases the risk of stroke or heart attack. The American Cancer Society found marked increases in the incidence of cancer of the uterus, gallbladder, kidney, stomach, colon, and breast associated with obesity.

It is estimated that osteoporosis, or low bone mass, affects 55% of men and women over the age of 50 in the United States (International Osteoporosis Foundation, n. d.). The loss of bone mass and bone strength as a result of this disease leads to broken hips, arms, and legs and to back injuries. Osteoporosis is often referred to as a "silent" disease. Few signs or symptoms appear until a bone breaks. Adding calcium to the diet, participating in a regular exercise regimen, and avoiding alcohol and smoking are key prevention strategies.

Other chronic problems that are frequent complaints of older people include constipation, urinary incontinence, and arthritis. Nutrition plays a role in each of these conditions. More information on nutrition is provided in Chapter 8.

Although one-on-one teaching may be easier, group learning that incorporates an opportunity for socialization and fun is much more likely to result in positive outcomes. You, as the LPN, may want to organize a group of elderly people in the community to participate in learning nutrition principles. One of the principles that should be taught is ChooseMyPlate, which replaced the food pyramid in 2011 (United States Department of Agriculture, n. d.) (see Chapter 8). This information, which is new to some people, replaces the food pyramid or the basic four concepts that many older people were taught.

Health-promotion activities aimed at altering a lifetime of eating habits must be reasonable, and the benefits need to be made apparent. Nurses should clearly understand what motivates the individual. In addition, nurses must be aware of the unique nutritional needs and problems that accompany later years.

Although there is no information regarding nutrition for Mrs. C., she may benefit from some nutrition guidance. Living alone and no longer having a routine schedule that was in place when she was working could affect her food choices. It was stated that she was 10 pounds overweight, and nutrition could help her reach a healthy weight.

Evidence-Based Practice

Kelley, K., Little, S., Lee, J.S., Birendra, K.C., & Henderson, K. (2014). Articulating meanings of positive adjustment to aging through physical activity participation among older adults. Journal of Park and Recreation Administration, 32(1), 63–79.

This qualitative study examined the meanings associated with physical activity participation by older adults in Senior Games. Physical activity has been encouraged as a way to reduce limitations that can occur as an individual ages, but aging brings age-related changes that can affect physical activity. This study demonstrated the ability and enjoyment obtained in the older adults when provided a wide range of activities. The social aspect of participation and even competition for some was found to be important and may assist in adjustments to age-related changes. The study also exhibited the ability of older adults to participate in physical activity challenges despite level of fitness.

Question

Which of the following inferences can you make? State whether the study summary provides extensive, limited, or no evidence to support each inference.

1. Older adults can enjoy physical activity.
2. Level of competition for older adults should be kept to a minimum.
3. Socialization during physical activity for the older adult will distract and keep them from participating fully.
4. Athletic abilities should not keep the older adult from participating in competitive activities.
5. As a health-care professional, encouraging and assisting older adults to participate in physical activity will help them to adjust to age-related changes.

This woman goes to Curves, a women's exercise club, three times a week to maintain her strength. This type of program has assisted her in losing weight as well as increasing her strength. Besides, she says, it is fun to socialize with the people there.

for older adults. Studies continue to emphasize the benefits of exercise and its importance to total health for all ages. The body's responses to exercise are fundamentally the same throughout life. Exercise stimulates the mind, maintains fitness, prevents or slows progression of some diseases, helps to establish social contacts, and generally improves quality of life.

Fatigue and lack of energy, poor sleeping habits, and poor circulation are common reports of older adults. These problems often result in inactivity. Inactivity leads to muscle wasting and weakening of the bones. This vicious circle results in disabling conditions and functional dependency. If exercise could be packed into a pill, it would be the most widely prescribed and beneficial medicine in the world. Chronic conditions such as heart disease, diabetes, osteoporosis, arthritis, obesity, and depression all have been shown to improve or

 EXERCISE AND FITNESS

In the 1970s, the fitness movement in the United States began. In the late 1970s and early 1980s, society begin to stress the importance of fitness

experience a slowing of progression with regular physical activity.

Physiologically, a regular exercise program can build and maintain muscle strength and endurance and can improve the capacity of the heart, circulatory system, and lungs. The commonly heard phrase "use it or lose it" is the overall theme for exercise and fitness in a person's later years. Exercise programs for people older than 60 should emphasize a regular routine of exercise to expand and increase strength, flexibility, and endurance. Such exercise programs can be developed for individuals with a wide range of conditions, from wheelchair-bound or bed-bound frail elderly people to physically active individuals. If an individual 65 years or older is in generally good health and generally fit, the Centers for Disease Control and Prevention (2014) (CDC) recommends 150 minutes of moderate intensity exercise per week with 2 days of muscle-strengthening activities for maximum health benefits. By-products of a good fitness program include increased energy, buildup of lean body mass, and increased self-esteem.

Regular, scheduled exercise for Mrs. C. would bring some routine back into her life, provide for some socialization outside her home, and assist her in reaching her ideal weight. In addition, the increased activity may help to decrease her complaints of fatigue and low energy while improving her sleep.

Strengthening

Strengthening exercises help build and maintain muscle condition by moving muscles against resistance. Simple strengthening exercises are needed to promote activity without tiring a person too easily. Muscle strength is also crucial to the support of joints and can help prevent problems related to arthritis. Improving muscle strength is a primary objective in slowing the progression of osteoporosis. Patients confined to bed lose muscle mass very

HEALTHY PEOPLE 2020

Goal

Increase the proportion of older adults with reduced physical or cognitive function who engage in light, moderate, or vigorous leisure-time physical activities.

(Healthy People 2020 [HP2020], 2013)

 Point of Interest

If an older person is able to meet life demands, it is unnecessary for the nurse to intervene. The only intervention necessary in this situation is to support the individual in what he or she is able to do.

quickly. It can be restored, however, when exercise is resumed. Something as simple as doing range-of-motion exercises while holding a soup can makes a difference in strength for most older adults.

As a nurse, you must be aware of the impact a short-term illness can have on an older person. Something as commonplace as the flu can cause significant weakness and inactivity. Weak muscles lead to falls, which can result in hip fractures and other injuries. If older adults are unaware of the importance of strengthening exercises, no incentive can return them to the normal level of function.

Strength-building exercises are also important for a person with diabetes because the exercises help regulate glucose metabolism by increasing muscle mass. The greater the muscle mass, the greater the glycogen level in the muscles, and the more energy will be available in reserve for periods of exertion.

Flexibility

Flexibility exercises involve slow stretching motions. Medical and fitness experts agree that stretching is the most important part of an exercise program designed to prevent injuries, reduce muscle tension, and maintain range of motion. As a result of the normal aging process, muscles tend to lose elasticity, and tissues around the joints thicken. Flexibility exercises can delay or reverse this process by preventing muscles from becoming short and tight.

All stretching motions should be done gradually and slowly, without any sudden force or jerking motion. You should encourage a variety of stretching exercises for different parts of the body, including arms, shoulders, back, chest, stomach, buttocks, thighs, and calves. All exercise routines should include warm-up and cool down with 5 to 15 minutes of stretching exercises. As the older person's range of motion increases, the individual will be able to reach, turn, and move in all directions with more grace and less pain.

Endurance

Endurance-building or aerobic exercises improve the function of the heart, lungs, and blood vessels. A frequent report from older people is "feeling tired." Endurance-building exercises help strengthen the heart to pump blood and the lungs to exchange oxygen and increase the elasticity of blood vessels. These functions are a vital part of fitness and feeling good. Walking, cycling, and swimming or water aerobics are excellent all-around exercises.

As stated earlier, the basic components of an exercise routine for older people include strengthening, flexibility, and endurance. In addition, attention must be given to breathing during exercising. Breathing is a vital part of an exercise program. As a person concentrates on the exercise, it is easy to forget to breathe. The correct breathing technique is to breathe out during vigorous effort or exertion and breathe in as the muscles relax.

A last comment on exercise is a caution for older adults who have not been exercising on a regular basis, who are frail, or who have cardiovascular problems. Anyone with heart problems or high blood pressure, who is overweight, or who has been told to be cautious in personal activity level should have an exercise program prescribed by a physician. It is important to have a check-up prior to beginning an exercise program and to maintain contact with the health-care provider.

Physical fitness is one component of life that enables people to live it to its fullest. As a nurse, you have a responsibility to understand and teach the importance of exercise and fitness to elderly patients. Remember to think holistically. What environment is best for the older person, who is there to be a support person, what is the incentive to make change? If you know these things and assist in making a plan that uses them, the program will be more successful.

Mrs. C. could possibly benefit from the inclusion of exercise, but she has told you she does not participate in regular exercise. Helping her to understand and believe in the benefits of may be first step to help gain incentive to include exercise as part of her routine.

Stress

Stress motivates people to act, forces them to think under pressure, and challenges them to be creative

---

Significance of strengthening exercises

Effects of Exercise	Exercise Plan Considerations
Builds and maintains muscle strength	Should be designed for the individual
Decreases arthritic pain over time	Should not be too tiring
Strengthens joints	Should promote activity
Slows process of osteoporosis	
The greater the muscle mass, the greater glycogen reserves, which means more energy	
Weak muscles lead to falls and possible fractures	

and resourceful human beings. The key is to be able to strike a balance between too much stress and not enough, between positive stress (*eustress*) and stress that is harmful (*distress*). As with all areas of health promotion, it is never too late to improve a technique. Failure to take a healthy approach to dealing with stress can greatly increase the risk of developing or worsening heart disease, cancer, and other chronic diseases (Sapolsky, 2004).

For most older people, stress is related to three basic areas: environment, body, and mind. Environmental stressors are weather, crime, crowds, time pressures, and the demands of others. The human body can experience stress because of illness, accidents, drugs, lack of sleep, and normal changes related to aging. The mind can create stress for people because of negative attitudes and perceptions, boredom, despair, and hopelessness.

Regularly occurring events such as trips to the grocery store, pain from arthritis, and fear of the unknown conditions of retirement all may create stress for older people. Stress-related problems and symptoms include ulcers (stomach pain), high blood pressure (no symptoms), arthritis (joint pain and muscle tension), heart disease (chest pain and difficulty breathing), cancer (increased susceptibility), headaches (constant worry), circulatory problems (cold hands and feet), and backaches (muscle spasm and chronic pain) (Sapolsky, 2004).

One of the most important strategies for health promotion is to help older people recognize their personal reactions to stress and their bodies' physiological responses. Tools used to recognize stress include a stress log or journal of daily stressful situations, life change inventory, and stress control inventory.

After an individual has recognized personal stress and his or her response to it, several interventions are available to help relieve it. As a nurse, you should understand and be able to recommend appropriate stress-reducing activities. These activities may be divided into the two categories: quick relaxers and long-term stress management skills.

A quick relaxer is something a person can do in 2 or 3 minutes to relax and counteract symptoms of distress. One of the most important, yet difficult, skills for some older people is learning simply to relax. Learning how to relax helps older people sleep better, control blood pressure, lower cholesterol, reduce headaches, relieve depression, reduce or eliminate use of drugs and alcohol, and smile

more. Examples of quick relaxers include roll breathing, progressive muscle relaxation, imagining a pleasant place or situation, eye relaxation, and exercise. The importance of exercise was discussed earlier in this chapter; however, it is worth emphasizing that exercise is the most natural way to relax. For the greatest calming effect, an elderly individual can combine fitness activities with breathing and other mental relaxation techniques.

For some older people, dealing with stress requires more than a few "stress-buster" quickie techniques. If stress causes continuous physical and mental discomfort that results in illness, learning how to deal with the source of stress needs to be a major goal. This assumes that the individual understands what is causing the stress.

Using the four stress management options listed here as a teaching tool is very helpful for many people. The four basic options are:

1. Attempt symptom relief (quick techniques).
2. Accept the stressor (change perception or attitude). *Example:* Your children frequently call you at the last minute to baby-sit your grandchildren. You may accept the stress and decide you really do not need much time to prepare, so say yes and enjoy! Another choice is to lovingly say no!
3. Alter the stressor (change or alter the source of stress so it is no longer there). *Example:* Make the decision that you will not be able to baby-sit unless they let you know 1 day ahead of time.
4. Avoid the stressor (remove yourself from the stressor). *Example:* Decide you will not be a babysitter for your grandchildren. After the source of stress has been pinpointed, the older person often can decide whether to accept, alter, or avoid it.

Stress management techniques may be unfamiliar to many older individuals, even though stress and recognition of stress have been in the spotlight for some time. Teaching older people stress management can be done very successfully through either group or individual activities.

Think of some symptoms recorded for Mrs. C. Could it be possible she is experiencing stress in her life from the loss of her husband and retirement? Stress management techniques may be another avenue to explore to assist her in being able to sleep at night.

🔲 LIFESTYLES

Maintaining a healthy lifestyle at any age involves more than getting fit, eating right, and coping with stress. Other challenging issues that people of all ages encounter are relationships, possible alcohol and drug abuse, and lack of self-care.

Relationships

Human life is constantly defined and redefined by our ties to others. The term *relationship* means any significant bonding in which a person feels a strong sense of responsibility toward the physical and emotional welfare of others.

As people grow older, the reality is that all relationships eventually end. Whether through divorce from a spouse or death of a spouse, child, family member, friend, or pet, the loss redefines one's life. An individual's ability to deal with the process of grief over the losses can result in significant personal and health changes and

This 65-year-old man goes fishing with his youngest grandson two or three times a week. Fishing always has been part of this man's lifestyle, but now he has the added close relationship with his grandson.

changes in dealing with others. How strongly these changes affect the rest of one's life depends on how well the individual, and those involved the personal life of the individual, cope with the loss. How people have coped with change and crisis in younger years predicts how they will deal with these same stressors later.

As years pass, life changes can become increasingly complex. Older adults must deal with changes caused by retirement, which can have major impacts on home life, health, finances, and role changes. In addition, the loss of relationships may be frequent and numerous. Mrs. C. has faced multiple losses in the last 2 years. Talking with her about these losses and discovering her previous coping skills may help her at this time.

As a nurse, you have an opportunity to help older adults gain insight into loss and life change. Chapter 11 contains a section on the stages of grief that may be helpful to you in understanding reactions of older adults to loss. You need to assess the effect that loss has on a person's ability to function with day-to-day activities. As an LPN, you must ask questions and allow the older person to share concerns. Health-promotion activities that focus on mental wellness can provide an excellent opportunity for older adults to express the concerns they face. The American Association of Retired Persons (AARP) offers resources to help lead discussions about the myths, fears, and reality of change as one grows older.

Alcohol, Drugs, and Aging

Abuse of alcohol and drugs among older men and women may be a more serious problem than most people realize. Until the 1990s, research on drinking and the health effects focused more on the younger generation (Holahan et al., 2014). Since that time more studies have focused on the effects in those 55 years of age and older. The inattention to this information occurred for the following reasons:

- The elderly population in the United States was small, and few older individuals were identified as alcoholics.
- Chronic problem drinkers (individuals who had abused alcohol off and on for most of their lives) often died before old age.
- Older people frequently have been able to hide drinking problems because they often are retired or have few social contacts.

Some families may unknowingly accept or encourage drinking in older family members. They may have the attitude that drinking should be tolerated because older people have only a limited time left to live and should be allowed to enjoy themselves. Sometimes the alcohol consumption seems to be an insignificant amount to the family, and they blame the resulting impairment on aging. (National Institute on Aging, 2012)

The amount, time, and place of alcohol consumption have little significance. The critical issue that needs to be addressed is what alcohol does to an individual's quality of life and functional ability. The substance use of a sleeping pill and wine before bedtime for Mrs. C. would warrant further investigation regarding her quality of life and functional ability. Despite studies indicating that older people consume fewer alcoholic beverages and have less alcohol-related problems than younger age groups, it can lead to a greater risk for health problems. It is important to screen for alcohol use because excessive drinking late in life, often in response to situational factors such as retirement, reduced income, declining health, or the deaths of friends and loved ones, may be a pattern of managing the stress. In these cases, alcohol is first used for temporary relief but later becomes a problem. (National Institute on Alcohol Abuse, 2005)

The physical effects of alcohol are significant for older people. Alcohol impairs mental alertness, judgment, physical coordination, and reaction time. These problems mimic and exacerbate the deleterious effects of other chronic conditions (dementia, depression, and arthritis) and increase the risks of falls and other accidents.

As people age, they seem to become less tolerant of even small amounts of alcohol, and the effect of alcohol on the body may be unusual. For example, the effects of alcohol on the cardiovascular system may mask the pain of an oncoming heart attack. Older people are the greatest consumers of prescription and OTC drugs. The combined use of alcohol and drugs increases the likelihood of a toxic or lethal effect.

Treatment efforts for older alcoholics have not been fruitful. It is easy to overlook or accept problem drinking because the drinking seems to offer enjoyment or comfort. It is much harder to create social alternatives to the life events that lie behind the increased use of alcohol or alcoholism.

As a health professional, you may be tempted to rush over or omit assessment questions referring to alcohol intake. Because nurses often play a key role in recognizing alcohol and drug problems, you cannot afford to avoid such questions. You always should ask what the impact of this problem may be on the older person's ability to function. It

---

QSEN

COMPETENCIES: Teamwork and Collaboration; Safety (Knowledge, Skills, Attitudes)

Respect Attributes of the Team

Mrs. Scott, an 82-year-old widow of 1 year, has been on the unit for management of her diabetes. She has been taking an oral hypoglycemic, but since the death of her husband 1 year ago she has been unable to regulate her blood sugar. She has spent the last few days as your patient and has been learning how to balance insulin, diet, and physical activity. She is preparing for discharge but is concerned about her care when she returns home.

During her time on the unit, she has had visits from a daughter and a son, and she tells you that she has another son that lives in another state who contacts her by phone at least once a week. Her chart indicates that a social worker has been in to visit with her, and she has agreed to have an assessment by a physical therapist before going home.

You have been assigned to prepare her for discharge.

1. Before discharge, it is advised that you have a meeting with those who will possibly be involved in her care at home. Recommend those individuals who should be in attendance at this meeting, and describe why they should be included.
2. Will it be important to include Mrs. Scott in any of the planning meetings? Why or why not?
3. Mrs. Scott lives alone and has had little physical activity during the past year. How would you encourage her to become more active?
4. What recommendations would you have for her safety in her home and her activities?
5. Would you give her any other education regarding activity, diet, and insulin?

becomes easy to see that the physical, mental, and social impact of drinking could contribute to alcohol dependency.

The primary health-promotion goal is helping older adults and their families recognize when alcohol is a problem. Second, straightforward information must be given to elderly adults regarding the effects of alcohol, especially in combination with drugs. The nurse needs to understand the older person's reason for drinking. Health-promotion activities that create alternatives should be made available to an older person with an alcohol problem.

Because of their critical importance, drug issues are discussed extensively in Chapter 21; however, emphasis on the problem of drug dependency and abuse is important. Drug abuse depends on the relationship of the individual to the drug in question. Harmful drug relationships are frequently termed *overmedication, dependency, abuse, problem usage,* and *habituation.* Regardless of the reason, if an older person misuses a drug or becomes dependent on it, the effects are similar to those of problem drinking. Physical and mental impairments resulting from prescribed or OTC drugs mimic disease states and increase the risk of falls, accidents, and dependency.

One role of health promotion is to offer education and screening regarding drug use. Promoting self-responsibility is the key component. Nurses must assess the impact of drug treatment on an older person's ability to complete ADLs. If a patient cannot afford a prescribed drug, he or she probably will not take the medication as ordered. If the older adult does not understand what outcomes are expected from the drug treatment, misuse of a drug may ensue by taking it for too long or taking too much of it.

SELF-CARE—TAKING CHARGE

Older adults are best qualified to keep themselves healthy and to know when they are ill. As a nurse, you need to respect and explore what the older person reports as the problem. Do not take charge and deny an older adult responsibility for personal health and health management.

Self-care, self-help, and *self-maintenance* are terms often used interchangeably to describe various aspects of an individual's efforts to maintain optimal health and functionality. When an individual cannot assume responsibility for self, the patient has the nursing diagnosis, Self-Care Deficit. Most individuals with this diagnosis need medical or nursing intervention.

From a nursing perspective, the focus is frequently on ADLs, which are the most basic self-care activities engaged in by older adults. It is common to see dependence in at least some basic ADLs for older people. Surveys show that people older than 65 years who live in the community are dependent in at least one ADL. In nursing homes, the prevalence is higher. In addition to ADLs, an older person needs to manage IADLs, such as food preparation, managing medications, and managing personal finances.

Regardless of whether an older adult is attempting to overcome a functional deficit in ADLs or IADLs, the same self-care skills are needed. Self-care involves the following:

1. Accepting personal responsibility for one's own health
2. Adopting healthy lifestyle habits with regard to fitness, relaxation, and nutrition
3. Learning how to make the changes you choose to accomplish the things you want to do

Can you understand how these three characteristics complement the concept of gerotranscendence? If you can't, discuss this with someone who is familiar with gerotranscendence, such as a classmate, and work to identify the relationships.

Accepting personal responsibility for health behaviors applies to the "why" of the decision more than the "what." *Self-responsibility* means that the older adult does not rely solely on spouse, children, physician, or nurse to determine "what to do to be healthy." The person must be allowed to think through the options and make each decision. This does not mean that a person should not seek the assistance of others, but rather that a need exists to work in partnership with the physician, nurse, or family (separately or together) to make the best decision.

The self-care concept emphasizes the need for encouraging individuals to take a more active role in maintaining or improving their health. Often, the patient does not understand this process, and it is not easy for older people to accomplish. Health-promotion strategies related to self-care must include helping the older adult understand how to be in charge of personal health decisions. Your efforts

---

Think Like a Nurse

You are taking care of 75-year-old woman who was recently discharged from a rehabilitation facility after a total knee replacement. She is unwilling to get up and walk, and she states that it hurts too much. How will you handle this situation? How will you apply your new knowledge of self-care?

---

should be focused on enabling an older person to be a wise medical consumer and to know how and when to work and communicate as a partner with the health-care team.

Your role as a health professional is twofold. First, you must offer activities to develop self-care skills, such as one-on-one or group activities that teach how to be an informed medical consumer, and you must provide information on prevention and screening guidelines, such as for a mammogram or a prostate examination. Second, you must ensure that the environment enables the older adult to use the skills to make choices and assume self-responsibility. If an older adult wants to be a partner with the health-care provider in a health decision, the provider should take the time to answer questions and ultimately let the treatment decision be made by the older adult. This same situation applies to nursing. If the older adult is expected to be involved in a self-care activity program, you, as a nurse, must be prepared to explain the benefits, procedures, and risks and be willing to let the older adult make the decision.

 ## CONCLUSION

Until more recently, the needs of older adults often have been ignored in the health-promotion movement. Health professionals mistakenly assumed that elderly people had no interest in health-promotion programs. As the United States has become more and more a home to an aging society, these views have changed.

As a nurse, you must understand the importance of promoting holistic wellness to all older adults, regardless of the presence or absence of disease. Attainment of a disease-free existence is not a xrealistic goal. Health-promotion efforts should be directed toward maintaining functional independence for older people.

Older Americans need information about how to lead healthy lifestyles. When information and opportunities are provided, older people often are willing to make the changes necessary to improve their health. Exercising regularly, maintaining a nutritious diet, managing stress effectively, taking medications safely, avoiding overuse of alcohol, and recognizing self-care as a choice are all behaviors that improve health and the quality of life. Pursuit of high-level wellness in later years is the responsibility of the individual and society.

CASE STUDY SOLUTION

1. Additional information in each category might include:

Nutrition

What are her daily eating habits? What type and amount of food and fluids does she consume? Does she eat alone?

Exercise

What is her normal daily activity level? How does this differ from her daily activity level before retirement?

Stress

What is her perception of coping with changes such as death and retirement? Has she stated any other physical
complaints, such as fatigue, headaches?

Relationships

What family or friends are important to her? In what social activities is she involved? Does she have any hobbies?

Substance Use or Abuse

When did she begin drinking wine every evening? When did her sleeping problems begin? Has she always taken sleeping pills?

Self-Care

Does she have a primary care provider? Does she understand the importance of exercise and disease prevention? Does she know the danger of combining drugs and alcohol?

2. Asking Mrs. C., "What is your biggest worry or concern in your life at this time?" would be a beginning. Although the nurse may see many areas of concern, Mrs. C.'s own concerns are more critical.

3. If the nurse begins by focusing on what Mrs. C. considers most important, it is easier for Mrs. C. to understand her own motivation.

4. Some potential conditions include:

Excess weight, which may lead or contribute to high blood pressure and physical limitation

Lack of exercise, which may contribute to weight gain but may also worsen arthritis and its effects on mobility

Emotional stress, which may lead to depression

Relationship concerns, which also may contribute to depression, isolation, and abuse of drugs and alcohol

Combination of alcohol and OTC sleeping pills, which may lead to further sleeping problems, alcohol and drug misuse, depression, injury, and further isolation

5. If Mrs. C. has not seen a health-care provider for 10 years, she needs at least a baseline physical assessment. She has some significant conditions that need to be addressed, such as borderline high blood pressure, sleep problems, and weight gain. In addition, she should have a basic screening related to disease prevention.

REVIEW QUESTIONS

1. Incentives for older persons to participate in health-promotion behaviors include:
   1. The belief that they will find the Fountain of Youth
   2. The belief that activities will help them die well
   3. The belief that activities will help keep them independent
   4. The belief that it will please their physician

2. Health-promotion programs appropriate for older people should focus on:
   1. Maintaining functional abilities
   2. Advancing youthfulness
   3. Enhancing chronic illnesses
   4. Developing dependence on others for care

3. Basic components of an exercise routine for older people are:
   1. Strengthening, endurance, and flexibility
   2. Strengthening, dieting, and power walking
   3. Strengthening, dieting, and aerobics
   4. Strengthening, aerobics, and ChooseMyPlate

4. Age-related changes that affect nutrition include:
   1. Increase in the ability to taste a wide variety of foods
   2. Increase in body fat
   3. Increase in lean body mass
   4. Increased metabolic rate because of aging thyroid

5. It is important to include an assessment of alcohol use in the older adult because alcohol in the elderly:
   1. Decreases the effectiveness of many OTCs and medications
   2. Masks symptoms of other serious health conditions
   3. Increases socialization opportunities but decreases family interactions
   4. Increases dietary intake, leading to weight gain

REFERENCES

Agency for Healthcare Research and Quality (2002). Research in action: Preventing disability in the elderly with chronic disease. *Research in Action,* 3, 1-7. U.S. Rockville, MD: Agency for Healthcare Research and Quality. AHQR Pub. No. 02-0018. archiv.ahrq.gov/research/findings/factsheets/aging/elderdis/elderdis.pdf

American Heart Association (2013). About cholesterol. www.heart.org/HEARTORG/Conditions/Cholesterol/AboutCholesterol/About-Cholesterol_UCM_001220_Article.jsp

Centers for Disease Control and Prevention (2014). How much physical activity do older adults need? www.cdc.gov/physicalactivity/everyone/guidelines/olderadults.html

Eliopolous, C. (2014). *Gerontological nursing* (8th ed.). Philadelphia, PA: J.B. Lippincott. National Vital Statistics Report (2012)

Holahan, C.J., Schutte, K.K., Brennan, P.L., Holahan, C.K., & Moos, R.H. (2014). Episodic heavy drinking and 20-year total mortality among late-life moderate drinkers. *Alcoholism: Clinical and Experimental Research,* 38, 1432-1438.

International Osteoporosis Foundation (n. d.). Facts and statistics. www.iofbonehealth.org/facts-statistics#category-23

Marcus, B.H., Williams, D.M., Dubbert, P.M., Sallis, J.F., King, A.C., Yancey, A.K., & Claytor, R.P. (2006). AHA Scientific statements: Physical activity intervention studies. *Circulation,* 114, 2739-2752.

National Institute on Aging (2012). Age page: Alcohol use in older people. https://www.nia.nih.gov/health/publication/alcohol-use-older-people

National Institute on Alcohol Abuse and Alcoholism (2005). Module I: Epidemiology of alcohol problems in the United States. pubs.niaaa.nih.gov/publications/Social/Module1Epidemiology/Module1.html

Recommended Adult Immunization Schedule-United States (2014). www.cdc.gov/vaccines/schedules/downloads/past/adult-2014

Sapolsky, R.M. (2004). *Why zebras don't get ulcers* (3rd ed.). New York, NY: Henry Holt and Company.

Stanton, M.W., & Rutherford, M.K. (2005) The high concentration of U.S. health care expenditures. *Research in Action* 19. Rockville, MD: Agency for

Healthcare Research and Quality. AHRQ Pub. No. 06-0060. http://www.ahrq.gov/research/findings/factsheets/costs/expriach/index.html

United States Department of Agriculture (n. d.). ChooseMyPlate. www.choosemyplate.gov/

Werner, C.A. (2011). The older population: 2010. 2010 Census briefs. Issued November 2011, pages 1-19. https://www.census.gov/prod/cen2010/briefs/c2010br-09.pdf

WEB RESOURCES

Centers for Disease Control and Prevention. Adult vaccination. www.cdc.gov/vaccines/adults/

Centers for Disease Control and Prevention. Healthy aging. www.cdc.gov/aging

Centers for Disease Control and Prevention. Physical activity for older adults. www.cdc.gov/physicalactivity/basics/olderadults/

United States Department of Agriculture. MyPlate www.choosemyplate.gov/

Safety

KATHLEEN PACO CADMAN

LEARNING OUTCOMES

1. Identify potential fall risks based on diagnosis, medication, and environment.

2. Give examples of measures that can be taken to promote optimal skin integrity.

3. Compare and contrast the manifestations of hyperthermia and hypothermia in the older adult.

4. Apply knowledge of behavioral patterns to help identify potential mental health concerns.

5. Analyze whether concerns for LGBT persons are being addressed with resources in their area.

6. Compare and contrast possible indications of the various forms of elder abuse.

7. Predict what emergency situations may arise in the older adult's community, and evaluate what resources are available for each situation.

8. Assess what safety issues are present for older adults in the home environment.

CONCEPTS

Safety

Advocacy

Violence

CASE STUDY

As a nurse, you are heading out to meet Mr. Paco, a retired accountant who has recently been discharged from the hospital to home health care and who is in need of extra assistance during recuperation. He is a 72-year-old Guatemalan gentleman, 5 feet 9 inches tall and weighing 147 lb, and he recently had a ground-level fall. In addition to various minor injuries, he also sustained a broken femur, which was surgically reset. After his wife of 42 years passed away 3 years ago, he has lived alone, sharing his spacious two-story home with his dog, Cloe. Until this accident, Mr. Paco was functioning independently with occasional assistance from friends, neighbors, and his grandchildren. Aside from hypertension and occasional lower back pain, both of which are managed with medication, he states that he is in good health. Following his surgery, the physician prescribed analgesics, muscle relaxants, and anticoagulants and insists that he use crutches around his home and a wheelchair when out of the house. As you are talking to Mr. Paco about taking his medications, he mentions that when he falls asleep while watching television in the evenings and forgets to take his pills, he adds them to the pills he takes the next morning. While doing a skin check on Mr. Paco, you notice that he has quite a few new skin tears on his arms and legs. When you ask him about them, he says that getting around with the cast on sometimes makes him bump into things.

Discussion

1. How would you explain to Mr. Paco that taking his medications in this manner places him at an increased risk for falls?

2. What items could be causing the tears in Mr. Paco's skin, and how can you best modify them?

3. Because Mr. Paco lives alone, what measures can you take to help prevent an emergency in his home? How can you help prepare for a disaster? What steps can be taken to ensure that he is as safe as possible in case of a health emergency?

 ## INTRODUCTION

Although safety is a key component in patient care for all ages, there are specific concerns that disproportionately affect the older adult population based on physiological as well as psychosocial needs. This chapter addresses key concepts for safety considerations.

 ## FALL RISKS

Each year, approximately one-third of older adults will have a fall. Of these, nearly 20,000 falls will have fatal outcomes, and more than 2.3 million elders will be taken to the emergency department for nonfatal injuries, with more than a half million injuries resulting in hospital admissions (Centers for Disease Control and Prevention [CDC], 2013b).

Even if the outcome is nonfatal, falls can result in fractures, breaks, lacerations, sprains, organ damage, traumatic brain injuries (CDC, 2013b), or other conditions causing severe disability. Once an older adult is disabled, even temporarily, he or she runs a greater risk for further impairment of overall health outcomes (HP2020, 2013). Although falls are the most prevalent cause of death resulting from unintentional injury among older adults, much can be done to prevent them.

HEALTHY PEOPLE 2020

Goal

Reduce the number of fall-related emergency department visits among older adults by 10%.

(Healthy People 2020 [HP2020], 2013)

Contributing Factors

Changes in physiology as the body ages place older adults at higher risks for falls and for injuries, both fatal and nonfatal, that result from falls. The primary contributory changes are related to the following (National Institutes of Health [NIH], 2013):

- **Musculoskeletal:** As muscles and bones progressively weaken, the ability to maintain a steady gait decreases. Body weight extremes affect this factor. Muscular atrophy and osteoporosis are more common in thin patients and places these patients at an increased risk for breaks. Obese patients, who may have stronger bones from weight-bearing activities, are at a great risk of sustaining injury from the impact of their own weight on their frame. High levels of discomfort during mobility may further decrease range of motion for mobility, which also increases the likelihood of falls.
- **Neurological:** Neuropathy and other neural changes can lead to poor balance and a shift in proprioception. This is particularly prevalent in persons with diabetes or those who have sustained spinal injuries. Inversely, arthritis or chronic back pain may result in increased painful sensations during ambulation. Both varieties of neurological changes can increase the risk of falls if they result in an abnormal or stuttered gait and impaired reflexes.
- **Sensory loss:** Often vision (macular degeneration, glaucoma, cataracts), hearing, and neurological function decrease as a person ages. This loss may be dangerous to the patient if he or she cannot see obstacles, listen to surroundings, or feel items that may be in the way. Vision and tactile losses are potentially progressive and particularly profound in patients with unmanaged or poorly managed diabetes.
- **Cardiovascular:** Orthostatic hypotension, which can be associated with dehydration (hypovolemia) or various cardiovascular abnormalities such as dysrhythmias, results in dizziness on standing. Initiation or changes made to administration of cardiovascular medications, such as those for hypertension, may increase the likelihood of orthostatic hypertension.
- **Genitourinary and digestive:** Urinary and bowel urgency or frequency for continent older adults promotes increased need for frequent trips to the restroom and thus increases the opportunity for injury. When these urges are present at night, and the patient may be maneuvering to the restroom when thinking can be hazy and the environment is darker, the risk for falls is greater.
- **Cognition:** Slowed reaction times, as well as confusion and short-term memory loss involving one's ability to self-ambulate, not only increase the number of falls sustained, but often also decrease reflexes, thereby increasing the magnitude of an injury.
- **Nutrition and hydration:** Fluctuations in blood sugar, as well as dehydration, can cause feelings of dizziness, which increases the risk for falls.

Fall Prevention Measures

Although it is not possible for the licensed practical nurse (LPN) to eliminate all risk for falls, various measures can be taken to help decrease the likeliness of a fall.

- **Wardrobe**: Ensure that clothing selected for the patient (by the LPN, patient, family, or certified nursing assistant [CNA]) fits properly.

Footwear that fits properly, does not slide or rub, and has good grip or traction is important. Millie, at 99 years old, proudly shows off her favorite shoes. She says that they help her feel safe when she walks, and they have enough grip to let her propel herself in her wheelchair.

Special attention must be directed to the length of pants, robes, or skirts worn by the patient, to ensure that the patient will neither trip over them nor get them caught between assistive devices, such as canes and walkers, and the floor. Properly fitting footwear is also crucial; footwear should have thin rubber soles and a method for comfortably yet securely fastening the shoe to the foot so it cannot inadvertently slide out of place. Also, if the patient needs glasses or hearing aids, the LPN must ensure, directly or through delegation, that these are in place and functional as part of the patient's overall wardrobe.

- **Medication:** Administration of all medications must be done according to the physician's orders. The LPN must monitor the potential effects of the medication on ambulation and report any risky manifestations to the charge nurse, or supervisor, so that the primary care provider may assess whether the administration times need to be adjusted. Medications that cause drowsiness or dizziness, such as sedatives, blood pressure medications, and narcotics, are often best given at night, as the patient is going to bed and will not be ambulating as much. Conversely, diuretics and laxatives, which both increase frequency for toileting, are best given during the day, to decrease injuries that may be sustained by rising too quickly from a lying position or moving through a dark room.
- **Nutrition and hydration:** Encouraging ample nutritional intake on a regular basis can help regulate blood sugar levels, to decrease the chances of dizziness. This is particularly important for diabetic patients. Also, encouraging adequate amount of fluid intake can help prevent dehydration.
- **Transitional posturing:** Whether caused by dehydration (hypovolemia), medication, or various medical conditions, orthostatic hypotension is common among older adults. The LPN must transition unsteady patients slowly from lying to sitting upright, then pivot them until their feet are on the ground, and then assist them with standing, by allowing ample time between each step, to decrease the effects of orthostatic hypotension.
- **Durable medical equipment (DME):** Although physical therapists generally assess the need for and order DME for patients, it is within the nurse's responsibility to monitor whether there are new or changed needs for DME, based on a change in condition. If so, the LPN should pass this information on to the supervisor for referral. Although DME such as single-point canes, four-post canes, two-wheel walkers, and four-wheel walkers can help decrease the chance of a fall, improper selection of the DME may inversely increase the chance of a fall. As posturing changes, a patient's DME may need to be reevaluated for proper size as well. Positioning and quality of grips for both comfort and form are also important to note.
- **Physical therapy:** If the floor or home health LPN notices decreases in mobility or increases in contractures, he or she should report this to the supervisor for possible referral to physical therapy. Interventions to prevent falls may include strength training to build muscle, increased walks to build endurance, and range-of-motion exercises to encourage flexibility. Range-of-motion exercise options include active low-impact exercises such as tai chi or yoga, as well as passive range of motion done by the LPN and other direct care staff.
- **Environmental issues:** Alterations can be made to the environment in which the older adult lives, whether he or she is in a home or an institutional setting.
  - **Primary living area:** Ensure that the living area for the patient is free of unnecessary obstacles or hazards. Check for adequate lighting, including night lights, to increase visibility. Also, assessing and adjusting tubing (oxygen, nasogastric [NG] tube, and intravenous [IV] lines) and DME location, when possible, decrease the chance of a patient's becoming entangled or tripping while ambulating.

Home health nurses should check the patient's house to be sure that walking areas are free of loose rugs, cords, planters, boxes, newspapers, toys (from pets or grandchildren), and other debris that could cause the patient to trip or lose balance while walking. It is also best practice to ensure that the patient has a telephone and lamp that are user friendly next to his or her bed and primary chair. This decreases risks associated with ambulating to the bed in low-light conditions or getting up in the dark to receive or place a call.

Having commonly used items within easy reach helps reduce the chance for falls that may occur in frequent ambulation and bending to find items. Glen's safety is improved by having a table with good light and his glasses, handkerchief, television remote, and telephone next to his favorite seating area.

- **Restroom:** Because many falls occur going to, from, or in the restroom, this area needs particular focus for safety. When applicable, rails should be in place next to the toilet and showering area. Furthermore, ensure that if the patient requires an elevated toilet seat, or a shower stool, this equipment is in place. Nonslip surfaces on the shower floor and a well-anchored shower door or curtain (not on a tension rod) are also imperative in promoting safety. Bath mats must be adhered to the floor to reduce the chance of falls while stepping into or out of the bathing area, and a towel should be easily within reach.
- **Other home setting recommendations:** Walkways to and from the home should be free of leaves, snow, or ice. Lighting outside the home, such as motion sensor or timed lights, can help increase safety not only by reducing falls when going in and out of the home, but also by increasing security from potential invaders. Furthermore, hand rails and skid reduction surfaces should be in place anywhere steps are present, both indoors and outdoors.

Increased safety precautions to prevent falls not only reduce the chance of injury, but also may help improve both the duration and quality of life for older adults. Fall injuries frequently result in broken bones and sometimes a near-paralyzing fear of falling. These factors often contribute to a more sedentary lifestyle, which may lead to further muscle atrophy, progression of osteoporosis, and pneumonia. This combination of outcomes decreases the chance for recovery and often proves fatal for older adults (Currie, 2008).

HEALTHY PEOPLE 2020
Falls

In addition to the initial injury, falls for elderly patient may result in:
- Fear of falling
- Sedentary behavior
- Impaired function
- Lower quality of life

(Healthy People 2020, 2013)

 SKIN INTEGRITY

The aging process causes skin to lose much of its elasticity, thus making it more fragile and prone to abrasions and lacerations. Although this is a natural physiological phenomenon, there are measures the LPN can take, both directly and through supervision of the CNAs, to help increase safety by reducing the frequency and magnitude of skin-related injuries. To ensure that breaches in the integumentary system are addressed quickly, the LPN must perform skin checks to assess for abrasions, lacerations, or breakdown, and communicate regularly with CNAs regarding the importance of reporting findings from skin checks performed during bathing.

Injury Prevention

Providing activities of daily living (ADLs) movement of the patient should be done gently, so as not to tear or shear the skin as a result of friction. Patients with particularly frail skin should be dressed in comfortably loose, lightweight, soft fabrics that are generally full length, to increase protection of skin. Clothing should have no sharp areas such as rough edges to elastic bands and broken zippers, buttons, or bra hooks that could damage the skin. The LPN should ensure that anyone in close contact with the patient also does not have any sharp edges, such as long fingernails, jewelry, and lanyards, which could injure patients with impaired skin integrity. As the LPN removes adhesive surfaces, such as tape for bandages or lines, he or she must be cautious to remove the surface gently, by pulling skin taught and cautiously lifting the adhesive little by little. Otherwise, tape and other adhesive surfaces can tear the skin. A further safety measure to prevent skin tears is assessing for and addressing object edges that are in the patient's environment. This includes looking for particularly rough surfaces, such as a ragged edge to a wooden table, as well as sharp corners or edges. Particularly in the home situation, the LPN must look for heavily worn or broken items that may be hazardous, such as a broken spring protruding through a bed or chair. Breaches in skin integrity may occur from hot water burns or scalding.

There is increased risk for the older adult if hot and cold water faucets are not clearly labeled or if the water heater is set too high. Scalding from hot water is particularly prevalent in this age demographic, as a result of thinner skin, and it causes approximately 1,500 hospitalizations each year. Evidence indicates a decrease in burn risk if water heaters are set to less than 120°F (Johns Hopkins, 2013).

Breakdown Prevention

As skin becomes more fragile, patients are also at increased risk for skin breakdown, including pressure ulcers. Breakdown can lead to infection, which can be detrimental and potentially fatal to the patient if not prevented or treated. The following measures can increase safety by decreasing the chance for breakdown.

- Use of foam pads or pillows to help redistribute weight on bony prominences can help prevent breakdown. This is particularly true in regions such as the hip bones, shoulders, and heels.
- Regular repositioning of the patient, as well as any foam pads or pillows, should be done at least once every 2 hours to redistribute areas of pressure and increase circulation.
- Routine application of emollients such as lotion helps to maintain skin integrity. Proper levels of moisturizer allow the skin to be less fragile, or not to tear as easily, compared with when the skin is either too dry or too moist. This includes application of specialized barrier emollients used for incontinent individuals, to decrease breakdown from excessive moisture (Voegeli, 2012). Because older adults often have a decreased immune system as well, the primary care provider may recommend antimicrobial lotions or creams, particularly in areas where the skin is still largely intact but with some abrasions.

EXTREME TEMPERATURE CONDITIONS

Exposure to extreme temperatures can cause adverse, and sometimes fatal, health reactions in the older adult population. Both excessive heat and cold, in combination with natural changes in the body's physiological functions and medication side effects, can cause profound changes in internal temperature regulation, as well as the circulatory and nervous systems.

Risks Associated With Heat

As people age, they often have decreased responses to temperature in their extremities, and they may have less adipose tissue to help insulate them. This combination often leads older adults to feel cold in temperatures that younger individuals may feel are comfortable. As a result, older adults often cover themselves with blankets, even when the temperature is quite warm. This practice, combined with decreased sweat production in older adults and a decreased sense of thirst, may cause internal temperatures to rise to unsafe levels (CDC, 2012).

To help increase safety and decrease risk from extreme heat, the LPN should evaluate the home for an adequate supply of clean water, as well as air conditioning or a fan. If an air conditioning unit is present, to increase safety the patient should not be seated or lying directly in front of it, to avoid the risk of hypothermia from exposure to the cold air.

The LPN should also provide education and demonstration regarding ways to lower body temperature safely in extreme heat. This includes adequate hydration as well as tepid, not cool or cold, baths for 10 to 15 minutes, or the use of a cool cloth around the patient's neck. When temperatures exceed 90°F, the LPN should be sure the patient is checked twice a day, either personally or by a primary caregiver (PCG), for signs and symptoms that indicate the onset of heat stroke, or hyperthermia (CDC, 2012) (Box 7.1).

Risks Associated With Cold

Older adults are often more prone to sedentary lifestyles, which may decrease the body's ability to generate heat. This situation, partnered with decreased insulation from adipose tissue, may lead to excessive heat loss during cold temperatures. For those living in cold environments, even if the

---

BOX 7.1 SIGNS OF HYPERTHERMIA

- ■ Body temperature higher than 103°F
- ■ Abnormal confusion
- ■ Headache
- ■ Heavy sweating or hot dry skin with no sweat
- ■ Pallor
- ■ Tachycardia
- ■ Fatigue
- ■ Dizziness
- ■ Muscle cramps
- ■ Nausea
- ■ Rapid, shallow breathing

(CDC, 2012)

---

patient does not or is unable to verbalize that he or she is cold, the LPN should regularly assess the patients for potential signs and symptoms of hypothermia (CDC, 2013a) (Box 7.2).

To help decrease the chances of hypothermia, the LPN can encourage the patient to wear multiple layers of comfortable clothing and have blankets accessible to further provide warmth. If the older adult is using a fireplace or heating unit, extra precautions should be taken to ensure that blankets or loose clothing are not near enough to ignite and that the patient is not close enough to sustain burns.

BOX 7.2 SIGNS OF HYPOTHERMIA

- ■ Shivering
- ■ Rapid breathing
- ■ Increased heart rate
- ■ Increased blood pressure
- ■ Memory loss
- ■ Slurred speech
- ■ Decreased responses
  - • Mental
  - • Physical
- ■ Increased lethargy or fatigue

(CDC, 2013a)

Another risk that is particularly dangerous in cold temperatures is the increased chance of heart attack as a result of strenuous activity, such as shoveling snow. This is based on the physiological response of the cardiovascular system to cold. Scientists at the London School of Hygiene and Tropical Medicine found that for every 1°C the ambient temperature drops, the chance of a heart attack increases 2%, particularly in individuals older than age 75 years (Bhaskaran et al., 2010). The nurse may need to help coordinate services for the patient, so that labor-intensive tasks, particularly those that are outdoors, are performed by other organizations or persons.

 MENTAL HEALTH AND SAFETY

One of the primary safety concerns for older adults is associated with cognitive difficulties or other mental health issues. These alterations in thought process may unintentionally or intentionally place the patient in dangerous situations.

Dementia and Delirium

The cognitive difficulties associated with dementia, including but not limited to Alzheimer's disease, as well as delirium, increase the chances of accidents as well as wandering (NIH, 2013). If an older adult suffers from cognitive disorders, yet is still physically able, he or she should not be left alone for any duration of time. This includes patients whose baseline cognition is fairly sound but who are having increased cognitive difficulties from delirium, often manifesting as a result of urinary or upper respiratory tract infections.

Those supervising the older adult, including the LPN, and potentially CNAs, family, friends, neighbors, and those affiliated with community services, should pay particular attention to hazardous areas such as the kitchen, where the patient may cook and forget to turn off the oven or stove, and the garage, where sharp, heavy, or toxic items may be stored. Also, precautions need to be taken to decrease the chance of wandering, or the risk of getting lost as a result of wandering. This may include a silent alarm system or ample scheduling of individuals to be present in the home. Supervision is particularly important in the evening hours because "sundowning" may exacerbate cognitive function impairment.

Furthermore, a "memory-impaired" identification bracelet that includes the patient's name and a reliable contact number, and a recent photograph of the patient with information such as height, weight, and full name indicated on the back in case it is necessary to contact police for a missing person's report, should be placed on the patient.

Mental Health Disorders

Older adults should be assessed regularly for verbalization or behavior patterns that may indicate a need for proper psychiatric evaluation. If the LPN notes any of the following potential indicators, he or she should promptly report it to the supervisor. Among the major mental health issues affecting older adults are depression, anxiety, post-traumatic stress disorder (PTSD), and substance abuse (World Health Organization [WHO], 2013).

- **Depression** may be indicated through verbalization of sadness, decreased socialization, increased sleeping, and verbalization of suicidal ideations, which may include frequent mentioning of wanting to be with loved ones who have passed away.
- **Anxiety** may manifest as increasing insomnia, verbalization of worry, and increasing apprehension about the world around them. Apprehension may be demonstrated by lessening of ambulation based on fear of falling or injury, a frequently stated distrust of others, both individual persons and society as a whole, or verbalization of fears related to death and the dying process.
- **PTSD**, particularly among veterans of foreign wars, can be amplified by dementia. The memories, or flashbacks, of traumatic situations suddenly becoming more frequent and lifelike, may they place the patient at great risk for injury to themselves or others.
- **Substance abuse** is reported to adversely affect approximately 1% of older adults, and it greatly increases the risk for both unintentional and intentional self-harm, including suicide and overdose.

Social and physical isolation can be common among older adults, and they may be cyclical. One common manifestation of decreased cognition or mental health issues, including depression, anxiety, PTSD, and substance abuse, is isolation from those around them. This isolation may be based on self-perceptions of shame, embarrassment as patients feel their memory slipping and think that others will notice, a lack of wanting to connect with others,

> ### Think Like a Nurse
>
> You have been taking care of a resident in your facility for several months and she has always been in good spirits, but today she's sullen and appears to have been crying. When you ask her what's wrong, she becomes withdrawn and looks away. You know that this past week was the 5-year anniversary of her husband's death. What mental health concern do you suspect, and how can you address this issue?

guilt felt for socializing in the absence of those who have passed away, or an increasing lack of trust of the world around them.

As a patient begins to isolate himself or herself, it can often cause mental health to decline more rapidly, which may lead to further isolation, and the cycle continues. Any abnormal change in attitude, behavior, or interaction level, including isolation, that varies from the patient's baseline should be noted and continually monitored (WHO, 2013).

SEXUAL SAFETY MEASURES

Often, little attention is focused on sex and sexuality in regard to the older adult population. The LPN, when obtaining the patient's social history, should inquire what the patient's gender identity and sexual orientation are, whether the patient is sexually active or not, and if so, whether the patient is using proper protective measures or not. Although these questions may seem uncomfortable, the answers should never be assumed. Sex and sexuality are a part of life for people of all ages, and safety should be addressed.

Sexuality

The homosexual, bisexual, and/or transgender (lesbian, gay, bisexual, and transgender [LGBT]) population in the United States is estimated to include as many as 7 million older adults (Hospice Foundation of American [HFA], 2013), but according to the CDC, more than 20% have not disclosed this information to their doctor, often because they have not been directly asked. Of those who have disclosed their sexual or gender identity, 13% have either been denied health care or believe that they received inferior health care as a result (CDC, 2013c). Many more LGBT older adults, particularly

Point of Interest

Discussions about sex and sexuality with your older adult patients may initially feel a bit awkward or personally invasive. Answers to these questions, however, should never be assumed based on the age of your patient, and addressing these topics may help focus much needed patient education.

Ask your supervisor whether your place of employment has set protocols for this line of inquiry, and if not, you can help initiate a discussion about the importance of health related to sex and sexuality for patients of all ages.

One possible conversational approach with older adult patients includes the following questions:

"I need to ask you a few questions that may feel very personal in nature, but they are simply part of helping us understand you in a more holistic way, so that we can best address your overall health needs. None of the questions are meant as an accusation, and some of the answers may feel very obvious, but asking them is merely standard practice. If there are any that make you are truly uncomfortable, you do not need to answer them."

1. As what gender do you identify yourself (male, female, other)?
2. What is your sexual orientation (heterosexual, homosexual, bisexual, asexual)?
3. Are you currently sexually active or have you been within the past year?
4. [If "yes" to question 3] How many sexual partners have you had within the past year?
   a. [If one partner] Is this a mutually monogamous relationship?
   b. [If multiple partners or not in a mutually monogamous relationship] Have you and your sexual partner(s) ever been tested for sexually transmitted infections?
      i. "Yes": Have you [or they] ever tested positive? [If "yes," then...]
         1. What sexually transmitted infection was diagnosed?
         2. What year was the diagnosis (and month if current year)?
         3. What treatment was given?
      ii. "No": Educate about the importance of regular testing.
5. Do you and your partner(s) always use condoms or other safety precautions? If "no," educate about the importance of contraceptive use.

those in same-sex unions, have been denied housing, in both public and institutional settings, based on their sexual orientation (Equal Rights Center [ERC], 2014). Box 7.3 lists some concerns for the LBGT older adult.

BOX 7.3   CONCERNS FOR LESBIAN, GAY, BISEXUAL, AND TRANSGENDER OLDER ADULTS

■ Denial of or inferior health care
■ Bullying, both physical and emotional
■ Societal alienation
■ Partner visitation rights
■ Partner rights in end-of-life decisions

(Chatburn, 2013)

One safety concern specific to this community includes physical and/or emotional bullying from peers and staff, particularly in clinical settings such as assisted living or long-term care facilities (Chatburn, 2013). LGBT older adults may also have faced bullying or alienation from family members, which could potentially result in lack of a social support system (U.S. Department of Health and Human Services [HHS], 2012b). Second, aside from the impact on their psychosocial needs, this may also place these individuals in a vulnerable position legally, in regard to end-of-life decisions, visitor privileges, and distribution of assets (Chatburn, 2013), particularly in states where same-sex unions are not legally recognized.

As a patient advocate, the LPN should provide protection for the older adult in regard to physical safety, psychosocial needs, and enforcement of legal rights, including division of assets and other end-of-life decision making. There are many resources available for the LGBT older adult at a national level and frequently also at state and community levels (Box 7.4).

Sexual Activity

Although pregnancy is not an issue among older adult women, it may still be a concern for older adult men with younger partners. Also, sexually transmitted infections (STIs) can be passed regardless of age, when protection measures are not taken. The CDC has reported that syphilis and chlamydia rates have nearly tripled within the older adult population within a decade (CDC, 2011), and the National Institute on Aging reports that nearly 25% of the human immunodeficiency virus (HIV) and acquired immunodeficiency syndrome (AIDS) cases in the United States are in patients over the age of 50 (National Institute on Aging [NIA], 2009). Meanwhile, a nationwide survey indicated that only 12% of male and 32% of female older adults who reported to be sexually active state that they always use safety precautions such as a condom during intercourse (American Association of Retired Persons [AARP], 2010).

Evidence indicates a direct correlation between an increase in erectile dysfunction medications and an increase in STIs in the older adult population (Jena et al., 2010). A study in the *New England Journal of Medicine* indicated that pharmaceutical interventions were reported to be used by 14% of older adult males, and others in this population had sought out non-pharmacological interventions as well (Lindau et al., 2007). As with patients of any age, sexually active older adults should be educated on the importance of using safety precautions during sexual intercourse.

Evidence-Based Practice

Jena, A., Goldman, D., Kamdar, A., Lakdawalla, D., & Lu, Y. (2010). Sexually transmitted diseases among users of erectile dysfunction drugs: analysis of claims data. *Annals of Internal Medicine, 153(1), 1-7.*

Linking between the use of erectile dysfunction drugs and increased rates of sexually transmitted infections in men over the age of 40 was supported based on evidence collected retrospectively on nearly 1.5 million men. The research team indicated that practice, based on this evidence, should include providing education about sexually transmitted infections to men when they are prescribed erectile dysfunction medications.

1. As the nurse providing patient education to a gentleman receiving erectile dysfunction medications for the first time, what information would you provide on sexually transmitted infections?
2. What do you anticipate to be barriers in this patient education? Are those barriers associated with the patient's outlook or your own discomfort?
3. What safety measures could you include in your teaching to help decrease the risk for sexually transmitted infections?
4. What impact do you feel this correlation would have on society? What populations would be most highly affected?
5. What are different possible causes for the link between erectile dysfunction medications and sexually transmitted infections?

BOX 7.4   ONLINE RESOURCES FOR LESBIAN, GAY, BISEXUAL, AND TRANSGENDER OLDER ADULTS

LGBT Aging Center: www.lgbtagingcenter.org

Services and Advocacy for Gay, Lesbian, Bisexual, and Transgender Elders: www.sageusa.org

Think Like a Nurse

You are taking care of a 74-year-old man who will be discharged the next day. While talking to him, he mentions that he has been divorced for 5 years and has decided to start dating again. His doctor even prescribed him erectile dysfunction medication. What safety issues should you discuss with him?

ELDER ABUSE

Elder abuse is an increasing risk facing the older adult population. Recent statistics indicate that 10% of older adults in both home and institutional settings have been the victim of abuse. However, current statistics are thought to be highly conservative estimates because most elder abuse goes unreported. It is estimated that only around 20% of cases are reported to and substantiated by Adult Protective Services (APS) because many forms of abuse are difficult to confirm if not directly witnessed (CDC, 2013d). Although often people think of physical harm when they hear abuse, there are multiple categories of elder abuse (WHO, 2002):

- **Physical abuse** involves damage or injury to the older adult's body. This may include broken bones, lacerations, malnutrition, welts, and bruises caused by another individual, and it includes injuries at all levels, not only those warranting medical attention. Injury from abuse may result in exacerbating existing health problems, disability, and premature death.
- **Psychological or emotional abuse** includes yelling or swearing at, belittling, insulting, intimidating, isolating, or manipulating the older adult. It may increase depression, anxiety, PTSD, fear, withdrawal from others, and feelings of helplessness.
- **Financial or material abuse** is the taking of money, possessions, or property from older adults without their permission. This also includes the misuse of funds, such as Medicare, Medicaid, and Social Security, which are allocated for care of the older adult.
- **Sexual abuse** includes forced participation of the older adult in any sexual act, whether he or she is giving or receiving the act. This also includes inappropriate touching of a sexual nature while providing care to the older adult. Persons with dementia are particularly vulnerable to sexual assault because perpetrators often believe that there is less chance of being reported.
- **Neglect and abandonment** are purposeful failures of providing the older adult with basic needs, including medical care, psychosocial needs, housing, nutrition, and assistance with necessary ADLs. This can include leaving an older adult alone for extended periods of time when he or she is unable to provide self-care.

Risk Factors

The risk of elder abuse is increased in situations where the older adult and the PCG have little social support, are highly dependent on others, are unable to care properly for themselves, have drug or alcohol dependency, lack coping skills, are prone to hostility, are under a lot of stress related to other aspects of their life, or have mental health issues (CDC, 2013d).

Prevention Factors

Communication is one of the first steps to preventing elder abuse. The LPN should listen for cues in conversations that may indicate the risk for abuse by others. This includes statements made not only by the older adult, but also by any others involved in their care or living environment. If the older adult is in the home setting with a live-in PCG, it may be necessary for the LPN to assess the PCG's social support infrastructure, ability to physically provide care, knowledge of financial management, and awareness of community resources that can train or aid them in areas where they are still learning (CDC, 2013d).

Reporting Suspected Abuse

Nurses, in most states, are considered "mandated reporters," which means that it is compulsory for them to report evident and suspected mistreatment or abuse. The LPN must report the findings to his or her supervisor and follow through to ensure that it has also been reported to the police, a long-term care facility ombudsman, or APS, depending on the patient's life circumstances and living environment (National Center of Elder Abuse [NCEA], 2014). LPNs caring for older adults should be aware of available resources for the prevention and management of elder abuse within the community (Box 7.5).

BOX 7.5   NATIONAL CENTER ON ELDER ABUSE: ELDERCARE LOCATOR

The Eldercare Locator is a public service of the U.S. Administration on Aging that connects users to services for older adults and their families. It can be used by calling 1-800-667-1116 or visiting www.eldercare.gov on the Internet.

SAFETY IN EMERGENCY SITUATIONS

Older adults are at an increased risk for injury or death in an emergency situation, often because of physiological or cognitive difficulties (AARP, 2006). It is estimated that 80% of the more than 41 million older adults living in the United States have been diagnosed with a chronic health condition, many with multiple comorbidities (HHS, 2012a). Although there is no way to prepare an older adult fully for all 21 emergency situations indicated by the Red Cross, and not all emergency situations are applicable to each place, basic measures to decrease the impact of an emergency can be taken (American Red Cross, 2014), and resources such as Ready.gov can be used to see which risks are greatest for each area (Ready.gov, 2013).

Preventable Emergency Situations

Many emergency situations can occur in the home, but it can be possible to prevent, or at least reduce, the risk of occurrence. Among the most prevalent are fire, flooding, carbon monoxide poisoning, and food poisoning (American Red Cross, 2014).

- **Fire** in the home setting is most frequently caused by cooking, but it may also be the result of heating or electrical malfunction, smoking, or an open flame. It is important for the LPN to be aware of fire risks in the older adult's living environment. Heat sources should be surrounded by a clear area, stove and oven knobs should be easy to maneuver, timers on cooking devices should be operational as a reminder, electrical outlets should not be used over their specific parameters for plugs, and the older adult should be incredibly cautious if smoking (U.S. Fire Administration [USFA], 2013). The home or facility should be equipped with functioning smoke detectors, as well as ample fire extinguishers for the living space, and an evacuation strategy should be discussed and demonstrated in case of a fire.
- **Flooding** most often occurs in the home setting as a result of frozen pipes in the winter. This can be decreased by allowing faucets to have a slow drip during subfreezing conditions, particularly for fixtures on an outer perimeter wall.
- **Carbon monoxide poisoning** is most common with fires (USFA, 2013), but it may also be present with gas leaks in the living environment. Because carbon monoxide is colorless and odorless, it is often undetected before causing fatalities. A carbon monoxide detector may be used in the environment to alert the older adult or the PCG to the presence of the gas.
- **Food poisoning**, as well as medication toxicity, may occur in the home setting, especially with older adults who suffer from dementia. The ingestion of spoiled foods or beverages, as well as improper consumption of medications, may cause illness or potential death. The LPN in the home setting should check the house for rancid or spoiled food and beverages, as well as ensure that medications are properly labeled and appear to be taken in the proper quantity for the time that has passed. If the LPN, older adult, or PCG suspects poisoning from food, beverage, or medication, Poison Control should be called (Box 7.6).

Natural and Human-made Disasters

In the case of a natural disaster, many older adults are unable to evacuate themselves. A recent nationwide study found that 59% of adults age 50 to 74 years and 85% of adults older than 75 years reported that they would be unable to evacuate themselves in case of a natural disaster (AARP, 2006). Regardless of the nature of the disaster, many preparation and response actions are similar, such as having a safety bag, knowing whom to contact, and registering the older adult with emergency services (HHS Administration on Aging [AOA], 2014).

It is recommended to create a safety bag for the older adult, regardless of whether he or she is in a home or a long-term institutional setting. This bag

---

BOX 7.6   AMERICAN ASSOCIATION OF POISON CONTROL CENTERS

The American Association of Poison Control Centers supports the nation's 55 poison centers in their efforts to prevent and treat poison exposures. Poison centers offer free, confidential medical advice 24 hours a day, 7 days a week through the Poison Help Line at 1-800-222-1222. This service provides a primary resource for poisoning information and helps reduce costly emergency department visits through in-home treatment.

should be equipped with the supplies necessary to sustain health for at least 72 hours, in the event that the older adult were to be trapped in the living quarters until help arrived (Box 7.7). The items in the bag may vary depending on the environment, but the LPN should check to be sure that they are properly stocked with up-to-date items, remove any clothing that may no longer fit, and remove any food or medications that may have expired.

The older adult should have access to an easy-to-operate telephone, when possible, that he or she can use to call emergency services, the LPN, the PCG, or others, as well as receive calls. Having an

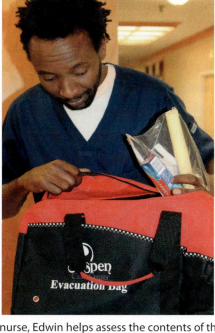

As a nurse, Edwin helps assess the contents of the patients' evacuation bags to be sure that everything is in place, functional, and up to date. This way, in case of emergency, the facility can be sure that each patient has the basic necessities to keep him or her safe and comfortable until more supplies arrive. This facility also has protocols in place for ensuring that the medication carts are part of the evacuation process. For those in a home setting, medications can be included in the bag.

easily readable list of emergency contact numbers near the phone is helpful, including name, role, and number for each person. This allows responders to know whom else they need to contact. It may also be beneficial for the older adult to wear a life alert system, in case of disaster or personal emergency. Emergency services have registries for older adults, so that responders know which facilities house those who are unable to evacuate themselves. Registration contact information can be found by contacting Eldercare Care Locator Services.

Health Emergencies

Whether because of illness, injury, or other health problems such as heart attack or stroke, older adults in the home setting are at a significant risk for health emergencies. If the older adult is in an institutional setting, the LPN must ensure that the call light is within reach and that the patient is able to use it. If the older adult lives alone, or with a PCG who is often away from the home, it may be wise to obtain a life alert system that the patient would wear while

---

BOX 7.7 ITEMS FOR SAFETY BAG

- Clothing (including jacket and sturdy shoes)
- Up-to-date list of:
  - Medications
  - Diagnoses
  - Allergies
  - Contacts (physician, power of attorney, family)
  - Necessary equipment
    - Glasses
    - Hearing-aid and batteries
    - Dentures and care products
    - Walker/wheelchair/cane
    - Pacemaker serial number
- 10-day medication supply (not expired)
  - Prescription medications
  - Over-the-counter medications
- Flashlight and radio with batteries
- First-aid kit
- Hygiene items
- Cash
- Whistle
- Blanket and/or sleeping bag, and pillow
- Copy of physician orders for life-sustaining treatment, if applicable, and insurance documents
- Nonperishable food and water (for at least 3 days)
  - Not past expiration date
  - Able to be easily opened
  - Include necessary utensils
- Cell phone with charger

(AOA, 2014)

alone. This would allow others to be alerted in case of an emergency. Also, having telephones and contact lists in easily accessible places may help the older adult get help in a health emergency.

Critically Examine the Following:

You notice that the facility where you have just been hired does not have any emergency preparedness kits for the residents living there. When you mention to your supervisor that you would like to participate actively in addressing this concern, he schedules a meeting for both of you to pitch the idea to your administrator the following Monday. What resources and information would be good to access before your presentation to her next week?

QSEN

COMPETENCY: Safety (Knowledge, Skills, Attitudes)

Promoting Safety for the Older Adult

As an LPN, it is your responsibility to provide a safe environment for your patients. Evaluate the CNAs to make sure they are performing tasks correctly; if not, provide the necessary instruction to ensure safe care. Assess the environment and watch for equipment or other items in the way that may cause falls. Also, make sure that a patient's equipment is functioning properly. If not, have it repaired or replaced.

If you notice unsafe care performed by another member of the health-care team or a family member, be sure to communicate your concern to the registered nurse (RN) or nurse manager. If you are aware of errors made, it is your responsibility to report the errors to the RN or nurse manager.

As a member of the health-care team, it is important that you value vigilance and monitoring of care by other members of the health-care team. It is also important to listen to your patients and their families if they voice a concern about the care being provided. By valuing other people's concerns, you will help provide a safer environment for your patients.

SAFETY ISSUES TO CHECK ON DURING HOME VISITS

Many LPNs work in the home health setting, and they can assess their patient's living environment for the aforementioned safety concerns. First, the most important step to ensure safety is communication. It is important for the nurse to hear what the older adult has to say; use keen observation skills to listen for potential indicators of safety breaches, and then follow up on these. Second, beyond communication, it is within the LPN's role to survey the environment visually in a way that maintains privacy. Third, the nurse should be aware of community resources that may be able to also help in the multidisciplinary efforts to promote safety for the older adult. These steps allow the LPN to implement holistic, safety-focused, care for the patient.

Listening for Safety Concerns

While communicating with the older adult, direct questions can be asked regarding safety, but it is also important to listen for other cues such as the patient's perceptions of the physical environment, as well as the interactions the patient has with others.

- **Fall risks.** Has any change in mental and physical function been mentioned by the older adult? If so, does this affect his or her ability to ambulate safely? Has the patient mentioned feeling more tired, confused, forgetful, or weak lately? Does the patient mention having to get up in the night to use the restroom more often, or with more difficulty, than before?
- **Skin integrity.** Has the older adult mentioned bumping into things recently? Has he or she recently acquired a new pet? Does the older adult mention itching or dryness? Has the patient mentioned any broken or rough edges in the home?
- **Extreme temperature.** Does the older adult mention how chilly he or she has been lately, or how warm it seems to be getting? Has he or she mentioned gardening outdoors in the summer, shoveling snow off the walkway in the winter months, or walking his or her dog during either season? Is there any change in speech ability or cognition that may indicate hyperthermia or hypothermia?
- **Mental health and safety.** Has there been a negative change in outlook from normal conversations? Is the older adult more withdrawn than usual? Has the older adult mentioned a

change in perception about himself or herself or others? Is the patient talking much more about those who have already passed away, and how much he or she misses them? Has the older adult stopped talking about the future, even the near future? Is the older adult more fearful than usual?

- **Sexual safety.** Did the patient mention a new relationship? If the patient is sexually active, has he or she mentioned symptoms that could be associated with an STI? Has the older adult mentioned feeling excluded from social situations based on sexual orientation?
- **Elder abuse.** Has the older adult mentioned people who have not been nice lately, or with whom he or she does not get along, who may be a safety threat? Did the patient mention feeling uneasy around someone? Has the older adult mentioned being left alone for long periods of time or being hungry or soiled for extended periods?
- **Emergency situations.** Does the older adult know whom to contact in case of emergency? Does he or she know the numbers for those people? Has the older adult mentioned neighbors or family who check on the patient regularly? Has the older adult mentioned any change in physical or mental ability, or has his or her speech changed in a way that may indicate there has been a health emergency?

Visually Inspecting the Environment

It is important to maintain the older adult's privacy when assessing the living environment. It is also imperative to remember that the patient maintains the right to live in a different level of cleanliness than is comfortable for the LPN and make lifestyle choices different from those than the LPN may prefer. The living environment of the older adult, both in a facility or home setting, may take on many different forms and styles, but if it is truly unsafe, to the point of being physically harmful or fatal to the patient, then the LPN should report this to a supervisor and ensure that it is followed up by any applicable authorities. The following information pertains to individuals living in either a facility or a private home, or both.

- **Fall risks.** Is the older adult wearing any clothing that would put him or her at an increased risk for falls? Does all of the DME appear to be in good repair and properly sized for the patient? Are nonslip surfaces in place

where applicable? Are there any broken or missing steps or railings? Is there adequate lighting, including night lights? Are there piles of papers or toys on the floor? Are walkways safe and clear, free from clutter or area rugs? Are there floor-level pets in the home?

- **Skin integrity.** Does the LPN see any rough or sharp edges in the home that may cause abrasions or lacerations? Has a skin check been performed? Is any injury or breakdown present? Has lotion been used regularly? Has the water heater been set to a temperature to prevent scalding? Does water coming from the faucet feel incredibly hot?
- **Extreme temperature.** Is there an operational heating and/or cooling system in the home? Does the older adult know how to operate it safely? Is he or she dressed appropriately to be comfortable in the current ambient temperature, or does the patient's skin feel abnormally cool or warm? Is there an ample supply of clean water in the home?
- **Mental health and safety.** Does the home seem to be in more disarray than usual? Is there a pile of newspapers in the driveway? Are any areas of the home filled with soiled dishes or clothing, more so than is the patient's baseline for living conditions? Are there large quantities of empty alcohol or medication bottles? Are any psychotropic medications missing, as if they have run out early? Does the older adult's hygiene seem in accordance with the baseline, or has there been a decrease in self-care? Is the patient more tearful, withdrawn, or agitated than normal?
- **Sexual safety.** Are there any changes to the skin around the genitalia that may indicate contraction of an STI? If the older adult is sexually active, and not in a mutually monogamous relationship, are condoms present?
- **Elder abuse.** Is there bruising or tearing of the skin on the inner thighs, genitals, or breast that may be the result of forced sexual acts? Are bruises or skin tears located other places, or are there any fractures or breaks of unknown origin? Does the older adult appear more frightened than usual, such as being increasingly jumpy around sudden movements? Does the patient report that he or she cannot find money that had been placed in the home? Are there signs that a PCG may have been absent for quite a while? Does the older adult seem fearful of a family member or a health-care provider?

• **Emergency situations.** Is a safety bag present and up to date? Can the older adult demonstrate ability to contact necessary people in the case of an emergency? If the patient has a life alert system, can he or she demonstrate proper use? Is an easy-to-use telephone, contact list, and light near the areas where the patient resides the most, such as the bed or a chair? Is there a clear path for evacuation in case of disaster? Are smoke and carbon monoxide detectors in place and functional? Are fire extinguishers present? Is there an ashtray near the areas where the patient most commonly resides, and if so, is it overfilled? If the outside temperature is below freezing, are faucets on outer perimeter walls set to drip slowly? Is the kitchen free of expired, rancid, or spoiled food and beverage products? Do counts on medications seem accurate for the amount of time that has passed since the medications were refilled, and are the medication properly stored, labeled, and current?

Contacting Resources

Preventing safety concerns can be done in part by constructing a solid support team for the older adult, consisting of friends, family, neighbors, health workers, and those from social circles such as church or other community groups. Communication among the support team members is crucial to help provide a safe situation for the patient.

Resources can be found in most communities to help address safety concerns that may be noted in the older adult's environment, particularly for those in the home setting who may be underserved. If the LPN believes that there is a safety breech present for the patient, he or she must act. If it is an issue that places the patient in immediate danger, then action must be taken, with consideration for the LPN's safety as well, to rectify the situation. This may include the need to call police or other emergency services, including 9-1-1. If no immediate danger is present, then the LPN's next steps would be to report any concerns to a supervisor and educate the older adult in applicable situations.

The supervisor or employing agency will most often have a list of area resources that are available for the older adult. This may include food delivery services, organizations that do home repairs and chores for those in need, LGBT legal assistance, support groups, and disaster response registries. On discussing safety concerns, the LPN can ensure that interventions are being properly implemented in response. Preventing safety concerns can greatly improve the health and overall quality of life for the older adult.

 CONCLUSION

Whether working with older adults in the community or in the facility setting, focus on safety is important. When safety measures are implemented, they decrease the chance of accidents and adverse health outcomes and increase the quality of life.

CASE STUDY SOLUTIONS

1. Mr. Paco is currently taking several medications that may cause dizziness as a regular side effect. When he takes several doses at the same time, there is an increased chance of dizziness. Because he is also unstable as a result of the use of crutches, Mr. Paco is at an increased risk for falls. It is also a concern that he is taking double doses of his anticoagulant because this may increase the chance of bleeding. Mr. Paco should be instructed that it is not safe for him to take two doses of medications at the same time. If he misses a dose, he should just skip the dose and take the next dose as scheduled. You will want to notify the registered nurse (RN) when doses are skipped. You may also want to check with the RN or primary care provider to see whether any of his medications can be taken earlier in the evening.

2. To avoid skin tears, you should make sure that his crutches and wheelchair do not have any sharp edges that can scrape his skin. It may be necessary to place some padding on his equipment. You may also want to make sure that his dog's nails are clipped and that the dog's collar does not have any sharp edges. Finally, you will want to make sure that Mr. Paco's clothes do not have a zipper or other closures that may tear his skin.

3. Because Mr. Paco is living alone, there is a concern for his safety. You should discuss with him the possibility of obtaining an alert system that he can use in the event of a health emergency. You will also want to make sure he has a telephone that is easy for him to use and is with him at all times. The contact information for friends and family members should be either programmed into the phone or listed on a sheet of paper next to his chair. The contact information for the home health agency should also be readily available. In the event of a disaster, Mr. Paco should have a safety bag packed with supplies as mentioned in the chapter. It is important to make sure he has a 3- to 4-day supply of his supplies in the event he needs to leave his home quickly.

REVIEW QUESTIONS

1. You recognize that your patient may be an increased risk for falls when she states, "I've felt so dizzy today." You know this dizziness could be directly linked to (select all that apply):
   1. Weather
   2. Hydration
   3. Mild dementia
   4. Nutrition
   5. Medication
   6. Infection
   7. Drug or alcohol misuse

2. As your patient is brought back indoors he seems confused, less responsive than normal, is breathing quickly, has a rapid heart rate, and is slightly slurring his speech. In addition to alerting your supervisor, which initial intervention do you perform?
   1. Check to see whether his extremities feel cold to the touch, and place a few extra blankets on him.
   2. Remove his light jacket, and turn the air conditioning up to high.
   3. Seat him in front of the fan, and bring him a glass of ice water.
   4. Instruct the CNA to keep an eye on him, and then take his vitals again in 1 hour.

3. All of the following may lead to increased anxiety in older adults, except:
   1. A ground-level fall
   2. Death of a spouse
   3. Alcohol consumption
   4. Beginnings of short-term memory loss

4. On an initial home visit your new patient, Sheila, frequently speaks about a woman named Elizabeth who lives with her. As you look at the mantle you notice many pictures of the two of them, so you:
   1. Figure they must be a lifelong friends who moved in together for companionship after their husbands passed away.
   2. Know that Sheila and Elizabeth must be lesbians in a relationship together.
   3. Redirect the conversation back to health-related questions because the ambiguity of the situation makes you feel uneasy.
   4. Ask Sheila to tell you more about Elizabeth's role in her life.

5. Abuse may manifest as all of the following:
   1. Lacerations, bruises on the face, broken bones
   2. Increased tearfulness, withdrawing from others, feelings of worthlessness
   3. Bruising on the genitals, increase in pressure ulcers, weight loss
   4. All of the above
   5. 1 and 3 only

REFERENCES

American Association of Retired Persons (AARP). (2010). Sex, romance, and relationships: AARP survey of midlife and older adults. assets.aarp.org/rgcenter/general/srr_09.pdf.

American Association of Retired Persons (AARP). (2006). We can do better: lessons learned for protecting older persons in disasters. assets.aarp.org/rgcenter/il/better.pdf

American Red Cross. (2014). Recovering after a disaster or emergency: Tools and resources. www.redcross.org/prepare/disaster-safety-library

Bhaskaran, K., Hajat, S., Haines, A., Herrett, E., Wilkinson, P., & Smeeth, L. (2010). Short term effects of temperature on risk of myocardial infarction in England and Wales: time series regression analysis of the Myocardial Ischaemia National Audit Project Registry. *BMJ*, 341, c3823.

Centers for Disease Control and Prevention (CDC). (2013a). Emergency preparedness and response: Winter weather. www.bt.cdc.gov/disasters/winter/faq.asp

Centers for Disease Control and Prevention (CDC). (2013b). Falls among older adults: An overview. www.cdc.gov/HomeandRecreationalSafety/Falls/adultfalls.html

Centers for Disease Control and Prevention (CDC). (2013c). The state of aging and health in America 2013. www.cdc.gov/aging/pdf/state-aging-health-in-america-2013.pdf.

Centers for Disease Control and Prevention (2013d). Understanding elder abuse. www.cdc.gov/violenceprevention/pdf/em-factsheet-a.pdf.

Centers for Disease Control and Prevention (CDC). (2012). Emergency preparedness and response: Heat stress in the elderly. www.bt.cdc.gov/disasters/extremeheat/elderlyheat.asp

Centers for Disease Control and Prevention (CDC). (2011). Sexually transmitted diseases: Interactive data 1996-2011. http://wonder.cdc.gov/std-std-race-age.html

Chatburn, A. (2013). *LGBTQ:* Care at the end of life [PowerPoint slides]. www.slideshare.net/andichatburn/lgbtq-special-care-at-the-end-of-life

Currie, L. (2008). Fall and injury prevention. In Hughes (Ed.), *Patient safety and quality: An evidence-based handbook for nurses*. New York, NY: Agency for Healthcare Research and Quality.

Equal Rights Center (ERC). (2014). Opening doors: An investigation of barriers to senior housing for same-sex couples. www.sageusa.org/files/lgbtSeniorHousingreportFINAL.pdf.

Healthy People 2020 (HP2020). (2013). Older adults: Injury prevention. www.healthypeople.gov/2020/topicsobjectives2020/overview.aspx?topicid=31#

Hospice Foundation of America (HFA). (2013). Aging and end of-life challenges in the LGBT community. http://changingaging.org/blog/hospice-brings-focus-on-lgbt-end-of-life-challenges/

Jena, A., Goldman, D., Kamdar, A., Lakdawalla, D., & Lu, Y. (2010). Sexually transmitted diseases among users of erectile dysfunction drugs: analysis of claims data. *Annals of Internal Medicine, 153*(1), 1-7.

Johns Hopkins University: Bloomberg School of Public Health. (2013). Home hot water temperatures remain a burn hazard for young and elderly. www.jhsph.edu/news/news-releases/2013/shields-home-hot-water-temperatures-burn-hazard.html

Lindau, S., Schumm, L., Laumann, E., Levinson, W., O'Muircheataig, C., & Waite, L. (2007). A study of sexuality and health among older adults in the United States. *New England Journal of Medicine, 357*, 762-774.

National Center of Elder Abuse (NCEA). (2014). Reporting abuse. www.ncea.aoa.gov/Stop_Abuse/Get_Help/Report/index.aspx

National Institutes of Health (NIH): Senior Health. (2013). Falls and older adults. https://nihseniorhealth.gov/falls/causesandriskfactors/01.html

National Institute on Aging (NIA). (2009). Health & Aging: HIV, AIDS, and older people. https://www.nia.nih.gov/health/publication/hiv-aids-and-older-people

Quality and Safety Education for Nurses (QSEN). (2014). Pre-licensure KSAS: Safety. http://qsen.org/competencies/pre-licensure-ksas/#safety

Ready.gov. (2013). Plan for your risks. www.ready.gov/plan-for-your-risks

U.S. Department of Health and Human Services (HHS). (2012a). A Profile of Older Americans. www.aoa.gov/Aging_Statistics/Profile/2012/docs/2012profile.pdf.

U.S. Department of Health and Human Services (HHS). (2012b). Recommended actions to improve health and well-being of lesbian, gay, bisexual, and transgender communities. www.hhs.gov/lgbt/health.html

U.S. Department of Health and Human Services Administration on Aging (AOA). (2014). Just in case: Emergency readiness for older adults and caregivers. www.aoa.gov/AoARoot/AoA_Programs/HCLTC/Caregiver/docs/Just_in_Case030706_links.pdf.

U.S. Fire Administration (USFA). (2013). Residential building fire causes. https://www.usfa.fema.gov/downloads/pdf/statistics/res_bldg_fire_estimates.pdf.

Voegeli, D. (2012). Understanding the main principles of skin care in older adults. *Nursing Standard, 27* (11), 59-68.

World Health Organization (WHO). (2013). Mental health and older adults. http://www.who.int/mediacentre/factsheets/fs381/en/

World Health Organization (WHO). (2002). World report on violence and health. www.who.int/violence_injury_prevention/violence/world_report/en/

WEB RESOURCE

Emergency Preparedness http://ready.gov

Nutrition for Older Adults

TAMARA DAHLKEMPER

8

LEARNING OUTCOMES

1. Perform a nutritional assessment on an older adult.

2. Develop a nutritional plan using MyPlate as a guide.

3. Identify the influence carbohydrates, proteins, and fats have on maintaining a healthy body.

4. Identify the influence vitamins and minerals have on maintaining a healthy body.

5. Discuss therapeutic diets for older adults with special nutritional needs.

6. List four basic causes of electrolyte imbalance.

CONCEPTS

Metabolism

Nutrition

CASE STUDY

Mrs. Salvador is a 75-year-old Hispanic resident who enjoyed good health until about 6 weeks ago, when she fell and fractured her left hip and left elbow. A week after her surgical procedure, Mrs. Salvador was transferred to a rehabilitation facility for care. She will need physical therapy before she will be able to care for herself at home. You have been caring for Mrs. Salvador for the past 3 weeks. You noticed Mrs. Salvador has lost 6 lb since her admission to the unit.

Discussion

Consider the following questions you should ask when evaluating Mrs. Salvador's weight loss:

1. Was Mrs. Salvador losing weight before her accident?

2. Are there any cultural needs that may affect her nutrition?

3. After reviewing the nutritional risk assessment on page 145, are there any questions from the assessment you should consider?

4. What information should you report to the RN?

INTRODUCTION

A nutritious intake of food is essential at any age to achieve optimal health. Good nutrition is a major contributor to feeling well. Healthy eating provides the body with energy to do things, such as work or play. It promotes clear thinking, fights disease, and usually tastes good. I often think of children (and adults) in third world countries who go to bed hungry and wake up to nothing or very little to eat. It is appalling that so many people die of malnourishment in this world. Nurses are key to teaching and supporting older persons in their care to understand and use the vast nutritional choices available in the United States. Nutrition is a crucial behavior for positive health in every aspect of living.

The amount and type of food necessary to promote health generally change as people age. Younger people can "get away" with eating donuts

---

Evidence-Based Practice

Boaz, M., Rychani, L., Barami, K., Houri, Z., Yosef, R., Siag, A., Berlovitz, Y., & Leibovitz, E. (2013). Nurses and nutrition: A survey of knowledge and attitudes regarding nutrition assessment and care of hospitalized elderly patients. Journal of Continuing Education in Nursing, 44(8), 357-364.

This study measured the association between nutrition knowledge and attitudes about nutrition care and feeding in nurses working in hospital settings. The study participants were employed at two hospitals in central and southern Israel. The sample size consisted of 106 nurses working in internal medicine and surgical departments. As part of the study, nurses ranked 11 nursing tasks based on importance; the lowest-ranked tasks included performing nutrition assessments, feeding patients, and providing appropriate food to patients. Most nurses did not think it is necessary to include nutrition status as part of medical rounds. The findings of this study suggest that providing nutrition education to nurses could increase nutritional knowledge and improve the use of nutritional assessments.

Questions

1. How can you apply the results of this study to your nursing practice?
2. What additional information do you need to learn to feel comfortable addressing your patients' nutritional needs?

or candy, whereas older people generally cannot eat such things without a weight gain or an increase in their blood sugar. This is because of their slower metabolism and other normal aging physiology. Foods that contain carbohydrates, proteins, fats, vitamins, and minerals in the appropriate amounts must be included in dietary planning for older adults.

As a licensed practical nurse (LPN), you need to be aware of physical changes related to aging that affect food intake. Examples of these changes could be gastric disorders caused by normal gastrointestinal (GI) changes and chronic diseases or illnesses that impact nutritional requirements. In addition, certain foods and medications can cause adverse drug reactions. Older adults may have difficulty chewing or swallowing food because of disease or poor dentition. Sensory changes in seeing, smelling, and tasting foods may influence an older person's appetite. Loss of appetite can occur as psychosocial changes bring on depression, dependency on others for meals, and changes in cognitive skills. Physical changes can also impact an older adult's ability to access or prepare food. As you perform nutritional assessments on older adults, you need to think about reasons why they may have nutritional deficits and ways you can assist them and their family in overcoming the problem (Box 8.1).

NUTRITIONAL ASSESSMENT

The place where you work may or may not have a nutritional assessment tool, and assessment tools may vary from nursing home to hospital. In many facilities, a dietitian does the nutritional assessment, but that is not always true. You need to be mindful of the basics of a nutritional risk assessment so that you can perform one successfully wherever you are working. The basics are as follows (Tabloski, 2013):

1. Has an illness or the person's condition been responsible for a change in eating patterns?
2. Does the person eat fewer than two meals a day?
3. Does the person's diet include fruits, vegetables, meat, and milk products?
4. Does the person's diet frequently include alcoholic drinks?
5. Does the person have difficulty chewing or swallowing food (known as *dysphasia*)?
6. Does the person have the resources to purchase food?
7. Does the person eat alone most of the time?
8. Does the person take three or more medications, either prescribed or over-the-counter (OTC), each day?
9. Has the person lost or gained more than 10 lb in the past 6 months?
10. Is the person able to shop, cook, and feed himself or herself?

Any of these nutritional risks can lead to malnourishment and can compromise health. You need to report the nutritional risks you identify to your supervisor. Good nutrition is essential to good health. The reconciliation of the basic problems listed is critical to improved health.

The objective in gerontological nursing is the best health possible for the best possible quality of life. Good nutrition is a powerful tool in making that happen.

BOX 8.1 RISK FACTORS FOR MALNUTRITION IN OLDER ADULTS

Physical immobility

Sensory changes

Poor dentition

Pain

Inability to acquire or prepare food

Depression or loneliness

 ## MANAGING WEIGHT

Monitoring weight also is an effective tool in assessing nutritional status. You need to be attentive to any changes in an older adult's weight. If there is weight gain, perhaps the person needs to become more active. It also is wise to check for edema because the weight gain could be caused by a greater physiological problem. If there is weight loss, this needs to be reported to the registered nurse (RN) to assess for possible causative factors.

Most of the common reasons older adults lose weight are related to physical or socioenvironmental

These older adults are enjoying the socialization that comes with dining together.

Priority Setting

The priority you need to set, to ensure good nutrition for the older adults in your care, is your commitment to their health. First, learn the information in this chapter. There is quite a bit of detail, but these are only the basics. They are the minimum you need to learn to be effective in promoting nutritional health. Then:

1. Apply the information to your own life.
2. Work with team members to see that effective nutritional assessments are done on admission for all patients.
3. Support your nurse manager or volunteer to assist in putting the pertinent information from the assessments into the care plans.
4. Go further and put up signs so the staff will know what assistance and encouragement each person needs. Examples are: "Offer fluids or juice every 2 hours and record." "Cut up fresh fruit for Mrs. Jonas." "Stay and visit with Mr. Tanaki while he eats. Encourage him to eat more food." "Mr. Welling has a food journal at the desk. Please record all food consumed."

As a caring professional, you are one member of the health-care team who can work with others to identify and manage nutritional problems that exist with older adults.

changes. Older adults generally have less mobility and may be unable to prepare meals efficiently or go shopping. Older people generally don't like to eat alone so they are less likely to eat complete meals. Some elderly people are forgetful and may neglect to prepare meals.

Older adults often have a decreased income, so they may not have the money or transportation to obtain adequate food. I remember an elderly woman who attended a gerontological clinic and asked me if it was "OK" for her not to take her antihypertensive medication so she could buy food. This is a serious problem because standard Medicare does not cover medications, so without a supplemental insurance, medications are very expensive for someone on a set income. A thorough and caring interview should reveal many of these problems and others that are age related.

There are several disease-related reasons why an older adult may lose weight. Are there changes in health that could cause weight loss, such as a prolonged illness? Does the older adult have metabolic changes that affect food absorption, digestion, or elimination? Have you noticed the older adult experiencing chewing or swallowing difficulties, or an inability to self-feed or even to see the food? Perhaps the person is depressed, or maybe the food does not taste good. If you are doing home care, there could be reasons the older adult cannot purchase, prepare, or eat the food. Be sure to ask about any problems related to nutrition. Part of a good assessment would be to ask the older adult why, in his or her opinion, the weight loss is happening.

Reasons for weight gain can be related to the process of aging. Weight gain is a problem for people of any age but seems worse for elderly persons who often have health conditions that can decrease their activity level such as arthritis or heart disease. In addition, as the human body ages, it has less lean body mass (muscle), and an equal amount of increased fat tissue (adipose tissue), which leads to a decrease in the basal metabolic rate (BMR). Unless people compensate for that normal physiological change by eating less, they gain weight. Because adipose tissue metabolizes more slowly than lean body mass, it does not burn calories as quickly.

TRACKING NUTRITIONAL INTAKE

During an illness, nutrition performs a vital role in the body's ability to heal. The critical foods—foods that provide energy and nutrients—are divided into three groups: carbohydrates, proteins, and fats. Each food group is necessary to maintain and repair the body during health and illness. It is important for you to have the knowledge to assess the inclusion of these food groups in a person's diet. This assessment can be done by evaluating if the person's diet includes a variety of fruits and vegetables and meats or other protein-rich foods, including grains. The assessment can be done by observing what the older adult is eating during mealtime or by keeping a food journal. If you have observed a patient or resident eating minimal amounts of food or showing signs of listlessness, you should talk to the RN about the problem and perhaps suggest a food journal. A food journal is a designated place where the person removing the food tray writes down not only the percentage of the food eaten but also the actual food. Then someone, such as a dietitian, is assigned to determine if the person is eating enough calories and specific nutrients. It may be helpful to complete a food journal for Mrs. Salvador in an effort to see exactly what she is eating at each meal. The journal needs to be kept for only 3 to 5 days. It is a great way to gather the detailed information needed to assist an older person with good nutrition. The dietitian is an excellent resource when there is a problem with someone not eating nutritious foods.

A review of the food groups, carbohydrates, proteins, and fats, can help you in your ability to assess and evaluate nutritional needs of older adults. Carbohydrates, proteins, and fats are found in various fruits and vegetables, meats, milk, and breads and cereal foods. It is important for older adults to eat a variety of foods with these nutrients to ensure that the body can maintain and repair itself.

NUTRITIONAL NEEDS OF OLDER ADULTS

Regardless of the health status of an older adult, he or she needs to have food that provides calories for energy and nutrients to maintain body functions. A person's food needs for optimal health change with age, physical activity, and health status. In 2011, the United States Department of Agriculture debuted a new visual depiction of suggested daily food intake called MyPlate, thereby replacing MyPyramid. Scientists at Tufts University introduced MyPlate for Older Adults that describes the nutritional needs for individuals as they age. The modified graphic shows a plate divided into four sections; vegetables and fruits, whole grains and breads, protein and fats, oils and spices. The size of the section represents which types of food should be consumed in what quantity. Each section displays pictures of the types of foods that can be eaten each category. The graphic also includes a section representing physical activity and liquids that can be consumed as part of a good nutrition plan.

The new MyPlate food guide is important to your knowledge base for teaching and supporting older people in their quest for nutritional health. Frequent use of the food guide will assist you in mastering the information necessary to give meaningful nutrition information to your patients. The food guide will be helpful to you in teaching Mrs. Salvador what she should be eating.

Carbohydrate Foods

There are two types of carbohydrates: complex and simple. Complex carbohydrates are those that the body breaks down slowly and that sustain energy over a longer period. Simple carbohydrates differ from complex carbohydrates in that they are easier for the body to digest and they provide a source of quick energy.

You need to know which foods provide carbohydrates that promote health. Carbohydrates come from grains, beans, nuts, milk, meat, fruits, and vegetables. Honey, molasses, sugar, and syrups also contain carbohydrates. The more carbohydrate foods are processed, the more the dietary fiber will be broken down, and some of the carbohydrate nutritional value will be lost. Simple carbohydrates come from milk and foods high in sugar content, and they are a source of quick energy. MyPlate provides a visual representation of the sources of carbohydrates that need to be included in a healthy diet.

Protein Foods

Sources of food rich in proteins come from plants and animals. Plant sources of proteins come from grains and include breads, rice, cereals, and pasta. Dried beans and dark green, deep yellow, and starchy vegetables are considered good sources of plant proteins. Animal sources of proteins come from milk, cheese, yogurt, meat, fish, and poultry. Refer to the MyPlate food guide for a visual representation of the

MyPlate for Older Adults

MyPlate for Older Adults. With permission of the Tufts University School of Nutrition.

This couple has learned the value of healthy nutritious food. Their meals focus on fresh fruits and vegetables, sodium restriction, calcium intake through dairy products, and low-fat proteins.

Critically Examine the Following:

To help you to be effective in assessing the nutritional status of others, you need to evaluate your own eating patterns and nutritional condition. This will help you be more understanding of the potential difficulty of managing a nutritious menu for older people in your care. Go to http://www.choosemyplate.gov/. Explore the site to see how you are doing. Keep a food diary for 3 days. How would you assess your eating habits? What do you need to change to make your diet healthier?

QSEN

COMPETENCY: Patient-Centered Care (Knowledge, Skills, Attitudes)

Providing Patient Education on Nutrition

Eating nutritious diets is important for older adults. However, many older adults may not know how to eat in a healthy way. For patients newly diagnosed with a chronic illness, such as diabetes, they may not know what foods to eat—or not eat—that will help with the management of their illness. Nurses play a key role in providing patients with nutritional education. You can use the MyPlate guide to show patients which foods to eat for a healthy diet in general. For patients on a special diet, you can work with the nutritionist in your facility to develop individualized plans for each patient. It is important to take the time to sit with the patient and a family member to review the diet plan answering any questions.

1. What is the process you will use to develop a diet plan for an older adult?
2. How will you assess whether a diet plan is meeting the nutritional outcomes for an individual?

Most older adults eat healthier meals and eat more of the meal if they are eating with family members. This daughter and her son have dinner with grandma three times a week. This assures the grandma of good food and company. She says she really looks forward to these dinners.

Proteins are divided into structural and functional categories. Structural proteins contain the amino acids that make up the hair, muscles, tendons, and skin. Functional proteins help the body perform the activities that keep the body alive, such as moving oxygen through the circulatory system. Hemoglobin; insulin; and myosin, which is found in muscle tissue and is the reason the muscles can contract, are functional proteins. The body requires a supply of proteins to repair worn-out or damaged tissues and to build up new tissue. They also play an important part in maintaining the body's water balance in metabolic activities and the body's defense system (U.S. National Library of Medicine, 2014).

When using the term *protein*, you need to remember the term *amino acids*. There are thousands of different proteins, and they all are made of various combinations of amino acids. The two classifications of amino acids are essential and nonessential. You should not confuse the terms *essential* and *nonessential* amino acids with their value to the body because both kinds of amino acids

sources of proteins that need to be included in a healthy diet.

Proteins are the building blocks of the body. They are necessary for building and repairing body tissue and are important for Mrs. Salvador as she recovers from her accident and subsequent surgery.

are important for good health. Nonessential amino acids refer to amino acids that the body can make itself. Essential amino acids are the amino acids that the body cannot make itself and must be part of the diet. Essential and nonessential amino acids are necessary for the body to function properly.

The terms *complete* and *incomplete proteins* refer to the foods that supply proteins to the body. A complete protein comes from animal sources and contains essential and nonessential amino acids. Incomplete proteins come from plant sources, but plants do not include both essential and nonessential amino acids. By eating different plant sources during the same meal, the body gets a supply of complete and incomplete proteins that provide the essential and nonessential amino acids for building, maintaining, and repairing the body. Think of eating beans and rice in the same meal. Each of these foods is an incomplete protein food. When they are eaten in the same meal, however, the body is able to use them as a complete protein. This way of obtaining protein for the body is used by millions of people who either prefer rice and beans instead of meat or cannot afford fresh meat to eat.

Age, gender, chronic diseases, fevers, infections, surgery, and traumatic injury are factors in determining the need for added protein for the body's maintenance and repair. The primary care provider (PCP) may order a laboratory test to measure the nitrogen level of a recovering older person to determine how well the body is maintaining its tissue. In malnutrition or an illness, the body may not have the proper nitrogen balance to support health. A positive balance of nitrogen indicates that there are adequate sources of protein for the body to use to build and repair tissues. A negative nitrogen balance indicates wasting of muscle tissues and impairment of body organs and their functions.

Urine tests measure protein metabolism. An increase in nitrogen level indicates that excess body tissue is being broken down. A serum albumin measurement helps diagnose protein deficits (Nix, 2012).

When you are collecting urine for laboratory tests that include *creatinine, albumin, transferrin, prealbumin,* or *retinol-binding protein,* and BUN, you will know the urine is being tested for nitrogen balance. The RN will give you instructions on how the urine should be collected. Dietary adjustments may be ordered after the laboratory results have been reviewed by the PCP.

Fat Foods

Fats are a group of foods that, when absorbed into the body, serve as a support and protection for the internal organs. Adipose (fat) tissue serves as a buffer or cushion from an external injury. Fats help to sustain the body's temperature. Certain vitamins—A, D, E, and K—are fat-soluble. The body must have foods containing fats to absorb these important vitamins. Some fat is required by the body to maintain health, but excess fat may lead to a change in the body's hormonal system that can suppress the immune system and leave the person at risk for an infection (Insel, et. al. 2012). Excess fat can also increase the risk of diabetes, heart disease, stroke, and even dementia.

Fats are found in plants such as beans and nuts and in oils produced from plants. Fats also are found in meat, poultry, fish, shellfish, and eggs. The food guide MyPlate provides a visual representation of the sources of fats that are heart healthy, are vital for a healthy body, and should be included in the diet.

Vitamin Foods

Vitamins are classified as either water-soluble or fat-soluble. Water-soluble vitamins are absorbed in water. As mentioned earlier, fat-soluble vitamins require fats for the body to absorb them. The names of vitamins are taken from the alphabet, letters A through K. With one exception, which you will see shortly, vitamins are not produced by the body and must be extracted from foods (or nutritional supplements).

Vitamin A is a fat-soluble vitamin that comes from animal and plant sources. Plant sources of vitamin A are dark green leafy vegetables and deep yellow or orange fruits and vegetables. Vitamin A is necessary for good vision, growth, and immune system function. Studies are ongoing to determine the role of vitamin A in cardiovascular diseases and cancers (Dudek, 2013). You should follow the research on the role of vitamin A in the diet and encourage the people in your care to eat foods that are rich in vitamin A. This information will help them improve or maintain their health. Vitamin A can be stored in the body's fat; a deficit in vitamin A may not be noted for some time. Some older adults take megadoses of vitamin A, which may become toxic. A symptom of excess vitamin A is a yellowish orange skin color. Always ask about the consumption of food supplements and carefully document what is being taken. This is especially important to do with vitamin A intake.

There are several classes of B vitamins, and they all are water-soluble. The B vitamins are listed as the B vitamin complex. Vitamin B_1 (thiamine) is necessary for the nervous system to function correctly and to help older adults have an appetite. Older adults who drink excess alcohol or have had a poor nutritional intake may need to have thiamine supplements. Foods rich in thiamine come from whole grains or enriched cereals, nuts, organ meats, and legumes.

Vitamin B_2 (riboflavin) is essential in building and maintaining healthy tissue. Foods rich in riboflavin are milk products, whole-grain and enriched breads and cereals, eggs, meats, and leafy green vegetables.

Vitamin B_3 (niacin) is essential in maintaining a healthy nervous system and skin and in preventing dementia. Foods rich in niacin are whole grains and enriched breads and cereals that are high in proteins. It is possible, however, for older people to have too much niacin in the diet. Symptoms of niacin toxicity are diarrhea, vomiting, gastric ulcers, and liver damage.

Vitamin B_6 (pyridoxine) assists in the metabolism and use of glycogen that has been stored as a fuel. Pyridoxine is required for brain activity and normal functioning of the central nervous system. Pyridoxine promotes healthy skin. Food sources of pyridoxine are eggs, whole-wheat products, peanuts, walnuts, and animal sources. Pyridoxine can be lost during processing of frozen foods, luncheon meats, and cereal foods. Toxicity from pyridoxine can occur with the inclusion of megadoses from dietary supplements. The classic symptom of toxicity is lack of muscle coordination. An overdose of pyridoxine has the potential for nerve damage as well.

Vitamin B_{12} (cobalamin) is essential for the production of hemoglobin and for proper nervous system function. Anemia and GI and neurological changes can result from insufficient amounts of vitamin B_{12}. The best foods containing vitamin B_{12} are from animal sources. Older adults who do not eat many animal products may require a supplemental source of vitamin B_{12}.

Folate is the most naturally occurring form of folic acid, which is rarely found in foods but is a supplement in vitamins and in fortified foods. Folate is essential to the formation of body cells and hemoglobin. Folate can be found in green leafy vegetables, dried beans and peas, organ foods, and orange juice. Folate from foods cannot be used well by the body; foods enriched with folic acid should be included in the diet (Dudek, 2013).

Low folate blood levels are associated with poor cognitive performance; taking a supplement may prove beneficial. However, there is no indication that a person with a normal folate level will see an increase in cognitive performance or resistance to

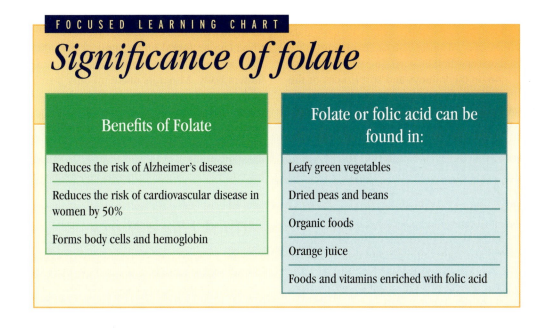

FOCUSED LEARNING CHART

Significance of folate

Benefits of Folate	Folate or folic acid can be found in:
Reduces the risk of Alzheimer's disease	Leafy green vegetables
Reduces the risk of cardiovascular disease in women by 50%	Dried peas and beans
Forms body cells and hemoglobin	Organic foods
	Orange juice
	Foods and vitamins enriched with folic acid

Alzheimer's disease by taking a folate supplement (Takahashi, 2011).

Vitamin C is also known as ascorbic acid. Vitamin C is water-soluble and is easily lost in cooking. Vitamin C cannot be stored by the body, so there must be a daily intake of food containing vitamin C. The body needs vitamin C to build and repair body tissues and bones and to keep teeth and gums healthy. Lack of vitamin C causes wounds to fail to heal, bones to weaken, and muscles to degenerate and puts the older adult at risk for infections and falling. Many foods are good sources of vitamin C. Citrus fruits, strawberries, kiwi fruit, tomatoes, cantaloupe, and dark green vegetables are only a few of the fruits and vegetables that are rich in vitamin C.

Vitamin D is one of the fat-soluble vitamins. vitamin D is not actually a vitamin because it is produced naturally by the body. The body can produce its own vitamin D if there is enough exposure to the sun. However, the ability to synthesize Vitamin D decreases with age. Few people have enough sun exposure, however, to produce sufficient vitamin D. Vitamin D is necessary for the absorption of calcium and phosphorus to maintain bone tissue and many other body functions. Without vitamin D, calcium cannot be absorbed. Older adults are at risk for vitamin D deficiencies if they are not eating enough fortified foods. Older women who have vitamin D deficiency are at risk for bone loss, which puts them at risk for fractures owing to osteoporosis. Vitamin D occurs naturally in very few foods. The sources of vitamin D are the sun, fish oils, and foods fortified with vitamin D. Excessive amounts of vitamin D supplements increase the risk of older adults absorbing more calcium than their bodies need. Increased calcium puts a strain on the kidneys and soft tissues of the body (Dudek, 2013).

Vitamin E (alpha-tocopherol) is a fat-soluble vitamin. Vitamin E provides protection for many body tissues and prevents red blood cells from being broken down. There is evidence that vitamin E aids in wound healing. Studies are ongoing to determine the role of vitamin E in preventing cancer and heart disease. Foods rich in vitamin E include peanut butter, nuts, seeds, wheat germ, and vegetable oils. Vegetable oils have been found to be the best sources of vitamin E. Leafy vegetables and animal sources also provide the body with vitamin E. Large doses of vitamin E may interfere with blood clotting (Dudek, 2013).

Vitamin K is a fat-soluble vitamin. The main roles of vitamin K are blood-clotting functions, aiding in bone development, and regulating blood calcium. Foods that supply vitamin K are leafy vegetables, cabbage, broccoli, cauliflower, fruits, and animal sources. Vitamin K is extracted by bacteria in the intestine from food sources that contain vitamin K. While vitamin K deficiency is rare, it can occur due to long-term antibiotic therapy. Antibiotics prevent the absorption of vitamin K from the intestinal tract. Hemorrhaging can be a complication of vitamin K deficiency, so individuals taking blood thinners should be monitored closely. If a person is taking blood thinners, he or she should limit intake of vitamin K and foods containing vitamin K. (MedlinePlus, 2013).

Think about all the vitamins and how the body requires these vitamins to build, maintain, and repair itself. Older people need to be assessed for vitamin supplements in their diets and encouraged to seek counsel concerning the consumption of megavitamins because of the multiple toxicity possibilities (Dudek, 2013). Consider the body's need for vitamins in helping Mrs. Salvador recover from her accident and subsequent surgery. Which vitamins will be the most most valuable in her recovery?

Mineral Foods

Along with the necessity of vitamins in the diet, you need to recognize the importance of the minerals people require to maintain a healthy body. Minerals are inorganic substances that are found in nature and in the human body. The 54 inorganic substances, called elements, that have been identified can be found on a chemical periodic table; 25 of these elements, or minerals, are found in the human body. Minerals make up only a small part of the body but are found in all body tissues and fluids. Minerals are classified according to the amount needed to maintain a healthy body. Macrominerals, or major minerals, are needed in greater amounts than microminerals, also called trace minerals. Macrominerals and microminerals

Think Like a Nurse

Design a daily meal plan for an older adult taking a blood thinner. Which foods will you include? Which foods will you suggest the person does not eat?

are essential for the body (Dudek, 2013). Included in the macrominerals are calcium, phosphorus, sodium, magnesium, chloride, and potassium. These minerals are known as electrolytes and can be lost as a result of vomiting, diarrhea, excessive sweating, or urination. The electrolytes must be kept in balance, or the older adult is at risk for complications.

Calcium is the most prevalent mineral found in the body. Bones and teeth are composed primarily of calcium. In older adults, additional calcium is necessary for the maintenance of bones and teeth. Calcium also is required for many other body functions, including blood clotting, muscle and nerve activity, digestion, and maintenance of blood pressure. Calcium is best absorbed in connection with vitamin D. Calcium is found in milk and milk products, leafy vegetables, legumes, and fortified food products. Osteoporosis can occur if there is a calcium deficiency. Calcium kidney stones are a risk if the body has too much calcium. Mrs. Salvador's calcium intake should be assessed to ensure she is getting the appropriate amount to aid with bone regeneration.

After calcium, phosphorus is the most common mineral in the body. Phosphorus combines with calcium in the maintenance of bones and teeth. Phosphorus is found throughout the body and is required for metabolism and cell membrane maintenance. Phosphorus helps maintain the body's chemical balance and is necessary for vitamin absorption. It is readily available because it is found in all meat products, whole grain products, fruits, and vegetables. Low phosphorus levels are usually not a concern because it is so available in food. High phosphorus levels may be seen in people with severe kidney disease.

Magnesium is necessary for energy, maintaining cell membranes, muscle and nerve function, blood glucose control, and blood pressure regulation. Sources of magnesium are whole grains, green leafy vegetables, dried peas, beans, and nuts (Dudek, 2013). Magnesium deficiencies occur with alcohol abuse and diabetes. Older adults are also prone to magnesium deficiencies because of decreased intake of magnesium and poor absorption in the stomach. Older adults are also more likely to have chronic diseases or take medications that cause magnesium depletion (National Institutes of Health, 2013).

Sodium is responsible for maintaining the water balance in the body. Sodium is necessary

This homeless man has learned where to go for the best meals possible. Some restaurants (e.g., fast-food places) discard their uneaten food at specific times of the day. This assures their customers of fresh food. It also provides this man with a good burger that is reasonably fresh. He also goes to the Salvation Army for lunch and the homeless shelter for dinner. Most of his day is spent outdoors, even on cold days like this one.

for glucose activity and nerve and muscle functions. Sodium deficiency is rare unless an older adult has chronic diarrhea, vomiting, excessive sweating, or kidney disease. The body usually excretes excess sodium through the kidneys. Excess sodium (hypernatremia) may cause hypertension in some people and edema in people with kidney disease, congestive heart failure, and cirrhosis of the liver.

Sodium is found naturally in foods such as milk, beets, and celery. Sodium is also found in processed foods and is often added during cooking and at the table. To lower sodium levels, an older adult may be advised to limit salt intake and to reduce processed foods in the diet.

Chloride, is found in the body's tissues and fluids. Despite the fact that the body contains only a small amount of chloride, this mineral is important in digestion and in maintaining water balance. Chloride partners with sodium (sodium chloride) in the diet. Chloride deficiency is rare but can occur with excessive perspiration, vomiting. or diarrhea. Too much chloride can result in hypertension and cause edema in people with congestive hearth failure and kidney disease. (Dudek, 2013).

Potassium is found in body fluids. Potassium is responsible building muscle, metabolic activities, electrical activity of the heart, and regulation of acid-base balance. The best sources of potassium are all meats and fish, milk and yogurt, and unprocessed fruits and vegetables. Potassium is water-soluble and can be lost when vegetables are cooked in water. An older adult who has a potassium deficiency (hypokalemia) may have muscle weakness or abnormal heart rhythms. Decreased amounts of potassium can be caused by diuretics, excessive use of laxatives causing prolonged diarrhea, and certain kidney disorders. Increased levels of potassium (hyperkalemia) can cause severe heart arrhythmias. Excessive amounts of potassium can be caused by certain heart medications, poor kidney function, and severe infection (MedlinePlus, 2012).

Minor minerals, which are called trace minerals, in the human body include iron, zinc, iodine, and fluoride. Iron is part of hemoglobin, carries oxygen throughout the body, and aids in metabolism. Deficits in iron may be caused by poor absorption by the body or health conditions that cause blood loss. Deficits caused by poor absorption or health conditions that cause blood loss reduce the effectiveness of the immune system, and cause anemia, which may cause weakness and fatigue. Excess iron may increase risk of infections, organ damage, and joint disease. Foods rich in iron are fortified breads and cereals, red meat, and legumes (Dudek, 2013).

Zinc is essential for wound healing and it aids in metabolic and immune functions. Zinc comes from animal sources, legumes, whole grains, and dairy products. Deficits in zinc may cause abnormal glucose tolerance, impaired wound healing, weight loss, loss of night vision, and diarrhea. Too much zinc can cause anemia, vomiting, renal failure, malabsorption of calcium, dizziness, and muscle pain (Dudek, 2013). Research has found that zinc can decrease the severity and duration of the common cold and can delay the progression of age related macular degeneration (National Institute of Health n.d.)

Iodine is needed for metabolism, normal thyroid function, and the production of thyroid hormones.

An iodine deficiency can cause hypothyroidism or an enlarged thyroid. Excess iodine is rare and may decrease the function of the thyroid gland. Sources of iodine are iodized salt, dairy products, and seafood (Dudek, 2013).

Fluoride has a role in bone and dental integrity. Fluoride's main source is water, to which it has been added as a supplement. The main concern with lack of fluoride is dental caries. Excess fluoride in the diet may cause damage to bones and joints (Dudek, 2013).

The quality of foods containing minerals is related to the soil where the foods are grown. Fruits and vegetables that are grown in soils rich in a particular mineral contain more of that mineral. The mineral content of foods is hard to determine because fruits and vegetables are grown in various areas of the world (Dudek, 2013).

Water

Fluids are considered an essential component of the older adult's nutrition plan. Water is the most plentiful and easiest dietary means of fluid intake. How much water or fluid the older adult should consume is determined by gender, age, chronic diseases, physical activity, metabolic activity, and heat exposure (Dudek, 2013). Older adults are at risk for dehydration because they often neglect drinking adequate amounts of fluids during the day.

Water is the main component of the body and has a vital role in maintaining body temperature. It serves as a transport for nutrients and wastes, is a lubricant to body parts, is a solvent for the body's chemical processes, and gives form to the cells and tissues of the body. Water can be found in soft drinks, juices, coffee, tea, milk, and foods containing high contents of water (Dudek, 2013).

Water helps maintain the body's temperature. Heat may be lost from the body by physical activity or an increase in temperature in the environment. The water lost by sweating during an activity or the increase of environmental temperature serves as a coolant to maintain a normal temperature. When fluid is lost through the cooling process, older adults need to increase fluid intake (Nix, 2012).

Blood and other body and tissue secretions are transported or circulate through the body. The circulated fluids carry oxygen, nutrients, and other materials to all body cells. Circulating fluids also

Point of Interest

It is best to check skin turgor over the forehead or sternum in older adults. You check the skin turgor by softly pinching the skin and then observing how fast the skin returns to normal. If it is slow to return to normal, the person is dehydrated.

carry waste materials from the cells. Fluids provide for smooth joint activity. Fluid also cushions the contact between the organs (Dudek, 2013).

Water is essential for the chemical processes in the body. Water is the necessary solvent the body uses for producing the chemical solutions required for health maintenance. It is vital for the body to maintain a water balance. Older adults are at risk for dehydration because of inadequate fluid intake, not feeling thirsty, medications, perspiration, and chronic diseases. You must remember to assess the older adult for oral fluid intake.

Body Electrolytes

As mentioned earlier in the chapter, the particles (minerals) in the body's solutions are made up of electrolytes and plasma proteins (Nix, 2012). The minerals that make up the body's electrolytes are calcium, phosphorus, sodium, magnesium, chloride, and potassium. Each of these minerals carries a chemical charge. Some have a positive charge, and others have a negative charge. You may decide to do a quick review of chemistry to understand better the chemical processes that happen in maintaining an electrolyte balance. For now, you need to be aware that all of the electrolytes must be maintained in a chemical state of neutrality. Any imbalance puts a person at risk for complications. These electrolytes are moved through the body by fluids. Consider fluids and electrolytes lost as a result of vomiting, diarrhea, excessive perspiration, or urination, and then consider the person's potential for electrolyte imbalance.

Plasma proteins consist of protein and globulin. They are the major substance in blood circulation and control the water movement in and out of cells. With this understanding, you should realize that blood volume is strongly influenced by plasma proteins. Electrolytes and plasma proteins must be kept in balance to maintain healthy body functions (Nix, 2012). Plasma proteins were discussed earlier in this chapter.

DIET PLANS

As the LPN, you need to be aware of the various diet plans that can be used to meet the nutritional needs of the people in your care.

A regular diet is given to older adults who are healthy, have no special nutritional needs, and are capable of making nutritious food choices. Amounts of foods depend on the person's appetite, and selections of foods are made by personal likes and dislikes.

A modified diet is given to older adults if they have a prolonged illness and have not eaten or if they have difficulty chewing or swallowing food. Foods in the modified diet range in consistency from clear liquids to soft foods.

Clear-liquid diets are foods that are liquid at room temperature and can be seen through. The PCP or dietitian needs to write directions about what foods are to be included in this diet. Clear or strained juices, teas, carbonated drinks, clear broths, and gelatins are some of the choices. Most clear-liquid diets do not provide adequate nutritional requirements so should be used for the shortest period of time possible. Patients receiving clear-liquid diets are moved to a full-liquid diet as soon as their health condition allows.

Full-liquid diets are composed of the foods included in the clear-liquid diet with the addition of foods that are liquid at room temperature but are not necessarily clear. This includes custards, ice cream, milk, some strained cereals, fruits, and vegetables. The full-liquid diet meets more of the person's dietary requirements but not all nutritional requirements. The dietitian gives you instructions on the food to include in a full-liquid diet.

Foods in the soft diet include those from a regular diet that have been modified for people who have difficulty chewing foods because of improperly fitting dentures or sore gums. Foods in this diet are mashed, chopped, or ground.

A therapeutic diet may be ordered for people who need tailored nutritional choices. The person may need more calories or fewer calories in the diet. There may be an order to increase or decrease the amounts of carbohydrates, proteins, or fats in the diet. The person may need dietary restriction on foods containing sodium, potassium, iron, or micronutrients. Examples of therapeutic diets are a diabetic diet or a low-sodium diet for a person with hypertension. Fluid restrictions may be necessary for some patients with chronic kidney disease. Older adults may have food allergies or may be unable to tolerate some foods; such foods should not be included in the diet.

There are health conditions in which a person's GI system can digest food but the person may be unable to consume food. Enteral, or tube, feedings are required for these people. Commercial or blended formulas are used to provide nutritional support by using a nasogastric or gastronomy feeding tube placed directly into the GI tract through the abdomen. The physician and dietitian determine types and amounts of formulas to be used.

Older adults with more extensive illnesses or injuries may require parenteral nutrition (PN). PN is administered intravenously. An RN is responsible for the maintenance and monitoring of this type of therapy. (Dudek, 2013). The RN instructs you, the LPN, on your responsibility in monitoring a patient receiving PN. If you need specific information on this therapy, be sure to ask. Do not pretend you know what you are doing if the opposite is true.

It is the responsibility of the nurse to assure the older adult is receiving the appropriate meal plan to meet his or her nutritional needs. By working with the PCP and a nutritionist an appropriate meal plan can be determined.

> ## Think Like a Nurse
>
> You are assigned to care for Mrs. Pearson, an 81-year-old woman who has had abdominal pain, nausea, and vomiting. Which type of diet most likely will be ordered for her? Explain why.

 ## CONCLUSION

Good nutrition is important for older adults as they age. As a nurse, it is important to assess your patient's diets and eating habits on a regular basis. Providing the older adults you care for with the appropriate nutrients in his or her diet can ensure a strong immune system, aid in healing, and help in the management of chronic conditions. Regardless of the type of diet the older adult you are caring for may be eating, you must remember to provide a pleasant atmosphere to encourage eating. Clear the area where the food will be set and open food containers as needed. Be unhurried and pleasant, and talk to each person. It may be necessary for you to assist the person in eating the meal. If so, be patient and kind as you perform this aspect of your job. Spending time with the person and sharing a pleasant conversation is a good time for you to educate, support, and assess the older adult's dietary needs.

Not all older adults for whom you will be caring for are in frail health. People are living longer and may have chronic diseases such as arthritis, heart disease, or diabetes. Many older adults consider themselves to be healthy, however, even with these chronic conditions. Under the supervision of the RN, you will have the opportunity to teach older adults about proper nutrition.

CASE STUDY SOLUTIONS

1. If Mrs. Salvador was losing weight before this current admission, you will want to consider doing the full nutritional risk assessment. Any problems identified on the assessment will need to be addressed before Mrs. Salvador goes home. If the weight loss occurred since her admission, you will want to address issues directly related to the care and treatment provided to her. Pain medications and a decrease in physical activity can decrease appetite. If Mrs. Salvador is eating her meals in her private room, you may want to encourage her to eat with the other residents or have family members visit during meal times. You will also need to make sure the food that is served is to Mrs. Salvador's liking.

2. Mrs. Salvador may have foods specific to her culture that are not being served at the facility. If this is the case, check with the facility dietitian to see whether these foods can be provided.

3. Additional areas you will want to address from the assessment are the effects of the current illness on eating patterns, issues with chewing, and medications affecting diet. If the weight loss began before admission, you will want to address all 10 questions.

4. Any identified risks should be documented and addressed with the RN.

REVIEW QUESTIONS

1. You are completing a nutritional assessment on an older adult. Which of the following statements should be of concern?
   1. "I eat at least three meals a day."
   2. "I have access to food."
   3. "Because of my arthritis I find it difficult to prepare my meals."
   4. "My husband and I eat our meals together."

2. Consider an older adult with bone and soft tissue injuries from a fall. Which diet would be the most effective for this type of person?
   1. High-carbohydrate diet, which would assist in giving the person enough energy for physical therapy.
   2. 1000-calorie diet, which would assist in weight reduction and make ambulation easier.
   3. High-protein, high-carbohydrate diet, which would assist in cellular rebuilding and energy.
   4. TPN, which would provide all nutrients and save energy for the older person.

3. Which of the following diets would be appropriate for an older adult who has problems with blood clotting?
   1. Diet low in sodium
   2. Diet low in potassium
   3. Diet high in vitamin A
   4. Diet high in vitamin K

4. All of the following can cause electrolyte imbalances *except:*
   1. Vomiting
   2. Diuretics
   3. Diarrhea
   4. Antibiotics

5. You admit a man who is very lethargic. Through your admission interview, you identify that he is a chronic alcoholic. He is thin and has poor skin turgor. You are concerned about his overall nutrition. He states that he *never* eats green and leafy vegetables. What nutrient do you recognize he needs and is not receiving?
   1. Magnesium
   2. Chloride
   3. Sodium
   4. Phosphorus

REFERENCES

Dudek, S.G. (2013) *Nutrition essentials for nursing practice*. (7th ed.). New York, NY: Lippincott Williams & Wilkins

Insel, P., Ross, D., McMahon, K., & Bernstein, M. (2012). *Discovering nutrition* (4th ed.). Sudbury, MA: Jones & Bartlett Learning.

MedlinePlus (2012). Potassium in diet. https://www.nlm.nih.gov/medlineplus/ency/article/002413.htm

MedlinePlus (2013). Vitamin K. Retrieved from https://www.nlm.nih.gov/medlineplus/vitamink.html

National Institutes of Health (2013). Magnesium. http://ods.od.nih.gov/factsheets/Magnesium-HealthProfessional/#h5

Nix, S. (2012) *Williams' basic nutrition and diet therapy*. (14th ed.). St. Louis, MO: Mosby.

Tabloski, P.A. (2013). *Gerontological nursing*. (3rd ed.). Upper Saddle River, NJ: Prentice Hall. Takahashi, P.Y. (2011). www.mayoclinic.org/diseases-conditions/alzheimers-disease/expert-answers/folic-acid-supplements/faq-20058055

U.S. National Library of Medicine (2014). What are proteins and what do they do? http://ghr.nlm.nih.gov/handbook/howgeneswork/protein

WEB RESOURCES

Choose MyPlate: http://www.choosemyplate.gov/
MyPlate for Older Adults: http://hnrca.tufts.edu/my-plate-for-older-adults/

Culturally Specific Care

9

DIANE LEGGETT-FIFE

LEARNING OUTCOMES

1. Define the differences between culture and ethnicity.

2. Identify health-care needs of black Americans.

3. Identify health-care needs of Asian Americans.

4. Identify health-care needs of Hispanic Americans.

5. Identify health-care needs of European Americans.

6. Identify health-care needs of Jewish Americans.

7. Identify health-care needs of Native Americans.

CONCEPTS

Advocacy

Ethics

Communication

Caring Interventions

Diversity

Family

Culture

CASE STUDY

During the genetic cleansing that took place in the former Yugoslavia, numerous refugees came to your community to live. Many of them had watched their family members be raped, tortured, and killed. They had nothing of material value and often no family.

You were assigned, as a volunteer, to work with one family. That was amazing in itself because it was an entire family! You met them at the airport and took them to their roomy and fully furnished apartment. You showed them how the bathroom worked and the shiny new oven and refrigerator and were pleased that there were enough bedrooms for them to sleep comfortably. Supper had been brought in by a local church group, so you left them in their new home and confirmed that you would be back in the morning to assist them in any way you could. It all felt good to you.

The next morning you were at their home bright and early because you were excited about what you would do with them that day. After knocking several times, you let yourself in and were shocked by what you found. No one slept in the beds, no one used the new sheets and blankets, and it appeared that no one used the toilet or shower (the new towels were unused on the racks). You found the family in the living room all sleeping together in a big knot of people. Also, there was a stack of small pieces of wood by the oven. You knew by what you saw that you had missed something major when you oriented these people to their new surroundings. After finding the family in the situation described, what are you going to do?

INTRODUCTION

I was raised in a state where 75% of the population is white, and 75% to 80% is Christian. Utah is a farming state, and I knew many Latinos who traveled through as they worked in the fields, but I didn't see a black person until I was 16. (I saw them on television, but not in person.) Because there are two reservations in Utah, I knew about Native Americans, but I did not actually know any because they lived and went to school on the reservations. My ancestors were Utah pioneers who sacrificed much to live where they had religious freedom. I feel confident in saying that unless you were born and raised in Utah, our cultures are very different.

The concept of culture is complex, but I have a definition that you should find useful. Culture consists of the nonphysical traits we inherit. I am referring to the stories our parents and grandparents tell us (for me it was the pioneer stories of my ancestors) and the traits we learn from simply being in our family or community groups. For me, it was a strong Scandinavian work ethic, family closeness, and a desire to better one's life. My Danish and Swedish emigrant ancestors were very poor, and each generation has worked to provide a higher standard of living for their children. Religion often is considered a significant aspect of one's cultural identity as well.

One common problem with culturally specific care is the tendency for each of us to be ethnocentric. This means that we, as people, think

⏱ Priority Setting

The priority for this chapter is clear: for you to give culturally specific care. That requires the skills of holism and caring and the ability to use the nursing process. This chapter gives you a basic background for several different cultural and ethnic groups. You need to focus on the individual, however. Talk to the person; take the time and make a genuine effort to understand the individual's personal needs based on culture and ethnicity as well as the more routine information you need to gather such as health and medication history. What you discover as personal needs for the individual may amaze you. Your responsibility is to meet those needs to promote healing.

that our "way" is the best way. When one thinks that his or her culture is superior to all others, there is a tendency to dismiss the cultural needs of other people—the thought being that each person should want to be just like you and your culture! This is an act of human nature. For example, when Christian missionaries traveled to the Pacific Islands, they tried to turn the natives into "proper" English men and women. The same thing happened to the Native Americans. Children were taken from their parents during the 9-month school year and were placed in the homes of "proper" white families in an effort to acculturate them. Hitler and others displayed their ethnocentric behavior by killing the "lesser" culture.

As a soon-to-be professional nurse, you need to be aware of any tendencies you have at ethnocentrism and squash them when you are in the clinical setting. As a professional nurse, your objective—your priority—needs to be cultural sensitivity that results in culturally specific care.

Culture is related to ethnicity, but it is not the same thing. Culture is our nonphysical inheritance, whereas ethnicity is the physical inheritance. I have blonde and blue-eyed sisters (you guessed it!); they got those physical characteristics from the Swedes and Danes on my family tree. When you discuss ethnic and cultural aspects of people, you are talking about transcultural nursing. This is a specialized arena of nursing in which cultural awareness is a priority of care. Nurses can earn a master's degree in transcultural nursing; however, you are not expected to know that body of information on such a high level. You simply need to recognize that ethnic and cultural aspects of older adults are an important concept of care.

A basic principle of transcultural nursing is being aware of the need to focus on it to give the best care possible. The other concept reinforced in this chapter is the common sense needed to give transcultural or culturally specific care to others that also addresses ethnic needs. For example, it just does not make sense to assist a Christian out of bed five times a day to face east and pray, just as it does not make sense to require a Muslim to stay in bed when what he wants is to get out of bed, face east, and pray five times a day. You need to be sensitive to the cultural needs of others in all aspects of their lives. Promoting the cultural values of any person assists them in achieving the developmental task of gerotranscendence, which

is a concept you should recognize as essential to aging well. In this chapter, your common sense will be enhanced as we discuss ethnicity and culture in several different ways.

ETHNICITY AND CULTURE AS CARING BEHAVIORS

There are multiple aspects to ethnicity and culture. Following is a story from an experienced nurse that addresses ethnicity and culture:

When I was younger and unmarried, I wanted to travel and still use my nursing skills. My ancestors were from Denmark, so that was a place I wanted to spend some time. I finally found a hospital that was eager to take me even though I did not speak Danish. I got my passport and traveled to the land of my ancestors. It all was very exciting. When I reported to work the first day, I realized I had entered a world totally unknown to me as an American citizen. The name of the hospital was exotic and quite beautiful when it was written in Danish. However, the translation to English was something like "The Torture Victims' Hospital." I was confident in my nursing skills before leaving for Denmark. I had worked for 3 years in a high-level intensive care unit (ICU) and knew my way around the system of health care. However, nothing had prepared me for my new job.

Torture victims? There was nothing like that in the United States! I was stunned when the nurse orienting me toured me through the building. The lights were turned low, and everyone walked quietly and spoke in semi-whispers. There was not an overhead public address system, nor were there visitors milling around. It was a building filled with men and health-care providers who moved about in the semi-darkness in a quiet and surreal manner.

I learned that the men, mostly former soldiers and spies from across Europe, were victims of torture from the Communist regimes of Eastern Europe. These were men who had fought or spied in places with danger that was absolutely unknown to me. My entire life changed because of the 6 months I was there. I learned much more than simply discovering the land of my ancestors. The men there often could not be touched because it brought back memories and/or fears of their torture. It took months for a patient to develop trust with any of the hospital employees. They didn't even trust each other because so many of them had been spies and felt that others were spying on them. It was a place of no laughter. The low lighting and diminished sound were to avoid startling the men, as they had the basic "fight" reaction to being startled. They were, after all, soldiers.

Because most of the men had been spies, they spoke English, as do most Danish citizens, so the language was not a problem for me. I spent my 6 months there quietly serving those men in any way I could. In addition, I learned a harsh reality concerning the price of freedom.

The ethnicity of the patients in this story would indicate that they inherited high IQs; healthy, strong bodies without chronic diseases; and strong will or self-concept that allowed them to survive torture without any apparent mental illness. The cultural aspects of the men indicated that they were patriotic and loyal, self-disciplined, and tenacious (they didn't give up).

The ethnicity (physical changes) of the United States is ever changing. The 2010 Census (2010) indicated that 74% of the U.S. population was white (United States Census Bureau, 2011). The prediction is that in 2050 that number will decrease to 47%. The prediction also indicates that the Hispanic population will grow from 14% to 29%; Asian, from 5% to 9%; and black will remain unchanged at 13% (Passel & Cohn, 2008). I realize that 2050 is a long way into the future; however, these numbers relate an ethnic trend. As you work in health care, the number of older people will increase, and the cultural diversity of those older adults will become even more diverse. The challenge is to be able to give culturally competent care to a greater number of older adults who are more and more diverse. To do so requires learning about different cultures and paying attention to people and their cultural needs as you give them care. Culturally competent care is a basic concept of administering holistic care to others. It is impossible to do this unless you understand and respect the ethnic and cultural core of each person in your care.

One of my nephews was 20 when he left his small rural community to visit other countries. His first real experience was in Latvia, a small country between the Baltic Sea and Russia. He flew into the capital city, Riga, and stayed there for a year.

He spoke the native language (he studied it before going to Latvia) and took the time to meet individuals and families. He was a teacher and spent a great deal of time with people outside of class as well. While in Latvia, he learned about the cultural and ethnic traits of the society. It was fascinating!

Think about the family in the case study. They came to a new area and appeared to be prepared to live the same life as they had been living. The individual working with the family did not ask questions and assumed the family knew about the living conditions. It is important to ask questions whether you are caring for someone culturally different or if you are a visitor in another culture.

This chapter contains a brief overview of the ethnic and cultural traits of several different groups found in the United States. You may be familiar with many of these groups already, but if you aren't, this is a good time to sit down and be "fascinated" by what you are learning. An example of what I mean is in the following story:

I remember one occasion when the daughter of one of the families in Latvia had a bad cold. Her mother called me and asked me to go to the hospital to visit her. I was amazed that her daughter had gone to the hospital and was admitted for a cold. The young lady was in the hospital for 4 days! I also met people (more than one) who took the standard 3 weeks off from work for the flu. I know I wouldn't have a job if I took 3 weeks off for the flu in the United States. The Latvian people look at sickness in a very different way from most Americans. From my personal experience of having a cold, I can say that all I got was cough syrup and my Dad telling me to buck up and get to school. The people of Latvia were responding to their illnesses in the way that was standard for their cultural norm.

 ## BLACK AMERICANS

I will be referring to people whose ancestors came from Africa as blacks or black people. This phrase refers to people who have origins in any of the black racial groups of Africa predominately, but it also includes people from other nationalities with skin that is black in color. Most members of black communities in the United States descend from people who were brought here as slaves from the west coast of Africa. The largest importation of slaves occurred in the 17th and 18th centuries, which means that black people have been living in the United States for many generations. In modern times, numerous black people have immigrated to the United States voluntarily and have traveled from Africa, the West Indian Islands, the Dominican Republic, Haiti, and Jamaica.

Blacks live in all regions of the United States and are represented in every socioeconomic group. They are disproportionately poor, however, with 25.8% of all black people living in poverty (Macartney, Bishaw, & Fontenot, 2013). In addition, a large number of black people live in urban areas surrounded by the symptoms of poverty—crowded and inadequate housing, poor-quality schools, and high crime rates. The living conditions and poverty of many older black adults are considered major contributors to the fact that black men and women die at a significantly younger age than white men and women. Life expectancy for black males in 2010 was 4.7 years lower (71.8 years) than white males (76.5 years), while life expectancy for black females was 3.3 years lower (78.0 years) than white females (81.3 years) (Kolchanek, Arias, Anderson, 2013, Office of Minority and Health Disparities 2007).

Black people have closer family ties when compared with other cultural groups and hold older members of their communities in high esteem because they value the wisdom and knowledge that comes with aging. This valuing may result in fewer black older adults in nursing homes than white older adults. It is unknown if difficulty accessing the health-care system also contributes to this fact.

Older black people often embrace the customs and traditions of their ancestors. The core of their health-care beliefs is often based on being in favor with God or a higher power. This group may express the belief that they do not have much control over their health because it is part of a greater plan. When you give care to older black adults, take the time to determine how you can support the person's health beliefs. That can involve a religious practitioner, the need for family presence, or a traditional healer (Shannon & Hassler, 2014).

The religious beliefs of this group vary, but the majority belong to the Protestant or Muslim religions (Shannon & Hassler, 2014). Some are descendents of Muslims who were brought here as slaves, and others have chosen to convert to Islam. Religious beliefs are an important part of the Muslim lifestyle, and as a health-care provider, you need to be familiar with them. Practicing Muslims eat a Halal diet, which means they do not eat pork or any pork products. You should work with the dietitian to ensure that the food of a Muslim patient is not "contaminated" with pork. There is a potentially serious problem with diabetic Muslims as well. If the individual is prescribed an insulin that is made from pork pancreas, a practicing Muslim will refuse to take it. Consult with the pharmacy to obtain nonpork insulin, and then assure the patient that the insulin is *not* made from parts of a pig so that there will be compliance in taking this critical medication.

Sickle cell anemia is an inherited disease that affects a high proportion of the black population (University of Maryland, 2013). It is genetically inherited, and scientists have concluded that it originally was an adaptation to fight the disease malaria. Sickle cells result in hemolysis and thrombosis of the red blood cells because the deformed cells do not flow properly through the blood vessels.

The symptoms of sickle cell anemia include hemolysis, anemia, and severe pain in the areas of the body where the thrombosed red blood cells are located. Statistics indicate that life expectancy has increased to age 50 years for children diagnosed with the condition. This is an increase from a 1973 life expectancy of only 14 years (University of Maryland, 2013). Some children develop complications that exist for the duration of their lives. The only way to prevent

Critically Examine the Following:

Imagine that you are in a part of the United States where you never have been previously. While there, you encounter the ethnic groups listed in this chapter. Read about the people, and then think about the information. See if you agree with what is written, as I know you have your own experiences with different ethnic and cultural groups. Consider the health-care implications of what you read. Always keep in mind that the information is not designed to stereotype people but to give a general background to different groups of people. Do your best thinking and come to class prepared to discuss your insights and ideas for this chapter.

FOCUSED LEARNING CHART

Poverty is defined as a family of four with an income of $24,230 or less per annum

Government Assistance	Living Conditions	Impact on Health
Public housing	Overcrowded housing	Tuberculosis
Government loans for school	Poor sanitation	Spread of infectious diseases
Medicaid	Homelessness	Diminished personal space
Aid to families with dependent children (AFDC)	Poor nutrition	Diseases of the GI system
Food stamps	Higher crime rates	Emotional detachment from society
Head Start programs	Crowded schools	Nonproductive life
Free school lunch		Malnutrition
		Obesity
		Diabetes mellitus
		Frequent homicide and suicide
		Violence in the streets
		Lack of personal safety
		Poor education with less opportunity for achievement

Note: In 2014, the Census Bureau added the supplemental Poverty Measure, which takes into account other expenditures and placed 10% of those older than age 65 years in the poverty level.

sickle cell anemia is to provide genetic testing and counseling to adults before they have children. This often does not happen because of the prohibitive cost of genetic testing.

The leading causes of death are similar for black and white populations; however, black mortality rates are higher. Blacks die of heart disease, cancer, and strokes at higher rates than whites. Unintentional injury is increased in black men 15 to 34 years old (although these are not elderly men, older men do live in the communities with high homicide rates).

There are many conclusions you can draw from the information you have just read that will assist you in understanding the needs of older

These black older adults have a strong religious background that assists them in the quality of their lives. Would their religion be considered ethnicity or culture?

Point of Interest

Black American infants have the highest infant mortality rate for mothers 20 years of age and older. The percentage of live births to teenage mothers is double that of other ethnic groups. Consider how these facts affect the lives of older black adults.

black adults in your care. My purpose is to inform you so that you can apply the information to your nursing practice. Your purpose is to learn the information and then determine ways, based on the needs of each individual, to increase your sensitivity to the person's personal health-care needs.

 ## NATIVE AMERICANS

American Indians, Alaskan Natives (Eskimos), and Aleuts (who also live predominately in Alaska) are included in the category of Native Americans. In this chapter, *Native American* is the inclusive term used because the aforementioned ethnic groups all were on this continent long before any other people. They were well established before the Europeans came here. In A.D. 1010, they repulsed the Vikings. The Vikings were here for a decade and then left in frustration. As more and more people came to the Eastern shores, the natives of this country were pushed by force west into the wilderness. They died because of exposure to disease brought by the Europeans, which their bodies did not have antibodies to fight, and they died in war trying to defend their homeland.

As Native Americans migrated westward against their will, they carried with them fragments of their culture. Their lives were disrupted, their lands were lost, and many of their leaders and teachers were killed. Yet much of their history and culture remain. Native Americans essentially live in most states, including Alaska, with most of them living in the Western states. Although many Native Americans live on reservations, others live in rural and urban areas.

The Indian Health Service recognizes 566 tribes of Native Americans in the United States (U.S. Department of the Interior, 2014). Each tribe has its own culture, folklore, and folk medicine. To tell you about 1 tribe is to leave out the specifics of 565 other tribes. All tribes have traditional beliefs in Mother Earth and the necessity of having harmony with nature, however. If a person is ill, it is thought to hurt Mother Earth, just as when Mother Earth is hurt by disrespectful behavior (such as pollution and litter), it hurts people. Many traditional Native Americans believe there is a reason for every sickness and pain that relates to their behavior. They often believe that illness is the price to be paid for something they have done in the past or something they are going to do in the future. Often, traditional Native Americans who are ill believe that the illness is the best possible price they can pay for what they have done or will do. Native Americans believe in treating illness despite the person's behavior having been the cause.

Traditional tribes have a medicine man or woman. For some tribes, this person is referred to as a shaman. The shaman is someone who should be welcomed into the room of the person who is ill. There may be dancing and chanting; family members may gather in the room and perform a healing "sing" with the shaman; or there could be incense or healing sand paintings. All of these traditional healing methods need to be respected. It is important for you to provide privacy to the people who come to participate, treat them and what they are doing with respect, and obtain any items they request. Working with a person in this manner is truly practicing holistic health care.

Native Americans often are caught in limbo in terms of modern health care. They are caught between their traditions and modern treatment—the shaman and the physician. Finally, they often are "lost" between the Indian Health Care Services (free access to care for people who live on reservations) and services in the community. It is estimated that 27% to 31% of all Native Americans live in abject poverty (Domrzalski, 2013, United States Department of Commerce [n.d.]). With such destitution comes poor living conditions and the problems that follow such situations. Native Americans have the diseases of the poor, such as malnutrition, tuberculosis, and high maternal and infant death rates. They also have a greater incidence of diabetes mellitus: 2.2 times higher than non-Hispanic whites (American Diabetes Association, 2013). At the beginning of the 20th century, diabetes was very rare in Native Americans. Why the change in a manageable disease? Some say diet and exercise changes from the traditional lifestyle were the causative factors. I was surprised to learn that the cancer survival rate among Native Americans is the lowest of any group in the United States (Native American Cancer Research Corporation, n.d.). Scientists do not give an explanation for this occurrence. Now that you know this fact, you have an obligation to take extra time to promote health screening and to perform health education related to cancer to assist older Native Americans in reducing their risks and identifying health problems early.

The seven leading causes of death, in order of frequency, among Native Americans are (Minority Health, 2012):

1. Heart disease
2. Cancer
3. Unintentional injuries
4. Diabetes
5. Chronic liver disease and cirrhosis
6. Stroke
7. Suicide

Close family bonds are typical in Native American groups, with elderly persons being treated as people with wisdom who are to be respected. It is becoming common for younger people to feel that the advice of their elders is no longer relevant to their modern lives, and they tend to ignore older adults.

Evidence-Based Practice

Kim, G., Ford, K.L., Chiriboga, D.A., & Sorkin, D.H. (2012). Racial and ethnic disparities in healthcare use, delayed care, and management of diabetes mellitus in older adults in California. Journal of the American Geriatrics Society 60(12), 2319-2325.

Diabetes affects a large portion of the population of the United States, and it results in disability or death. This study examined a sample of adults 60 years of age and older from five racial and ethnic groups in California who had self-reported a diagnosis of diabetes mellitus. The sample included non-Hispanic white, African-American, Hispanic, Asian, and American Indian and Alaska Native adults. From these groups it was found that African Americans were less likely than whites to seek care or see a care provider and were more likely to visit an emergency department for diabetes care. Hispanics were less likely to take medication for high cholesterol but were more likely to follow the American Diabetes Association guidelines for regular blood glucose testing. Asians were less likely than whites to perform regular blood glucose tests or have feet examined. American Indians/Alaska Natives were less likely to take heart attack prevention medications, but were more likely to use insulin or oral diabetic medication.

Questions

1. What factors may contribute to the differences in access and use of health care for the management of diabetes?
2. What information is provided through this study that would assist in increasing the use of health care for the management of diabetes in the various ethnic or racial groups?

Think Like a Nurse

What are the first five causes of death in your cultural or ethnic group? If you don't know, make an intelligent guess and prepare a list. Is suicide, homicide, or alcoholism on the list? What does it mean to a society when deaths of that nature are on the list of the most common causes of death? What does it mean to have so many people dying from tuberculosis and diabetes? Do you know any Native Americans? If so, perhaps you could talk with one of the elders in the family and ask them what they think of modern health care. You also should learn about traditional healing methods from them.

Many traditional Native Americans may find the questions asked during an assessment or history taking offensive. Asking personal questions can be seen as probing and being disrespectful. You may find it necessary to develop a relationship with the older person before asking the questions you need answered. It would be wise to ask younger family members (adult children) for much of the history, so that you will be seen as less intrusive by the older person. Be sensitive to the nonverbal reactions of the person, and use your common sense based on your knowledge of the culture, communication, and the disease process.

 ## ASIAN AMERICANS

There are nearly 14.7 million Asian Americans in the United States. As a population group, Asian Americans have grown at a faster rate than any other group (Hoeffel, Rastogi, Kim, & Shahid, 2012). Asian Americans come from many different countries. The category of Asians includes people from China, Japan, Korea, Cambodia, India, Malaysia, Pakistan, and the Philippine Islands. The term *Asian* refers to people with origins in the Far East, Southeast Asia, and the continent of India.

The different groups of Asians came to this country for various reasons. The Chinese migration began in the mid-1800s because of a severe drought in China. The Chinese workers were hired for cheap wages to assist in the gold rush and to build the transcontinental railroad. They were victimized and generally treated poorly by Americans who were concerned about them taking their jobs. Many Chinese lived in Chinatowns, which were neighborhoods within larger cities where they went as a place of refuge from the abuse they received from others.

Japanese immigrants started to arrive at about the same time as the Chinese. Similar to the Chinese, they took any job offered to them so that they could support their families. This resulted in a strong prejudice from men who also were afraid of losing their jobs. Restrictive laws were passed that limited immigration and did not allow a person from Japanese descent to marry native-born Americans. The greatest indignity occurred during World War II, when 70,000 American-born Japanese were confined to relocation camps. Immigration laws also restricted Japanese people from coming to the United States at that time.

Filipinos began to immigrate in the 1900s and were employed as farm workers. Koreans began to immigrate in the early 1900s to work on plantations, predominately in Hawaii. Another group of Koreans came to the United States with their husbands, American servicemen, after the Korean War. After the Vietnam War, there was an influx of Vietnamese and Cambodians seeking political refuge.

Asian Americans have the highest median income of any foreign-born group, are well educated and are more likely than other immigrant groups to obtain resident status (Taylor, 2013). All of these factors assist them in being healthier people. Yet they are from a variety of cultures, each with definite concepts and opinions.

The following story from an experienced nurse may help you to understand the involvement of traditional elders in many Asian cultures:

The nurse was working on the pediatric intensive care unit (PICU) and was the primary nurse for a 6-year-old boy who had been hit by a car. He and his parents were of Japanese descent and were American citizens. He had severe injuries and faced a prolonged treatment and rehabilitation regimen. Every day there were new decisions that needed to be made regarding his treatment plan. It was the nurse's responsibility to talk to the parents and explain all options to them for every decision. On the very first day, the nurse became concerned about the parents' inability to make decisions regarding their son's care. The nurse, Roger, needed answers and had concerns that could not wait until the next day as the parents requested. Roger wondered if language was a problem but learned that the parents were born in the United States and had university educations. The nurse shared his experience with the doctor, who also became concerned about the management of the little boy and his multiple problems. Delays were not a good idea based on the criticality of the boy's condition.

It was 2:00 p.m. before the parents came to Roger with a decision. With them were the father's parents. They were immigrants to the United States and were dressed in traditional Japanese clothing. The son was quite formal when he introduced Roger to his father and mother. Something in the way he did the introductions indicated to Roger that it was more than a simple courtesy. Roger invited the four of them to the unit's counseling room for privacy and sat down with them. What he learned in the next few minutes was of priority importance to the care of his young patient. In the traditional culture of this family, the oldest male made all important decisions for family members. If the grandfather was deceased, the grandmother would make the decisions for everyone. This process is based on the traditional Asian respect for the wisdom of older people. The parents wouldn't make decisions that they believed should be made by their parents.

Roger obtained the necessary contact information for the grandfather, introduced the grandparents to the physician and other nursing staff, and felt relief over the management of the care for the little boy. It was clear on the care plan to contact the grandfather for all decision making, and the process worked well. The grandparents always notified the parents about what had or was going to happen, and the family structure was kept intact. Most important, the little boy received the best care that could be given, and there was no communication frustration or distress.

This little boy's name is Youta. He is dressed in traditional Japanese clothing in honor of his grandfather's birthday.

The previous story indicates how most Asian people feel about their elders. Similar to the black and Native American cultures, there is a great deal of respect for older people and their wisdom. As you give care to people from these cultures, *be sure* you address the older person with his or her formal name, such as Mr. Fudano or Mrs. Begay. Do not assume a casual relationship with any older adult. I believe that older people from all cultures deserve the highest level of respect they can be given. This includes how you speak to them, preserve their modesty, and listen to them because it is their wisdom that is so highly valued. You should never give a command to an Asian older adult because it is a definite insult.

In traditional Asian families, older family members are cared for at home. This decision is based on the value the family members place on someone older. Another story that emphasizes this concept happened to a doctorally prepared nurse who was visiting the People's Republic of China in an official capacity:

One evening she had dinner with Madame Chou, the President of the Chinese Nurses Association. This is a very powerful position and one that is appointed by the government. Madame Chou was in her early 60s, and the conversation was done through a Chinese interpreter. Madame Chou asked the American nurse what type of nursing she did in the United States. The nurse, who loved old people and her work in nursing homes, explained with excitement where she did her clinical practice in nursing homes. Madame Chou visibly reacted negatively to what was being said. She even pulled back from the table. The nurse quit talking and apologized for anything she said that had been offensive. Madame Chou responded that she was concerned that the nurse was so happy to be cruel to the older people in her country. The dinner did not end on a pleasant note. The next morning the two women were to have breakfast together and then part, as the American nurse was moving on to another part of China. At breakfast, the American nurse apologized again and asked Madame Chou about nursing homes in China. Madame Chou thought for a few seconds and then said there are five. Keep in mind that this is a country with one-fifth of the world's population, and there were five nursing homes! She said they existed for those older people who did not want to be around little children or who had no family with whom they could live when they needed help. Then she made arrangements for the nurse to visit a rural nursing home.

I tell this story to emphasize that you must always be sensitive to the older person in your care; this is a time to develop good common sense based on information about older adults.

Asian Americans born in the United States have the same general good health and similar health problems as other citizens. People from most Asian cultures are comfortable with a physician being in charge of their health management for acute conditions. It is common, however, to use traditional remedies for chronic illnesses. These remedies may include herbs, acupuncture and acupressure, cupping, and spirituality. Allow and support their personal remedies and assist in any way that is appropriate. Always inform the registered nurse (RN) about what is taking place.

 ## EUROPEAN AMERICANS

Most European Americans have white skin and are easily mistaken for someone who has lived in the United States throughout his or her life. Many of them speak English, and, depending on how long the European has spoken English, there may or may not be an accent of the person's country of origin. European immigration started with the Pilgrims and has continued since that time.

Each European country, similar to each Native American tribe, has its own individual culture from its region of the world. European Americans are as diverse as the people of the United States because all European countries have experienced constant immigration. The following story makes a point about the need for your sensitivity and thoroughness in giving nursing care to Europeans:

I remember being assigned an older white man who was admitted to the surgical preoperative area. The man was there for abdominal surgery that day; his wife accompanied him. The couple was well dressed and knowledgeable about the surgery. All went well until I came back on duty early the next morning and noted that Mr. Swensen had not received any pain medication since his late return from the recovery room. Being a firm believer in the

concept that pain must be managed for optimum healing to take place, I went to his room immediately. He was pale; however, his dressing was secure and without drainage, his vital signs were within normal limits, and when asked if he wanted anything for pain, he simply stated, "No, thank you."

I felt concern for this man but also believed in the adage that "what a patient states is his pain level is his pain level." Within an hour, his wife came to visit him and then rushed to the nurse's station screaming with frustration. When I listened to her I learned a valuable lesson. She was very upset because her husband had not received any pain medication since his surgery. According to her, he had severe pain, and she couldn't bear to see him so uncomfortable! I gently took her with me to a quiet place to talk after I asked another nurse to give Mr. Swensen the appropriate pain medication. Mrs. Swensen, an American citizen, had only recently married Mr. Swensen, a native of Sweden. In the Swedish culture, it is considered rude for a person to accept something the first time it is offered. Mr. Swensen was a very proper gentleman who was waiting for the nurse to make to him, the mandatory second offer of the pain medication. When she did not, his upbringing required him to endure the pain unnecessarily. This very unfortunate situation would not have happened if I had known more about his culture, talked with him in more depth about his pain, or talked with his wife. I feel that I missed this critical aspect of Mr. Swensen's health care because I did not use the principles of holistic nursing care.

One of the major differences in health-care delivery between most European countries and the United States is the understanding each has about the responsibility and delivery of health care. Because many European countries have national health-care plans with socialized medicine, there is an expectation that the federal government is responsible for each person's health care. This is in sharp contrast to the United States, which is more individualistic in terms of health care. Health care in the United States is seen as being reliant on family or extended family groups. This change is often a challenging one for older European adults to accept. It definitely makes working within the health-care system challenging. As the nurse, you need to be aware of this potential problem and refer the person or the family to a social worker for more information. Assist the individual by making an appointment with the social worker if necessary.

 ## HISPANIC AMERICANS

The 2010 census indicates that the Latino and Hispanic populations made up more than half the growth of the United States population from 2000 to 2010 (Ennis, Rios-Vargas, & Albert, 2011). The terms *Hispanic* and *Latino* are used interchangeably throughout this section because they are the terms recognized by the U.S. government. These terms refer to people, or their predecessors, who immigrated from Mexico, Puerto Rico, Cuba, Central and South America, Spain, and other Spanish-speaking communities to the United States. This group has the following characteristics:

1. Hispanics live in family households that are larger than those of non-Hispanic whites and have a median age of 27 years.
2. Among the 18- to 24-year-olds, 14% did not complete high school in 2013, which is a decrease from previous years.
3. Hispanics who make it to college are less likely to complete college than whites.
4. The Hispanic jobless rate in 2009 was 12.5%; for whites it was 8.7% and for Asians it was 7.5% (United States Department of Labor, Bureau of Labor Statistics, 2011).
5. Hispanics are more likely than non-Hispanic whites to live in poverty (Ennis, Rios-Vargas, & Albert, 2011; Macartney, Bishaw, & Fontenot, 2013; Maxwell, 2012; United States Department of Labor, 2011).

The previous facts allow us to make several general assumptions. First, the median age of 27 years for this group indicates that there are not as many older people in the Hispanic population. Many of them live in multigenerational homes, which is a positive thing. They probably are poor and do not have a high school education. There are people who are the opposite of this generalized picture, however. As with all ethnic and cultural groups, you need to avoid stereotyping people while still meeting their needs. It is a challenge.

For older Hispanics, traditional beliefs concerning health do not readily work well with modern health-care treatments. Some traditional Hispanics

think that good health is "good luck." When their health is not good, that is simply a mechanism of the "bad luck" they are experiencing. Other traditional Hispanics believe that good health is a gift from God, and as such, it is something not to take for granted. People with this philosophy are expected to maintain their own good health by eating nutritious food, exercising, and getting enough rest. It is the person's responsibility to maintain his or her balance in the universe. Illness may be seen as a punishment for wrongdoings. This belief may

---

QSEN

COMPETENCY: Patient-Centered Care (Skills, Attitudes)

Effective Communication and Valuing Differences

A Hispanic couple has brought Mr. Hernandez, their 73-year-old father, to the emergency department. He is cyanotic and dyspneic, yet he refuses to take oxygen. Neither the children nor the father speak English well, and you know only elementary Spanish. Mr. Hernandez is irritable when you take his vital signs and won't let you finish. He keeps repeating a phrase that you do not understand: "Es mala suerte! Es mi mala suerte!" ("It is bad luck! It is my bad luck!"). The family hovers around Mr. Hernandez, stroking his hand and face and asking you in broken English what could be wrong with him. It is difficult to move around the room with the number of family members arriving to be at the bedside. You leave the room, notify the RN of the situation, and contact an interpreter for the family. You return to the room, try to make Mr. Hernandez comfortable, and offer any assistance for comfort to the other family members.

Patient-centered care means communicating effectively and valuing the differences of individuals (ethnic, cultural, and social backgrounds).

1. Is it appropriate to allow the family members to remain in the room with Mr. Hernandez when he is so irritable and in distress? Why or why not?
2. How did you show respect for the patient and family?
3. What values and needs are important to this family at this time?

result in less compliance with treatments and more involvement of traditional healers, methods, and family members. Those that are acculturated to the United States will be more likely to follow the health practices of the United States. It is important to ask and be aware of the beliefs of those with whom you are working (Mauk, 2014).

Overall, Hispanic cultures assume the responsibility of caring for elderly persons. There are so few older adults that those who live to be older are treated with respect and love. Hispanic people generally do not admit an elderly person to a nursing home; they try to avoid hospital admissions as well. They keenly feel the responsibility to care for older adults in the home surrounded with family. As a culturally aware care provider, you need to assume the role of patient advocate and inform the nurse and appropriate others of the desire for the older person to be cared for in the home, if that is true. In many situations, a hospital admission can be avoided with a strong home health-care plan. This approach requires effective teaching for the family members who are assuming responsibility for the care, and teaching can be a challenge when English is the second language for the people you are teaching. Read the following story from an experienced nurse, and consider how you will teach people with minimal English skills:

I always have been a coronary care nurse and enjoyed the challenge of family and patient teaching very much. There was one situation where I did not feel successful until I did something drastic. Mr. Lopez, a 73-year-old Hispanic man, was admitted to the unit with a massive heart attack. He had a charming wife and three adult children. None of them spoke English well, and I did not speak any Spanish. Because of the language problem, I felt I was not being successful with the teaching. This man had a strict medication regimen, was scheduled for cardiac rehabilitation (a supervised rehabilitation program at the hospital) three times a week and for an echocardiogram (ultrasound examination of the heart), and had critical follow-up appointments with the physician. I had pictures of the medications with their time and dosage, a picture of the supervisor for cardiac rehab (I had the supervisor meet Mr. Lopez earlier in the week) with times and dates, and the appointments written down with directions on how to get to them.

I went over the information for the last time on the day the man was to be discharged. In his broken English, he kept saying, "You have fixed me." I would respond, "No" and would explain again the regimen he needed to follow. He seemed to think that because he was feeling so much better, he was healthy again. I sensed that he would not be following his discharge instructions and was very concerned. This went on for several minutes until I stopped and drew another picture. It was a stick figure of his family. He recognized who they were and was smiling. Then I took a marker and "Xed" out the figure of him and nearly shouted, "You will be dead!" He was taken back by what I said. Then he looked at the picture of his family and the teaching pictures and information I had made for him. He turned toward me and said, "I understand." For the first time, I felt that he did. With his new understanding, I went over the teaching plan again, and he really listened. He took out his pocket calendar and wrote things on it in Spanish. He spoke to his wife in his own language and explained things to her. I felt like there was a future for this man and his family.

I don't know if shouting "You will die!" at someone is the best teaching approach. In this situation, it was effective, although unconventional. For you to be good at teaching people who speak

---

▶ Point of Interest

Envidia, or envy, is considered to be a cause of illness and bad luck. Many traditional Hispanic people think that to succeed actually is a failure. This is based on the idea that people envy a successful person. When friends, family, and neighbors envy a person in the community who has achieved success, that person will blame the envy for any illnesses. Several social scientists have determined that the low economic and success rates of some Hispanic groups can be attributed to belief in Envidia.

English as a second language, you need to focus on your skills and awareness. It is imperative to have access to an interpreter when working with those who do not speak English; you or your facility need to have a list of people with language skills who can be called in such situations.

Another concern to address when caring for older Hispanic people is the weather, especially if this is the first year they are in the United States and your winter climate gets cold. Many Spanish-speaking countries have warm climates, and cold weather is nonexistent. These people need to be taught about Pneumovax and the annual flu shot. You also should check to be sure they have or can afford fuel for warming their homes. The federal government has assistance programs for household heat. You should refer a person in need to a social worker for information.

Another barrier to health care that many Hispanic people encounter is poverty. Similar to so many others we have discussed in this chapter, Hispanic people tend to be poor. Along with poverty are the diseases of poverty, including malnutrition, heart disease, and diabetes. Knowing this should cause you to check the person's laboratory work to determine if any of these conditions are a problem.

It is important to ask older Hispanic adults if they feel safe in their neighborhood. Do they go out for walks? Do they visit a local recreation center? Do they visit with their neighbors? If they do not feel safe doing these things, they may be staying in the house for prolonged periods and should be assessed for depression, muscle disuse, and loneliness. Be creative and use your common sense based on knowledge to assist in resolving such problems. Could a group of elders go for a walk together and, perhaps, be safer? Does the senior center have a bus that could pick the older person up routinely? Including the older adult and the extended family in a discussion of such problems may result in creative solutions.

A serious barrier to receiving modern health care is time orientation. To most Hispanics, time is a relative event because minimal attention is given to the exact time of day. This attitude toward time becomes a problem when the Hispanic person leaves the folk healer and goes to see a physician because of worsening health. The folk healer comes to the patient's home 24 hours a day, 7 days a week. The physician can be seen only if the older adult goes to the office and waits a long time to be seen. It is ironic to these older adults that they cannot be late (which they often are), but the physician can be very late without criticism. Older Hispanic adults often are slow in coming into the health-care system; by that, I mean that their disease is well developed by the time they get there. This often is because they have gone through all of the folk healers and their suggestions in their local community before coming to a physician. It is important to understand this behavior rather than criticize it.

Traditional Hispanic people, especially older people, have a belief system based on treating "hot" diseases with "cold" remedies or vice versa. An example is that penicillin, a "hot" prescription, may not be taken for diarrhea, constipation, or a rash because they also are "hot" diseases. The only way you will know what is "hot" and "cold" is to ask. Write down the pertinent items and add them to the care plan. You also should tell the nurse or team leader verbally so that the information can be shared with the members of other shifts. Another example

This 63-year-old man is an illegal alien from Mexico. He does not have health-care insurance or a steady job. He stands, sometimes for hours, on a specific street corner where people who want day help come to hire him, which will allow him to buy food and pay his other expenses. As he ages, how will his lifestyle affect his overall health? Consider that he has no insurance, no guaranteed income, and minimal finances for essentials and that he stands on a cold (or hot) street corner each day hoping for work.

relates to the use of diuretics. When a diuretic is prescribed, along with encouragement to eat more bananas and raisins for potassium replacement, the bananas and raisins may not be eaten. They are considered "cold" foods and cannot be eaten with a "cold" disease. The resolution to this problem is to determine what the "hot" and "cold" diseases are and decide if there is a way to word the current illness so that it is a "hot" disease (never lie, however). The purpose of mixing "hot" and "cold" diseases and treatments is to find and maintain the individual's personal balance.

JEWISH AMERICANS

The strength of the Jewish religion binds Jewish people together. Jews from many parts of the world have immigrated to the United States. It is estimated that a greater number of Jews live in the United States than live in Israel, which is approximately 6.5 million (Sheskin & Dashefsky, 2013). There were several waves of immigration, most of them resulting from the horrors of prejudicial behavior from dominant societies. The most significant example of this behavior is the death of 6 million Jews during Hitler's "ethnic cleansing" of Germany. I recall doing an evaluative visit to a large Jewish nursing home on the East coast. While there, I met several survivors of the Holocaust. I listened to their stories and touched their tattoos (numbers tattooed on the wrists of all prisoners as a form of identification), and my life was changed forever. Despite the insults they endured, many lived to a wonderful old age.

When Jewish immigrants arrived, they were forced to work in factories and live in tenement housing, while experiencing prejudice from many people. Yet, they have shown excellent leadership in business, arts, and sciences and have made major contributions to American society. A high percentage of all Jewish Americans have a college education. When you have an older Jewish adult as a patient, you need to recognize their personal strength and motivation and that they may have more education than you do. Although Yiddish is a traditional language for Jewish people to use with each other, essentially everyone speaks English as well.

Traditional Jews recognize two aspects of health: the spirit and the body. Maintaining good health is an expectation. The use of modern medicine is encouraged; however, a rabbi (religious leader) may be consulted when transplantation or life-and-death issues need to be decided. Prayer is used to ask God for improvement of a condition or healing of one's body. The Torah (the holy book of the Jews) teaches Jewish people to visit and assist the sick. Most elderly Jews have a strong family and community support system.

Traditional Jewish people follow a kosher diet; they avoid mixing meat and dairy products, and eating shellfish and pork are forbidden. The Jewish culture has many holy days that are observed in a formal manner. You are responsible for assisting older Jewish adults to maintain their healing process as well as meet their need to observe any holy day that may occur while they are in your care.

The following story happened to an experienced nurse who successfully managed what could have been a very negative situation:

One day I was assigned an older woman who was recovering from surgery for a ruptured appendix. She was doing well considering what had happened. I had not been assigned to her before, but I noticed that on the previous day she was bright and pleasant. I was excited to spend time with her. You can imagine my surprise when I went into her room and found her arguing with the certified nursing assistant (CNA). I invited the CNA out of the room and asked her what had happened. After I listened to her identify the problem, I explained to her that she must never argue with the patients and that she should bring all problems that might cause an argument to me, as the licensed nurse. Then I went in the room to talk to the patient, Mrs. Goldstein.

The argument was based on the fact that Mrs. Goldstein would not eat or drink anything. She asked the CNA to remove her water pitcher and her breakfast tray, as well as cancel her meals for the rest of the day. Then she asked the CNA to see to it that she not be disturbed throughout the day. You can see the problem with these requests. Mrs. Goldstein was recovering from a very serious peritonitis caused by the ruptured appendix. She should not be NPO (nothing by mouth), and the staff would need to check on her and assist her with ambulation, administer pain medication, and check her vital signs and dressing. Also, when the body is recovering from something serious, it does need nutrients. I had a problem, and it was critical that I resolve it well.

I went into the room and sat down by Mrs. Goldstein. I asked her to tell me what the problem was. I felt it was essential that I get her version of what had happened. I reached out and touched her hand and made sure I was close to the bed so we both could see and hear each other. Mrs. Goldstein simply and clearly told me that she was Jewish and that it was Yom Kippur, the Day of Atonement. She went on to explain that Yom Kippur was the High Holy Day of the Holy Days for her religion. It was sacred to her. Yom Kippur was a day of repentance. No one drives; therefore, her family would not be visiting. And she needed to fast, so she would not be eating or drinking during the day. She felt that this would allow her to be cleansed spiritually and enable her to repent of her sins. I was very concerned.

It was obvious Mrs. Goldstein was a devout Jew and that the sacredness and traditions of Yom Kippur were deeply embedded within her. How could I meet her needs within the framework of respecting her body, mind, and spirit? I talked to her and listened, and then we made a plan.

Mrs. Goldstein agreed that God would understand if she did not observe Yom Kippur in the manner she usually did after I explained the importance of fluids to her healing body. As a result, she agreed to drink water only. Then we talked about nutrition and the work her body cells were doing to heal her. She agreed they needed fuel and said light meals would be satisfactory. I promised her that the staff would come in only for essential activities so she would have time to meditate and ask forgiveness of her sins. She seemed happy with our decisions.

I spent nearly an hour with this wonderful older woman working out a satisfactory solution that would meet her needs holistically.

Then it took another 30 minutes to make the necessary arrangements for the day. Fortunately, I work with a team of nurses who "covered" my other patients while I worked with Mrs. Goldstein. I called dietary and organized her meals, including another breakfast. I put a note on her door that said she was not to be disturbed without consulting me. Then I asked the CNA to take the water pitcher back into her room and coached her on a way to apologize for her aggressive behavior and express understanding for the sacredness of the day for Mrs. Goldstein. Fortunately, the CNA was willing to do as I suggested, as she felt badly about her previous interaction.

It was a hectic but satisfying day. Mrs. Goldstein's needs were met on every level without endangering her body. She had a wonderful day and expressed her gratitude to everyone she saw on the following day. I was appreciative to the staff for understanding her needs and assisting me to meet them; it really took a team effort.

 ## CONCLUSION

Giving culturally competent care in a caring and holistic manner requires a great deal of attention, sensitivity, and knowledge. This chapter gives you a basic background about common minority groups in the United States. Ethnic and cultural aspects of care were discussed. As the number of aging people in the United States increases and their diversity expands, it is crucial that you become familiar with the needs of older adults from all backgrounds. When you learn to do this, you will be giving culturally competent care, which is the goal.

Ask questions of older adults and partake of their wisdom as you learn about them and their lives. Advocate for them as they live their culture and religion. Provide them with the items they need to practice their health beliefs. Respect them for the lives they have lived and the reasons they have lived them.

CASE STUDY SOLUTION

First, you would control your surprise and that bit of criticism that some people may feel. Then you would think about what you know about the culture of these people because the problem seems to be one of cultural differences. The following is what I would have done. You may have other ideas that also would work. Remember that my thoughts are not the only answer, or even the best answer. Value your own thinking.

I hope I would have thought to bring breakfast. I would have had the family gather around the table and eat. Because I wouldn't have known their religion or preferences regarding blessing the food, I would have asked them what would be appropriate. While we were eating, I would have listened to what happened after I left them. Remember, they were refugees from a war-torn country where the military government had tried to kill everyone of their ethnic background. They would have told me stories of how they had to live to survive. They were poor and oppressed people to begin with and had been homeless for several months; they were accustomed to living off the streets or stealing to eat. They were from a very poor country and did not know what the oven and refrigerator were designed to do. The children had gathered the stack of sticks so they could be put into the oven to cook. The bathroom was another complete mystery to them. (They had gone outside to take care of their elimination needs.) They thought the towels and sheets were too pretty to use! Why were they sleeping on the floor? That was how they slept to keep warm and to be together if soldiers came.

By listening to these people, really taking the time to listen, I would have learned where to begin to acculturate them to modern Western society. I would have patiently explained the details of the items in their apartment, and then I would have demonstrated how things worked and let them do what they emotionally could. My only rule would have been that they could not build a fire inside the oven! It might have taken weeks before they could sleep in beds and even longer before they could sleep in separate beds.

With support and respect, this family could make a successful transition to their new lives. It might take more time than I originally planned, but it all would be very rewarding. I would have continued to work with them until the father got a job and the mother learned to shop and cook in her new country. English-as-a-second-language classes would have been a priority for everyone, and when the children seemed adjusted to the new culture, I would have assisted the family in getting them into school.

REVIEW QUESTIONS

1. Increasing diversity of the population requires that nurses become:
   1. Culturally proficient
   2. Culturally sensitive
   3. Culturally awakened
   4. Culturally desirous

2. When caring for an individual from another culture it would be important for the nurse to:
   1. Provide hot drinks because cold drinks are forbidden in other cultures
   2. Maintain eye contact and touch the patient frequently
   3. Educate the patient on the facility's expectations
   4. begin the interactions with questions regarding the culture

3. Some factors can be attributed to culture while others are more likely to be attributed to personal characteristics. Which factors would be attributed to personal characteristics? (Select all that apply.)
   1. Intelligence
   2. Nonverbal gestures
   3. Gender roles
   4. Diet
   5. Mathematics skill
   6. Value for older adults
   Answer: 1 and 5

4. A client is being admitted to the facility. During the admission assessment you discover the client speaks and understands very little English. To provide optimal care you will need to:
   1. Contact a trained interpreter to assist
   2. Request the family member to translate
   3. Write the instructions in large letters
   4. Locate someone in the facility to interpret

5. The kosher diet would strictly follow which basic rule?
   1. No pork, shellfish, or white flour products
   2. No dairy products served with meat, and no beef or shellfish
   3. No white flour products, pork, or dairy products
   4. No dairy products served with meat, and no pork or shellfish

REFERENCES

American Diabetes Association (2013). Treatment and care for American Indians/Alaska Natives. http://www.diabetes.org/living-with-diabetes/treatment-and-care/high-risk-populations/treatment-american-indians.html

Domrzalski, D. (2013). Nearly a third of NM's native Americans live below the poverty level. *Albuquerque Business First,* February 20.

Ennis, S.R., Rios-Varga, M., & Albert, N.G. (2011). The Hispanic population: 2010. www.census.gov/prod/cen2010/briefs/c2010br-04.pdf

Grady, A. M. (2014). Enhancing cultural competency in home care nurses caring for Hispanic/Latino patients. *Home Healthcare Nurse 32*(1).

Greenberg, S. (2011). Administration on aging: Profile of older Americans. U.S. Department of Health and Human Services. www.aoa.gov/Aging_Statistics/Profile/2011/docs/2011profile.pdf

Hoeffel, E.M., Rastogi, S., Kim, M.O., & Shahid, H. (2012). The Asian population: 2010. www.census.gov/prod/cen2010/briefs/c2010br-11.pdf

Kochanek, K.D., Arias, E., & Anderson, R.N. (2013). How did cause of death contribute to racial differences in life expectancy in the United States? Centers for Disease Control and Prevention: NCHS Data Brief 125. www.cdc.gov/nchs/data/databriefs/db125.htm

Macartney, S., Bishaw, A., & Fontenot, K. (2013). Poverty rates for selected detailed race and Hispanic groups by state and place: 2007-2011. U.S. Census Bureau. www.census.gov/prod/2013pubs/acsbr11-17.pdf

Maxwell, L.A. (2012). A demographic imperative: Raising Latinos' achievement. *Education Week,* 31(34), 4-5.

Minority Health, Centers for Disease Control and Prevention. (2012). American Indian and Alaska Native populations. www.cdc.gov/minorityhealth/populations/REMP/aian.html

Native American Cancer Research Corporation (n.d.). Native Americans and cancer. www.natamcancer.org/page12

Office of Minority and Health Disparities, Centers for Disease Control and Prevention. (2007). 10 leading causes of death white population, U.S., 2007. www.cdc.gov/omhd/populations/White.htm

Passel, J.S., & Cohn, D. (2008). U.S. Population projections: 2005-2050. Pew Research Center: Social and Demographic Trends. Retrieved from http://www.pewhispanic.org/2008/02/11/us-population-projections-2005-2050/

Shannon, M.A.P., & Hassler, L.J. (2014). Culture and spirituality. In Mauk, K.L. (ed.). *Gerontological nursing: Competencies for care* (3rd ed.). Burlington, MA: Jones & Bartlett Learning.

Sheskin, I., & Dashefsky, A. (2013). Jewish population in the United States, 2013. Berman Jewish Databank. http://www.jewishdatabank.org/Studies/details.cfm?StudyID=737

Taylor, P. (ed.) (2013). The rise of Asian Americans. Pew Research Center. http://www.pewsocialtrends.org/2012/06/19/the-rise-of-asian-americans/

United States Census Bureau (2011). 2010 Census data. http://www.census.gov/2010census/data/

United States Department of Commerce (n.d.). Poverty thresholds by size of family and number of children: 2013. United States Census Bureau. http://www.census.gov/hhes/www/poverty/data/threshld/index.html

United States Department of the Interior (2014). Indian affairs: Tribal entities list. *Federal register 79*(19). www.bia.gov/WhoWeAre/BIA/OIS/TribalGovernmentServices/TribalDirectory/index.htm

United States Department of Labor, Bureau of Labor Statistics (2011). Unemployment rates by race and ethnicity, 2010. www.bls.gov/opub/ted/2011/ted_20111005.htm

University of Maryland Medical Center (2013). Sickle cell disease. http://umm.edu/health/medical/reports/articles/sickle-cell-disease

WEB RESOURCE

Bureau of Labor Statistics: http://www.bls.gov/
Pew Research Center: www.pewresearch.org
United States Census Bureau: www.census.gov

Activity, Rest, and Sleep as Criteria for Health

TAMARA DAHLKEMPER

LEARNING OUTCOMES

1. Express an understanding of the importance of activity for all older adults, including the most disabled.

2. Discuss the significance of activity for people with and without chronic diseases.

3. Describe normal rest and sleep patterns for older adults.

4. Identify older adults who are most at risk for developing rest and sleep disturbances.

5. Apply nursing interventions to older adults who are experiencing problems with activity, rest, or sleep.

CONCEPTS

Comfort

Mobility

Stress and Coping

CASE STUDY

Mrs. McDonald is an 86-year-old woman who lives with her eldest son and his active family of five children. Mr. McDonald died the previous year of heart disease. After his death, Mrs. McDonald became less and less able to care for herself. She cried a great deal and refused to walk to the kitchen to prepare food. She said it was "too much work." She complained of not being able to sleep, yet whenever her son, Sean, came over to see her, she was sleeping in her chair. Being concerned about his mother, Sean moved her into his home with his wife and five children.

Mrs. McDonald had her own room but had to walk a short distance to the bathroom. She often was incontinent because it was "too hard" to get to the toilet. She always was tired and napped four to five times a day. Sean had two teenagers who often had friends over to the house. They were noisy and tended to stay until 9:00 or 10:00 in the evening on the weekends. There also was a 5-month-old baby who woke up crying twice a night. All of the bedrooms were on the same floor, so each noisy incident awakened Mrs. McDonald.

Sean's wife, Mary, began to complain of having to wait on the children (baby, toddler, 5-year-old, and the teens) and Mrs. McDonald. "She won't get out of her chair or do anything for herself. I can't stand the incontinence; my house smells," Mary told Sean one day as she was crying. Sean felt caught between the needs of his mother and the needs of his wife and children. He was committed to not putting his mother in a nursing home because she was adamant about not going to "live in the county poorhouse." Sean called a local home-care agency to see if they could help him with his problem. You are the nurse assigned to Mrs. McDonald. What are you going to do? This is a holistic problem because the entire family is involved, so approach your solution with that in mind.

INTRODUCTION

Activity promotes life physically and psychologically. Even minimal activity has several physical benefits. See Box 10.1 for a list of benefits. Frail health in older adults is associated with inactivity. The psychological benefits include the sense of well-being that comes with having the freedom to move from one place to the other and to take care of oneself, even if that care is minimal. Rest is a luxury that I assume you do not get to experience a great deal because you are a student who probably also is working and taking care of a family. The peaceful feeling that comes from an afternoon nap is a wonderful thing.

Adults have to work at getting enough rest, which leads us to sleep. I feel confident that there are days, perhaps even right now, when you feel sleep deprived. It is a difficult way to go through your life, isn't it? I am hopeful that this will not be

 Priority Setting

The priority for this chapter is for you to allow all older adults to do as much for themselves as possible. It is that simple. The challenge is that the person may not want to do all he or she can do. Perhaps the person's family members have pampered and waited on him or her more than is healthy for the older person. Perhaps he or she needs good pain management so that moving is not so painful. Whatever the challenge, you need to use the information in this chapter to determine what is keeping the person from doing everything possible as independently as possible. Be clever, be smart, be caring, and be holistic. But you must get the job done!

BOX 10.1   BENEFITS OF PHYSICAL ACTIVITY FOR THE OLDER ADULT

Decreased risk for obesity, diabetes, and cardiovascular, respiratory, musculoskeletal diseases

Improved quality of sleep

Preservation of muscle strength and endurance

Increased aerobic capacity

Greater bone density

Greater mobility and independence

Better bowel control

Better appetite control

Improved balance

Improved joint function

Decreased risk of falls

Improved memory and learning capabilities

Increased sense of well being

with them into their later years. Other older adults participate in sports as a spectator only and spend a great percentage of their free time watching television or sitting with a computer. For them, it is as if exercise is a luxury instead of a necessity for good health. With the growing obesity problem in the United States, the lack of exercise as a normal part of one's day should be a serious concern for you as a health-care provider.

It is a delight to me to see older persons golfing, mowing their lawns, or walking their dogs. In my mind, I simply say "yea!" What I see are people who are using the health they have and are working to maintain it. I even get excited when I see someone with a cane and oxygen zooming around the grocery store in an electric cart. Even though they are not walking, I appreciate the effort it took for them to get to the store. They had to get up, eat, dress, and manage getting to their car and then the store. They are interacting with an environment different from their home and have to stretch and move to get the items they need from the shelves. It is wonderful to see people moving at whatever their physical activity level is. The idea of exercise, for all of us, is if we keep moving, we *will* keep moving!

Advantages and Disadvantages of Exercise

As a nurse giving care to older adults, you have several complex concerns to manage in terms of activity and exercise for older adults. The number one problem often is managing an older person's chronic conditions (Box 10.2). Degenerative arthritis makes it difficult to walk; pulmonary disease makes it challenging to move at all. With the aging of society, many old-old people use canes, walkers, wheelchairs, and oxygen that add to the need for planning when exercising. Nevertheless, elderly people need to exercise.

When people exercise, they are assisting all of their major systems. Exercise improves the functioning of the heart and lungs, the musculoskeletal system, and the digestive and excretory systems, and it provides feelings of self-satisfaction. Setting goals and having meaningful things to do, all of which require some activity, combats depression, insomnia, and boredom.

When older people do not exercise, they are subject to osteoporosis; joint immobility; indigestion; constipation; pneumonia; weakened cardiac

a permanent condition for you. There should be a time, when you are through with school, when you will be able to get more sleep. I want you to consider, however, what it would be like to be an older adult whose sleep patterns have changed from what they always have been and whose sleep definitely has diminished in quality and quantity. Sleep deprivation in older persons can be a very serious consideration when planning nursing care. The importance of managing activity, rest, and sleep is critical in giving care to older people.

 ## ACTIVITY

Activity for people in the United States has changed over the years. As society has moved from an agrarian (farming) society to an industrial one, the natural activities that dominated society, such as farming, have changed as well. To accommodate the change in activity, many people now go to gyms or join organized community sports groups to get enough exercise to be healthy. In their younger years, many baby boomers have developed good exercise habits that will continue

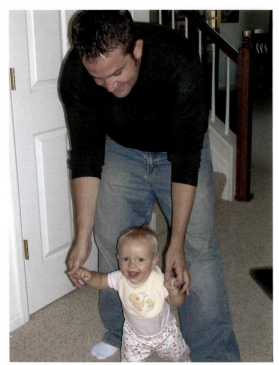

When this child was learning to walk, she needed assistance from her parents. She would walk and walk and walk until she learned to do it independently. Can you draw an analogy from this child to an older adult who has experienced an injury that limits mobility?

and other muscles; pressure ulcers; and the depression, insomnia, and boredom mentioned. The aging process is a challenge to maintaining a healthy lifestyle. The instrument for avoiding the

BOX 10.2   TEN MOST COMMON CHRONIC CONDITIONS IN PEOPLE OLDER THAN AGE 65 IN THE UNITED STATES

1. Arthritis
2. Hypertension
3. Problems hearing
4. Heart conditions
5. Visual impairment
6. Deformities or orthopedic disability
7. Diabetes
8. Chronic sinusitis
9. Hay fever and allergic rhinitis
10. Varicose veins

pitfalls of inactivity in older adults is the care given by you, as a licensed practical nurse (LPN), and the members of the family, who you are responsible to teach.

How to Keep Older Adults Active

The first rule when working with older persons and their exercise needs is to allow them to do as much for themselves as possible. This sounds very simple; however, in the real world of your clinical practice, it is not. There is pressure to get everyone to the lunch room in a nursing home in a timely manner, and walking residents to meals is more time-consuming than putting them in wheelchairs to transport them. Yet, walking residents to the lunch room is an excellent way to give them some exercise despite the time crunch. This could become problematic for you as you organize your time. It is critical that you and the people you manage (the nursing assistants) organize yourselves so that everyone can be assisted in walking to their meals, if possible. Once there, the residents can use their time to visit with each other, discuss the day's events, and compliment or complain about the food. The difference between getting them to lunch at your convenience and ambulating them to lunch with time for socialization is one of quality of care and caring.

In the hospital, you may need to assist an older adult to a chair so that meals can be eaten while sitting upright (better digestion, less acid reflux). Assisting someone to the toileting room, without the use of a wheelchair, promotes bowel elimination, and the walking is important for muscle strengthening (including the heart) and the avoidance of increased osteoporosis.

The "allowing people to do as much for themselves as possible" rule extends to all of the care you render to people in a nursing home, hospital, or home. Allow individuals to brush their own teeth, comb their own hair, and dress themselves as much as possible. All of these actions take time but are excellent for range of motion and self-esteem building. Teaching this principle to family and friends further enhances the quality of life of older adults. Tell them what you are doing and explain the "why." You need to role-model safe and caring ways for assisting the person in your care. During the time you are assisting older persons, talk to them, listen to what they have to say, and value their wisdom and experience. This valuing behavior helps build self-esteem, and it is a caring and wise way to use the time you are spending in activity with your clients.

While planning exercise for specific older adults in your care, be aware of their physical ability. Consider Mrs. McDonald in the case study. Although she has no physiological reason for why she does not walk on her own, because she has been somewhat immobile for several months, she will need to start slowly with her activity. It is not helpful to put persons in a situation that makes major demands on their bodies that could be unsafe. For some people, sitting in a circle and throwing a ball from one to another is good use of their upper body and is fun. For other persons, it could be boring and beneath their physical abilities. Begin with a conservative plan, and increase it if it does not physically stress the person (Box 10.3).

These older adults are getting their physical activity for the day.

HEALTHY PEOPLE 2020

Goal

Increase the proportion of older adults with reduced physical or cognitive function who engage in light, moderate, or vigorous leisure-time physical activities.

BOX 10.3 TYPES OF EXERCISE FOR OLDER ADULTS

Endurance

Muscle strengthening

Balance training

Flexibility

 REST

Rest is something most people want to experience more than they generally do. I am sure you would like some time off to do nothing but rest; I do find that to be common among busy students. When dealing with older adults, you have a specialized group of people who have specialized rest needs.

Because of the number of chronic diseases older people tend to have, they may be unable to rest owing to pain or stress over their diseases. In another scenario, the person may feel that all he or she does is rest! The key to managing the rest needs of older people is to identify what their needs are.

Pain

A common reason people cannot rest is because they have pain that keeps them awake. Pain needs to be identified and managed. It not only inter-feres with rest and sleep, but it also decreases activity. Chronic pain may leave a person totally fatigued and unable to participate properly in a restorative care program. In addition, some behavioral problems in institutionalized older adults stem from ineffective pain management. A psychiatric evaluation may be requested for screaming or abusive behavior on the part of a resident of a nursing home who in fact is experiencing physical pain. A failure to identify pain as a factor affecting behavior and function may result in poor medical management. Pain in older people is frequently either overtreated or undertreated simply because it is difficult to assess. Some older adults want every ache treated with a drug, whereas others maintain a stoic attitude: "Why bother? There is nothing that can be done, anyway." Older people often perceive pain differently. Some pain receptors may not be as acute as they were in the past. Medical journals document clinical cases describing "silent" myocardial infarctions or "painless" intra-abdominal emergencies. These cases may not be silent or painless but may reflect an older person's normal aging situation. Cognitive impairments, delirium, and dementia are some barriers to pain assessment. People who have a dementia process or a stroke and become aphasic may be unable to give an accurate pain history. They may be unable to describe when the pain started or at what point in the day the pain becomes most severe.

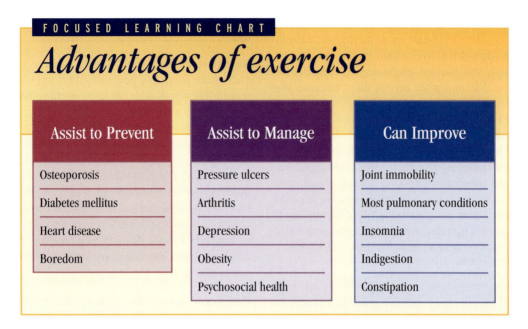

FOCUSED LEARNING CHART

Advantages of exercise

Assist to Prevent	Assist to Manage	Can Improve
Osteoporosis	Pressure ulcers	Joint immobility
Diabetes mellitus	Arthritis	Most pulmonary conditions
Heart disease	Depression	Insomnia
Boredom	Obesity	Indigestion
	Psychosocial health	Constipation

Most people describe the pain in the here and now. A person in pain is often self-absorbed and inattentive to activities in the environment. A sensitivity to other medications that results in delirium makes pain management difficult for older people. Delirium may also be one manifestation of an attempt to treat a person's pain. An assessment for delirium should be made whenever there is a change in cognitive function after the start of any new pain medication. Refer to Chapter 18 for information on assessing delirium. Multiple chronic disease processes and acute processes compound the difficulty. There may even be an acute exacerbation of a chronic problem. These multiple sources of pain make diagnosis difficult, and pain management becomes a challenge.

There are two myths regarding pain in older adults. One myth is that pain is normal. As body systems begin to wear out, one might expect an increase in pain. At any age, pain is the most common symptom of a disease process, however, and should be investigated and treated. Another myth is that pain and sleep are incompatible. Nurses often disbelieve a patient's complaint of pain when they bring a pain pill and find the person asleep. The wrong conclusion is drawn. It is believed that an individual really in pain could not possibly sleep. The exhaustive feature of pain is seldom considered in the assessment process. The last myth is that narcotic drugs are not safe for older people. Narcotics provide effective pain relief for some chronic conditions and terminal illnesses. These drugs should be used on a scheduled basis, such as every 4 hours or every 6 hours. Use of a narcotic on an "as needed" basis does not provide effective pain management. Some nurses believe that narcotics dull an older person's LOC. They fear that an older adult would be unable to benefit from the support of family or friends in the time remaining before death. Effective relief of pain actually promotes interaction, and the initial drowsiness soon wears off.

Although pain is a highly subjective experience, there are two methods for assessing it. Simple observation from a nurse who knows the person well can be very effective. A grimace or clutch of the chest provides a vivid picture of pain. Assessment questions may follow these observations. Clinical practice guidelines for acute pain management identify the quantifiable measures of pain that should be considered in an assessment, including the intensity of the pain, the duration of the pain, the quality of the pain, and the personal meaning this pain has to the older adult. The impact on the person's functioning is also included. Assessment tools are available. A good tool addresses the older person's pain history and coping strategies for dealing with pain and medications in the past that have been effective. It is important to ask questions that help to describe or define the pain. Noting the

QSEN

COMPETENCY: Patient-Centered Care (Knowledge, Skills

Individualizing Activity

You have the knowledge to determine a safe and meaningful activity for each individual. Think of the person holistically—for example, what the individual can do and what he or she enjoys—and then plan accordingly. Washing dishes in warm water is a successful way to exercise arthritic hands and fingers with less discomfort. Encourage arm and ankle exercises while watching television or ankle exercises while working at the computer. A walk outside to the sidewalk and back may not seem like much unless you are the person with pain or dyspnea doing the walking. Suggest a pet if it seems appropriate. The value of pet therapy is well published, and taking care of a pet requires physical movement.

All exercise plans for older adults in your care need to be ordered or approved by a primary care provider. In addition, all reputable nursing homes, hospitals, and home-care agencies have access to physical therapists. Use the physical therapist to teach you and the family the best approaches and techniques to use with each individual.

1. Consider the older adults in your life? What forms of activity do they incorporate into their daily lives?
2. Discuss what you can do to help them become for active.

Point of Interest

For a healthy older adult, the Centers for Disease Control and Prevention (CDC) recommends a minimum of 2 hours and 30 minutes of moderate aerobic exercise each week and muscle strengthening activity 2 or more days a week working all major muscle groups (CDC, 2014). The exercise can be divided into smaller increments of time as long as each session is at least 10 minutes long. However, for older adults who are in poor health, just keeping them moving is important. For example, having the older person walk to the kitchen to get a drink of water is better than having someone getting it for the person. Having the older person do two or three arm extensions while holding a soup can in each hand is better than not doing any. As you plan your care, think of ways you can involve older adults that make movement necessary

Critically Examine the Following:

Look at your own busy life and holistically plan an exercise program for yourself.

What are you currently doing for exercise?
What do you want to do (lose weight, walk further, play ball better)?
How can you do it?
Do you already have an exercise program that works for you?

intensity and duration assists in providing an objective measure to a highly subjective experience. Simply asking "How is your pain today?" may prompt the response, "Well, it is there." The simplest method of pain assessment is the use of a pain intensity scale. You, as the nurse, can draw a line indicating that the far left (L) end of the line defines no pain and the right (R) end represents the most pain the person has ever experienced. The person can point to the place on the line that reflects current pain level. Another commonly used method is to ask the older adult to rate the pain on a scale from 1 to 10, with 10 being the worst pain imaginable. It is your responsibility, as the LPN, to identify the pain and share that information with the registered nurse (RN) or health care provider. It is the responsibility of the RN or health care provider

to do a comprehensive assessment to determine the causative factors related to the pain. Your responsibility, besides reporting the pain and its impact on the resident or patient, is to check for more common possible causes of the pain. Is the individual positioned properly? Are position changes made often enough to prevent pressure ulcers from starting? Have you checked the medications to see if there is a drug reaction or interaction? Listen to the person experiencing the pain and carefully describe it when you chart. Providing adequate pain relief is part of giving holistic care to your older patients.

Evidence-Based Practice

Chen, Q., Hayman, L.L., Shmerling, R.H., Bean, J.F., & Leveille, S.G. (2011). Characteristics of chronic pain associated with sleep difficulty in older adults: The Maintenance of Balance, Independent Living, Intellect, and Zest in the Elderly (MOBILIZE) Boston Study. Journal of the American Geriatrics Society, 59, 1385-1392.

More than 765 persons age 64 years and older participated in the Maintenance of Balance, Independent Living, Intellect, and Zest in the Elderly (MOBILIZE) Boston Study. The study found that widespread moderate to severe pain is strongly associated with sleep difficulty in older adults.

Question

With this new understanding about the relationship between pain and poor sleep, what can you do to prevent pain from being a deterrent to good sleep in your older patients?

Critically Examine the Following:

Look carefully at your life and identify the three major stressors you currently are experiencing, then (1) list the stressor, (2) state whether it is "good" stress or "bad" stress, (3) describe how you are managing it, and (4) indicate whether your management of it seems to be successful. If you feel you are not managing the stressors satisfactorily, indicate a plan that would assist you in more effective management of the stress.

Stress

Every person has his or her own personal ability to manage stress. This is very important because stress is a normal part of life. Think of the stress in your own life. Without deadlines, you would not be stressed enough to get your school papers or care plans written and prepare for your tests. Every day people manage the stress of weather changes, worldwide events (war, hurricanes, floods), interactions with others, time constraints, and other physical and emotional stressors. For some people, getting up and getting dressed in the morning are major stress points. Stress is part of everyone's life, and it will not go away. The key to stress is not elimination; it is management.

Life is a series of stressful events. Much of the stress actually enhances our lives (getting up in the morning and getting dressed). Some stress assists us in achieving our goals and other stress simply makes us feel alive and assists us in avoiding boredom. The problem with stress is that there can be too much of it; this is called "distress" and can be damaging to our lives physically and emotionally. The potential for the negative effects of distress is why stress management is crucial to understand. The informative section in the chapter on promoting wellness (Chapter 6) would be valuable for you

to reread. The content supports the principles of achieving rest by managing stress. Refer back to Chapter 6 and apply the information to the concept of appropriate rest for older adults.

"All I Do Is Rest!"

If you hear this or similar comments from your elderly clients, you need to assist them and their family members to understand the information in the activity section of this chapter. All people need to move to the extent of their ability. The movement works their muscles, and that encourages the body to rest. One of the main considerations when planning activity and rest is to assist the older person to alternate them throughout the day. Many older people have worked for most of their lives and consider daytime the right time to "do their work" or activities, and they rest in the evening.

As most of us age, we have less stamina for prolonged activities, such as working for 8 consecutive hours. It is important to teach older people and their families to modify the level of activity in a day to what works best for the individual. A combination of activity and then rest, activity and then rest again is generally the best way to stay healthy and happy as an aging person. The older one becomes, the more common this tends to be. It is common for older people to take one or two naps a day. Napping is perfectly natural because of the aging body. Encourage naps that are intermingled with episodes of activity throughout the day. You need to be aware of the possibility of oversleeping because of boredom or depression, however.

Take a moment to consider if the person is bored. If so are, find out what interests the person has and then find an avenue to help the person to pursue their interests. Is he or she interested in volunteering for an organization? Or interested in participating in the activities at the senior citizen center? If the person is unable to leave his or her home, are there activities that can be brought into the home? Do the neighbors need to know that their visits are very welcome, or is there an adopt-a-grandparent program at the local high school? An adopt-a-grandparent program is where teens volunteer to be with one particular older person. Generally, this arrangement results in a very satisfying relationship for both individuals.

Keeping older adults engaged in life is important. Take the time to talk to the older adults to whom you give care and learn about their life interests.

The older adult is taking a nap during her busy day.

SLEEP

Sleep is the most significant activity people can participate in for quality health. Every person, at whatever age, needs sleep to function normally. During sleep, the body physically repairs body tissues and emotionally resolves the issues of the day. Some people need only 6 hours of sleep, whereas many need the traditional 8 hours. Generally when people age, they feel less rested, and many need more sleep than they get.

What Is Sleep?

The central nervous system controls sleep-wake patterns. There are two types of sleep: rapid eye movement (REM) and nonrapid eye movement (NREM). Every individual of every age needs to experience both types of sleep every night. The sleep cycle has four stages of NREM and one stage of REM. The NREM stages go from relaxation to deeper and deeper sleep. The REM stage is the deepest sleep and is essential for a good night's rest. People often go through this sleep cycle four times a night, with each cycle allowing for deeper and more restful REM sleep. If the person's sleep is interrupted, the cycle starts over again from the beginning, and much of the deep sleep needed for optimal health is lost. This deep sleep is the healing sleep. When you wake up from a night's sleep and feel really great, you have, in all probability, had uninterrupted cycles of sleep.

Another aspect of individual sleep patterns is the person's circadian rhythm. This is the body's response to the day-night cycle of the sun. Within this cycle, people develop personal responses to their sleep needs. A common problem is that as

people age, they wake up earlier. As a result, they get tired during the day and need one or more naps. The daytime fatigue comes from normal physiological changes in the person's circadian rhythm. Research indicates that circadian rhythms change over time, resulting in younger people sleeping late in the morning (think of your own teen years) and older people awaking earlier. This normal physiological change causes many older people to want to stay up late so that they do not wake up at 4:00 or 5:00 in the morning. Getting up early also reinforces the need for naps throughout the daytime hours (Box 10.4).

BOX 10.4   MEASURES TO ASSIST WITH SLEEP

Balance daytime activity and rest.

Provide activity during the day.

Provide socialization.

Limit number and length of naps during the day.

Maintain bedtime routine.

Provide 2 to 3 hours of uninterrupted sleep during the night.

Think Like a Nurse

Now that you know about normal sleep patterns and changes in circadian rhythms, what have you observed that indicates nursing in general does not consistently address this problem when giving care to older adults? Make a list of three nursing care approaches that could be altered to meet the personal sleep needs of older people.

1. In nursing homes, residents often are put to bed between 7:00 and 9:00 p.m. Putting people to bed so early does two things that have negative consequences. The first consequence is that putting adults to bed at the same time as one would put children to bed does not focus on the residents' needs but rather on the needs of the staff and the tasks they must complete by a certain time. All adults with normal mental capacity should be able to determine their bedtime, rather than being put to bed like children. This behavior is demeaning to older persons. In addition, it forces the person to lie in bed awake for lengthy periods during the night and early morning because he or she simply cannot sleep that long at one time. Remember that their circadian rhythm has changed as a normal part of aging. It may be inconvenient for the staff to allow people to go to bed at the time they wish to go to bed, but it provides autonomy for the individual person in a system that does not always allow for individual decisions.

2. In most hospitals, it is noisy at night, and older people, who generally are lighter sleepers, just cannot stay asleep once they get to sleep. This constant awakening disrupts their NREM and REM sleep cycle. It is essential that nursing staff make regular rounds, take vital signs, and do other things such as checking dressings and intravenous fluids. For most older people, all that movement and noise interfere with sleep. It also is helpful if the activities that need to be done in a patient's room all are done at one time so that there are fewer sleep interruptions. Could the IV or dressing check be done when medication is administered? Staff always should use flashlights rather than turn on the room lights. Noise in the hallways and at the nurses' station should be kept to a whisper level so as not to disturb the patients.

3. If older residents or patients do get up early, is there a place for them to go to read, watch the early morning news, or have a cup of coffee? Because early awakenings are normal physiology, the staff should have a way of managing this occurrence in a positive manner.

Sleep Disorders

There are various sleep disorders diagnosed, but the end result tends to be the same. Older adults often have trouble falling asleep and staying asleep, and they awaken fatigued, which can last throughout the day. As you probably know from personal experience, people who do not get enough sleep are often irritable, and in older adults, that can lead to confusion (Saccomano, 2014). The management of sleep disorders is an important aspect of the care you need to be giving to elders.

A common sleep disorder is insomnia (Reeve & Bailes, 2010). Insomnia occurs when people have difficulty getting to sleep or remaining asleep, or they simply feel that they do not get enough sleep. Insomnia is not a disease, but rather it is the result of some other condition. Imagine the pain from arthritis without effective pain management. You may be too young to know how devastating arthritic pain can be, but it definitely is enough to keep a person awake.

Another common cause of insomnia is sleep apnea. Sleep apnea occurs when a person's airway is partially obstructed during sleep. The classic symptom is fatigue on awakening and throughout the day. People with sleep apnea are very tired *all* of the time. They often snore throughout the night, which can result in insomnia for their sleep partner. People with sleep apnea are frequently obese.

Sleep apnea is treated with continuous positive airway pressure (CPAP) while sleeping. The CPAP machine eliminates the airway obstruction by forcing air into the trachea throughout the sleep period. This is done through a mask that is strapped to the person's nose. Untreated sleep apnea can lead to right-sided heart failure and eventually pulmonary hypertension. You need to pay attention to people who complain of constant fatigue. It is your responsibility to report such complaints to the RN or physician rather than dismiss the complaint.

Other common reasons for insomnia include frequent urination, gastroesophageal reflux disease (GERD), chronic obstructive pulmonary disease (COPD), congestive heart failure (CHF), depression and anxiety, and medication side effects. These medical conditions should be treated by the PCP. It is your responsibility, as the LPN, to report symptoms related to these conditions and their management to the RN or PCP. Then, as the excellent nurse you are or will become, go a step further by applying nursing interventions where applicable.

Critically Examine the Following:

Nursing interventions often bring the needed information and comfort to patients and residents experiencing insomnia. Take the situation of frequent urination as a causative factor for insomnia. There are nursing actions that theoretically can improve this situation. Make a list of things you can do and the reasons why. Focus on nursing knowledge and not medical knowledge, such as medications. I will write one action and rationale for you as an example; then you need to complete the list. Be prepared to submit your plan to the faculty person.

1. ACTION: If possible, terminate drinking fluids at 6:00 p.m. This is a challenge for anyone accustomed to drinking throughout the evening, but a worthwhile behavior. The nurse will need to give sips of fluids with medications at bedtime. Be pleasant and supportive to the person giving up the fluids. It is hard!

   RATIONALE: It is simple. If the kidneys do not have fluid to process, there is minimal urine. Remember how important it is that any person sleeping has continuous sleep? If not, then refer back to the previous section. This action may be all that is necessary to stop nightly urination. You should write three more nursing actions that can assist this type of patient.

People with COPD and CHF sleep better if the head of the bed is raised. The same is true of someone with GERD. Provide a calming environment for someone with anxiety and monitor medications for possible side effects.

Nocturnal movement is another physiological condition that causes insomnia. There are two common types of nocturnal movement. The most common is restless legs syndrome (RLS), which is an irresistible urge to move one's legs. This can happen several times a night, and each episode is capable of awakening the person experiencing the situation. RLS can be managed with medication.

For some people, heat application also helps the legs to relax. Be sure to report this disruptive complaint to the RN or PCP so that it can be effectively treated.

Another disruption to sleep is nocturnal myoclonus, which is sudden moving or kicking movements of the lower extremities. This happens without warning and is very disruptive to sleep. Again, report it rather than ignore it as "just another complaint" because medications can assist in managing the disorder. These problems are legitimate concerns when considering sleep patterns and, subsequently, the overall health of the people to whom you give care.

Dementia is a deterrent to effective sleep for the person with dementia and his or her sleep partner. Sleep patterns are altered in someone with dementia, which often results in being awake and wandering at night. This is very disruptive for the caregiver, who most often is the spouse of the individual with dementia. The result is two people who are sleep deprived and having difficulty because of fatigue. This is one reason that many communities have respite programs for caregivers of persons with dementia. The person with dementia is taken to the respite center for constant care, and the caregiver has a few hours or a weekend to rest, visit relatives, or engage in other activities important to a quality of life.

Psychological conditions often are detrimental to effective sleep patterns. People who are depressed often awake early and have hypersomnia, which is sleeping during the time people normally are awake. Anxiety often is related to difficulty falling asleep and frequent awake periods during the night. Psychiatric disorders can be treated with medication and therapy. Several disorders interfere with sleep and other life issues. Be diligent in your awareness of what is going on with the people to whom you give care. Talk to family members to gather information and an accurate past history. Share what you learn with the RN and PCP so that a psychiatric assessment can be made and treatment can be started. The benefits will be much more than a good night's sleep (Box 10.5).

As you evaluate and teach the patient and the family about healthy sleep, keep the following deterrents to good sleep in mind as part of your teaching plan. The following contribute to poor quality sleep: sedentary lifestyle, alcohol, tobacco, caffeine in the evening, disrupted sleep patterns, noise, and light in the sleeping environment. It is

BOX 10.5   RISK FACTORS FOR SLEEP IN OLDER ADULTS

Nocturnal urination

Urinary frequency

Health conditions

Medications

Lifestyle changes

Environment

 CONCLUSION

The care of older adults requires a special sensitivity to their health needs. Their health is the main factor in determining their quality of life. To have maximum health, all people need activity that fits their physiology, rest that accommodates their lifestyle, and sleep that allows them the ability to function without fatigue. You, the nurse, are the key to these things happening for older adults. The ageist stereotype that the United States has for older adults leads many people to believe that lack of activity, taking several naps a day, and complaining of fatigue are simply factors that accompany aging. You now know that when these problems are recognized and documented, they can be managed through an interdisciplinary team approach (you, the RN, the PCP, and the family). Many of the problems can be resolved through good nursing care approaches and family involvement. It is your responsibility to facilitate this type of care.

your responsibility to make the environment conducive to sleep, to teach the patient and family members about what disrupts sleep, and to report any medical conditions appropriately so that they can be treated. Carefully examine and talk to any person in your care who seems fatigued. Fatigue is *not* a normal outcome of aging; it is a problem.

CASE STUDY SOLUTION

Gathering Information

You ask the admitting RN if you can accompany him on his first visit. He agrees that you should be there. While the RN does the admission, you ask Mary to show you Mrs. McDonald's room and the bathroom. While you are walking down the hallway, you talk to Mary about the problems she is having. It is obvious the entire family needs help if you are going to assist Mrs. McDonald. The following items need your attention.

Depression

Mrs. McDonald's behavior indicates that she could be depressed and has been since the death of her husband. You use the Beck Depression Scale as an assessment tool on Mrs. McDonald; the results indicate that she is clinically depressed. You talk to her and observe her to see if what you hear and see support the results of the test. Your observations lead you to talk to the case manager, who contacts the physician. After talking to Sean, the physician orders a mild antidepressant for Mrs. McDonald. You will observe her closely for the next 3 weeks to determine if there has been a change. If the medication does not relieve the depression symptoms, you may need to suggest some psychological therapy sessions to assist her in managing her feelings regarding the death of her husband. You know that if the depression is managed, Mrs. McDonald will sleep better and be better able to care for herself during the day.

Strengthening

Mrs. McDonald needs more activity to become stronger. You arrange your first visit to be when the entire family is at home. Mrs. McDonald also is present at this family meeting. You explain the "first rule" of activity for older adults: It is for the person to do all activities possible for himself or herself. Mrs. McDonald is not doing that because she has the 5-year-old and the toddler running errands for her frequently during the day. She refuses to go to the bathroom—hence her incontinence—and she seldom leaves her room "because she is so tired."

Mrs. McDonald likes the idea of being more independent, so she agrees to listen to your plan, which follows. You also explain to everyone that the more activity Mrs. McDonald has during the day, the better she will sleep at night.

1. She will come to the dining room for all meals. (Mary has been feeding her in her room, which contributes to Mrs. McDonald's depression.) Mary agrees to walk her to the dining room for breakfast and lunch in time to enjoy eating with the family. The teens agree to take turns walking their grandma to the dining room for dinner.

2. The 5-year-old volunteers to "work out" with grandma while she does arm exercises with a soup can in each hand twice a day. You need to evaluate how many lifts she can do with her current muscle strength. You will reevaluate this frequently.

3. The teenagers agree to take turns taking grandma for a walk each day. You demonstrate how to get her out of the chair and how to use a walking belt (you brought one from the agency that will be left at the home) and emphasize that "a walk" initially will be a short trip in the hallway. You will monitor Mrs. McDonald's strength and add to the distance traveled as is appropriate.

Incontinence

This is a major problem that often is the reason families place their older family member in a nursing home. It is unpleasant for the caregiver and the person experiencing the incontinence. The smell tends to bother the entire family. You see this as an urgent matter. You explain to the family that the exercise will assist Mrs. McDonald in becoming strong enough eventually to

continued on page 194

CASE STUDY SOLUTION *continued*

ambulate to the bathroom. In the meantime, something must be done to make the situation manageable.

You talk to Mary and Mrs. McDonald privately and suggest adult briefs. Mrs. McDonald is able to change them herself, and their use would diminish the smell in the house and stains on the furniture and floor. You suggest a tight-lidded container as the place to dispose of the briefs. This will help control the smell as well. The container needs to be emptied every day. Mrs. McDonald is excited to have this type of autonomy, and Mary is visibly relieved.

You should advise other methods of bladder control, but because they are not the focus of this case study, they are not discussed here.

Sleep and Rest

Mrs. McDonald naps four to five times a day and still feels exhausted. You should ask her to keep a log (with Sean's help, if necessary) about her sleep. What time does she go to bed? What time does she wake up? How many times a night does she get up or become fully awake? What causes her to awaken? This information should be shared with the RN or the PCP so that decisions can be made about medical and nonmedical interventions for Mrs. McDonald's fatigue.

In the meantime, you can get to work on basic nursing interventions. Is the room quiet at night without disruptive lighting? Does Mrs. McDonald avoid alcohol, smoking, and caffeine, as they are things that can disrupt her sleep? Is the room warm enough, and is the bed comfortable for her? Does she need more pillows or a bed that is elevated because of COPD or CHF? Does she need a new nighttime ritual, such as reading a large-print book with a 100-watt lamp? Would she like the family to come into her room and have family prayer at bedtime? There are several interventions you can investigate.

It would be an effective idea for Mrs. McDonald to try to have only two naps a day. She needs to be tired when she goes to bed. Staying awake, if it is reasonable, along with her new strengthening program will help her sleep.

There are other plans you could work out for Mrs. McDonald and her family. Consider at least two more and write them as part of this case study solution.

REVIEW QUESTIONS

1. When considering activity for older adults, the greatest challenge is:
   1. Getting them up and about without hurting your back
   2. Keeping their weight within normal limits so that it is easier to move them
   3. Managing their chronic diseases
   4. Doing as much for them as possible as a pain management intervention

2. The normal sleep cycle for older adults:
   1. Has four NREM cycles and an extra REM cycle. This occurs approximately four times a night
   2. Is not affected by the interruption of the NREM/REM cycles
   3. Has a built-in mechanism, which develops as people age, that makes awakening more difficult
   4. Does not change or adapt as people age

3. The normal circadian rhythm:
   1. Changes as people age
   2. Does not change as people age
   3. Protects older adults from sleepless nights
   4. Causes significant disruptions in normal sleep patterns in older adults

4. Older adults who are most at risk for rest/sleep disturbances include all but the following:
   1. Older adults with sleep apnea and obesity
   2. Older adults with depression or dementia
   3. Older adults with RLS or myoclonus
   4. Older adults who are underweight and confused

5. Many sleep/rest problems can be managed with effective nursing interventions. Choose from the following list the activity that is not based on nursing knowledge:
   1. Sleep apnea testing
   2. Appropriate toileting pattern
   3. Strengthening program
   4. Administering the Beck Depression Scale

REFERENCES

Bureau of National Health Statistics (2008).
Centers for Disease Control and Prevention (2014). How much physical activity do older adults need? www.cdc.gov/physicalactivity/basics/older_adults/index.htm

Reeve, K., & Bailes, B. (2010). Insomnia in adults: etiology and management. *Journal of Nurse Practitioners,* 6(1), 53-60.
Saccomano, S. (2014). Sleep disorders in older adults. *Journal of Gerontological Nursing.* 40(3) 38-45.

WEB RESOURCE

NIH Senior Health: http://nihseniorhealth.gov/

End-of-Life Issues in Older Adults

TAMARA DAHLKEMPER

LEARNING OUTCOMES

1. Define the essential characteristics of a hospice organization.

2. Identify the five stages of grief as outlined by Kübler-Ross.

3. List the qualities necessary for a nurse to give end-of-life care.

4. List the eight signs of imminent death.

5. Use knowledge of palliative care to provide information to a patient and family.

6. Differentiate between a living will and a durable power of attorney.

11

CONCEPTS

Grief and Loss

Stress and Coping

CASE STUDY

Mr. Reed is an 80-year-old patient with terminal pancreatic cancer. He has received treatment in the past, but his physician has decided that further treatment will not benefit him. Mr. Reed lives alone and has no one to care for him, so he is being admitted to a long-term care facility. He has two daughters who both live out of state but have come into town to help Mr. Reed with his transfer to the facility. Since his admission, Mr. Reed has been very quiet and has not said much about his current physical condition or shown any emotion. On meeting Mr. Reed's daughters, Liz and Joyce, you find they are concerned about their father's rapidly declining physical condition. Liz doesn't understand why the cancer is not being treated and wants to contact the physician to start treatment for the cancer. Joyce is saying that it is time to let their father die and maybe they should consider hospice. The suggestion of hospice makes the one daughter angry and she states "Dad is not ready to die yet. If you put him on hospice he will just die sooner."

Discussion

1. How will you handle the disagreement between the daughters?

2. How will you bring Mr. Reed into the discussion regarding his thoughts about his death?

INTRODUCTION

- *End-of-life (EOL) issues* are vital issues in health care throughout the United States. Americans want to experience a "good death" without being burdened by symptoms or technology. Nurses have an essential role in maximizing EOL care by improving symptom management; communication; and education about choices, referrals, and psychosocial treatments. You, as the care

provider, have the responsibility to explain to older adults and their family members all of the options, referrals, and resources available. As you review some of the options in this chapter, it is very important that you examine your own attitudes, values, and beliefs regarding death. You need to consider what happens if your personal beliefs conflict with the choices and decisions made by an older adult in your care. The focus of this chapter is to explore how to assist older adults to die well through the excellent care and support you provide them as they approach the end of their lives.

This nursing assistant is helping this man to enjoy the last few months of his life.

THE MYSTERY OF DEATH

As all people know, death is an inevitable and natural human experience. It has, however, been shrouded in mystery and envisioned as an experience of great suffering, generally contemplated with fear. Dying, on the other hand, is an unpredictable event. The exact moment or situation in which someone will die is never known. As a person moves through the dying process, they and their family members will experience many emotions ranging from acceptance to denial as well as fear, anger, joy, and confusion.

Those emotions are real and will be emotions that you, the nurse, will experience as you encounter family members of a dying person. People need to be allowed to cope with death in their own way, even if it is to deny death's reality until the end. As the caregiver to older adults, you need to be prepared to be a positive influence for appropriate EOL issues. First, you need to be educated in EOL issues and learn to communicate them. Then, you need to provide the older adults in your care with a high quality of life and a good death. You need skills in working as a team with other caring professionals, families, and the dying person, understanding and applying the guiding principles of gerotranscendence for yourself and your patients. Finally, you need to maintain a positive work environment. Without skills in these areas, the quality of EOL care for older adults is diminished.

 ## STAGES OF GRIEF

Grief is the normal reaction to a catastrophic loss. What defines the catastrophe? The person experiencing the loss has that responsibility. A catastrophe to one person may not be one to another. Understanding and compassion are essential when relating to people experiencing losses.

Dr. Elisabeth Kübler-Ross, a Swiss psychiatrist, spent much of her life defining the stages of grief.

Priority Setting

This chapter describes the role of an EOL nurse. It talks about what you need to learn and explains many things you should work to understand. Caregivers cannot apply information regarding EOL in an effective way unless they have come to an understanding within themselves about death. That is your priority for this chapter. Take the content you read and internalize it. Think about people who have died who were important to you. How did you feel, react, and grieve? If you are confused or uncomfortable with death experiences, where can you go to get more information? Who can you talk to about the death of someone who was close to you? Do you have religious beliefs that comfort you or friends who can assist you to accept the death? Do you understand gerotranscendence, through which individuals plan for their own good death and accept it? Do you apply gerotranscendence to your own life?

To give effective EOL care, you need to be at peace with death and its complexities. You should see it as the personal, meaningful, unique experience it is and then be able to share that with the patients, residents, and families with whom you work.

Critically Examine the Following:

Now that we have discussed various aspects of EOL issues, it is time for you to express some of your thoughts on the topic. Take a few minutes to contemplate and consider your perfect death. The purpose of this exercise is to have you apply the information you have just read. Some of the questions you should answer are listed. Answer them and then add more detail. Consider this a "free write," where anything you say will be respected.

How old will you be when you die?
What will be your general health condition?
Who will still be alive and be with you as
    you die?
How will you die?

Add other comments you want to make.

Now consider your ancestors and how and when they died. You have described your perfect death, but few people get to experience such an event. By looking at your parents' and grandparents' health and the death of family members, you will see your genetic predisposition. What do your genes indicate as a possible death?

Do you have any potentially dangerous hobbies such as skydiving or car racing? Do you drive an excessive number of miles in a year? Do you have poor health habits? What do these lifestyle behaviors indicate about your eventual death?

You will die. By trying to understand your own death, you will be able to give better care to people who are at the end of their lives.

Death, the greatest personal loss a person can have, was the focus of her grief work. If you understand the five stages of grief, you can recognize them within yourself, the older adults to whom you give care, and their families. It is important knowledge to acquire.

Death is hard. It is a one-time experience, which makes death a unique and powerful experience. When a person dies, that individual loses everything they ever had. The dying person loses friends and family members, home, pets, beauty—everything. The stages of grief demonstrate the normal human reactions that people can have when facing a loss. Perhaps the person grieving is a family member of the person dying. His or her loss is also great. In addition to death, the stages of grief are valid with the loss of an extremity through amputation or loss associated with a stroke or divorce; for a young girl, the loss of a date to the prom can result in a brief grieving process.

Kübler-Ross (1969) identified the five stages as follows:

>   Acceptance
>   Depression
>   Bargaining
>   Anger
> Denial

Think of these terms as steps in the process of resolving grief. The person experiencing the loss can go from one stage (or step) to another and then move back up or down the stages. There is no exact formula or prescription to follow because people are individuals and manage their grief in very personalized ways. Nurses need to allow this type of independent grieving.

Denial

When a catastrophic loss occurs, a person's psyche has difficulty accepting it. Consider a young mother who leaves her aging and confused mom outside for "only a moment" while she goes in the house to get her baby. When the young mother comes out of the house, her mother has wandered out into the street, is hit by a car, and eventually dies in the hospital. Some denial behaviors are shock, praying for it to not be true, walking about, or standing and saying, "No, not Mom" over and over again.

Denial is the psyche's way of protecting itself from the harsh, bitter truth. It is as if the young mother were wrapped up in a soft, protective cocoon. This psychological protection is there

until the person's psyche can deal with the loss. You have heard of people who "were in a daze" during the funeral of a loved one. That is denial. There is no reason to try to force people out of denial. They will move to the next stage when they are able. During this time, people need to be protected from neglect, injury, and financial abuse. Family members need to understand this stage of the grief process and be willing to take care of other children, prepare meals, and protect the grieving person.

Anger

When the psyche has developed the strength to face the situation, it comes out in a way that tends to keep people away, which saves the person grieving a great deal of energy. What else does it do? This is the one time that anger should be encouraged in a person and supported as a healthy behavior when it occurs. Can you think of some of the advantages of the grieving person showing anger?

Anger demonstrates an awareness of the loss and its consequences. This is one step toward adjusting to the loss. It is also an outlet for the outrage the person feels. Assist the grieving person not to hurt himself or herself or others with the anger. The family needs to understand the advantages of the anger so that they can accept what is happening and support the behaviors that occur.

Bargaining

The anger is as if the psyche wants to "scare away" the bad thing that has occurred. As we know, that does not work. When the grieving person realizes that the "bad thing" will not go away, he or she often turns to God or another higher power. This behavior often is demonstrated by bargaining.

Bargaining is seen as something like prayers to a higher power stating that the person will donate a great deal of money to a charitable organization, will never sin again, or will actively do good for others. The thinking is that if one trades something of value, like goodness, with a higher power, then a miracle will be performed. This is very heartbreaking for family and friends. Many say they prefer anger over the wrenching episodes of bargaining. The negotiation process is the final chance to change the situation. If the higher power cannot "fix things," then no one can. This time in the grieving process requires patience and gentleness. People are often exhausted in their efforts to support the grieving person. They do not have much more to give. Yet, more is asked of them. When you teach families about the bargaining stage, reassure them that this is often near the end. Praise them for staying with the grieving person throughout the entire experience. Try to give them strength and courage to see the experience to its conclusion.

Not everyone believes in God or a higher power. Work with grieving people in whatever way they are bargaining. The principles are the same for all forms of grief bargaining.

Depression

Depression never is an easy condition. In the grieving process, it definitely shows progress. When a grieving person is depressed, it means that the individual does not accept the loss but accepts the fact that nothing can change it. The denial, anger, and bargaining did not work. It makes sense that the grieving person would be depressed.

As with all forms of depression, actively assess for suicidal thinking. If you identify it, keep someone with the grieving person and contact the registered nurse (RN). Suicide is a preventable outcome, so be sensitive to its possibility. Depressed people cry, they sleep a great deal, and they have low energy. Teach this to the family members. Ask them to support the grieving person through this last hurtle to acceptance.

Depressed people do not need to be told, "Everything is all right." For them, nothing will ever be all right again. They need quiet love and support while they find a way to continue on with their lives.

Acceptance

When the grieving person reaches acceptance, there is a sense of relief. The individual still is searching for life structure without the loved one who died. The point is that the grief process is over,

This woman has accepted that she is going to die. As is common with so many people, she does not want to interact with the world anymore. She is done; she has accepted the fact that she is close to death. Notice that she has her call light in hand "just in case." She also must have slowing circulation, as indicated by the afghan, blanket, and oxygen.

and living has started again. The grieving person still may call out the name of the deceased person, be found crying after finding a piece of clothing of the loved one, or just sit quietly contemplating the life of the person who died. This is normal.

The grieving process is difficult for the person experiencing the loss and the family members. The management of the experience can be improved when you, the LPN, know the stages of grief and readily share them with appropriate people.

After reading this last section, consider the daughter Liz from the case study. What stage do you think she is in currently? As a nurse, what can you do to support Liz during her grieving process?

QUALITIES FOR A NURSE TO BE A PROVIDER OF END-OF-LIFE CARE

Many nurses have difficulty talking about EOL matters with patients. You need to learn new skills and acquire new knowledge to improve the care of older adults who require EOL care (Box 11.1). Some of the new knowledge you need may be communication skills and knowledge of resources and available services.

You, as a nurse, have a tremendous potential to change the care of dying older adults and the support given to their families. It is crucial that you understand human nature as you give care to people who are dying. You need to be able to identify the stages of grief and translate those stages to family members. Because the stages are expressed individually by different people, you need to be able to comprehend the impact on specific individuals and understand the nature of the people involved.

Tolerance and Empathy

Each individual you encounter in your work is unique. As the care provider, you will need to gain an understanding of people and their differences. This requires that you learn to become tolerant and empathetic to those with whom you associate. Synonyms of tolerance are *compassion, endurance, patience, impartiality,* and *open-mindedness.* Synonyms of empathy are *understanding, sympathetic, identifying with the patient,* and *providing insight and feeling in your care.* To provide appropriate tolerance and empathy, you must strive to create an environment that meets the physical, emotional, social, and spiritual needs of each dying person. You will also need to show tolerance and empathy for the family members of your dying patients. The two daughters from the case study are both dealing with the reality that their father is going to die and will need care and understanding as they support their father through a difficult time.

Sense of Humor

Having a sense of humor with the dying person is a simple way to assist in relieving, reducing, and soothing the symptoms of a disease. You must know the personality and mood of the older adult in your care before making jokes about the situation. You must make sure that it is done at the right time and in the right situation. Think about a time and place when you were suffering and laughter helped with the cure.

Communication

Communication is the key to most situations. When it comes to death and dying, this situation has the possibility of being discussed in a context of hope, meaning, and opportunity. With strong communication skills, uncertainty is replaced with certainty, hopelessness is replaced with faith, and despair is replaced with empowerment.

Good Listening Skills

Being a good listener is the greatest skill any nurse can have. Take time to listen to older adults' stories about their children and grandchildren, stories about falling in love, and possibly stories about losing their loved ones. Older people enjoy sharing their life experiences. It is important to remember when talking to an older person that you need to speak in a voice that he or she can hear. Move in close to the person, touch his or her shoulder, smile, and listen to what he or she has to share.

BOX 11.1 QUALITIES TO DEVELOP BEFORE WORKING WITH DYING PEOPLE

- *Motivation*
- *Emotional maturity.* Death is serious and individualized and happens only once for each person.
- *Tolerance and empathy.* Nothing goes according to a formula or procedure. This is true of the dying process and people.
- *Communication skills.* You need the ability to empathize with all people involved in the death experience.
- *Confidentiality.* A sense of discretion and respect for patient and family privacy is essential.
- *Flexibility.* You must be willing to do what patients and their families need, not what you think is best.
- *Dependability.* Dependability turns into trust.
- *Good listening skills.* Listening is a wonderful gift you can give to someone who may be feeling frightened and alone.
- *Sense of humor.* Humor in difficult situations can be a plus. It is okay to laugh with patients and families.

FOCUSED LEARNING CHART

Understanding tolerance and empathy

A care provider's goal is to understand the needs of people experiencing an end-of-life situation.

Tolerance	Empathy
Compassion	Understanding
Impartiality	Identify with person
Endurance	Sympathetic
Patience	Be insightful
Open-mindedness	Allow self to feel situation

To listen, you must be fully present and attentive to the other person. You are not listening if you:

- Are in a hurry
- Are thinking about yourself
- Interrupt
- Ask the same question twice
- Do not ask any questions
- Assume that you know what the other person is going to say

A good listener is one who does not think about what to say until after the other person has finished speaking. When talking to Mr. Reed about his concerns regarding his death, it is important to listen quietly while he talks and ask questions for clarification.

 ## CULTURAL ACCOUNTABILITY

In addition to the previously mentioned qualities that are needed to care for individuals nearing the end of their lives, it is important to be familiar with the cultural diversities of the older adults in your care. A person's culture influences the decision-making process in regard to various treatments.

In many cultures, a family's interdependence, harmony, duty, and obligation to an older family member are obvious. Some cultures believe that it is inappropriate to tell someone that he or she is dying because it would create a sense of hopelessness and sadness. Some cultures believe that a sick individual should not be allowed to make any decisions about EOL care but rather have the family or the eldest son make those decisions. Cultural needs should be addressed immediately on admission to any facility for you, as the LPN, to be aware of the family's and the individual's diverse needs.

 ## END-OF-LIFE DECISIONS

As a care provider for individuals who are nearing the end of their lives, it is crucial that you recognize the importance of being aware of the decisions a person has made about his or her current and future medical care and to honor his or her preferences. Discussing EOL issues can be difficult for many older adults and their families. As a nurse, it is your role to guide the patient through this discussion and make sure the patient's wishes are documented. Having the patient make these decisions provides the health-care team the information they need to provide the best care to the patient. It also helps family members understand the wishes of their loved one so they can provide support to the patient during a difficult and stressful time.

Gaining an understanding of all of the issues surrounding EOL care is a daunting task. You will run into challenges about knowledge and skills in assessing and managing pain in cognitively impaired older adults. You will experience frustration about primary care providers being unwilling to consider a nurse's assessment and recommendations. You will find it difficult to deal with the strong emotional attachments that are formed with older adults at the EOL stage. These are all reasons to learn and study EOL issues.

Palliative Care

Palliative care is the term used to describe care that is no longer aimed at a cure or active treatment of a certain medical condition. Instead, the goals of palliative care are to provide older adults with comfort and to manage their symptoms. This could include treating an infection that is causing a dying person discomfort while not treating the terminal illness.

Palliative care is not limited to a hospital setting because an older adult may receive palliative care in a long-term care or assisted living setting. Palliative care is the art and science of quality EOL care. It is your opportunity, as an LPN, to take the initiative in providing palliative care that ensures comprehensive, holistic EOL care for all older adults who are experiencing life-threatening, progressive illness. It is the opportunity to be sensitive and respectful to the older person's values, religious beliefs, family traditions, individual cultures, and beliefs. It is a tremendous amount of responsibility.

Hospice

Hospice comes from the term hospitality and can be traced back to medieval times, when there was a need to find a place of rest for weary and ill travelers. Today, hospice organizations are located all over the United States. Although hospice services are being used more widely, most hospice organizations report being underused. This is poor use of a potentially tremendous service. The hospice team provides care to the patient as well as support and education to family members. Hospice care can be provided in a care facility or home setting.

Often, referrals to a hospice come "too little, too late" to be most effective. Only 30% of dying patients are referred to hospice, and some of these patients are referred in the last hour or day of their life (Quill, 2012). An example of providing successful care is that of patients with Alzheimer's disease. Providing them with palliative care may be the primary long-term mode of care. When death is imminent, generally around the last 6 months of life, a hospice team should be called on to provide their specialized knowledge to the palliation plan of care for the transition from dying to death. Providing Mr. Reed's daughters with information about hospice is important. They have many decisions to make regarding the best care for their father, and hospice workers can provide assistance in making those decisions.

BOX 11.2   ESSENTIAL COMPONENTS OF HOSPICE PROGRAMS

The following qualities can be found in an excellent hospice program:

- Serves patients, families, and the community with sensitivity to different cultures, values, and beliefs
- Provides interdisciplinary teams of palliative care experts educated to give competent, compassionate, highly skilled, state-of-the-art care to dying people
- Has a low patient-to-worker ratio
- Is responsive 24 hours per day, 7 days per week
- Elicits and responds to patient and family needs and wants and encourages involvement of patient's own physician
- Produces accurate, reliable data about care, outcomes, and costs
- Earns community support

Adapted from St. Christopher's Hospice. (2001). http://www.stchristophers.org.uk/.

QSEN

COMPETENCY: Patient-Centered Care (Knowledge, Attitude)

Respecting Patient and Family Needs

John has been taking care of a 75-year-old patient with terminal cancer who is receiving chemotherapy and is on home-care service. The patient's wife, Ann, has provided the majority of his care while he has been ill. For the last week, she has been voicing to John her concern about her husband's recent decline and increased need for pain medication. Ann is concerned that her husband is not comfortable and worries that the chemotherapy is not helping him and wants to stop all treatment. She states that she is physically and emotionally tired. She also states that she feels guilty about "giving up" on her husband. John spends the next hour listening to Ann while she tells him how she doesn't want her husband to suffer anymore. John then talks to her about hospice care and the services it can provide and suggests she make an appointment to see about getting her husband on a hospice service.

Patient-centered care means providing support to family members and diversity of their needs.

1. Do you feel the patient's wife is "giving up" on her husband?
2. What emotions is Ann struggling with at this time?
3. Do you feel John was inappropriate in suggesting hospice care to Ann? Why or why not?
4. What services can hospice provide Ann?

 ## ADVANCE DIRECTIVES

One of the most difficult situations that health-care professionals face when caring for older people is how to assist patients and families who are trying to make decisions about whether to start, continue, or stop life-sustaining treatments. Elderly people as a group account for 73% of deaths each year, making EOL treatment decisions far more prevalent among them. Documents that assist the health-care team in making such complex decisions are advance directives. There are two types of advance

directive documents available: the durable power of attorney for health care (also called health-care proxy) and living wills.

The health-care proxy has the authority to make health-care decisions if the individual loses the ability to make decisions or communicate personal wishes. The proxy can make decisions as the need arises and is not restricted to a decision that was made previously without knowledge of the current situation.

The other type of advance directive is known as a living will. This is a legal document that allows individuals to share their opinions and wishes regarding their death. The living will can list in detail the types of treatments a person wants to receive such as mechanical ventilation, cardiopulmonary resuscitation (CPR), or a feeding tube. Or the living will may state that a person wants everything done to sustain life. Despite the importance of an older adult's completing an advance directive, many

 # Evidence-Based Practice

Hickman R.L., & Pinto M.D. (2013). Advance directives lessen the decisional burden of surrogate decision-making for the chronically critically ill. Journal of Clinical Nursing, 23, 756-765.

Despite federal legislation supporting the use of advanced directives, most aging persons do not complete advanced directives. As the person becomes more incapacitated by illness, there is a need for someone to make health-care decisions on that person's behalf. This is considered surrogate decision making. This study looked at the relationship between advanced directive status and the burden put on surrogate decision makers. The study found that when an advanced directive existed, specifically a living will, it did decrease the burden associated with surrogate decision making. This study supports the need for patient and family education about advanced directives.

Questions

1. As an LPN, what education can you provide to your patients and family members regarding advanced directives?
2. For a patient without an advanced directive, how can you support the family as they make life and death decisions for their loved one?

This family is discussing end-of-life issues with their parent and completing an advanced directive.

aging Americans are reluctant to complete the appropriate forms (Camhi, et al. 2009). The legal statutes that govern the use of advance directives vary from state to state. You, as an LPN, must clearly understand the advance directive laws where you work. For more information about legal issues related to advance directives, refer to Chapter 5. You can also refer to Appendix A for an example of an advance directive.

 ## IMMINENT SIGNS OF DEATH

As an LPN, it is important for you to know the imminent signs of death. It is easy to assist someone in his or her preparation to die if the person has received a diagnosis of a terminal illness. A terminal diagnosis allows individuals to realign their priorities, mend various relationships, and say goodbye to loved ones. In addition, a terminal diagnosis allows staff the opportunity to prioritize their care and assist persons in meeting their goals and achieving a peaceful life closure.

Critically Examine the Following:

Have you considered what you would like written in your living will? Do you want to be pain-free? What about use of antibiotics? What about use of mechnical ventilation? What about a feeding tube? Use Part 2 of the advance directive in Appendix A to begin writing your living will.

When death is near, bodily functions slow, and certain signs and symptoms occur, including the following:

• Rapid, weak pulse
• Decline in blood pressure
• Dyspnea and periods of apnea
• Slower or no pupil response to light
• Profuse perspiration
• Cold extremities
• Bladder and bowel incontinence
• Pallor and mottling of skin
• Loss of hearing

One of the last senses lost is that of hearing.

One clear sign of imminent death is terminal restlessness (TR), another term for agitated delirium. This is a common occurrence for individuals nearing the end of their lives. It may appear as involuntary muscle twitching or jerks, thrashing or agitation, tossing and turning, or yelling and moaning. Reports indicate that more than three-fourths of dying patients experience this condition. TR occurs in the last hours of life. It is the spiraling down of physiological functions and can be very distressing to the older adult who is dying and to family and staff members. At this time so close to EOL, there is a crucial need for careful and thoughtful intervention to provide the dying person with comfort and to be able to control his or her symptoms.

Dying is an individualized experience. It is something that has never happened to the dying person before, and the individual may need your assistance in making the death a good one. One thing you can do is talk to the person to identify individual attitudes and knowledge regarding death, disease, and support systems already in place. Formal assessments are done by the assigned RN; however, you, as the LPN, are giving the bedside care and need to be prepared to respond to questions that are asked after the RN's assessment. The goal of your assessment is to be able to gain a clear understanding of the older person's experiences with his or her illness. In addition, you need to be able to identify distressing symptoms that need management, convey your concern and empathy to the persons involved, and evaluate any risk that may be expressed owing to current distress or feelings. It is important for you to take immediate action when a problem is detected.

To begin an appropriate assessment or interview with the dying person, you should ask various questions about discouragement or distress. For example, "What hurts or distresses you most, and how can I help?" Another good opening question to ask is what the person worries about most when the illness is at its worst and what has been most difficult throughout the process. Your assessment should review the older adult's various abilities to cope with stress and anxiety. For example, "During periods of discouragement, some people wish all this suffering were over. Have you felt this way? Tell me about it." "You seem to feel as if life is not worth living. Are you thinking of doing something to hasten your death? Tell me about it." "No one thinks about ending their life without a reason; tell me how you are feeling."

 ## CONCLUSION

Now that you have read this chapter, I hope you understand the importance of giving meaningful EOL care to all people but especially to older adults. Dying is a unique experience for everyone. The hallmark of a professional nurse is one who can support the dying person and the family in their personal uniqueness of that special event.

I admire your desire and passion for working with older adults. They are at a fragile time in their lives when they are in need of people who care about them. As the LPN who will provide older adults who are dying with positive EOL experiences, you are one of those individuals.

CASE STUDY SOLUTIONS

1. As an LPN, you need to assess what Mr. Reed understands about his cancer and the fact that his physician has decided to stop treatment. You also need to identify his attitude toward his own death and any concerns he may have about the dying process. As part of this assessment you will want to identify any cultural needs that may have an impact on Mr. Reed and how the nursing staff could support Mr. Reed and his daughters during the dying process. This discussion needs to be a private conversation between you and Mr. Reed at a time when he is rested and comfortable. During this discussion, you need to be willing to answer all of Mr. Reed's questions honestly. If you are unable to answer specific questions about his cancer, you will need to make sure there is an opportunity for Mr. Reed to address these questions with his physician. Once you know what Mr. Reed thinks and feels about his cancer and eventual death, then you will be able to advocate for his needs.

2. You will want to encourage Mr. Reed's daughters to discuss with their father what he is thinking and feeling about his death. They need to have an open discussion about their father's wishes regarding his death.

3. As part of this process, you will want to contact a hospice agency to talk to Mr. Reed and his daughters regarding the services hospice can offer. You will want to identify whether Mr. Reed has completed an advanced directive. If not, you will want to discuss with Mr. Reed and his daughter's the importance of having an advanced directive. You need to provide the appropriate forms for their review and signatures.

REVIEW QUESTIONS

1. When an elderly client experiences TR, he or she will display symptoms such as:
   1. Involuntary muscle twitching or jerks
   2. Extreme fatigue
   3. A sudden energy for life
   4. A calm affect causing the body to have no reactions

2. Palliative care is described as:
   1. The type of care aimed at a cure or active treatment of a certain medical condition
   2. The type of care that provides comfort and management of symptoms
   3. The type of care that allows the family to make all of the decisions
   4. The type of care that provides bereavement support to the family for 1 year after death

3. The stages of grief in order are:
   1. Denial, anger, bargaining, depression, acceptance
   2. Denial, communicate, pain, sadness, joy
   3. Denial, affection, bartering, acceptance
   4. Denial, anger, acceptance, joy, peace

4. When speaking to an elderly dying patient, it is important to:
   1. Never talk to the patient, but rather communicate all decisions through family members
   2. Communicate clearly, possibly with a sense of humor, in a manner that the patient will be able to hear what is being said
   3. Explain your frustrations with the patient and his or her care in front of the patient and the family
   4. Be sympathetic rather than empathetic with the patient and the family

5. Four of the eight signs of imminent death are:
   1. Increased blood pressure, warm extremities, bowel and bladder incontinence, and pallor and mottling of the skin
   2. Loss of hearing, dyspnea and periods of apnea, and increased bowel and bladder control
   3. Increased sexual drive, slow pupil response to light, increased awareness of surroundings, and more communicative
   4. Rapid weak pulse, profuse perspiration, loss of hearing, and decline in blood pressure

REFERENCES

Camhi, S., Mercado, A., Morrison, S., Du, Q., Platt, D., August, G., & Nelson, J. (2009). Deciding in the dark: Advance directives and continuation of treatment in chronic critical illness. *Critical Care Medicine, 37,* 919-925.

Kübler-Ross, E. (1969). *On death and dying.* New York, NY: McMillan.

Quill, T.E. (2012). Physicians should 'assist in suicide' when it is appropriate. *Journal of Law, Medicine and Ethics,* 40(1), 57-65.

WEB RESOURCES

Caring Connections: http://www.caringinfo.org/
Hospice and Palliative Nurses Association: https://www.hpna.org

Hospice Foundation of America: http://www.hospicefoundation.org/
National Hospice and Palliative Care Organization: http://www.nhpco.org/

Environments of Care

12

KATHLEEN R. CULLITON

LEARNING OUTCOMES

1. Discuss the role of the licensed practical nurse (LPN) as an environmental manager.

2. Describe at least two components of the physical environment that nurses need to consider.

3. Discuss the aspects included in a climate of caring.

4. Identify at least four settings in which nursing care for older adults is provided.

5. Describe how nurses in various care settings meet the needs of older adults.

6. Discuss relocation stress and ways in which a nurse can help an older person adjust to a new environment.

CONCEPTS

Collaboration

Care Coordination

Health-care Organizations

CASE STUDY

Your neighbor, Sally, asks your advice about finding good care for her 80-year-old grandmother. The grandmother, Mrs. Gilmore, lives at home alone in an isolated section outside the city limits. She recently was discharged from the hospital after injuring her right arm in a fall at home. Her right arm is in a full cast from fingers to upper arm, which makes it difficult for Mrs. Gilmore to cook and perform other self-care activities. Your neighbor is unable to visit her grandmother daily because of work and child-care commitments. Sally is worried about her grandmother's ability to remain at home. She invited her grandmother to move in with her for at least a month, but Mrs. Gilmore insists on staying in her own home. Sally asks for your advice. She ends the conversation with the statement, "I just don't know what else we can do to make sure Grandma is safe and taken care of in her home."

Discussion

Based on the previously described situation and your reading of this chapter, what advice would you offer Sally?

 ## INTRODUCTION

One of the most important tasks for a nurse is to manage the patient-care environment. Florence Nightingale saved the lives of hundreds of soldiers during the Crimean War simply by cleaning the wards, opening the windows, and providing the soldiers with daily hygiene. Nightingale and her nurses also provided direct, caring, "hands-on" nursing to the soldiers under their care. Before Nightingale's interventions, there were more soldiers dying in the hospitals because of the lack of hygienic conditions than there were dying in the battles. Improved health for the men fighting the Crimean War required environmental management and quality nursing care.

The role of a nurse is not that of a housekeeper but that of an environmental manager. To be effective caregivers, nurses must be aware of the influence of environment on the health and functioning of the patient. Nurses are responsible for the manipulation of environmental conditions to improve patient care. In Florence Nightingale's era, environmental management included such tasks as opening windows to clear the patient's room of stale, potentially illness-producing air; managing raw sewage because plumbing was not available; and controlling the population of mice and rats in the hospital. Modern nurses also must understand the effect that the environment can have on enhancing or impeding the progress and functioning of older adults.

 ## ENVIRONMENTAL MANAGEMENT

Providing care to older adults must include environmental management. Assessment of the environment is the first step. As a licensed practical nurse (LPN), you need to examine the total environment starting with where the older person is living. There are multiple environments of care in which an older adult might live. If the person lives at home, you might ask the following questions: What is the neighborhood like? Is it a safe neighborhood for an older person? Is there a security system in the home or building?

If an older adult lives in a nursing home or is receiving care in a hospital or rehabilitation center, you might ask the following questions: What is the staffing ratio? Is the environment clean and free of odor? Is there a place where the older adult can socialize with family and friends?

If an older adult lives in an assisted living environment, you might ask: How far is it to the dining room? Are there activities that interest the person? Is there a nurse available 24 hours a day?

Assessment of the physical environment includes all aspects of the older adult's living situation that can be seen, heard, touched, or smelled.

This nursing home resident with dementia and generalized weakness has found herself in a climate of caring. Notice how her clothes match and appear well cared for? Her hair is nicely done, and she is smiling. The LPN kneeling next to her demonstrates a basic symbol of caring. She got down to the older woman's wheelchair level so that she could be seen and heard.

Each of the physical items in the environment can either contribute to or detract from the optimal functioning of the older person. A room that is too hot may make the older person tired, lethargic, and unwilling to participate in personal-care activities. A room that is too cold may likewise result in lack of activity because the older person is unwilling to get out of bed or to come out from under the cover of an afghan.

A crucial question to ask throughout the assessment of the physical environment is how well the older person functions in the living areas. Is the environment as barrier-free as possible? Can the older person walk unencumbered or wheel a wheelchair through the entire setting? Are there features in the environment to promote physical function? These may include grab bars in the bathroom by the commode, shower, or bathtub seat and handrails by stairs. When assessing how the older person carries out activities of daily living, be aware of possible alterations that may improve function. Lowering a mirror or moving a storage

Think Like a Nurse

People do everything better when they are in a caring environment. Remember Dr. Jean Watson's theory of human caring? She has spent her career researching and documenting the significance of caring in our lives. When a nurse and a patient connect in a caring way, Dr. Watson refers to it as "transpersonal caring." This happens when you, as the nurse, relate to the older adult in a holistic manner that is based on caring, or, in other words, you care about every aspect of the person's life, including his or her environment.

area below shoulder level may improve safety and convenience. The risk of falling can be decreased with adequate room lighting and the use of night-lights. The room where the older person reads should have high-intensity illumination. When assessing Mrs. Gillmore's home you will want to keep the safety of her current environment in mind.

Climate of Caring

Another important part of the environmental assessment is evaluating the climate of caring. The climate of caring involves the people in the environment and the environmental tone and atmosphere. The people in an older person's living environment may include family members, neighbors, friends, and paid caregivers.

The people in an environment are extremely important to the older adult's potential for improvement and optimal function. Families, staff members, and visitors can be encouraging and uplifting or depressing and discouraging. A climate of caring includes persons who present a positive but realistic outlook. An older adult's personal space is respected in a caring climate. Such an atmosphere also affords opportunities for privacy, encourages activity and involvement, and facilitates independence.

Safety

In any setting, safety for the older person is a primary concern. Are there any environmental hazards, such as frayed extension cords, malfunctioning equipment, or broken furniture? Falls among elderly people are common. Although not all falls can be avoided, one thing that can be done is to keep the environment free of fall risks. Such risks include clutter, throw rugs, wheelchair leg rests, and poorly fitting shoes or slippers. A pet sometimes can be a fall risk as well. Refer to Chapter 7 for other safety issues.

Stimulation and Personalization

Opinions vary on whether environments for older adults with cognitive impairment should be very stark and nonstimulating or should contain eye-catching and stimulating components. What is more important is a personalized environment for the older person. Personalized items help older adults relate to the environment and maintain a sense of identity. A special picture can be displayed in a hospital room or nursing home. In some settings, such as nursing homes and retirement communities, the entire bedroom or apartment can be personalized with cherished furniture and decorations.

A climate of caring facilitates optimal independence and autonomy for each older person living in the setting. Sometimes the routines and regulations necessary to operate a large health-care facility such as a hospital or nursing home cannot accommodate the individual needs or desires of older adults. The nurse must assess, however, which rules and routines are absolutely necessary and which are the result of a controlling institution or individual staff member. Although a nursing home may need to serve meals at particular times because of regulations and staffing, the rule that all residents must be dressed for breakfast may be unnecessary. This rule does not allow for each resident to take the time personally to do as much of the dressing as possible. Such a rule can force a resident to be dependent on staff for dressing. A climate of caring provides multiple opportunities for individual choice in the environment and encourages the older person to function as independently as possible.

Personal Space and Territoriality

Personal space and territory are important to every human being. Personal space is the area around a person. Some individuals define their personal space very close to their bodies, whereas others define it as a broader area. It is viewed as an intrusion for someone to invade another individual's personal space. In providing nursing care, nurses must frequently invade the personal space of the patient. Nurses must be conscious, however, that they do not do so unnecessarily.

Territory is the space used by a person and seen as owned by the person. Think about a current class. Do the students tend to sit in the same seats during each class session? Technically, you and your classmates do not own the seats, but the tendency exists to define a territory and return to it habitually. The seating arrangement in a dining room in a nursing home or retirement community is frequently consistent for each meal. This consistency tends to occur whether or not seats are assigned. Individuals defend their territory if an unwanted person intrudes. An older person who has a favorite chair at home or in the nursing home may fiercely defend it from others.

Privacy

All human beings need time to be alone. People need to have opportunities for privacy and for human contact. It is difficult sometimes for an older person living in a health-care setting to find opportunities for privacy. Many hospitals and nursing homes have multiple-occupancy rooms so that the patient may never have a chance to be truly alone. As a nurse working with older persons in a congregate setting, you must be aware of the older person's needs for privacy. You should respect that right to privacy by knocking on the door before entering, pulling cubicle curtains during care, and arranging private time for the older adult.

Activity and Involvement

As a person ages, the number of social roles fulfilled tends to diminish. An older woman who was once a daughter, a wife, a mother, a neighbor, an accountant, a Scout leader, and a bridge player may hold none of these social roles at 90 years of age. Because of aging and disability, these roles may no longer be possible. Involvement with others is still a need, however. A climate of caring affords each individual multiple and diverse opportunities for activity and involvement with others.

As a nurse working with older people in multiple health-care settings, you can help to provide important opportunities for active involvement. It is important to find out the older person's prior social roles, particularly the ones he or she most enjoyed. Activities that include tasks associated with these roles should be encouraged. It also is important to create opportunities for social interaction. By introducing the older person to others in the setting who may share similar interests and

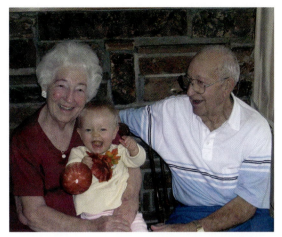

This grandma and grandpa are both past 80 years of age and have lived in their current home since they were a young married couple. They have made it clear to their children that they do not want to leave their home if they become ill. They have a large extended family, and they want to be around them until they die. Many older people have a strong aversion to leaving their homes, which is why home care is such a valuable resource to older adults.

by arranging seating for natural conversation rather than against walls, the nurse can be instrumental in encouraging social exchanges.

 RELOCATION TRAUMA

Moving from one environment to another is stressful. Anyone who has ever moved from one house to another or from one city to another can appreciate the stress of relocation. It takes time to adjust to and become familiar with a new setting. During times of crisis or illness, one has less energy available to deal constructively with stress. Older adults are particularly susceptible to being overcome with the stress of relocation. Such stress also is referred to as transitional stress. This term refers specifically to the emotional stress that occurs during the time a person is changing from one phase of life to another.

Older people use a considerable amount of energy coping with chronic illness and disabilities. The onset of an acute illness or some other major crisis requires additional coping. If the crisis or illness results in the need to move to another living situation, the older person's coping abilities may be exhausted. A crisis, superimposed on the day-to-day stresses of living with disability and dysfunction, frequently leaves the older person with little coping reserve to deal with the stress of relocation and transition. When the stress is overwhelming, and the older person is unable to cope with the situation, signs of decompensation appear. These may include disorientation, agitation, acting out, and hallucinations. It is common for an older adult newly admitted to any of the health-care settings described in this chapter to exhibit some of these signs. The movement from one environment to another can be extremely disruptive to the older adult; this disruption has been termed *relocation trauma*. You will want to consider the possible impact of relocation trauma on Mrs. Gillmore when assessing her situation.

In addition to identifying and understanding relocation trauma, the nurse can help to relieve relocation stress. Relocation trauma is temporary, and the behavioral signs of decompensation should diminish as the older person becomes familiar with the new environment. You can accelerate the process of adjustment, however.

Limit stimulation and the introduction of new activities and people on the older person's first day in the setting. Orient the older person to the environment slowly so that he or she can incorporate new areas and routines gradually. On the first day, introduce only people and places that are absolutely necessary. For example, placing an older person in the dining room of a nursing home with 20 other residents shortly after admission may be overwhelming.

Look for ways to provide links between the old environment and the new one. The more familiar the new environment is to the older person, the easier the transition is for the person. Bringing favorite furniture and objects, such as pictures, to the new setting increases its familiarity to the older person. Including the older person in planning for the move is ideal. This is not always possible, however, if the move occurs because of an acute illness. If it can be arranged, involve the older person in selecting the items to take to the new location.

 SETTINGS OF CARE

Older persons may receive health-care services in a variety of settings. This chapter does not discuss all such settings or services but reviews some of the most commonly used settings of care.

FOCUSED LEARNING CHART

Relocation trauma

Symptom of Decompensation	Nursing Care
Disorientation	Temporary condition
Hallucinations	Familiar items such as furniture and photos
Agitation	Involve family and friends
Acting out	Be caring
	Limit stimulation (people, places, and activities) for the first few days

---

QSEN

COMPETENCY: Teamwork and Collaboration (Knowledge, Skills, Attitude)

Using Teamwork to Provide Patient-Centered Care

Mrs. B. was moving from her home of 40 years to a retirement community. She had some short-term memory problems and walked with a slow gait. To help with the move, Mrs. B.'s son packed for her and sorted through all of her belongings. He identified what items to take and what to give away. Because many of her things were very old and worn, her son decided to purchase all new furniture and decorations for her new apartment. The new apartment looked beautiful. After moving, Mrs. B. became extremely disoriented and paranoid, and she accused everyone of stealing her belongings.

Her son was very upset, and the evening desk clerk reported that the son was trying to figure out what to do next. Because there is minimal interdisciplinary team staff at a retirement facility, you contact the administrator and the nurse consultant to arrange a meeting with the resident and her son. In the meeting the son is allowed to express his concerns about the dramatic change in his mother's demeanor and behavior. The group allows Mrs. B. to talk about the move from her home and her concerns and distress in the new apartment. The group discusses how nice the new furniture and items are in Mrs. B.'s apartment but how the lack of unfamiliar things may be contributing to her confusion and paranoid behavior. The group agrees that the son will bring some old family pictures, the anniversary clock, and some of Mrs. B.'s handwork to give the apartment some familiar touches.

In some care areas you will have to enlist the help of different individuals assigned to the care of a resident. Administrator and nurse consultants may not have direct patient-care responsibilities, but the well-being of the resident is their job. They have the resources and connections to ensure the best outcome for this resident and her son.

1. As the nurse in the retirement community, what would you have taught Mrs. B.'s son about preparing his mother for relocation?
2. What suggestions would you have to avoid this problem with future residents?

Adult Day Services

Adult day services (ADS) are available in many communities to provide supervised activities for older adults. Day treatment centers for older people with psychiatric problems and day hospitals for older persons with considerable physical disability are available in many localities. Day treatment centers and day hospitals focus on a particular type of older person and provide specific services to meet their physical and psychiatric needs. Many ADS provide transportation for the older person to and from the center. Fees for day care may be charged on a sliding scale, according to the ability of the older adult to pay. Some ADS are private pay while others may participate in a Medicaid waiver program. As a general rule, Medicare does not pay for ADS. Generally, the older person or the family must pay for these services personally.

A typical day in this care setting includes planned activities such as group discussion, current events, exercise, snacks, and lunch. Volun-teers may visit a center to speak on community affairs or health-promotion topics or to present entertainment programs that encourage group participation. Many centers have activity directors who plan and schedule events that are appealing, offer a variety of choices for the older adult, and promote group interaction.

Nurses working in ADS provide numerous services, according to the needs of the individual. Assessment of the older person's physical, psychological, and emotional functioning is a critical component of the nurse's role in the day-care center. Health teaching to older persons and their families also may be included in the nurse's role.

Some older people may need assistance with mobility, toileting, or eating. Other older adults may need help in taking medications. Still others simply need encouragement to participate in center activities. Nurses in adult day-care centers need a solid foundation in gerontological nursing to help them in their daily interactions with older people. This foundation ensures that subtle physical or emotional changes are not disregarded or blamed simply on "old age."

Acute illnesses in older adults can manifest in atypical fashion. A nurse who knows and appreciates normal aging is better prepared to assess subtle changes in older persons and to be alert to the possible implications of these changes. Because so many older adults have chronic illnesses, medication administration often becomes a major responsibility for the nurse in an ADS. The nurse

needs to be skillful at administering medications and needs to know their expected effects and possible side effects. The nurse also can use knowledge of medications to teach the older person and family members the importance of safe and accurate medication use. Do the older adult and family members know which medications are being taken and why they are prescribed? Are the older adult and family members aware of possible side effects, potential drug interactions, and the necessary steps to take if problems are suspected? The nurse, as teacher, has an important role in this setting.

Ongoing assessments of ADS participants are especially important. Frequent contact with the older person allows nurses to see subtle changes in function that may signal serious underlying physiological problems. The nurse's powers of observation and knowledge of the aging process are crucial in detecting actual or impending illness. Is an older person experiencing mobility changes? Are you seeing decreased participation in formerly active participants? Has an older person had changes in weight or affect? If you are making these types of observations, the next question to ask is why are you seeing these changes? Good communication skills may uncover a change in family living conditions, changes in medication, or exacerbation of the effects of a chronic illness.

ADS provide opportunities for socializing and staying involved in the world. Many families use day care to give respite to the main caregiver for the older adult. The stresses of caregiving can have a strong effect on the older person, caregiver, and family. Respite allows caregivers some time to

---

Think Like a Nurse

You are the licensed nurse at an adult day service. Mrs. Y. attends the center every Monday, Tuesday, and Wednesday until after lunch, when her husband picks her up. This Tuesday you notice, for the second day in a row, that Mrs. Y. has been unsteady when she walks. She stops to rest frequently when moving around the center and has been falling asleep during group activities. These behaviors are unusual because Mrs. Y. normally ambulates well, participates enthusiastically in center activities, and often encourages others to "join the fun." What further assessment do you now want to make? What types of questions would you ask her husband?

attend to their own needs. Grocery shopping, housekeeping, socializing with friends, and participating in enjoyable activities for the caregivers can often mean the difference between continued home care versus institutionalization for an older adult. Nurses in ADS are able to use their assessment skills to identify the older person's strengths and weaknesses, help elders to continue to participate in daily living activities, and provide information for older persons and their families about community resources.

Although ADS nurses may perform few technical nursing procedures, they use a variety of different nursing skills. ADS nurses must have particularly strong physical and psychological assessment skills. They also must be adept in communication and teaching. An ADS nurse also must have a thorough knowledge of community resources and be able to refer older persons and their families to appropriate services in the area.

With the increasing awareness and concern about care for people with dementia, some programs are now available to provide ADS specifically for older persons with cognitive impairments. These ADS are designed to give care that takes into account the abilities and safety needs of patients with Alzheimer's disease or other dementias.

Home Care

Home health-care agencies provide numerous services for older adults in the home. These agencies provide nursing services, given by licensed nurses and nursing assistants, and therapy services, such as physical, occupational, and speech therapy. Many agencies also provide medical supplies and equipment. Most agencies are licensed and eligible for state or federal reimbursement for services. Medicare, Medicaid, and community funding may pay for limited home health-care services if the older person qualifies for such reimbursement.

Home care may be provided on a daily basis or intermittently, according to the needs of the patient. Nursing care provided in the home has become more complex in the past two decades. It is not unusual for people who need help during their recovery to be discharged from the hospital "quicker and sicker." Older adults with a chronic illness may be receiving home care to avoid frequent hospitalizations.

The LPN in home care works under the supervision of the registered nurse (RN) case manager.

Evidence-Based Practice

Borowiak, E., & Kostka, T. (2013). Comparative characteristics of the home care nursing services used by community-dwelling older people from urban and rural environments. Journal of Advanced Nursing, 69(6), 1259-1268.

Over the years 2006 to 2010, the researchers visited 935 older adults living in an urban area and 812 older adults living in a rural area in Poland. Of the randomly selected older adults in the urban area, 4.1% were receiving home care and 6.5% of the rural living older adults were having nursing care in their home. The assessments of all of the older adults found that the significant risk factor for requiring nursing care in both the rural and urban setting was declining functional status. One of the biggest differences found between the urban and rural older adults was that a significantly larger number of urban older adults lived alone. More of the rural older adults had a family member or neighbor available to assist if they needed care support.

Questions

1. This is a Polish study. What do you think would be a difference between home-care nursing use in urban and rural areas of the United States?
2. Do you think that finances, education, insurance, and social support are different for urban and rural older adults?
3. As a home-care nurse, how would you incorporate these results in your practice?
4. How is care different for home-care patients with decreasing function?

In the home-health role, the LPN is assigned basic nursing care, medication administration and teaching, and dressings and wound care. The LPN often is asked to work with a certified nurse assistant (CNA) in coordinating care for the patient.

A certain amount of creativity is needed in home-care nursing owing to limitations in the type of equipment and supplies that are available. As in other settings, it is helpful for the nurse to be aware of resources available to the older adult and of ways to gain use of those resources. Nurses who

Think Like a Nurse

As an LPN for a home-care agency, you are assigned Mrs. E. Mrs. E. is 75 years old and lives with her husband in their home. Mrs. E. was just discharged from the hospital after surgery to pin her broken right hip. She is not capable of weight-bearing, and the physical therapist is scheduled to visit her at home twice a week. Mrs. E. has mild dementia and frequently forgets that she is not permitted to walk. Her husband, Mr. E., wants to keep her in bed to remind her not to walk. What care do you need to teach Mr. E.?

choose home-care nursing can expect a variety of older persons and conditions. Caring for older adults in the home can be very rewarding and challenging. Because a home-care nurse generally visits the older person on a less-than-daily basis, patient and family teaching is very important. Teaching may be needed to help the family ensure a safe environment for the older adult. Education about fall prevention, medication safety, positioning, and transferring techniques for older persons and families may be needed. A family also may need to learn more complex procedures, such as how to change dressings or give injected medications.

The amount of time spent with older persons is often limited by the nurse's workload and the reimbursement for care given. The nurse is responsible for assessing and documenting care needs and providing prescribed treatments. Good communication skills are important to ensure that all members of the health-care team are aware of the older person's needs and progress.

Community-Based Care

Nursing opportunities are available in various settings not linked to formal institutions such as hospitals or nursing homes. LPNs may provide care for older adults in a community clinic, dialysis center, or physician's office. In these noninstitutional settings, the nurse may practice under the direct supervision of a physician rather than RN. Practice in these settings often includes assisting with physical examinations and treatments, and nurses in these settings are frequently an important source of information and clarification for patients. The nurse uses assessment skills and provides information on resources available in

the community to meet the older person's needs. Contact with older adults in these settings may be more infrequent than in other care settings.

Hospice

Hospice care is designed to provide care for a dying person and the family. A team approach is central to the hospice concept. Team members include physicians, nurses, social workers, and nursing assistants as well as other ancillary workers. The goal of hospice care is to help dying persons remain at home, if possible, with all the support needed to ensure a "good death." In this case, "good" means that the older person is kept comfortable and able to receive the support of family and loved ones in a familiar setting.

Hospice work allows nurses to give direct patient care and develop a close relationship with the patient and family. As in the care settings previously discussed, the nurse's role as a teacher is especially helpful. Most families are not prepared to meet the needs of a dying family member. The hospice nurse can teach family members how to provide for the comfort of their loved one. The nurse also can identify hospice resources available to help families and older persons cope during this extremely demanding time. Nurses who have not worked in a hospice setting may be reluctant to try this type of nursing because all of the clients are terminally ill. Talking with nurses who work in a hospice often shows, however, that the team support and the closeness to patients and families provide a high degree of job satisfaction.

Assisted Living Environments

As people age, there is a tendency to simplify lifestyles and living space. The size of the home needed to provide adequate living space for a family can become more of a burden than an asset to older adults. Assisted living communities are an increasingly popular way for the elderly person to have a home without homeowner responsibilities. Not having yard work and other maintenance tasks associated with a large home relieves numerous burdens. Assisted living communities generally offer apartments with community dining and activity areas. They have a nurse, an activity director, CNAs, and housekeepers. The goal for these retirement communities is to appeal to a broad range of older adults by offering security and various conveniences and services. Although communities for retirees have been popular for quite a while, assisted living facilities that also provide services for older adults with physical care needs are now increasingly common. Many assisted living complexes have a satellite branch of a home health agency on site.

The goal of assisted living units is to provide older persons with help in performing activities of daily living. Frail older persons who do not require continuous care are able to have help in such activities as meal preparation, grooming and bathing, laundry, and housekeeping. Most assisted living programs require that the older person be ambulatory and fairly independent. Much of the care provided is done by nursing assistants rather than LPNs. The LPN in an assisted living program often provides supervision for nursing assistants, medication administration, basic documentation of care given, and assessment of the older person's ability to function.

The nurse in an assisted living community also must use creative talents to ensure that the environment is as homelike as possible. The nurse must be flexible in tailoring care to the individual needs of each older adult. The nursing assistant in assisted living care may be called a resident assistant and perform many functions that do not relate directly to activities of daily living. Nurses and nursing assistants working in assisted living care often are very involved in activities and social planning for residents.

Some assisted living facilities provide a continuum of care for older adults. Elderly adults can be admitted to their own apartments, but if their health changes, they can also be admitted to the nursing home for care.

For many older adults, the appeal of a continuing-care retirement community lies in the fact that adults are able to stay in a familiar environment regardless of their health status. Nursing in a continuing-care retirement community offers many opportunities. Home visits, health promotion or screening activities (e.g., blood pressure–monitoring clinics), health teaching, and direct bedside care to nursing home residents are a few of the opportunities available to nurses in continuing-care communities. As in assisted living situations, supervisory ability is a valuable asset for the LPN. Retirement community nursing allows nurses to work with older adults who have various needs and abilities. The ability to apply your knowledge of the aging process in this setting

helps you enhance the quality of life for the older persons there.

Nursing Homes

The nursing home is an area of practice that has been available to practical nurses for many years. With the growing number of frail elderly adults and old-old (85 and older) adults, the need for nursing home care is great. Some nursing home residents need a full range of nursing care; others may be independent physically but have cognitive changes that require a high degree of supervision to maintain their personal safety. Two categories of nursing home care are defined by federal regulation. The first category is the skilled nursing facility (SNF), and the second is the nursing facility. The nursing facility level was previously referred to as intermediate care.

All nursing homes must be licensed by the state in which they operate. If they wish to receive reimbursement from Medicare or Medicaid for the services provided to residents, they also must meet additional federal requirements and be certified by the federal government. A nursing home may choose not to accept Medicare and Medicaid funding and admit only private-pay residents.

In an SNF, licensed nurses provide care around the clock, and an RN is present at least 8 hours a day, 7 days a week. A SNF also offers the services of allied health professionals, such as speech, physical, or occupational therapists, at least 5 days a week. A nursing facility generally does not have the same level of staffing by RNs or therapists as an SNF.

Regardless of category, long-term care facilities offer a team approach to meeting the older person's needs over time. Facilities that receive federal funds are required to offer the services of a social worker and an activity director and dietetic consultant. Licensed nurses can gain input from various sources in planning and delivering care by being actively involved with the interdisciplinary health-care team.

In long-term care, the LPN has traditionally been responsible for supervising the nursing assistants who give hands-on care to residents; the LPN also gives medications and performs treatments.

A nurse interested in long-term care has the opportunity to get to know residents well over a long time. Because of the changing needs and physical condition of residents, the long-term care nurse

PATIENT EDUCATION

As an older adult anticipates transitioning from an acute care setting or an assisted living facility to a long-term care facility, he or she will have questions about how to choose a facility. Nurses can be instrumental in helping patients and families in the selection of a nursing home. The following is a list of some key elements that should be addressed when visiting a facility.

- The environment is clean, well maintained, odor free, and secure.
- There is a provision for private areas and the ability to personalize rooms.
- The overall atmosphere is calm and welcoming.
- Residents are well groomed, and personal equipment such as wheelchairs and walkers is clean.
- Staff are professional in appearance and are attentive to the residents.
- The schedule for daily cares is flexible to allow for individual needs.
- The facility provides restorative programs and resident and family councils.
- Meal schedules are flexible and provide a variety of options.
- There is an adequate number of staff members with low turnover.
- Restraints and safety equipment are used appropriately.

The person should visit several nursing homes for comparison. The visits should be done at different times of the day to ensure that patterns of care are consistent from shift to shift. If it is allowed, the person should ask questions of the staff, residents, and family members about the care that is provided. The Centers for Medicare and Medicaid Services has developed a checklist that can be used when visiting a nursing home. The checklist and other information can be accessed at http://www.medicare.gov/Pubs/pdf/02174.pdf (Centers for Medicare and Medicaid Services [n.d.]. Your guide to choosing a nursing home or other long-term care.)

These older women are healthy and able to volunteer at their community's local nursing home. They assist others with making the transition to a new environment and provide many services that otherwise would be unavailable.

needs very good assessment skills. Long-term care nurses use skills such as monitoring resident responses to treatments, observing for signs of decreasing function, and assessing subtle changes in condition on a daily basis. Accurate documentation; skillful use of the nursing process; and good interpersonal skills in working with residents, staff members, and family members are valuable tools in long-term care.

Care in a nursing home differs from hospital care in many ways. The skills required of the nursing home nurse are no less challenging and the tasks no less difficult than those of the hospital nurse. The goal for a hospital patient is to cure illness in a brief time. For a nursing home resident with multiple chronic conditions, cure is impossible. In the nursing home, care rather than cure is the primary focus. When you make the care given to residents transpersonal caring, the quality of that care improves remarkably.

Acute Care

The final clinical site for working with older adults is the acute care setting. Most hospital admissions are patients 65 years and older. Depending on the source used, it is estimated that 40% to 65% of hospital admissions include older adults. Nursing practice in a hospital setting presents many opportunities and challenges. Usually, LPNs are given responsibility for a set number of patients, and, depending on policy, they may perform various procedures. Most patients are hospitalized only briefly. The emphasis on cost containment and federal mandates means that reimbursement for care is often limited to a set period. Hospital-based practice requires all of the basic skills an LPN possesses. Acute care also involves brief contact with a large number of patients.

There are several challenges in giving nursing care to older adults in the hospital setting. These challenges include establishing a trusting relationship over a short period, dealing with problems secondary to relocation stress or medications, and resisting the tendency to stereotype patients because of their age. In addition, a major challenge for a nurse working with older people in the hospital setting is to create a safe and caring environment that facilitates independence; this must be done while the tasks required for the cure and treatment of the person are accomplished. Environmental management, as discussed earlier in this chapter, is the most difficult task to accomplish in the hospital setting. The short time frame and the urgency for treatment in many situations do not readily accommodate the slowed responses and

Priority Setting

As with the other chapters, everything mentioned in this chapter is important. The question is: What is the priority?

As a novice nurse, you need to know about the different environments of care, so that you can:

1. Recognize the best place for you to be employed. It is important to have a satisfying job that allows you to be the most effective caregiver possible.
2. Function most effectively as a member of the health-care team. By knowing about different environments of care, you have more information to share with the team where you are working. This is an important aspect of being a valuable member of the health-care team.

One of the positive things about being a nurse is the fact that there are so many opportunities for different types of work.

abilities of older persons. It is your challenge to slow things down so that the older adult can manage them.

As a gerontological nurse, it is important to understand the special needs of older adults. They have difficulty seeing and hearing. They move much slower, and they need clear explanations as to what is happening. When you recognize these needs of older adults, you have a responsibility to meet the needs and assist others involved in the care of the older adults to slow down and focus on those needs as well.

Think Like a Nurse

Mr. W. is a 90-year-old resident of a nursing home who was admitted to your floor at Hoover Medical Center for treatment of heart failure. He has significant dementia, is in-continent of bowel and bladder, and is very unsteady on his feet. As his primary nurse, what can you do to make his hospital environment more like home? What steps will you take to ensure that Mr. W. is receiving continuity of care between the nursing home and hospital? Who will you communicate with to assure Mr. W is receiving continuity of care between the nursing home and the hospital.

 CONCLUSION

This chapter has provided a brief overview of the nurse's role in environmental management and the various settings where older adults receive health care. Of special significance for the older adult is the opportunity to receive care from a nurse who is familiar with the aging process and uses that knowledge when giving nursing care in any setting.

CASE STUDY SOLUTION

When a nurse assesses her friend Sally's grandmother, Mrs. Gilmore, she finds that Mrs. Gilmore's home is all one level and has been remodeled to consider the needs of an aging home owner. Grab bars have been installed throughout the bathroom. The shower is a simple step-in model with a seat allowing Mrs. Gilmore to sit and operate the shower water controls. The toilet is a tall model and the sink is raised. Mrs. Gilmore has a wide step aerobics step next to her bed that she uses to get in and out of the bed. She also has an emergency alert system that is part of her home security system. Her neighbors have a key to her home if there is an emergency.

This is a pretty safe environment so the main concern is personal cares and meal preparation. Home care or private duty home health aids could be enlisted to help Mrs. Gilmore with personal cares and meals.

REVIEW QUESTIONS

1. Mr. D., 75 years old, is discharged from the hospital after a right-sided cerebrovascular accident. He requires at least 6 weeks of further nursing care and physical therapy. The facility most likely to meet these needs is:
   1. A continuing-care retirement center
   2. Hospice care
   3. An intermediate-care facility
   4. A skilled nursing facility

2. Hospice care provides a multidisciplinary approach to caring for people with:
   1. A chronic illness
   2. An acute exacerbation of a chronic illness
   3. A terminal illness
   4. A contagious illness

3. The major benefit of living in a continuing-care retirement community is:
   1. Low household maintenance requirements
   2. Services available for a continuum of health-care needs
   3. A safe environment for older adults
   4. The presence of a hospital in the complex

4. Mr. J., 83 years old, has Alzheimer's disease and has wandered from home on several occasions. Mrs. J. is concerned for her husband's safety and desires some respite services. You recommend that she investigate:
   1. A local nursing home
   2. The local senior center
   3. A home health-care agency
   4. An adult day-care center

5. In the home health-care setting, the LPN can expect:
   1. A limited amount of equipment and supplies to be available
   2. Intermittent contact with clients
   3. To care for clients discharged from the hospital with many physical care needs
   4. All of the above

6. When discharging (or transitioning) a patient from the hospital to a long-term care facility, it would be important for the nurse to include:
   1. A detailed description of the medications for the patient to review
   2. Contact cards for the patient of various therapies involved in the care
   3. All communication, contacts, medications, and therapies for the facility
   4. Detailed information regarding family involvement in the patient's care

WEB RESOURCES

American Association for Long Term Care Nursing:
Home Healthcare Nurses Association: http://www.hhna.org/
Hospice and Palliative Nurses Association: https://www.hpna.org

Long Term Care Nurses Association: http://www.ltcna.org/

Management and Leadership Role of the Licensed Practical/Vocational Nurse

13

SUSAN THORNOCK

LEARNING OUTCOMES

1. Identify the four management styles and determine when each would be effectively used in the gerontological setting.

2. Identify communication skills and techniques that can be effectively incorporated into your role as a charge nurse.

3. Identify delegation skills required for the LPN charge nurse in the gerontological setting.

4. Integrate decision-making skills into safe patient-care scenarios.

5. Recognize the use of the planning loop in setting priorities.

6. Identify three common errors made in doing employee evaluations.

7. Explain the importance of "total quality management" as it relates to the gerontological setting.

CONCEPTS

Professional Behaviors

Communication

Clinical Decision Making

Caring Interventions

Managing Care

Collaboration

CASE STUDY

Nurse White graduated as a Licensed Practical Nurse (LPN) 6 months ago and has been steadily employed at a skilled nursing facility (SNF) for 5 months. For the past 3 months Nurse White has functioned effectively in the role of charge nurse, on a 25-bed unit, on the 0600 to 1800 shift. This 25-bed unit is full and has one Certified Nursing Assistant (CNA), in addition to the LPN charge nurse, on the day shift.

As Nurse White arrives for his shift:

- He is greeted by the 10 students, the instructor, and the newly hired LPN, all eager to get their assignments.

- The charge nurse who works the 1800 to 0600 shift is not at the front desk, and Nurse White is anxious to receive report before delegating assignments.

- Passing of medications is to begin at 0630.

- Patient assessments are to be reported at the 1000 interdisciplinary meeting.

- As he goes to find the night nurse he sees the CNA coming out of a patient's room in tears. The CNA rushes by Nurse White and loudly exclaims "I cannot work with that family. They continually treat their mother like she is an idiot, and now they are treating me the same way. I'm done!" Nurse White goes into the room to find the patient crying and the patient's daughter insisting the medications have not been given correctly for the past 2 days. She wants to review her mother's medications immediately.

- The instructor of the students rushes down the hall to find Nurse White and tell him that Dr. Jackson just called and was in her usual uproar over her new admit in room 222. Evidently, the new admit was incoherent on admittance last evening, and the night nurse had called to report a fall and a possible fracture to the right lower extremity; the night nurse left a message for Dr. Jackson that this did not appear to be an emergency and the patient was complaining only of mild pain. Dr. Jackson is just returning the call and would like you to call her as soon as possible.

- A student nurse greets Nurse White and the instructor as they are exiting the patient's room and tells them that the night nurse is in the bathroom and is very ill.

- He also needs to attend a morning interdisciplinary care-planning session at 1000.

Discussion

Take a minute to reflect on this scenario. Make a list of your priorities, as though you are Nurse White, in order of importance. As you list your priorities, provide an explanation of your decisions for listing your priorities in this order. After you have completed the list with the explanation, provide a narrative that describes how you would implement the priority list. Keep in mind the focus of this chapter: management and leadership. It will be easier if you first list all of your priorities and then put them in order of importance.

 INTRODUCTION

Management and leadership, as they apply to the Licensed Practical Nurse (LPN) in the geriatric setting, are constantly changing to keep pace with changes in the health-care delivery system. Up to this point you have been educated through a directed program of study that incorporates the process of nursing with an emphasis placed on physical sciences and research. The basics of physiology, pathophysiology, pharmacology, and the basic medical and surgical procedures and skills have been your primary concerns. Somewhere along the line, leadership and ethics may have been touched on, but only briefly, and certainly not in the context of the LPN's role in management and leadership.

Entering into the position of a novice nurse, as an LPN, and being expected to understand your role as a manager and leader can be somewhat daunting. You may readily understand the role of a patient caregiver at the LPN level, and all of the accompanying requirements of being a safe patient caregiver, but may lack the full understanding of the management and leadership skills associated with this position. This is not to say the novice LPN is not a good manager or leader, it is just to point out there has, most likely, been no formal training to enhance what may or may not come naturally to you.

An important attribute to identify, as you read through this chapter, is how to motivate yourself to be a good manager and how to lead, inspire, and empower others whom you manage.

MANAGEMENT AND LEADERSHIP ROLES

Recognizing that the work of an LPN will always require management and leadership skills and that the scope of practice and responsibility may frequently change will go a long way in helping you recognize what your management responsibilities are in any setting. It is challenging to be an LPN prepared to assume the responsibility of management, but when it is done with skill it can add to the outcome of safe patient care in a multidisciplinary work environment.

In some nursing homes, LPNs are directors of nursing, whereas in some hospitals, they are not allowed to administer medications. This diversity in scope of responsibility is important to understand. If a registered nurse (RN) is on the healthcare team, the LPN is responsible to the RN. This is always true because of the dictates of licensure. It is possible for an RN and an LPN to have the same job description in an organization, just as it is possible for an LPN to be the director of nursing or shift supervisor. Even if you and an RN have the same job description, you have different licensure; the licensure and its scope of practice are critical for you always to follow.

At the time of employment, the LPN should clarify the scope of responsibility and role expected to be fulfilled. Determining that the duties assigned are not in conflict with the state nurse practice act also is important. As licensed nurses, all LPNs are responsible for knowing the law governing their practice. This responsibility should not be delegated to a supervisor or another nurse.

MANAGEMENT AND LEADERSHIP STYLES

In this chapter, the terms "management" and "leadership" are presented as synonyms. However, it is important for you to understand that you can be a leader without being a manager. In other words, you do not need to be appointed as a manager to become a good leader. Gaining an understanding of the different leadership styles will help you as you function in either role. As you read through this portion of this chapter, see if you can compare the traits associated with each of the management and leadership styles as they relate to the type of manager you would like to become. Most of you have worked with people you consider good managers. As you look at the different traits of each of the following leadership styles, make sure you identify those traits in people you have worked with or know well. Also decide what method you would like to use, in specific situations, as you develop your own leadership and management skills.

In this chapter, four basic styles of leadership will be compared:

- Authoritative (Autocratic)
- Permissive (Laissez-fair)
- Democratic (Participative)
- Multicratic (Eclectic)

Other leadership styles exist, and many leadership theories have been proposed. The LPN nurse manager needs to understand the basic styles and be flexible enough to incorporate other information as it becomes pertinent. The overall objective for comparing the basic styles of leadership is for the LPN to determine an effective but flexible leadership style for professional use.

Authoritarian

In the strictest sense, authoritarianism functions with a high concern for tasks done and low concern for the people who perform those tasks (Dahlkemper, 2013). The authoritarian style is a style that demonstrates control and overall direction from a boss or a manager. It is certainly not the preferred style in our day and in our society.

Many of us do not respond well to dictators. This style can be oppressing and decrease motivation among workers when the majority of the decisions are made by the manager and when the employees are allowed little feedback or recognition.

An authoritarian manager does not allow for creative thinking or new ideas. No opportunities are presented to try new concepts on a patient or resident care plan unless the idea is the manager's own. This type of manager is more interested in seeing that the work is done rather than that the patients are being lovingly cared for and their individual needs are being met. As an example of this type of management, the workload plan would require baths to be completed by 11:00 a.m. instead of treating the patients as individuals and allowing them autonomy in planning their morning care.

As in most things, the authoritarian has a purpose and a place. There are times when this type of management can and does work; it is usually situational. It is very effective in a code situation when one person needs to take charge to save a life. It can also be effective if there are time factors dictating a massive amount of work needing to be accomplished in a short period of time of if your level of knowledge is at ground zero and you need direction. You would not want to adopt this management style permanently, but it could be used effectively when necessary if you are skilled in knowing when to use it.

Situations exist in which this type of management style is crucial for success, such as during an emergency. If a visitor or older adult fell to the floor in cardiac arrest, this type of manager would take over, give orders, and, in all likelihood, save the life of the person. The problem with this management style is that life is not a constant series of emergencies. This style does not allow for the creative and caring approaches that are necessary for effective gerontological nursing. Often, older persons miss out on the best possible care, and the employees miss out on opportunities to learn and grow as they implement new care practices.

Permissive or Laissez Faire

The permissive style is either very effective or a complete disaster. There is no real direction displayed in this type of management. There is more delegation but not as much guidance; basically the employee needs to be able to function on his or her own. This can be very advantageous if your employees can function at a higher level and take responsibility for the outcome. The basic strategy is to allow the employees to make the decisions, do the planning, set the goals, and essentially manage the organization. This manager sees employees as ambitious, responsible, intelligent, and creative.

It is important to examine this type of management style in relationship to organizations involved in gerontological health care. For many people, especially those who need guidance, the permissive style can result in a feeling of no direction. It is not motivational or empowering for those who need direction and can actually create a sense of havoc. In some instances it can set up a situation detrimental to patient safety. Most care given to elderly adults depends on federal approval and on complex payment systems that go through state and federal government organizations. It is difficult to envision the federal guidelines for safety (Occupational Safety and Health Administration [OSHA]) or for nursing home licensure carried out in a permissive or laissez-faire manner. The same is true for quality-assurance programs in healthcare environments. Most facilities providing care to older adults require specific attention to the paperwork that keeps an organization in operation. It also is necessary to have layers of responsibility that ensure every person in the facility the best possible care with attention to detail.

In other environments, permissive management is very successful. An example is a group of highly motivated, professional people, such as a group of researchers, for whom independent thinking is rewarded. Conversely, it is difficult to imagine an effective nursing home or hospital unit being managed with this style of leadership.

Democratic or Participative

The democratic style is thought to be the preferred style in most situations. Allowing decisions and input from others and encouraging participation can help to create a highly functioning team. When we discuss communication later in this chapter, you will see that a democratic team approach is effective, and the synergism created allows for more to be accomplished.

The democratic management style places strong value on the people on the team. The manager gathers information from the other team members and presents it to the group. All suggestions from the group are considered before decisions are made by the group (Anderson, 2009).

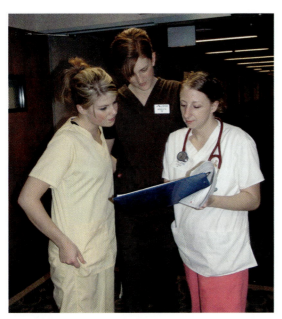

A democratic management style involves others in decision making.

This is a very open system of management, yet it identifies the individuals who are responsible for the various projects being managed.

The democratic style is thought to be the preferred style in most situations. Allowing decisions and input from others encouraging participation can help to create a highly functioning team. When we discuss communication, later in this chapter, you will see that a team is much more effective and the synergisim created will allow for more to be accomplished.

The advantage of this type of management is a great majority of the employees will buy into the decision because they have been part of the decision making. The disadvantage is this type of management takes longer for the decisions to be made. Generally, however, the results are positive, and the employees are very satisfied. This is a style that works well in gerontological environments because it is focused on people and includes the employee, the older adult, and the older adult's family members. It is a system that considers change and improvement continuously and assigns responsibility for such ventures.

Multicratic or Eclectic

Multicratic or eclectic is actually the best type of management because it allows you to use all styles of management. Different styles are certainly needed for individual situations. This style of management would allow for maximum participation and optimal outcome of most situations. The disadvantage of using multicratic is that you must be a very skilled manager. You would need to know and understand the different management styles and have the ability to assess what each person and/or situation needs to achieve optimal outcomes. The disadvantage would come if you were to misjudge a situation, an employee or peer, or a patient or patient situation.

As an LPN nurse manager, you need to evaluate yourself and determine which general management style is yours. Then consider whether it is a style that is best used in the care of older people. If it is not, you need to learn more about other management styles and, with that knowledge, consider making changes in yourself. You may need to find a mentor who has a management style you would like to learn more about and ask that person to assist you. This mentor could teach you, become a role model for you, and assist you in applying the management techniques you want in the real-world setting. Being a manager is a challenging facet of your professional life. Take the time to learn the skills and patterns of thought that you need to function at your most effective level.

 COMMUNICATION

The most important skill in any style of management in any situation is communication. Nurses in gerontological care spend 85% of their time communicating with a variety of people who are involved in the care of older adults. Mastering the skills of communication is essential for a successful LPN. Communication involves delivering messages that will be understood; listening to messages that may or may not be confusing; and properly interpreting messages that have been misdirected or are delivered with intense emotion, such as with anger.

For the LPN, the art of communication involves various groups of people. The LPN needs to be able to communicate successfully with the older adult, the family or other members of the person's support group, and the numerous members of the interdisciplinary health-care team. Being part of a team, especially a highly functioning team, is not an easy task; it requires effort on the part of every team member. Your communication skills, along with collaboration, credibility, compassion, and coordination, are important factors in demonstrating competence and respect to all, including the patients in your care. Expertise in communication is demanded every day from individuals who manage, direct, or administer care to older people.

Verbal Communication

Verbal communication is the exchange of ideas and understanding that occurs through the use of spoken words and phrases. For the message to be received, the sender must use words and phrases that are appropriate for the listener. The success of all communication is measured by the question: Was the message properly received?

It should be easy to remember sitting in a class and "listening" to a lecture or presentation when you did not "receive" the message. Perhaps you were too tired to concentrate, or the instructor was boring or had inappropriate content to share. For communication to occur, being present is not enough. The critical measure is whether the listener actually understood or "received" the message.

Nonverbal Communication

Nonverbal communication is the ability to share messages without using words. It refers, among other things, to a person's body posture (is the person tired and slouched over, or excited and alert), the tone and speed of the voice, the kind of clothes a person wears, and hand and facial movements. Nonverbal communication is considered to be the most honest communication a person can receive. Someone may say, "I'm having a great day. How are things for you?" in a cheerful-sounding way, but an examination of his appearance may indicate something different. The face is not smiling, and the posture is one of fatigue. The person's hands may be clenching and unclenching as a symptom of stress. Another classic example is a resident in a nursing home who is asked each morning, "How are you?" and each day responds verbally, "I'm fine." The person asking the question is busy with the breakfast tray or the linen and does not look at the sad and worried face of the resident who answers with the reply that is expected, rather than with the truth.

The ability to recognize honest communication and respond to it is crucial for a successful nurse manager. The nurse manager must learn to develop the refined skill of understanding nonverbal communication because it conveys valuable information about patients and employees. Nonverbal communication is an honest method of communication and allows the LPN to follow through on problems and concerns that otherwise might not have been recognized.

Communicating With Patients and Residents

The decision to work with elderly adults is a commitment to accept the normal physiological losses that accompany the aging process. That commitment requires knowledge of the normal changes that occur in elderly people (see Chapter 2) and the skill to work with them successfully. A tendency exists in our ageist society to judge older people negatively because of the normal aging processes they exhibit. Normal aging changes that might affect communication are slower speech, presbycusis (difficulty in discriminating sounds), presbyopia (difficulty seeing near objects), and overall slower movements or responses to what is being communicated. The knowledgeable LPN recognizes these as normal occurrences and responds to them with skill and compassion.

Some people are impatient and negative about the aging process. It is as if they were punishing people who had simply neglected to die young! This is ageist behavior and is unacceptable in any setting. The skills necessary for successful communication with older adults must be firmly based on respect for them as people. If that ingredient is missing, communication is unsuccessful. Consider the following strategies (not every older adult would need every strategy):

- Do not approach the person from the side because you may not be seen, and the person could be startled by your sudden appearance. Approach only from the front. This factor is important because of the gradual loss of peripheral vision that often accompanies aging.
- Place yourself on eye level with the older person so that a comfortable presence occurs during the communication process.
- Reach out and touch the person if it seems appropriate; this is often the bridge to a trusting relationship.
- Speak at a normal rate and do not shout, even if the older person is having trouble hearing. Shouting does not overcome the problems of presbycusis. Speak in a normal tone and speak slower than usual, but not so slow as to insult the person.

FOCUSED LEARNING CHART

Understanding nonverbal communication

Critical to learn, to recognize, and to respond to as a nurse manager	The most honest form of communication	Examples
		Posture
		Facial expressions
		Tone and speed of voice
		Personal hygiene
		Type of clothing being worn
		Hand and facial movements
		Symptoms of stress

- If the patient is having trouble hearing you, move closer and speak in a normal tone. Moving closer often allows for lip reading or the reading of facial expressions.
- Pleasantly repeat what is being said, if necessary.
- Do not be impatient or judgmental.
- Place yourself and the older adult in a setting where there is a bright light but no glaring of light.
- Use a setting without disturbing or distracting noises.
- If the older adult gets confused while speaking or responding to a question, give the person time to collect personal thoughts. Do not rush the person.
- Repeat questions or comments in a different sentence structure if the older person is having trouble understanding what is said. Do not keep repeating the same information in the same way.
- Reflect on what the older person has said by repeating it back in a different way; for example, "Do you mean that you are lonely because your wife is in the hospital and not able to visit you here in the nursing home?"
- Listen carefully to the words used and verify what they mean.
- "Listen" carefully to the body movements and other nonverbal communication and verify what they mean.

Your goal is to have the message successfully received. The use of these basic, caring strategies enhances your achievement of that goal and your relationship with the older adults in your care.

Communicating With the Families of Older Adults

Often, the family members of older patients or residents are worried, exhausted (if there has been extensive care given at home), and experiencing feelings of guilt over the condition of their family member or the necessity of admitting their loved one to a health-care facility. Successful communication with this varied group of people is challenging because of their emotional status. The issues involved often go beyond concern over an admission to a hospital or nursing home to such highly charged questions as the right to die, the decision

Point of Interest

Most of you have either played sports or watched sports being played, by your children or on television by the pros. In each sporting activity there is a certain etiquette that is followed if the game is played well. The etiquette, or the rules, are not the same for each sport, but the rules for each sport are equally important. For instance, in basketball, body contact denotes a foul. Depending on how many fouls or what kind of foul, the opposing team may be awarded an extra shot or two, which can culminate in a loss to the offending team. Soccer penalizes teams when players are "off sides." Baseball has a set of rules that readily change depending on your age, your gender, and your league. The rules for each type of sporting activity are somewhat different, and the penalties for each variation of the game rules also differ. The kicker is, if you are playing the game and you do not know the rules but you violate the rules you will still get the penalty. Ignorance is no excuse when you are playing the game. The better you are, the more you play, the more professional you become, the more you will understand the subtleties of the game rules or etiquette. The same is true for understanding the scope of practice or the appropriate etiquette for leadership and management for the LPN. Remember these words "ignorance is no excuse." Knowing there is protocol and that the protocol changes for each place of employment, or each unit or floor, at your place of employment is important. Know the rules and use them to your advantage as you maintain the highest level of safe patient care.

whether to do an amputation, or dealing with a diagnosis such as Alzheimer's disease.

It is crucial for the LPN to recognize the emotional environment of the family members before entering into any communication with them. The goal is still the same: You want the message to be received by the listener. Some communication strategies for families are as follows:

• Listen to them before you attempt to impart information. It is essential that you evaluate the emotional environment to determine if they are able to listen to you. Often, just listening allows for you to learn critical information that you otherwise would not learn.
• Plan to spend time with the family members. They have questions and concerns, and they deserve to have them addressed.
• Family members often feel guilty over some issue with their loved one and need to have that clarified. Families need not feel guilty unless evidence of elder abuse is found.
• Find a quiet place to speak to the family. It should be a place where they can sit comfortably and be together as a group. The nurses' station is never an appropriate place for meaningful communication other than the simple sharing of facts.
• As nurse manager, the LPN needs to facilitate the sharing of information with the family. This could mean arranging an appointment with the

social worker or assisting a family member to reach the physician.
• The older adult's family is as important as the older person. Generally, strong personal relationships that are interdependent exist. Always treat the family members with the high level of respect and concern that you use with the older adult.

Interdisciplinary Team Communication

As an LPN you will interact, on a daily basis, with an interdisciplinary team (IDT) that can provide services and knowledge to enhance the well-being of your individual patient, as well as provide a greater benefit to your organization as a whole (Lancaster, Kolakowsky-Hayner, Kovacich, & Greer-Williams, 2015). Working with a dietitian to help determine the best diet for your diabetic patient when the patient is discharged from your facility may ensure that your patient will better comprehend why you are asking him or her to check blood sugar three times a day and adjust diet and insulin accordingly. Involving a medical social worker to provide follow-up care for this same patient has the potential to increase your patient's compliance and safety once in their home environment. Including family members who can give encouragement as the patient with newly diagnosed diabetes learns to make life changes will provide

When working with a colleague on patient or resident care or other projects, be sure that your message is received. It pays to check and double check.

the support the patient needs to maintain compliance with this required change of lifestyle. The combined knowledge and skills of these team members provides a much better outcome than if any one of these team members were to try to go it alone. This type of collaboration in patient care is an active form of synergism that can significantly benefit safe patient outcomes and reflect positively on your organization. Generally, the care given to older people in all settings is based on the interdisciplinary approach. It is critical that the nurse manager be an active and contributing part of this team. Generally, nurses are with the patients 24 hours a day, or if the older person is a home patient, the nurse generally sees the individual more frequently than other members of the team. This constant attendance of the nurse to the patient provides a vast amount of personal and pertinent information. It is essential that the nurse manager be active in contributing to the knowledge base and planning of the IDT.

Concern arises over how to share information the nurse has gathered about the older person. It needs to be shared with skill so that the message is received. This process is different in a group setting than it is with an individual patient or family members. The group consists of professionals who have specialized knowledge regarding the older person. There is rarely sufficient time to discuss the patients in a thorough and relaxed manner. A time crunch often exists in IDT planning that establishes a unique atmosphere for communication. The following are strategies for communicating with an IDT:

• Come prepared! There is no time to waste in these meetings, whether in groups or one on one.

• Plan ahead and have priority concerns in your mind or on a piece of paper.

• This is not a team of nurses, and members of an IDT may not understand a nursing concept that is very familiar to you. Because nursing is its own specialty, you may be asked to justify your requests or concerns or to teach the team about a nursing concept.

In most situations, the nurse has the role of patient or resident advocate. This occurs naturally because of the amount of time nurses spend with patients compared with other disciplines. This time allows for personal information and concerns to be communicated. It is crucial that the patient advocacy role be accepted by the nurse so that the patient is protected from the system and its potentially depersonalizing effects.

 ## ADDITIONAL COMMUNICATION SKILLS

Very specific skills are necessary for successful communication, and each of these skills can be used appropriately in all settings. Such skills are necessary to clarify communication errors, or potential errors, and are commonly necessary in difficult situations. They are important for every LPN to add to the communication skills checklist, and their importance can be compared with that of being expert at cardiopulmonary resuscitation (CPR). You may not use the skills very often, but when they are necessary, you need to know how to use them.

Assertive Communication Skills

The normal physiological reaction to being attacked physically or verbally is "fight or flight." This reaction occurs without thinking about it; it is normal physiology. When a situation occurs in which you are being attacked verbally or feel threatened by what is being said or done, the normal response is to fight back (an argument) or to take flight (avoidance). In the framework of assertive communication, these two normal responses are more formally identified as *aggressive*—fight—or *passive*—flight. The third concept that belongs on a continuum between these two is *assertive*—dealing with the problem.

Ideally, you would use assertive behavior when someone has violated the rights of an individual either verbally or physically. Assertive behavior is the most effective response to that violation. The major rule regarding the concept of assertive communication is simply that the assertive response *must not* violate the rights of the person who just infringed on your rights. What does that look like? An argument is the best example. Someone comes to the nurses' station and criticizes you in an angry, loud manner. There are residents or patients, visitors, and co-workers in the area listening to this *aggressive* communication. It is embarrassing and humiliating to be the victim of a communication delivered in such an inappropriate way. The normal physiological response is either to run away, perhaps crying *(passive)*, or to scream back *(aggressive)*. Screaming back or starting an argument is a violation of the other person's rights. It does not matter if he or she deserves it; it is still wrong. The *passive* behavior, or running away, does not violate the other person's rights, but it does prevent a resolution of the problem.

Assertive communication requires that the person being violated not respond in a normal physiological fashion to the situation. Instead, it is necessary to resist the normal response and use the skills of communication to promote problem solving. This is done most effectively in a private area. Assertive communication often follows this response format:

"I feel" — Tell the other person how the aggressive attack made you feel. Perhaps you feel frustrated, devalued, angry, or frightened. Many other options are available for you to describe how you feel about what has been said.

"When you" — Describe for the person the behavior that has caused you to feel the way you do. It could be "when you raise your voice at me," "talk about private concerns in public," "demand things from me that I cannot do," "or criticize me in front of others." Many other statements could be used here. The statements used must not be personal statements that attack the other person.

"We should" — Together determine a solution to the problem. This is difficult to do because it is not one of the two normal and usual responses. Use it anyway. Take a deep breath and simply ask what the two of you can do to prevent this from happening again. Be open-minded and expect that there will be more hostility because of the discomfort that comes to the aggressive person with your unusual approach. It is hoped that the two of you can resolve the problem. If not, you still have done a good thing. Another

skill that may help you in this type of situation is active listening.

Active Listening

Another communication skill that complements assertive behavior is that of *active listening*. Most people respond to aggressive and negative remarks with defensive communication. While the aggressor is making comments, the person being attacked generally is mentally preparing the defense to the aggressor's attack. These are the defensive comments that often provoke an argument. They follow the script of "It is not my fault; now let me tell you why!"

Active listening requires that the person being verbally attacked listen to what is being said. Because of the natural inclination to prepare a defense, listening is a challenging thing to do. Just listen, and, while listening, try to determine the cause of the problem beyond the apparent anger.

The person who is out of control must be removed to a private setting, such as an office or the clean holding area. This prevents that individual from self-embarrassment in front of others, and it places you in an environment with fewer distractions.

After the angry person has finished saying all the aggressive things there are to say, he or she will take a deep breath and stop talking. This is where the person uneducated in communication skills presents his or her defense. You, the nurse manager, need skills beyond the ordinary person, however. Active listening is one of those skills. The deep breath is the signal to use the information you

---

Critically Examine the Following:

Think back to the last "failed communication" you either observed or took part in. Would it have helped to make the conversation successful if the skills of assertive communication had been used? Briefly describe the failed communication and then reword it using the assertive communication pattern.

Assertive Communication Pattern:
"I feel ..."
"When you ..."
"We should ..."

learned, while listening, to clarify the problem and negotiate a solution.

Comments such as "You seem so frustrated with…," "It is unlike you to be so upset," or "How can I help?" are effective ones to use. They are not what the aggressive person expects to hear and generally prevent the person from losing control again. They are helpful comments that show caring and problem-solving skills. These are hallmark behaviors for nurse managers. The next move is for the two people involved to sit down and look at the problem rationally and work on a solution. The whole process begins with the nurse being able to stop "self-defending" and focus on listening.

The format for active listening is as follows:

- Remove the conversation to a private setting.
- Listen.
- Do not prepare a defense.
- Listen for the deep breath that means the person has finished speaking.
- Show support for the other person's feelings.
- Negotiate how to resolve the problem.

Some LPNs reading this text may feel concern over being responsible for assertive communication and active listening skills. They are two of many possible communication skills that could have been discussed in this book. They are listed for a very specific purpose. LPNs, in management roles, have very challenging positions that may place them in serious situations that must be managed rather than ignored. Some people will say, "But I am just an LPN!" and feel that their role does not involve

Evidence-Based Practice

White, M.J., Gutierrez, A., McLaughlin, C., Eziakonwa, C., Newman, L.S., White, M., Thayer, B., Davis, K., Williams, M., & Asselin, G. (2013). A pilot for understanding interdisciplinary teams in rehabilitation practice. Rehabilitation Nursing, 38, 142-152.

This article reported on a pilot study that investigated the skills conducive to interdisciplinary teams interacting effectively to achieve a common goal. Questions related to barriers and facilitators of effective teams were asked of nurses, physical therapists, and occupational therapists involved in rehabilitative care. The most significant outcome of this pilot study, related to this unit, was the identification of the facilitators. Communication and collaboration were found to be imperative to the effectiveness of the team, with communication being the most significant.

Questions

1. Teamwork is a confirmed method to achieve a common goal and has been proven to increase patient-care outcomes. In addition to patient-care outcomes, identify two other benefits that your facility can expect when interdisciplinary teamwork is employed.
2. The Institute of Medicine (IOM) has identified interdisciplinary teams as one of five core competencies for improving patient care outcomes. White et al. (2013) identify that effective teamwork requires good communication skills. List three other skills that will help ensure effective team work.
3. Identify two of the four barriers to teamwork.

Critically Examine the Following:

During the next week, carefully observe yourself or others as they communicate in professional settings. Determine whether you observe the following actions. Record your thoughts and make comments regarding each communication technique.

1. Passive communication:
2. Aggressive communication:
3. Assertive communication:
4. Active listening:
5. Inactive listening:

managing and solving problems of this nature. If you are a nurse manager, however, you have an obligation to develop the skills necessary for managing these acute and potentially destructive problems.

 CARE PLANNING HOOP

Decision making is one of the most important skills you will use in nursing. When you think about the fact that nurses are the largest group of caregivers in our health-care delivery system, and that nurses provide the majority of care, then you have a better understanding of why good decision-making skills are so important. Your sound clinical judgment is central to your patient's well-being and optimal outcome. Your ability to assess a patient and identify all pertinent factors surrounding that assessment are of primary significance.

Every day, decisions must be made regarding the workload of the LPN and others that affect the scope of LPN practice. These are decisions that should be made with careful thought and planning, rather than casually and without attention to detail. The decision that may be required of you could be as simple as who will get the first bath as you give morning care, but even this decision may have serious implications for the patients or residents who are receiving your care. Other decisions that may be required of the LPN nurse manager could be counseling an employee whose behavior is unacceptable, making care assignments, confronting a physician or therapist with an alternate plan of care for a resident, or managing daily staffing. None of these tasks—or the many others that are required of a nurse manager—are easy or simple. They require the highest level of skill and attention to manage the process of making such decisions effectively.

To set priorities and make excellent decisions, the LPN nurse manager must understand the importance of planning, which is an intelligent process of thinking based on facts and information, rather than on emotion and wishes. An example is the holiday schedule. Staff members want Christmas Day off to be with their families. You, the manager, want everyone on your staff to be happy, but you have a clear picture as to what would happen if you granted everyone's wishes for Christmas Day! Instead, you need to make a rotation plan for the holidays, or perhaps draw names out of a hat, assign requests according to seniority, or determine some other way for the Christmas Day shift to be adequately staffed.

Planning is a process that never ends. It can be thought of as a hoop with notches where you stop and enter another phase of the planning process; then you continue going around the hoop over and over again. It is unrealistic to develop a plan and think that it will never change. It may be perfect for the moment, a week, or even an entire year; but the complexity of health care and the individuality of patients or residents and staff members require that your excellent plan be continuously re-evaluated. The planning hoop (Fig. 13.1) begins with an assessment.

FIGURE 13.1 The Planning Hoop. An effective nurse manager must determine that planning is critical to getting the total workload done effectively.

Assessment

What is the problem or potential problem that concerns you? You know how to do a physical assessment. This is a similar process. Look at the problem from "head to toe" and assess what really is wrong. If it is a staffing problem in a nursing home, look at the mix of licensed and unlicensed personnel. Is it right for the needs of the residents?

Is the problem a lack of knowledge? If it is, you need to assess where the lack is, who needs to know the information, and how to teach it most effectively. Do not be distracted by other issues as you do your assessment. Keep focused on the problem you are trying to resolve and learn all you can about it. Otherwise, it would be similar to trying to assess two residents at the same time. One does not get a clear picture of the problem unless a very focused effort is made. The next step in the planning hoop is to set goals.

Goal Setting

Now that you have a complete set of data regarding the problem, you have enough information to set goals. This is very similar to the nursing process. Instead of writing a care plan, you are preparing a plan to resolve a management problem. Make the goals reasonable and achievable. Not everyone can have Christmas Day off. If the problem is an unbalanced mix of licensed and unlicensed personnel, your goal could be to correct the mix through attrition and selective hiring within the next 6 months. If the problem is knowledge, your goal would be to have 100% of your staff attend a class on the information needed by a specific date. The goals should be meaningful and reflect your most careful and organized thinking.

Implementation

Implementation is the test of good planning. Was your assessment done accurately, and are your goals realistic? Perhaps the actual implementation requires you not to hire an RN or LPN when one applies because your staff has too great a proportion of licensed personnel. Or, implementation may mean that you need to find the budget money to pay the staff to attend the education program you determined they needed. In addition, you need a plan for getting everyone to attend. This could involve bonus money or other rewards, and in all likelihood, it would mean presenting the education program several times. Implementation is the actual performance of your plan.

Evaluation

Did your plan work? Was Christmas Day successfully staffed, and did the staff feel that the staffing decisions were made with fairness? Within 6 months, was your staff mix at the level where you needed it to be? How effective was your education program? Did it bring about the change you wanted? Such questions initiate the process of evaluation. A nurse manager cannot just do something and consider the problem solved. Instead, a careful evaluation must be performed so that the cycle of the planning hoop can begin again. That's right; once you have evaluated your plan, you need to do another assessment and begin the circle again!

Many people do not spend a great deal of time planning solutions to the unit's problems. The profession of nursing is filled with "doing" types of people. One of the critical skills of being a manager is to learn to quit "just doing" and begin planning "to do." It is a challenge to take the time necessary to plan because planning does not enter into the conventional description of a "good nurse."

When a person is planning, that person is sitting somewhere quietly thinking. The profession of nursing generally does not see that as productive because beds need to be made, and there are baths and treatments to be given. With those unfinished care issues, how can a real nurse take the time to sit and think? A real nurse manager soon learns that doing the thinking or planning is critical to getting the total workload done effectively. So, fight the urge to be busy when planning is needed. Teach the staff that the time you spend planning is critical to the overall picture of care for patients and job satisfaction for them. Be courageous enough to use the planning hoop to resolve problems and prevent new ones. Because if you do not, you will become a victim of crisis management.

Crisis Management

A crisis manager is a person who does not take the time to plan. This manager waits until the week before Christmas to resolve the problem of the staffing crisis. A great deal of hysteria, excess energy, and distress are involved in solving problems when they occur, rather than foreseeing them and taking the time to plan a solution for the problem. The phrase, "All I do is run around and put out fires!" is indicative of the crisis manager. It is not effective management and can be prevented by the implementation of the planning hoop into your management style. Look to the future and anticipate problems. Then devise a plan for solving them before a crisis happens.

Some situations still will become a crisis for even the best manager. Accept this, solve the problem, design a plan so it will not be a crisis the next time, and move on to the next situation.

Think Like a Nurse

Prioritizing is actually a highly learned skill that can become a great asset to you, as well as the people in your care. It is an art when it is done correctly. Keep in mind that if you do not learn to prioritize correctly, you could very well put you and your patient at risk. Refer back to the case study at the beginning of this chapter. The ability you demonstrate in prioritizing your tasks and implementation of patient care can make a huge impact on your patient's outcomes. You need to make sure that the order of your prioritization can create an optimal outcome for the patient in a safe and caring environment.

PRIORITY SETTING

Every LPN has learned how to prioritize the work of giving patient or resident care. Traditionally, the sickest patient receives the nurse's attention first, and the least seriously ill person waits until last. This concept assumes that each patient is assessed and observed frequently, rather than being ignored until his or her turn comes to receive care.

Priority setting in management situations has a similar format. The priority of each management problem is determined after the assessment of the situation has been completed. The method for determining priority problems generally is based on determining what is essential for the organization or the person at the time. Staffing for Christmas Day is essential, as is giving pain medications in a timely manner.

The nurse manager needs to think of the entire organization when determining priorities. They often are divided into two categories: (1) concerns that relate to patient or resident care and (2) concerns that relate to the process of running the business of the institution.

Each category should be considered separately, although a great deal of overlap of concerns occurs in implementing problem solutions. Each concern needs to be listed as a *need* or a *want*. Needs should be met before wants. It is helpful to use this method for categorizing your management concerns before prioritizing them.

Making Care Assignments for Older Adults

One of the day-to-day management skills used by LPNs is that of making care assignments for older adults. The skill of making effective assignments is crucial to any clinical area. The goal of making successful care assignments is to match the worker with the older person in a manner that allows for the best nursing care to be administered and received. As the manager, you also need to focus on an assignment that affords the highest level of employee satisfaction. This requires sensitivity, awareness of the skills and attitudes of others, and the ability to form a plan and to follow through on it. Several aspects of making care assignments should be examined.

When making care assignments, you must consider the personal skills of each person you are managing. You have learned how to assess older adults; now your question might be, "How do I accurately assess a nursing assistant's skills?" Dr. Patricia Benner (2001), who developed her nursing theory in her book, *From Novice to Expert*, describes a specific way to identify clinical skills. Benner's theory focuses on intensive care, RNs, and their clinical expertise along the five points of:

- Novice
- Advanced beginner
- Competent
- Proficient
- Expert

As a nurse manager, it is important for you to understand the five points of clinical expertise and how you can use them to identify skill levels for CNAs and other individuals who work under your direction. The five points are:

1. *Novice*—CNAs performing at this level have no prior experience with certain situations. They do not understand the detailed information regarding what is happening. They simply do not have the experience to understand what is going on in the situation. For example, a CNA may have several years of employment as a CNA but may not have any experience working on an Alzheimer's unit. As a nurse manager, you should be aware of such a lack of skill and may want to assign a novice CNA to work several shifts with a CNA who is experienced in caring for people with Alzheimer's disease.

2. *Advanced beginner*—CNAs functioning at this level can demonstrate limited acceptable performance. Advanced beginners generally have had multiple clinical experiences, independently or with a mentor, so that they have a general understanding of the clinical situation. Advanced beginners perform tasks using behavior that follows instructions only, rather than appropriate behavior for a specific situation.

As the nurse manager, you may ask a CNA to assist a resident into the shower. When the CNA enters the room, the resident is found confused and combative. Rather than gauging the situation and deciding that this may not be the best time to give this resident a shower, the CNA does everything possible to complete the

It is worth your time to consider the level of expertise that the CNAs who work with you have achieved. This knowledge influences your scheduling, educational programs, and, most importantly, the quality of care provided to older adults. It is your responsibility to identify and assist CNAs who need more education or experience.

task of giving the shower. The focus is on the task, not the aspects of the specific situation or the needs of the older person.

3. *Competent* — A competent CNA has an increased level of skill and ability. The knowledge is based on following the positive role-modeling of other CNAs and dealing with various situations in which clinical skills were learned. A competent CNA still focuses on organizing the assigned tasks, however. A competent CNA makes sure the time is managed well in an effort to complete the tasks on the list, instead of basing work decisions on the older person's needs.

As a nurse manager, it is critical that you ensure that the resident's needs are actually being met by the CNA in a timely manner. Otherwise, the individuals you manage may give care based on a schedule and a list rather on than the needs of older adults.

4. *Proficient* — A proficient CNA is much more comfortable with clinical skills and has the ability to deal with different situations as they arise. A proficient CNA engages more with the older adult and family members instead of focusing on required tasks. The focus of nursing care of a proficient CNA is on the needs of the older person rather than on a list. An advantage to working with proficient CNAs is their ability to reprioritize the workload based on patient or resident needs. As a nurse manager, you may delegate several things to a proficient CNA, who then decides in what order they should be completed.

5. *Expert* — An expert CNA has experienced many different situations and has learned from the experiences. These experiences assist the CNA in making decisions based more on intuition (referred to by Benner as "intuitive knowing") than on timetables and rules. An expert CNA knows the older adult's patterns of behavior and is able to anticipate the unexpected. This complexity of skill and thinking assists the CNA in making decisions based on the "big picture" or the holistic needs of the person receiving care.

An expert CNA walks into a room where an older adult is behaving differently and spends time with the person in an effort to identify the problem. The expert CNA takes vital signs and asks questions so there are data to report to the licensed nurse. The expert CNA knows what to do for this patient.

Are you able to identify where your CNAs fit in Benner's five points of clinical expertise?

Do you have a new CNA who is still working at the novice level? If so, that person should be assigned to older adults who require only basic skills that were learned in the CNA class. A novice CNA also should be assigned to an expert CNA who can assist with care when needed and serve as a positive role model. Novice CNAs should not be assigned to give care to challenging patients or residents. They could be assigned to work with another CNA who has the challenging patient or resident and, in that way, have experiences that eventually lead the CNA to the level of expert without hurting an older person in the learning process.

Do you also have a CNA who has worked at the facility for several years, is very familiar with the residents, and has excellent clinical skills? That is the CNA who should be assigned to the most challenging older adults so that these older adults can benefit from the CNA's skills and knowledge. This may not always be the sickest patient on the unit. The assignment could be to the latest admission, in which the older person and the family are having a difficult time adjusting to the transitional stress of the admission.

It is important when developing staffing patterns that a team should not consist of a novice CNA and a novice licensed nurse. A better staffing pattern would be an expert CNA with a novice nurse or expert nurse with a novice CNA. The mix of novice and the levels of expertise that lead to expert are important to acknowledge and use as you manage care.

When you, as the nurse manager, have identified the expertise levels of each nursing assistant, you should praise each one for their special skills and allow them to use those skills. Assist employees to develop skills related to their interests and abilities, and recognize them for the skills they develop. Assign staff members older adults who would benefit from their skill and knowledge. This assignment enhances quality of care and employee self-esteem, which enhance the entire organization.

When working with older adults, it is generally more effective to assign the same employee to an older person for several days in succession. This practice allows the caregiver to learn the personal needs and nuances of the persons receiving care and address them successfully. When a "new" person is assigned to an older person each day, it puts a demand on the older adult to need to explain again that he or she cannot hear out of the right ear, that the older adult wants two cups of coffee on his or her breakfast tray, or that it is the older adult's right knee that does not work very well. Generally, a comfortable camaraderie and sense of teamwork develop between the caregiver and the care receiver that enhance the work of healing when they work together over time.

Sometimes a difficult or demanding older person requires more energy and patience than most employees can provide day after day. When this occurs, the nurse manager should rotate the assignment in a direct effort to avoid burnout of the employees.

Another consideration for making assignments is that of physical demands. Often when caring for older adults or chronically ill patients, a heavy physical demand is made in turning, positioning, and assisting the older person to ambulate. When the nurse manager makes the assignment, the physical, muscular work of the care should be considered so as not to overwork a particular employee. Another consideration is the geographic placement of the rooms. It is unnecessary to make assignments that require an employee to travel to both ends of the hall or in other diverse patterns. Make a strong effort to group the room numbers assigned to avoid unnecessary walking. Most workdays are tiring enough.

Delegation

As the LPN manager, you need to know what is involved in delegating to CNAs. The goal is to delegate tasks while maintaining quality patient and resident care. Your first step is to familiarize yourself with the nurse practice act for the state where you work. This document defines the roles and responsibilities of a licensed nurse. You need to determine if the nurse practice act allows for delegation and, if so, whether there are any limitations as to what you can delegate to a CNA or unlicensed assistive person.

Your next step is to become familiar with the policy and procedures for your facility and the written job descriptions. Any job you assign must be within the employee's job description. After you have identified a task that can be delegated, you need to use sound delegation approaches. Also keep in mind how delegating this task would affect the safety of the older adult. Has the older person been accurately assessed, and are there any safety issues that need to be addressed? The National Council of State Boards of Nursing (NCSBN) has developed guidelines to help nurses ensure safe and proper delegation. The NCSBN has developed the Five Rights of Delegation, which provides a checklist that nurses can use when making delegation decisions. The Five Rights of Delegation are:

1. The right task
2. The right circumstances
3. The right person
4. The right direction
5. The right supervision

Generally, CNAs can do tasks that assist older adults with basic needs and activities of daily living. They cannot assess, plan, or evaluate any aspects of patient care. If an older person is taking digoxin (Lanoxin) for his heart, the nurse can delegate to the CNA the task of taking an apical pulse and notifying the nurse what the heart rate is when the pulse is taken. The CNA cannot decide if the older adult can have medication based on the pulse the CNA took. In addition, the nurse makes the decision as to when the pulse should be checked again. When working with CNAs, it is very important that the nurse give clear instructions regarding what time the task should be completed and whether the CNA needs to report back to the nurse directly after completing the task. It is wise to encourage CNAs to take notes as you are giving them the information regarding the delegated assignment. When delegating a task to a CNA, you still are responsible for the older adult's care. If you delegate a task to a novice CNA, and the task should have been delegated to an expert CNA, or if you do not give proper supervision, you may be held responsible for the outcome of the care. If you delegate to the appropriate person and provide appropriate supervision, the CNA may be liable for his or her own actions (Yoder-Wise, 2011).

As a manager, you should always be willing to delegate certain projects. As organizational needs arise, you may be assigned a project that would not allow you to complete your regular workload. This is a good time to delegate routine work that can be done by someone else.

In your role as an LPN, you will find it necessary to do effective delegation. Does that mean that you delegate the projects that you do not want to do? Does delegating make you a lazy person? The answer to both of these questions is "no." Delegation of routine tasks to someone else frees the manager to work on more complicated unit needs. Because delegation is crucial to effective management, you want to ensure you are doing it as efficiently as possible. When delegating to anyone, your responsibility as the manager is to identify if they have the basic skills or education necessary to complete the assignment. You also should ensure they have the time to complete the assignment by the deadline without requiring them to put aside their regular job responsibilities. Delegating to someone who is interested in the assignment is a good choice.

When the individual for the assignment is identified, you should give him or her clear, direct instructions on what is to be done, including why the individual is doing the assignment. How the person completes the assignment should be an individual choice. This is the really hard part. When you delegate a responsibility in the manner described earlier, just leave it and allow the person to do the work. You can "check in," determine whether the person needs something, or just observe so that you can step in if there is a critical situation. Giving the employee autonomy in deciding how to complete the assignment is a positive factor for the employee and the key to successful delegation. It also is important that you do not oversupervise the employee. If you are going to watch and participate in every step of the project, you may want to ask yourself why you chose to delegate it.

Definite time lines for completion of any delegated project should be discussed, and the manager should check in periodically to ensure that the deadline will be met. Monitoring the assignment periodically allows for questions and discussion regarding the project as the work is being done. Being available for interaction is an important concept. You always should be available to assist the employee if he or she is having difficulty. Taking the delegated project back would be a last-resort behavior because it makes the employee feel like a failure and "demotivates" rather than motivates. When the project is complete, you must evaluate the performance, giving praise and additional information to the employee. This feedback lets the person know what was done well and what may be done differently next time he or she is given a similar assignment. Delegation is an effective way to assist someone to move from novice to expert because of the opportunity to develop new skills and have new experiences.

Medication Aide – Certified

The Medication Aide–Certified (MA-C) is a developing role in health care, especially in the long-term health-care setting. The MA-C expands the education and knowledge of the CNA position by attending additional classroom and clinical hours in accordance to state regulations. It is the job of the MA-C to administer selective medications safely under the supervision of a licensed health-care provider.

Understanding appropriate delegation is important when working with this new health-care provider.

The MA-C must work at least 1 year, or 2000 hours, as a CNA before taking a MA-C course. Concepts the MA-C learns and incorporates into patient care include the basic principles and techniques this position needs to know about medication and medication administration. The MA-C does not have the expanded knowledge or education of the licensed caregiver, but he or she does gain an overview of common drugs, including their effects and side effects and common interactions. MA-Cs are taught medication use in a diverse population and how to avoid common medication errors. This knowledge greatly increases patient safety, as long as the licensed personnel understand what can and what cannot be delegated to the MA-C.

Drug classifications, basic principles, drug action, drug interactions, and general drug information are concepts covered in the MA-C course. Considerations to gender and age, including distribution, metabolism, excretion, and monitoring, will help the MA-C determine safe administration of medications in diverse health-care settings. Knowledge of how to work with a nurse to determine the correct drug order and ordering methods are among the skills taught in a MA-C course.

State laws and regulations associated with the role of the MA-C in the safe administration of medications in the health-care setting are important knowledge for the MA-C and for the licensed caregiver who delegates medication administration to the MA-C. There are legal and ethical aspects associated with the responsibilities of the MA-C and regulations that are identified for the licensed nurse in the delegation process. It is important for you, the LPN, to know and understand your state practice act as it is associated with this new position. Communication and accountability in giving safe patient care are extremely important skills for the licensed nurse.

The most important factor for the LPN is to always be cognizant of patient safety factors, the progression of delegation in the nursing process, and how the MA-C interacts and functions in this process. The skills discussed in this chapter on leadership will go far in helping you work in collaboration with the health-care team, including the MA-C, for optimal patient outcomes.

 MANAGING PERSONNEL

As a nurse manager, you will be involved in, if not responsible for, the hiring and evaluating of employees. This is a critical aspect of your job and one that requires the highest level of professional skill and performance. This work cannot be done by intuition or "best guess." All personnel decisions directly affect the lives of the employees of the institution. These people deserve as much care and attention as the patients.

The hiring process is where the employee begins a career with your organization or, if not employed, will leave with an impression that will be taken out to the community. It should be your desire to have that impression be a good one. Many legal issues are involved in the hiring process. Be sure to clarify them with your personnel manager or administrator. Laws exist that involve the advertisement of a job and how the interview is conducted, and federal rules identify questions that cannot be asked in an interview because of concern over discrimination. Be alert to these rules and follow them.

The purpose of interviewing someone for employment is to find someone who fits with the philosophy and image of your institution. The applicant needs the licensure or certification that the job description demands and the experience to perform the job at a satisfactory level. The interview also allows the nurse manager to determine the shift availability and whether the potential employee is available for part-time or full-time work. An effort should be made to learn the specific interests of the applicant so that plans can be made to use any special skills and knowledge the person possesses. The screening process of the personnel department presumably would eliminate anyone unqualified for the job. Unqualified people do not need to be interviewed.

Interview

The purpose of the interview is to exchange information. Be prepared to give positive information about your facility to all applicants whether they are to be employed or not. You want applicants to say favorable things about your organization even if they are not selected for the job. During the interview, the nurse manager is expected to determine the applicant's:

• Dependability
• Skill level

When interviewing someone for a position, establish a friendly and positive atmosphere. Be consistent in the interview process with all applicants, and be honest in your assessment of qualifications.

- Willingness to assume the responsibilities of the job
- Willingness and ability to work with others
- Interest in the job
- Adaptability
- Consistency of goals with available opportunities
- Conformity of manner and appearance to job requirements

The interview has definite purposes and should be conducted in a professional manner. It is not the place for social chitchat; however, some warm and friendly comments at the beginning of the interview should put the applicant at ease so that the interview can be emotionally comfortable.

The greatest predictor of the applicant's future success is past performance. Is this someone who has worked with older adults previously and enjoyed it? Has the applicant sought additional educational experiences that would enhance work in your type of setting? Was this person a desirable employee at the last place of employment or, if a new graduate, a good student? These crucial pieces of information should be noted on the application and verified in the interview.

It is your responsibility as the nurse manager to set the tone for honesty in the interview. Be specific and direct in your comments. It is helpful to have an interview guide available to use for every interview. This guide is a written document that contains questions, directions, and pertinent information to be shared with the applicant. The presence of an interview guide ensures you, the applicant, and the institution that the same process is being used in every interview. It avoids the gathering of prejudicial information and provides consistency in the interview process.

Questions on the interview guide should cover subjects such as which shifts the applicant is willing to work, whether part-time or full-time work is desired, and feelings about working with older people. It also could contain a brief case study or scenario about a gerontologically focused situation that requires a response from the applicant. The presence of two or three such questions gives you additional information about the potential employee. All applicants must be asked the same questions to avoid discrimination or the appearance of discrimination in choosing future employees. You also need to review the Title VII Civil Rights Act carefully before conducting any interviewing. This federal law prohibits discrimination in any personnel decision on the basis of race, color, sex, age, religion, or national origin. A comfortable format for an interview is as follows:

- Use an opening to establish rapport and put the applicant at ease.
- Share the interview procedure with the applicant.
- Discuss the applicant's interests in being employed at your facility.
- Obtain an educational history.
- Discuss future plans of the applicant, such as upward mobility and future education.
- Share case studies and situations and discuss them.
- Inform the applicant about the organization.
- Allow time for the applicant to ask questions and get answers.
- Close by clarifying how to reach the applicant after the interview, informing the applicant when the decision will be made, and thanking the applicant for considering your organization for employment.

Employee Evaluation

After the nurse manager has made a decision to hire an applicant, a very focused effort must be made to give that person a thorough and extensive orientation to the job, its standards, and its expectations. The quality of personnel hired and retained in the organization determines the success of the organization. The quality of the orientation directly determines the overall success for the organization and the employee.

After the employee has had the opportunity to work with other qualified employees and to establish an effective working routine, the new employee can be allowed to work independently. A resource person should always be available, in some way, to the new employee for the first 3 months of employment. This provision indicates that a sincere effort is being made to ensure success for the organization and the employee.

Each organization has an established process for evaluating employees. The first evaluation may come at 3, 6, or 12 months. Earlier and more frequent evaluations take more of the manager's time but also provide regular feedback for the employee. Overall, it is generally time well spent. Your organization also should have an established written form for evaluating employees. This process should be consistent for all employees to avoid discrimination.

For all employing organizations, a performance appraisal may be based on the following five basic realistic assumptions:

1. The appraisal is intended to help an employee improve the management of the workload.
2. Employee appraisal is a difficult process, but it is a skill that can be mastered with hard work.
3. Few people like the current form (a perfect one simply does not exist).

4. The employee's supervisor makes the appraisal.
5. Information must be gathered on a day-to-day basis.

The challenge to the nurse manager is that the performance appraisal must accurately reflect the person's actual job performance. It cannot contain prejudicial information, hearsay, or undocumented information. It is designed to be helpful to the employee, and by assisting the employee to improve, it is helpful to the organization.

Traditionally, potential evaluation problems can contribute to an inaccurate evaluation. The first one is *leniency error*. This occurs when a supervisor wants everyone to be buddies or to be the manager's best friend. It results when the manager "looks the other way" or gives an employee the "benefit of the doubt" rather than finding out what really happened.

A competent nurse manager cannot afford to be "best friends" with employees. The manager needs to be the manager. It is crucial to success for the manager to be an honest and fair person who does not lose the ability to be objective. The leniency error does not help an employee improve, and it does not contribute to the overall functioning of the organization.

The *recency error* is an indication of a manager who has forgotten the basic assumptions of evaluation and who has not kept records of employee performance over the year. Because of the lack of written record, the manager evaluates only on what is remembered most recently. All employees know when their annual review is scheduled and often find it easy to "look good" during the time just before their evaluation. This type of evaluation process enhances neither the performance of the employee nor that of the organization.

The *halo error* is allowing one trait to influence the entire evaluation. It could be either a strongly positive trait or a strongly negative one. Either way, it clouds the objective evaluation of an employee if only the halo behavior is remembered. Evaluations need to be fair and comprehensive regarding the employee's behavior and skills.

The evaluation process is critical to the growth and stability of the organization. Evaluation standards cannot be successful if they are ambiguous. The process of rewarding a strong employee and counseling a poor employee must be valid. This happens only if the manager maintains

Think Like a Nurse

One of the most effective habits you can develop as a manager who does performance evaluations is that of gathering evaluation information on a daily basis. With the use of computers, it is much easier than it used to be to get this organized. Simply have a disk for evaluation. Each employee's name or section should be on the disk. When something happens, you simply record it. It could be a compliment from a family member or a display of poor judgment. Making notes on your performance disk is something like doing your patient charting: It needs to be done every day. You won't make a note on every employee every day, but it is important to record the significant things that have happened for the day. This technique for organizing data will make your evaluation process a "breeze"!

a professional and consistent attitude toward the evaluation process.

Negative or probationary evaluations are very difficult for all managers to give. Use the same process you would use for a positive evaluation. Make it fair and comprehensive, and share the information you have in a professional manner. For all terminations, the process of counseling the employee must be carefully documented over time. This is an act of fairness toward the employee and a protection against litigation for the institution.

Providing Education for Employees

This chapter has discussed management concepts needed to supervise employees. Now the question is, "What is the nurse manager's role in providing continuing education to the staff?" What can the nurse manager do to move CNAs from novice care providers to expert care providers? Health care changes on a regular basis, and as licensed professionals, we all are trying to keep up with the changes. It is important for unlicensed health-care providers to keep up with health-care changes as well. As a nurse manager, you need to assist with this endeavor.

Several areas of education need to be addressed. The first is the orientation process for new employees. It is suggested that orientation programs for new CNAs should last at least 3 months. An orientation program should match, one on one, a new or novice CNA with a veteran or expert CNA. The program should provide the new CNA with the information needed to function as an effective member of the nursing team at the end of the orientation period. The orientation information should include the policies and procedures for the facility, information about the daily operation and schedules for the facility, and, most important, detailed information about the older adults and the specific skills needed to give excellent nursing care.

The expert CNA who is willing to be a role model and mentor for the new employee should be a valued employee who consistently demonstrates expert clinical skills and care behaviors. This is a CNA who demonstrates willingness to orient the new employees as well. It is appropriate to demonstrate valuing of employees who participate in the orientation program through some type of a reward.

Novice CNAs must have continuity of instruction throughout the orientation. If the facility has five units, the CNA should spend equal amounts of time on each unit. The time spent should be consecutive days so that the CNA can become acquainted with the staff and procedures on one unit before moving to the next. This approach also provides consistency of care for the older adults who are getting to know the new employee.

At the end of the orientation period, the new employee should be evaluated. The nurse manager must decide at this time if the employee is acceptable for the facility. If you are not satisfied with the employee's performance, a plan of action should be developed to assist the employee in meeting the requirements necessary for successful employment. This also may be the time when the nurse manager may make the difficult decision to terminate the employee.

When a nurse manager hires an employee, an effort should be made to increase and maintain the skills of the employee. There are various ways to accomplish this goal. Mentorship programs match individuals together when one person has the required skills and the other person needs to learn them. These programs generally last for a longer time than orientation and in most cases are less formal. A CNA who is interested in becoming an LPN may be matched with an LPN who is interested in helping the CNA be prepared for nursing school. Or, you may have an employee who works well with people with Alzheimer's disease and their families. This individual could work as a mentor for other employees who would like to possess the same skills.

Some facilities use clinical ladder models to increase employee skills. Different levels of knowledge and ways to obtain and document the skills

The LPN provides education sessions to staff to update their skills.

Think Like a Nurse

Your patient sees satisfaction and quality care as a subjective process, your facility sees satisfaction as an objective process, and you, the caregiver, are supposed to bring the two sides together to achieve the most optimal outcome for both sides. It sounds more difficult than it really is, because in reality, your facility has ways to determine their needs and act on those needs to help everyone, especially the patient, achieve patient customer satisfaction. As you become employed as an LPN and take on the role of the charge nurse, you will want to make sure you are cognizant of the cost of patient care, as well as the quality of patient care. If you are not cost conscious, the facility you work in may experience financial losses that will cause the facility to fail. It is your job to determine what quality management means to your facility and to your patient.

are identified. When an employee meets the requirements of one level or "rung" of the ladder, there often is a promotion. When employees have met the requirements for an advanced level, they often are recognized with a ceremony and a monetary award, an increase in pay or a set one-time dollar amount. Facilities have found that clinical ladders can assist with employee retention and improve employee morale. The benefit to the facility is better patient care. The improvement in care is a result of the facility seeking to prepare its own expert CNAs, LPNs, and RNs.

MANAGING THE QUALITY OF CARE

The process of managing and evaluating the quality of health care is not new. Florence Nightingale (1846) urged that all nursing care be carefully evaluated. Because of her innovative nursing-care practices and her ability to measure and evaluate nursing care, she was able to measure changes in the health of patients. At one hospital during the Crimean War, she measured a decrease in patient mortality from 50% to 20% after her nursing-care ideas were instituted. Different outside organizations measure the quality of care given in hospitals and nursing homes. The Joint Commission was founded in 1952 to evaluate health-care services. Two nursing organizations followed this trend in

the late 1950s. The American Nurses Association developed and published standards of care for the various nursing specialties, and the National Leagues of Nursing published standards that the public could expect from nursing education. Quality health care is the right of people who enter the health-care system. The aforementioned organizations provide outside evaluation of the health-care system. Other methods for making self-evaluation that involve the LPN also exist.

Total Quality Management

Total quality management (TQM) is a management philosophy that emphasizes a commitment of excellence throughout the entire health-care organization. The principles are widely used throughout many business organizations in addition to health care. The overall purpose of TQM is to improve quality of service and ensure customer satisfaction.

The four major characteristics of TQM are (1) customer/patient focus, (2) total organizational involvement, (3) use of quality tools and statistics for measurement, and (4) identification of key processes for improvement. The LPN is involved in all four aspects of the TQM process.

Most nurses naturally believe that their focus is the customer or patient. This is the overall theme of TQM and calls for all personnel in each department to focus on the needs of the patient. An example would be a smoother admission process, given that that process is often an area that provokes customer complaints. Another example is the housekeeper responding to the patient. This could simply be friendly visiting or putting aside the housekeeper's usual work to go get a nurse for a patient.

The customer focus of TQM is most effective when all employees in a hospital or nursing home respond to the challenge to focus on the needs of the patient. This philosophy eliminates the idea of "That is not my job!" Instead, everyone works toward the overall goal of satisfied customers. A nurse may need to assist the housekeeper in making beds because of the large number of admissions and discharges done in one shift. A physician may need to transport a patient from the emergency department to the unit; respiratory therapists may assist patients to the toilet; the unit secretary may need to transport patients who are being discharged to their cars.

The point is that everyone is committed to the idea of customer satisfaction and is willing to fulfill whatever role might be necessary and safe to meet that commitment.

The use of high-quality tools and statistics to measure the level of care that is being given is an important consideration. An organization cannot determine whether the quality of care is being improved unless accurate measurement occurs. This measurement generally is not the responsibility of the LPN but an upper-management or administrative assignment. The LPN may need to complete forms or make reports that contribute to overall measurement of the work being done, but such an assignment would be made by someone else in the system to you, the LPN.

The fourth component of TQM is identification of key processes for improvement. All activities in an organization can be described in terms of people working together. The term *identification of key processes* refers to the efficiency or effectiveness of the work people or teams do together. An example is the *PDCA* cycle. This is the *P*lan, *D*o, *C*heck, and *A*ct cycle. It defines the processes a group or team should be following as they do their work.

QSEN

COMPETENCY: Team Work and Collaboration

Working Effectively With Interprofessional Teams

Mr. Wise is a 69-year-old man recently admitted to a long-term care facility. He has been active all of his life but was recently in an automobile accident that left him paralyzed from the waist down. His wife is 10 years younger but she is unable to care for Mr. Wise at home because of her own health problems. When Mr. Wise is admitted, he is very upset and distraught. As the nurse goes in to begin the assessment, Mr. Wise is verbally abusive and screams at the nurse to leave him alone. He then turns to his wife and tells her to leave and never come back. He tells her she has abandoned him and he never wants to see her again. The wife begins crying uncontrollably but says she will not leave. Mr. Wise tells the nurse to help him prepare to return home immediately. The nurse has been on the job for only 3 weeks and does not feel that she is equipped to deal with a patient in this type of emotional distress. The nurse realizes that she has other members of the interprofessional team in the building and has identified that she will need some help with this patient.

Other members of the interprofessional team include her charge nurse, the physical therapist (PT), the nutritionist, the Certified Nursing Assistant (CNA), and the medical social worker (MSW). The nurse calls for help from the CNA and the MSW. Her rationale is that the CNA can help with the physical needs of this patient and the MSW can provided the emotional support and identify a support system for this family during this time of crisis. The nurse makes sure she identifies a caring CNA, even though this CNA is working in another wing of the facility. The CAN and MSW both arrive within minutes of one another.

The MSW is able to work with the patient and calm his fears. When the wife determines that the husband has settled down, she becomes more interactive and begins to help her husband settle into his new environment. The CNA begins to interact with the spouse and explains the layout of the building and the activities as she helps the spouse put away belongings and organize the room. Within a few minutes the MSW has calmed the patient and begins talking with the spouse about community support that would be advantageous for her well-being.

Think about it: The nurse had the knowledge to recognize the contributions of other team members; in this case it was the MSW. The nurse was able skillfully to request help from the MSW and demonstrated respect for the attributes that the MSW could bring to this situation as a team member in this patient-care setting.

1. What would the outcome have been if the nurse had tried to handle this emotional family situation on her own?
2. Why do you think it was a good idea for the nurse to integrate the skills of the CNA and the MSW into this family's personal and emotional crisis?
3. How do you feel the nurse demonstrated respect for the professional attributes of the MSW?

Priority Setting

How do you highlight one priority among a group of highly important nursing skills? For instance, understanding good leadership and management, fine tuning your delegation skills, implementing good decision making and critical thinking, setting priorities in safe patient care, implementing quality patient care, and following good communication skills are all significant parts of your job, which means they are all areas to prioritize.

To set a good example, a priority must be set. This chapter focuses on communication skills; the rationale for this is that becoming skilled at communication will highlight all of the other skills mentioned in this chapter. It comes into play when you implement good leadership, delegate, give instruction, and receive report; it is significant in accurately relaying the decisions you make, and it is essential for safe patient care. You need to learn good communication skills and incorporate them every day, in every interaction associated with your job.

Please reread the sections in the chapter referring to these skills. Then consider how you can become great at using them. You may want to read more about them in management books in the library. Talk to your faculty person about them. Discuss them with nurses (RNs and LPNs) where you work or during your clinical experiences. Observe people in all settings to see if and how the skills are used. I think you will find that many people don't use them, and then there are problems.

To be really good at active listening and assertive communication, you need to do what *does not* come naturally. You need to overcome your natural tendencies as a person. With attention to yourself and others, you can develop these skills, and they will be strengths to you throughout your career.

CONCLUSION

Having a clear understanding of our health-care system, including all of the the regulations and policies, is a challenge for you as an LPN. Keeping this in mind, you can imagine how challenging being a patient in the health-care system is, especially being a patient in a skilled nursing facility that he or she calls home. That is one reason it is so very important to fine tune your communication technique. Good management and communication skills are some of the most important skills you will learn in identifying and communicating the optimal outcome for your patients. Review the case study at the beginning of the chapter and identify how these skills could support you in your new position as an LPN charge nurse.

CASE STUDY SOLUTION

1. **Decision Making:** You must first make decisions on how you will accomplish all the tasks you have before you. This is where you will prioritize your list, keeping patient safety at the forefront of all decisions. Take a look at your priority list to make sure you have done this.

2. **Delegation:** If you take the first 10 minutes to delegate what you believe can safely be delegated, this will save you a great deal of time and stress and will contribute greatly to the quality of care your patients receive. What can safely and quickly be delegated to others so that you, as the charge nurse, may take on the most important issues as you work your way through the priority list? Priorities that can safely be delegated, in this instance, include the following:

   a. Using your communication skills, ask the student instructor to assign her students to the patients on your unit. She knows where the charts are because she has been in your facility many times. Tell her to use the charts and to make sure each student will cover two to three patients under the instructor's direction. Make sure she follows up with you to report her assignments.

   Consider: If the policies in your facility allow for LPN students to disperse medications under the direction of their clinical instructor, then you are set. If not, you may want to consider calling in a Medication Aide – Certified (MA-C) to make sure the medications are passed safely and on time. However, you will consider that this decision will certainly add to the expense of the day but will greatly add to the quality of patient care.

   b. Ask the new LPN to check on the night nurse. Have her report back to you on the night nurse's and availability to participate in report. After the new LPN has completed this task, you will want to keep her at your side, to observe, while you complete patient care and follow through with your list of priorities.

   Consider: You must receive report as soon as possible so you will know of any other patient problems you may be facing. You will want the LPN whom you will be orienting to be involved in report, but you would not want to have her take that report and then pass the information on to you. You have not worked with her yet, and you do not know her skill level at this point in time. Your concern will always be patient safety.

   c. Using your communication skills, acknowledge with the CNA that you will interact with the patient and family member that has caused her stress. Let her know that she does not need to return to that patient at this time. Assure her that you understand how she feels but that you are in need of her professional help and follow through in this immediate time. Schedule some time later in the day to discuss this situation with her and to listen to her side of the story. Ask her to begin ADLs for all patients.

3. **Actions/Implementation:** Now that you have efficiently made good decisions and safely delegated tasks, you have greatly decreased your stress and at the same time increased the quality and the safety of care that your patients will receive. The total amount of time you have taken to make these decisions and delegate these tasks is about 5 minutes.

   a. Because you are near the room of the irate family member, briefly step in again and communicate with the patient and the daughter. Let them know that you have an emergency and that you will return as soon as you have investigated and resolved this

continued on page 250

CASE STUDY SOLUTION *continued*

emergency. Let them know this may take an hour and that you will bring the medication list with you when you come. This conversation should take no more than 2 to 3 minutes.

b. No more than 10 minutes have passed since you walked in the door. You can now immediately and safely go to the new admit and complete an assessment of what has taken place. If the night nurse is available, then call her, from the patient's room, to receive her input on this particular patient. Determine in your communication with the night nurse and the patient:

Is the patient coherent?

What was the assessment on admit?

Did the patient fall?

Complete a new assessment on this patient with attention to the report of a possible fracture. Call the physician with the results of the assessment and your determination of a possible fracture. Implement care as ordered by the physician. Some of this care may be delegated, depending on the outcome of the assessment.

c. Receive report from the night nurse so that you can efficiently begin your rounds. Send the night nurse home.

d. Confirm the student assignments and that patients' medications are being passed by the students and instructors or that you have an MA-C called in to help.

e. Begin your morning assessments with the patient of the irate family member, and prepare to discuss the patient's prescribed medications and how they have been delivered. You will need to make sure that HIPPA is not being violated with this family involvement.

f. Begin your new LPN's orientation by having her follow you through your morning assessments. You can ask questions and learn more about her skills as you begin the day.

g. Complete your assessments, and be prepared for your interdisciplinary meeting by 1000.

h. After lunch, meet with your CNA, and use your leadership and management skills to initiate a productive conversation. As a manager you can mentor your CNA by modeling behavior and communication skills that will assist the CNA to learn to interact with irate patients and family members.

i. Follow up with those to whom tasks have been delegated.

j. Sit down with your new LPN to discuss the process of orientation.

This case study is not unlike a situation that you may be presented with every day that you work. If you can become skilled at communication, decision making, and delegation, you will accomplish a greater level of success as you interact with your patients and co-workers.

REVIEW QUESTIONS

1. As an LPN you must practice within the definition of your state's nurse practice act. The best way for you to determine whether the current job description is within the nurse practice act is to:
   1. Ask your co-workers
   2. Read the nurse practice act for your state
   3. Read the policies and procedure manual at your place of employment
   4. Discuss it with the personnel office during the hiring interview

2. The authoritarian style of management is not usually effective in the gerontological setting because:
   1. Authoritarian managers are not very person focused
   2. Most employees need much more guidance to perform tasks correctly
   3. It allows for a personable and caring approach to tasks, which is more time consuming
   4. Of the the high number of emergencies in this setting

3. As an LPN communicating with your patient while completing a patient assessment, you realize an important part of that assessment and the most honest form of communication is:
   1. Nonverbal communication
   2. Verbal communications with facial movements
   3. Sitting quietly and listening
   4. Your patient education skills

4. Generally, the best and safest patient care given to the older people in all settings is based on:
   1. The family's wishes
   2. The nurse manager's conflict management making skills
   3. The interdisciplinary team approach
   4. The permissive management style being used

5. You were hired 6 months ago as an LPN charge nurse for a skilled nursing facility. You are preparing for your first evaluation. You know that this performance review is not intended to:
   a. Improve the management of your workload
   b. Criticize your overall performance
   c. Discuss the manager's appraisal of your overall performance
   d. Assist you to improve your patient-care interactions

6. As a nurse manager you should be cognizant of your interactions with all employees. If you were to want to be everyone's buddy or make sure everyone is your best friend, you would be subject to the:
   1. Halo error
   2. Leniency error
   3. Recency error
   4. Partiality error

REFERENCES

Benner, P. (2000). *From novice to expert. Commemorative edition*. Upper Saddle River, NJ: Prentice-Hall.

Dahlkemper, T.R. (2013). *Anderson's nursing leadership, management, and professional practice for the LPN/LVN*. (5th ed.). Philadelphia, PA: F.A. Davis.

Lancaster, G., Kolakowsky-Hayner, S., Kovacich, J., & Greer-Williams, N. (2015). Interdisciplinary communication and collaboration among physicians, nurses, and unlicensed assistive peronnel. *Journal of Nursing Scholarship, 47*(3), 275–284.

White, M.J., Guitierrez, A., McLaughlin C., Eziakonwa, C., Newman, L.S., White, M., Thayer, B., Davis, K., Williams, M., & Asselin, G. (2013). A pilot for understanding interdisciplinary teams in rehabilitation practice. *Rehabilitation Nursing, 38*(3), 142-152.

Yoder-Wise, P.S. (2011). *Leading and managing in nursing* (5th ed.). St. Louis, MO: Mosby.

WEB RESOURCES

American Nurses Association. Nursing control over practice and teamwork. http://nursingworld.org/MainMenuCategories/ANAMarketplace/ANAPeriodicals/OJIN/TableofContents/Vol-18-2013/No2-May-2013/Control-over-Practice-and-Teamwork.html

American Nurses Association: Ten lessons in collaboration. http://www.nursingworld.org/MainMenuCategories/ANAMarketplace/ANAPeriodicals/OJIN/TableofContents/Volume102005/No1Jan05/tpc26_116008.aspx

Delegation National Council of State Boards of Nursing: https://www.ncsbn.org

Just for CNAs. www.justforcnas.com/blog/delegation-how-nurses-cnas-work-team

unit TWO

Clinical Practice

Infection

VICKIE ANDERSON

14

LEARNING OUTCOMES

1. Identify causes of infection in older adults.

2. Use appropriate environmental and hygienic measures that can reduce infectious diseases.

3. Develop a plan to assist an older adult in maintaining a healthy immune system.

4. Identify appropriate immunization protocols.

5. Identify infections that can be precipitated by chronic medical conditions and by the aging process.

6. Discuss the role of the licensed practical nurse (LPN) in the management of infections in older adults.

CONCEPTS

Infection

Immunity

CASE STUDY

Mrs. B. is 95 years old and was recently widowed. Mrs. B. and her husband immigrated to the United States from South America 45 years ago. She has been in generally good health and is being treated for osteoporosis and a mild elevation in blood pressure. Mrs. B. has reported a persistent dry cough for 1 month. Her health history does not reveal any other health problems. Mrs. B. uses a walker to help her ambulate. She enjoys a close relationship with her daughter and church friends. She has lived alone for nearly a year because her husband resided in an extended care facility until his death. Mrs. B. insists on being as independent as possible but does allow family and friends to visit her and help her with some personal and household tasks. Mrs. B. prefers speaking in her native language, which is Spanish.

Just before his death, it was discovered that Mr. B. had infectious TB. Mr. B. was plagued with a persistent cough and recurrent pneumonia for the last 5 months of his life. A full-scale contact investigation was initiated at the extended-care facility and among close family members.

A PPD (Mantoux) skin test was done on Mrs. B., and she was found to have a 16-mm induration. A chest x-ray revealed right upper lobe fibronodular calcification. It was suspected that Mrs. B. had a case of infectious TB. Medical orders were written for a sputum test to confirm the suspicion of TB, for a liver function profile laboratory test, and for medical treatment to be started. Results of the liver function test were normal. The sputum test came back 4+ for acid-fast bacilli. Mrs. B. did have active TB. The appropriate medications were started to treat the disease.

Mrs. B. is to wear a high-efficiency particulate air (HEPA) filter mask when in public places or anytime she is with other people. The mask is necessary only until her sputum smears become negative for acid-fast bacilli. You are the LPN assigned to Mrs. B. as her home health nurse.

Discussion

1. What nursing care should the LPN implement?

2. How can the LPN help Mrs. B. maintain social contact with family and friends?

 ## INTRODUCTION

Everyone wants to be healthy. Even a simple head cold is an irritating and inconvenient event in our lives. As a nurse, you know that there are many more serious infections than a head cold. When these infections attack older adults, the problems can be grave. This chapter is a challenge to you, the bedside nurse, to protect older adults knowledgeably from the reality of infection.

Natural immunity to infection may not be affected by aging in healthy older adults. Some infections tend to increase with the process of aging, however, and can be major health problems in older people. The physiological responses of older adults during an infectious illness differ from those of younger or middle-aged adults. The febrile response

in older adults is diminished. The basal temperature in older adults is generally lower, so it is important to understand that a low-grade fever may indicate an infection in an older adult. The nurse needs to assess for an increase in temperature based on a person's baseline temperature. The older adult may also show signs of physical and mental decline before an increase in basal temperature occurs. In addition, the course of illnesses leading to recovery or death is different.

This chapter provides information on the prevention of infection and the treatment of infections when they occur. Items to be discussed are as follows:

• Maintaining a healthy immune system by participating in health-promoting activities

This picture portrays a sharp contrast between the health of the immune system. The great-grandson is 19 and in perfect health. His grandmother is 84 and should not be around anyone with an infectious disease because of her compromised immune system.

- Preventing infections with scheduled immunizations, keeping a clean environment, and following good hygiene
- Knowledge about common infections

Infections can affect all the systems of the body and may be precipitated by chronic medical conditions.

As a nurse caring for older adults, you need to be aware of your own personal hygiene and become vigilant about washing your hands and taking proper care of soiled materials. Standard precautions should be used when there is a question about the spread of an infection. Infections can be carried from patient to patient on the hands of a nurse. As a dedicated caregiver, you want to avoid being a carrier of even the most innocent contaminant. The nursing role in the management of infection in older adults includes recognizing, reporting, and documenting signs and symptoms of infection, complying with medical direction for care, and preventing the spread of infection.

PATIENT EDUCATION

Older adults and their families should be taught the importance of maintaining current immunizations. The immunizations that all older adults should have based on the recommended schedule are Tdap, seasonal influenza, pneumococcal, and shingles. Older adults who travel frequently, especially outside the United States, should check with their primary provider before traveling for information about additional vaccinations that may be needed.

MAINTAINING A HEALTHY IMMUNE SYSTEM

One of the purposes of the immune system is to protect the body from the invasion of harmful bacteria, fungi, viruses, parasites, and other microorganisms. As the body ages, lymphocyte function and antibody immune responses become delayed or inadequate and put the older adult at risk for infections. The following are ways to support the health of the immune system.

Nutrition

The LPN is responsible for assessing and monitoring an older person's nutritional status. This is an important aspect of maintaining a healthy immune system. (Review nutrition and the reasons for poor nutrition in Chapter 8.) It is important to identify nutritional deficits and potential reasons for these deficits. The LPN must determine, through questioning and observing the person's nutritional patterns, why there may be nutritional deficits.

Lifestyle

The need for exercise, rest, and stress management and the need to avoid cigarette smoke and alcohol

 Priority Setting

This chapter discusses so many serious infections that, in my mind, there is only one overriding priority. It is described well in the chapter. I can summarize it by saying, "Wash your hands!"

Think Like a Nurse

Infections and *hand hygiene* are words often used at the same time. Hand hygiene—washing your hands with soap, water, and friction for a minimum of 15 seconds—is the CDC's recommendation. Teaching older adults this principle may save them many illnesses. As a health-care provider, it is important to remember to do appropriate hand hygiene between patient-care activities. In home health, extended care, or hospitals, there may be alcohol hand rubs. These products are safe to use and helpful in decreasing the spread of infections.

---

use are discussed in Chapter 6. Compliance with these activities heightens the abilities of the immune system. As an LPN, you need to assess compliance or noncompliance with these activities frequently and educate the person as necessary. Knowing older adults' lifestyles, living conditions, and economic situations is important when assisting them in maintaining a healthy immune system. Consider Mrs. B. from the case study. What can she do to strengthen her immune system to help her recover from TB?

Chronic Medical Conditions

Chronic medical conditions have an effect on an older adult's immune system. Chapter 15 discusses chronic medical conditions and the potential for infections. A classic example is a person with diabetes. You need to educate the diabetic person to take precautions to prevent infections by wearing appropriate shoes, observing for lesions that do not heal, and caring for skin cuts and abrasions.

Urinary Tract Infections

Preventing urinary tract infections (UTIs) is an important aspect of preventive nursing. UTIs are the most common nosocomial infections in older people with indwelling catheters. If a catheter is needed, the best practice is to remove it as soon as safely possible. Chronic bacteremia is also common in older adults and is caused by colonized bacteria in the bladder. Generally, there are no symptoms with chronic bacteremia. Older adults should be encouraged to drink adequate fluids and to empty their bladders frequently. Incontinence may be the initial symptom of a UTI.

If incontinence occurs, older persons should have their skin cleansed and soiled clothes replaced. Older adults' skin is sensitive and can break down, which invites infection. Changes in mental or physical status can also be a sign of a UTI and should be assessed by the nurse.

Respiratory Infections

Respiratory infections, especially pneumonia, may have a significant effect on an older adult. There are several risk factors that contribute to respiratory infections: decreased immune response, including age-related changes to the lungs; immobility; and increased incidence of hospitalization.

Pneumonia is one of the primary causes of death in the elderly population. Signs and symptoms of pneumonia can be altered in older adults, so patients should be watched closely to avoid a serious case of pneumonia.

Pneumococcal and influenza vaccines are encouraged in this population to prevent pneumonia and other respiratory infections. Encouraging mobility and proper nutrition and fluid intake can help decrease complications of respiratory infections. Mrs. B. will benefit from a nutritious diet and an adequate intake of fluids.

Integumentary System

Changes in the integumentary system accompany the process of aging. Many factors influence

---

QSEN

COMPETENCY: Safety (Knowledge)

Decrease Risk of Harm to Patients

Mr. Lowe is experiencing slight confusion and a decrease in physical strength as noted by his inability to get out of the chair on his own. He is also very unstable on his feet once he is standing. These are symptoms that are new for Mr. Lowe.

Changes in the mental and physical status of an older adult are a concern and should be assessed for an underlying cause in an effort to address the problem.

1. What could be causing the change in Mr. Lowe's mental and physical status?
2. As an LPN, what can you do to assist Mr. Lowe?

Point of Interest

The CDC changed the term *universal precautions* to *standard precautions* (CDC, 2007, 2007 Guideline for Isolation Precautions: Preventing Transmission of Infectious Agents in Healthcare Settings). This term means you treat everyone's blood and body fluids as if they are infectious.

changes in the course of aging. Exposure to the sun, diet, heredity, and general health affect the skin. Pressure ulcers and their potential for infection are discussed in Chapter 17. The LPN needs to be aware of other skin infections. Redness, swelling, pain, lesions, and discoloration are some signs and symptoms of skin infections. As an LPN, you must report all signs and symptoms of a skin infection to the registered nurse (RN).

Skin pathogens include the following microorganisms:

• Staphylococcal bacterial infections include impetigo, boils, carbuncles, and cellulitis.
• Streptococcal bacterial infections include impetigo and erysipelas.
• Fungal infections include the cause of "athlete's foot" and thickened nails on the fingers and toes.
• Viral infections include herpes zoster (shingles) and herpes simplex.
• Parasitic infections include scabies and lice.

It is impossible to protect people from the invasion of harmful microorganisms, but an older adult with a healthy immune system will have a better recovery if an infection occurs. Adherence to wellness activities, plus additional measures, can prevent infections and increase positive outcomes.

 ## PREVENTING INFECTIONS

Immunizations

Immunization recommendations change as people age, and health conditions affect immune responses. Some older adults were never vaccinated as children, especially those born outside the United States (American Geriatrics Society, n.d.). The need for an older adult to be immunized is not always recognized. Immunization histories may not be part of the person's medical record, or the information simply may not be noted, which is why immunization histories are an important part of the assessment that you, as the LPN, will perform. In addition, the older adult's immune system may need to be "boosted" for the body to continue to have the ability to resist certain infections. The LPN must consider the need for the older adult to have continued protection from preventable disease.

Immunizations should be continued throughout life for vaccine-preventable diseases. Based on CDC guidelines, the following vaccinations or boosters are recommended for all older adults:

Tetanus, diphtheria, and pertussis (Tdap)
Seasonal influenza
Shingles
Pneumococcal

Older adults with a weakened immune system should not receive the shingles vaccination (CDC, 2014). Also, older adults who travel extensively will want to check with their primary care provider to see if they need the following vaccinations: MMR, hepatitis A, hepatitis B, and yellow fever (American Geriatrics Society, n.d.).

These immunizations are generally available in PCP offices, senior centers, home-health agencies, public health departments, and some pharmacies.

Tetanus, Diphtheria, and Pertussis Vaccine (Tdap)

Tetanus, diphtheria, and pertussis are serious diseases caused by bacteria. Diphtheria and pertussis are spread from person to person, whereas tetanus enters the body through cuts or wounds.

Tetanus, diphtheria, and pertussis vaccines (Tdap) can help prevent these diseases. A single dose of Tdap is recommended for people 11 through 64 years of age. Another vaccine, called

Td, protects against tetanus and diphtheria but not pertussis. Td is recommended every 10 years for people age 7 and older.

Seasonal Influenza Vaccine

More than 60% of seasonal flu-related hospitalizations occur in people 65 years old and older (CDC, 2014). The influenza or "flu" vaccine should be given each year to all adults, unless contraindicated. Older adults who have lung disease, diabetes, kidney disease, or other diseases that affect the immune system should be particularly encouraged to get the vaccine. The seasonal influenza vaccine should also be given to residents living in long-term care, assisted living, or other long-term care facilities. Household contacts of high-risk older adults should also receive the influenza vaccination. The flu virus changes each year, so the formulation of the vaccine changes each year. In 2009, individuals were given a separate vaccine developed specifically for the outbreak of H1N1 that year. Currently, the standard flu vaccine provides protection for H1N1. In 2014, H1N1 was the most common flu virus causing illness in the United States (CDC, 2014). Vaccines should be given starting around mid-October.

Shingles (Herpes Zoster) Vaccine

This vaccination is newer to the list of preventable diseases through vaccinations. Shingles is a painful, localized skin rash (often with blisters) that is caused by the varicella-zoster virus, the same virus that causes chickenpox. Anyone who has had chickenpox can develop shingles. Shingles most commonly occurs in people 50 years old or older, people who have medical conditions that keep the immune system from working properly, people who receive immunosuppressive drugs, or people under a great deal of stress. An estimated 1 million Americans get shingles every year, and about half of them are 60 years old or older. Some people will have severe pain that can continue long after their rash clears up, or they may suffer from other painful complications that may last for years (CDC, 2014). The LPN accesses the need for the immunization and reports the findings. The primary care provider determines whether the immunization is needed.

Pneumococcal Vaccine

Pneumococcal disease occurs most frequently in older adults and those with a predisposing conditions such as pulmonary disease. Pneumococcal

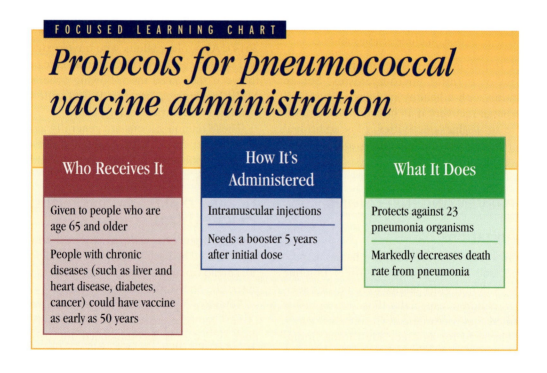

FOCUSED LEARNING CHART

Protocols for pneumococcal vaccine administration

Who Receives It	How It's Administered	What It Does
Given to people who are age 65 and older	Intramuscular injections	Protects against 23 pneumonia organisms
People with chronic diseases (such as liver and heart disease, diabetes, cancer) could have vaccine as early as 50 years	Needs a booster 5 years after initial dose	Markedly decreases death rate from pneumonia

vaccine provides protection against 23 pneumonia organisms. Only one dose is needed if it is given after age 65, but a booster is needed 5 years after the initial dose. When chronic health conditions, such as pulmonary disease, cardiac disease, diabetes, renal disease, alcoholism, liver disease, or cancer, are present, the vaccine should be considered at age 50 (CDC Guidelines, 2014). If pneumococcal vaccine was given before age 65, a second dose is required after age 65. The second dose needs to be given at least 5 years after the first dose. The primary care provider determines when the vaccine should be given.

 ## SAFE FOOD AND WATER

Food-borne diseases are very common in the United States. Millions of people become ill each year as a result of contaminated food, and thousands die. Microorganisms find food a great place to live and breed. The signs and symptoms of food-borne diseases may resemble a bad case of "stomach flu," and the older adult may delay seeking medical care. Most food-borne diseases have common signs and symptoms, which are abdominal pain, fever, vomiting, and diarrhea of sudden onset. Laboratory testing (stool culture) is required to identify the infecting organism. In your role as the nurse, you will want to note the following in a suspected food-borne illness: the time that signs and symptoms occurred, what the person ate in the last few days, where the food was served, and whether other people became ill. This information should be reported to the local health department. The health department investigates all potential food-borne diseases, and they take appropriate actions. Food-borne infections can be prevented by good hand washing, using safe foods, and keeping food preparation areas sanitary. You need to instruct older adults preparing food to:

• Store food correctly
• Protect food from insects, rodents, and animals

 ## Point of Interest

• About one-fourth of the U.S. population, including President Woodrow Wilson, got influenza during the 1918 pandemic.

 # Evidence-Based Practice

Inelmen, E.M., Sergi, G., & Enzi, G. (2007) When are indwelling urinary catheters appropriate in elderly patients? Geriatrics, 62(10), 18-22.

Indwelling urinary catheters (UCs) are used for elderly patients for many reasons, including incontinence, urinary retention, pressure ulcers, and, in some cases, ease of burden for caregivers. Although there are clinical reasons to use a UC, these devices should be used with caution because of the increased risk of infection. When the decision is made to insert a UC, it should be used for the shortest period of time. While the UC is in place, clean technique should be used when handling the catheter. Nursing staff should use clean gloves when touching the catheter and any part of the retention bag.

Questions

1. Once a UC is placed, what signs should the LPN watch for that could indicate a urinary tract infection in an older adult?
2. What will the LPN teach the CNA about caring for a patient with a UC?

• Cook food thoroughly
• Eat cooked food immediately
• Refrigerate uneaten food immediately
• Reheat cooked foods thoroughly
• Wash hands frequently
• Keep food preparation areas clean

Because of decreasing eyesight and sense of smell, some older adults may not be able to determine when food is spoiled, thus increasing their chances of becoming ill with a food-borne pathogen.

 ## ENVIRONMENTAL CLEANLINESS

Household Pets

Household pets are a source of friendship and companionship for older adults. Older people need to be aware, however, that pets also can become a source of infection. Pets may become infected and transfer their disease to household members. Animal waste can become a source of infection if it is not properly handled. A pet needs health and medical consideration to protect the older adult from a disease carried by the pet. An assessment of the home always should include mention of household pets and how care of the pet is managed.

Kitchens and Bathrooms

Kitchens and bathrooms are great harbors of infections. Household assessments need to include bathroom inspection of towels, tooth-care items, sinks, tubs, and toilets. Instructions by the LPN include not sharing personal hygiene items such as razors and tooth-care articles. Kitchen assessments involve reviewing food preparation and food storage as discussed earlier. Personal cleanliness and hygiene may need frequent reinforced instructions. When instructing older adults about hand washing, the LPN should include cleaning under the fingernails. Older adults who love and care for others in the household would not want to be the cause of a loved one's illness.

 ## SEXUALLY TRANSMITTED DISEASES

Many health-care providers are uncomfortable when considering sexually transmitted diseases (STDs) in older adults. A myth of aging is that older people cannot participate in enjoyable sexual activity. The reality is that they can, and many do. With the development of erectile dysfunction medications and various vaginal creams, there is the potential of increased sexual activity and sexually transmitted diseases in older persons.

Some people who have lived in monogamous relationships and have lost their companion may have sexual relations with one or more persons who have uncertain sexual histories. This factor can have a strong impact on an older adult's overall health. STDs about which you, as the LPN in the community, should have a working knowledge include syphilis; gonorrhea; chlamydiosis; hepatitis A, B, and C; HIV; genital warts; lice; and other viral and bacterial infections. These diseases generally are discussed in basic medical/surgical classes. Their impact and treatment in older adults do not differ from that in younger adults.

As the nurse, you need to teach older adults who are sexually active with more than one partner the signs and symptoms of STDs and to seek medical treatment for them immediately. Older adults tend not to discuss sexual matters with younger people. This is a barrier that you need to overcome through caring and sensitive communication skills. Older adults need to realize the variety of STDs and the symptoms of the most common ones. They should be able to report their symptoms clearly so that the appropriate tests can be performed for accurate diagnosis. Common symptoms are pain, discharge from the penis or vagina, abdominal pain, and genital lesions. Your responsibility is to teach the older adults in your care about STDs, their signs and symptoms, how to get appropriate care, and how to have safe sex. The initial intervention that you, as the LPN, need to undertake is sex education. People age 60 and older generally have not had the benefit of sex education on any level. They did not have the friendly chat with their mom, high school gym teacher, or a sex counselor. An intensive but sensitive interview may indicate that the older adult does not have a full working knowledge of his or her own reproductive system even after having multiple children. This is the place to start if your assessment indicates that there is a knowledge deficit in this area. Be careful to not patronize older adults, or, in other words, do not treat them as though you are the "all-knowing" parent. Be a colleague and a friend. Explore the information together. Share only what is essential for good health unless the learner indicates a desire for more information. Allow the older adult to share the wisdom that comes through the experience of having and raising children.

The second educational concept that you need to teach sexually active older adults is safe sex. Many older people no longer feel a need to protect themselves sexually because they are not concerned about becoming pregnant. Your responsibility is to teach them that safe sex also means protection against STDs, most critically HIV/AIDS. Many older adults have never used a condom. Older adults often associate condoms with birth control, something about which they no longer feel concern. It may be uncomfortable to teach someone old enough to be your grandparent how to use one. The easiest technique may be practicing putting a condom on a banana. It is acceptable to laugh and make the teaching fun. Laughter would assist the older adult who is uncomfortable with the exercise to relax and learn better. Make the point that the only truly safe sex is abstinence or monogamy. Then emphasize that condoms are next in terms of safety and should always be used.

Obtaining a Sexual History

Prevention of STDs in older adults is the reason for obtaining a sexual history. Some older adults are at little or no risk for STDs, whereas others may be at high risk. Health education, appropriate treatments, and stopping the transmission of STDs begin with the identification of at-risk behavior.

A sexual history is an integral part of a complete patient history profile. The right questions need to be asked to elicit responses that give key information about risk factors and patient behaviors. Open-ended questions are more likely to give responses that have the most pertinent information. "Tell me about your sex life" would give much more information than simply asking, "Do you have sex?"

Patients must be reassured that their responses are confidential. Developing a confidential relationship aids the LPN in building a rapport of trust and confidence with the older adult. It is important to remember that the patient's values regarding acceptable sexual behavior may differ from yours, and you should not make personal judgments.

Some specific questions need be asked and may cause you, as the interviewer, some discomfort.

This couple, both in their early 70s, recently married. They should be educated about safe sex practices.

Questions such as "How many sexual partners have you had in the past 3 months?" or "Do you prefer to have sex with men, women, or both?" can seem intrusive. These answers are very important, however, when identifying potential risks for STDs. A complete sexual history should be included on the history form.

HIV and AIDS

Older people are at increasing risk for HIV/AIDS and other STDs. In 2015, persons aged 55 years and older accounted for 24% of all people with HIV/AIDS in the United States and older. Because older people do not get tested for HIV/AIDS on a regular basis, there may be even more cases than those that are currently known.

Many factors contribute to the increasing risk of infection in older people. Older people in the United States generally know less about HIV/AIDS and STDs than younger people because elderly adults have been neglected by the individuals responsible for education and prevention messages. In addition, older people are less likely than younger people to talk about their sex lives or drug use with their PCP, and PCPs tend not to ask their older patients about sex or drug use. Finally, older people often mistake the symptoms of HIV/AIDS for the aches and pains of normal aging, so they are less likely to get tested (CDC, 2015).

Another point that needs to be explored with sexually active older adults is the type of disease HIV/AIDS really is, a chronic disease. The common association is with diabetes mellitus. People recognize diabetes as a disease for which there is not a cure and one that requires a careful medication regimen. It also is seen as something with which millions of people live successfully.

It is crucial that the older adults you teach understand that HIV/AIDS is a chronic disease. The main goal of HIV treatment with antiviral medication is twofold. The first goal is to decrease and slow the growth of the virus, and the second is to do this without causing extreme side effects, which can include fatigue, pneumonia, diarrhea, nausea or vomiting, dizziness, insomnia, skin rash, and dry mouth. Antiretroviral therapies (antiviral medication) have brought renewed hope for many people living with HIV. However, they do not offer a cure.

When caring for someone with HIV/AIDS, always use standard precautions. It is crucial that

Think Like a Nurse

Remember, transmission of HIV/AIDS is from blood to blood. The virus dies quickly when outside the body. Holding a hand, hugging, or sharing close air space will not spread the disease. You will be protected from this disease while working with patients who are HIV/AIDS positive by using standard precautions: do not touch blood or body fluids unless you are wearing personal protective equipment.

What should you educate the patient and family about the transmission of HIV/AIDS?

you follow the medication regimen closely and report any adverse reactions immediately. Good nutrition and hydration also are important; you can encourage this by sitting with the older adult in a nonrushed manner and providing encouragement to eat and drink. The intake and output in older adults with HIV/AIDS should be carefully noted.

The responsibility you have as the nurse is to educate the sexually active older adult in an effort to promote avoidance of all STDs, especially HIV/AIDS. If you are caring for a person with HIV/AIDS, you have a responsibility to assist him or her with management of the disease.

 TUBERCULOSIS

In the early part of the 20th century, tuberculosis (TB) was a major cause of death in the United States. In the 1940s, new drugs became available to treat TB. The United States, in contrast to many poorer countries, had the resources to treat all cases of TB, and the disease was almost eliminated in this country before the 1980s. Worldwide, TB is the cause of many illnesses and deaths, however. Resources for TB treatment have been lacking in poorer countries and continue to be problematic for world health organizations.

Few new cases of TB were reported in the 1970s in the United States because of the national "push" to treat the disease. This lack of reported cases resulted in TB services being cut from government funding sources in the 1980s. Suddenly, after this cut, new cases of TB began to occur. HIV was identified at that time, and TB was diagnosed

in some HIV-infected patients. Was lack of funding for treatment a reason for an increase in TB? This question continues to be debated by the public health service because treatment protocols for TB have been complicated by a TB strain that is drug resistant. The appearance of this drug-resistant strain coincided with a period of minimal treatment when individuals with TB were not finishing their prescriptions to the point that would have killed the infection. Drug-resistant TB is seen throughout the world.

The number of TB cases reported to the CDC represent a decrease in occurrence, because the the number of reported TB cases in 2012 was the lowest recorded since national reporting began in 1953. The TB case rate is 3.2 cases per 100,000; for a total of 9,945 TB cases in the United States.

Older adults have a high probability for exposure to TB compared with when they were younger. In many cases, older adults were exposed but never developed the disease. The TB bacterium may lie dormant in the body for many years and never cause active disease unless the immune system weakens, which can happen as people age. The signs and symptoms of an active TB case are night sweats, weight loss, low-grade fever, and chronic cough.

TB screening should be conducted on all nursing home residents to identify undiagnosed cases for treatment. Staff members and other residents need to be protected from TB if a case is identified. Family members may also need to be protected. Mrs. B. most likely contracted TB from her husband. Sputum smears also confirm a case of active TB. The LPN may be asked to collect a sputum specimen. The protocols at your facility dictate how the specimen should be gathered. Review the protocols, and ask questions if you are unsure of the procedure.

As a nurse, you need to follow the medical orders closely and watch for signs and symptoms of complications with the drug protocols. It is possible that you will be asked to watch the older person take the medications to ensure that the pills are consumed. The medications may cause some side effects in the older person, which is why the patient may avoid taking the medication. Directly observed therapy (DOT) has been found to be successful in ensuring that the medications are being taken as directed. The LPN may do this or choose a responsible family member to observe the medication therapy.

Point of Interest

Drug-Resistant Organisms

The misuse of antibiotics has caused drug resistance. This means that the organism has become familiar with the antibiotic, which cannot now kill a specific organism. The organisms that infect our bodies have a great ability to change to survive. They become familiar with the antibiotics that are in the bloodstream. If there is not enough antibiotic in the body or if a wrong antibiotic is used, the organism can change its shape or chemistry so that the antibiotic cannot adhere to the organism and kill it. This is what drug resistance is.

The following is the best advice to decrease drug-resistant organisms:

1. Take antibiotics only when prescribed. It is just as important that if you start the antibiotic, you also finish every pill. Doing so ensures the killing of the organism.
2. Do not take antibiotics if you have a cold or the flu. They will not do any good. Antibiotics do not kill viruses, which are what cause colds and flu.
3. Wash your hands. This decreases the spread of drug-resistant organisms to other people who may have weakened immune systems that could easily be infected by the organism.
4. Do not treat people who have a drug-resistant organism as though they have the plague. Your protection is to wear personal protective equipment when touching an ill person's blood or body fluids.

Let us look at an example: A research study was being done to see if older adults in a nursing home had methicillin-resistant *Staphylococcus aureus* (MRSA) colonized in their nose; if it was present, the symptoms and level of illness were recorded. An 85-year-old mother of six children and grandmother to 17 grandchildren agreed to be in the study.

The test came back positive that she had MRSA in her nose. She was not ill with this organism and did not have an infection. She was colonized. This mean that organism is present but has not caused the patient to become ill with an infection. After the study identified the MRSA, the nursing home placed her into solitary confinement. She could not go out of her room to participate in the daytime activities and had to eat all meals alone in her room. This was devastating to the woman, who was in the nursing home to enjoy friends and neighbors during the last years of her life. She was very social and enjoyed her time with her friends and with her large family. This woman was also instructed not to hold, touch, or kiss any of her children or grandchildren. She was horrified about having to live as she was being told. More important, this older woman clearly was given the wrong information.

When a person is colonized (not showing any signs of an infection) with a drug-resistant organism, the following principles should be taught:

1. Wash your hands before you leave your room. Basic hand hygiene with an alcohol hand rub kills drug-resistant organisms.
2. If you have a cold or a cough, you need to use tissues and good hand hygiene.

In this case, the proper teaching provided this woman with a return to her usual quality of life so that she could continue to enjoy her life in the nursing home and with her family.

The prevention and control of multidrug-resistant organisms (MDROs) is a national priority—one that requires responsibility from all health-care facilities and agencies. At some facilities, an infected person with an MDRO may be placed into contact isolation. The person caring for this patient needs to wear gloves. If you would like further information on this subject, go to: CDC.gov and look under "MDRO."

Make sure you understand the organism that a patient has and whether it can or cannot be spread. I am sure that having this woman out with her family and friends lengthened her life and added a tremendous amount of enjoyment. Correct education and information can take away the fear of drug-resistant organisms.

Medication regimens would be ordered specifically for persons with TB in your care. You need to be aware of medication doses, times to be given, and possible side effects.

As an LPN, you need to teach older adults with TB to wear a mask when in public or with people. You need to support the older person because the mask is uncomfortable to wear, difficult to use, may cause an imbalance in blood gases, and may cause the person to be sensitive about needing to wear the mask. The mask needs to be worn until sputum smears confirm that the person is no longer infectious.

Hospitals have special ventilation rooms for patients with TB to prevent the pathogen from being spread to other areas of the hospital. If the person is at home and weather permits, windows and doors should be opened to ventilate the home.

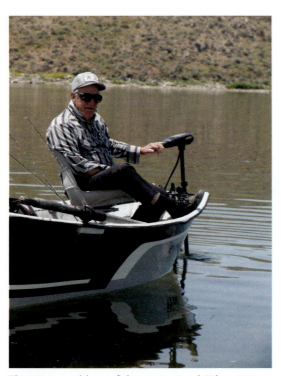

This 65-year-old man fishes year round. When it is "mosquito season," he protects himself with a long-sleeved shirt and an upturned collar. It still is possible to get bitten by a mosquito, but he is minimizing the danger by being cautious.

Sunlight destroys the TB bacteria, so excursions outside on a sunny day should be encouraged.

 WEST NILE VIRUS

West Nile virus is an infection that has caused older people to become very ill and can lead to death. The first case of West Nile virus was reported in New York City in 1999; it has now spread across the United States. The mosquito is the vector that transfers the infection from birds to humans. The symptoms are fever, chills, headache, aching bones, malaise, symptoms of respiratory infection, and muscle pain. Encephalitis or meningitis are complications of West Nile fever (CDC, 2015, West Nile Virus). The LPN should advise older adults to protect themselves against mosquito bites by wearing long-sleeved tops and long pants and insect repellent from dawn to dusk. Screens on windows and doors help keep the mosquitoes out of the house. In addition, because mosquitoes breed in standing water, all containers, such as a birdbath, should be refreshed often.

As an LPN, you need to teach older people that sufficient precautions against mosquitoes could help them to maintain their current quality of life.

 CONCLUSION

This chapter has discussed infections that have the potential to cause illnesses, including serious illnesses leading to death. The LPN has an important task to perform by assessing signs and symptoms of infectious diseases. The immune system changes with aging and may make it more difficult to recognize an infectious process. The LPN often is responsible for assessing older adults. Remember to consider the subtle signs and symptoms that could indicate an infectious process, including elevated temperature, lesion, redness, swelling, and pain. The LPN needs to consider other changes the older adult may exhibit, such as confusion, lethargy, and loss of appetite. It is important for the LPN to be a critical thinker while performing an assessment on older adults.

CASE STUDY SOLUTIONS

What nursing care should the LPN implement?

1. The LPN should incorporate appropriate respiratory isolation measures until Mrs. B. is no longer infectious. The HEPA filter mask is worn for personal protection. If the weather permits, windows and doors should be open for sunlight and ventilation. The sunlight kills the TB bacterium, and the ventilation can disperse any airborne bacteria.

2. The LPN should observe Mrs. B. taking all her medication. This is called DOT, or directly observed therapy. It means that the LPN would need to visit the home daily or designate a reliable family member or neighbor to ensure the medications are taken correctly. The objective of DOT is to ensure compliance with the medical regimen and avoid building any drug-resistant TB bacterium.

3. The LPN needs to educate Mrs. B. continually on the importance of taking all the medications. You need to teach Mrs. B. about the side effects of the medications. With any medication, you need to watch for generalized rashes, hypersensitivity, and shortness of breath that are associated with medication dosing. You are responsible for medication compliance and for observing for complications. Immediately report all changes to the RN case manager.

4. How can the LPN assist Mrs. B. with maintaining social contact with her family and friends?

   1. As the LPN, you need to help Mrs. B. to not feel socially isolated because of the need to limit visitors for infection control measures. You do not want her to become depressed or lonely. Make your own visits unhurried and pleasant. Make the effort to bring stories that would interest her. Reinforce the fact that this is a temporary situation, and she can expect to return to her usual activities as soon as her sputum smears return negative. When appropriate therapy begins, Mrs. B. could become noninfectious within 2 weeks.

   2. You need to instruct Mrs. B. on how to wear a filter mask when in public or with others. The mask is uncomfortable when worn, even for short periods. It can impair ease of breathing and may promote feelings of claustrophobia. Changes in blood gases may occur when the mask is worn for any length of time. Mrs. B. may feel self-conscious when wearing the mask in public. She may prefer to stay at home until she is no longer infectious. As her nurse, you need to listen to her and support her in her feelings. Teach her the importance of wearing the mask despite the discomfort. Ensure that she has access to the telephone and telephone numbers of her family and friends. (The numbers may need to be written in large print.) Does Mrs. B. have access to the Internet? E-mail is an effective way to communicate with people. If her communication needs are met, she would only have to wear the mask minimally.

   3. Mrs. B. may experience feelings of anger, loss, guilt, or uncertainty or a host of other feelings associated with her disease. You need to be sensitive to her feelings. In many cultures, TB is a "taboo" disease because it is seen as a disease of the poor. TB is an emotionally charged disease, and you are the person to give social support to Mrs. B. to assist her in managing her feelings.

   4. With the exception of the specific treatment for TB, the care of this patient will be similar for other individuals with infectious diseases.

REVIEW QUESTIONS

1. Mrs. R. is 80 years old and is in good health. On a recent visit, her daughter noticed that her mother seems confused and has decreased energy. Mrs. R. may have developed:
   1. Dementia
   2. A urinary tract infection
   3. An intolerance to food she recently ate
   4. Insomnia

2. This vaccination should be given annually to every resident in a long-term care facility.
   1. Influenza
   2. Pneumococcal
   3. Shingles
   4. Tdap

3. Mr. Z. is discussing his immunization history with the nurse. He mentions that at age 63 he received a pneumococcal vaccine. When does Mr. Z. need another dose of the vaccine?
   1. He does not need another dose
   2. 5 years after his first dose
   3. 10 years after his first dose
   4. Only if he gets pneumonia

4. You are admitting Mrs. J., 75 years old, to your rehabilitation facility after her knee replacement surgery. As part of the admission assessment you:
   1. Ask all of the assessment questions in front of the man she has introduced as her partner
   2. Skip the sexual history part because you assume that at her age she is not sexually active
   3. Ask her partner to leave the room before asking her questions about her sexual history
   4. Stop asking about her sexual history when she becomes embarrassed

5. When discussing HIV/AIDS with an older adult, that person needs to understand:
   1. With newer drugs, HIV/AIDS can be cured
   2. When taking the medications, you do not need to practice safe sex
   3. If you are older than 65, you do not need to be concerned about contracting the disease
   4. HIV/AIDS is incurable and is considered a chronic disease

REFERENCES

American Geriatrics Society (n.d.). A pocket guide to common immunizations for the older adult (≥65 years). www.americangeriatrics.org/files/documents/AGS_PocketGuide.pdf

Centers for Disease Control and Prevention (2014). 2014 recommended immunizations for adults by age. www.cdc.gov/vaccines/schedules/downloads/adult/adult-schedule-easy-read.pdf

Centers for Disease Control and Prevention (2013). Trends in tuberculosis—United States, 2012. http:// www.cdc.gov/mmwr/preview/mmwrhtml/mm6211a2.htm

Centers for Disease Control and Prevention. (2015). West Nile virus. http://www.cdc.gov/westnile/symptoms/index.html

Centers for Disease Control and Prevention. (2015). HIV Among people aged 50 and over. http://cdc.gov/hiv/group/age/olderamericans/index.html

WEB RESOURCE

Centers for Disease Control and Prevention: www.cdc.gov

Common Medical Diagnoses

15

KRISTIANN WILLIAMS

LEARNING OUTCOMES

1. Explain differences between acute and chronic stages of common medical problems in older adults.

2. Describe at least two common physiological changes in each body system that are normal aging changes.

3. Demonstrate nursing care appropriate for long-term care of an older adult who has one or more of the common pathologies discussed in this chapter.

4. Apply the concept of gerotranscendence to the common medical diagnoses of older adults (Healthy People, 2014).

CONCEPTS

Perfusion

Oxygenation

Mobility

Sensory Perception

Metabolism

CASE STUDY

Mrs. O. is an 82-year-old widow who has lived alone since the death of her husband last year. She was able to care for herself with all activities of daily living and had help with light house-keeping, shopping, and banking. During the past 6 months, her energy and endurance have lessened and she has gained 10 lb. Her appetite has not changed, and her food intake is reported to be the same. Her social activities include church and contact with her four children and grandchildren at least once a week. Mrs. O. has been told that she has beginning cataracts in both eyes, which need to be checked every 2 months. The only symptoms she has noted are blurring of vision and increased glare, especially at night. She has been treated for several medical problems, including osteoarthritis, HTN, and CHF. Her current weight is 175 lb, and her height is 5´6˝.

Her mental status has been intact, and she takes pride in her good memory. She has lived a successful life and seems prepared to manage her illnesses and eventual death as she talks about them freely.

An appointment with her physician resulted in hospitalization for 4 days. The following were reported on admission: BP = 187/98 mm Hg; P = 90 (apical) irregular beat; R = 24 with some dyspnea on exertion. The physician heard inspiratory crackling in both lower lung bases (posterior) up to the mid-scapular area. He made a tentative diagnosis of acute CHF with atrial fibrillation. After 4 days in the hospital, she was sent home. Digoxin (Lanoxin) was ordered at 0.25 mg q.d., and Mrs. O. was given a no-added- sodium diet and was told to decrease the amount of fat in her diet.

Case Study Discussion

1. What nursing approaches, especially monitoring through home care or physician office visits, can you suggest that may have helped to prevent this acute attack and hospitalization?

2. What chronic health-care problems might interfere with total self-care?

What activities needing increased assistance might you anticipate?

3. What positive characteristics of Mrs. O. could be used to help her monitor her own health condition?

4. What referral sources can you think of that could be helpful to Mrs. O.?

 INTRODUCTION

Congratulations! You now are at the point where you will learn how to enhance and personalize the bedside nursing care you will give to older people. The points of emphasis are specifically on the physiology and psychology of older adults. You will recognize what makes gerontological nursing a specialty after reading this chapter and the following chapters. Be open to the uniqueness of giving holistic care (care that involves the entire person) to older adults. Frame the care that you give within a transpersonal caring format. The knowledge you will learn will be valuable to you throughout your entire career.

Older people develop multiple health-care and medical problems that often complicate nursing and medical treatment plans. Older adults statistically have at least two chronic diseases or health-care problems by the time they reach 65 years of age (Centers for Disease Control and Prevention, 2014a). In contrast, younger people frequently see a physician or enter a hospital with a single health problem.

This chapter provides information in the following four areas:

- The differences between the acute and chronic states of a problem or medical diagnosis. More emphasis is placed on problems related to

Priority Setting

This chapter provides an excellent explanation of chronic disease. The priority here is for you to focus on the chronic disease information and learn and understand it. Because you will spend much of your career caring for older adults and because older adults statistically (on average) have two chronic diseases, you need to know about them. Learn the information in this chapter and build on it as you spend time in clinical areas. Ask questions of other nurses and the older persons with chronic diseases. Learn to understand how the diseases affect older people and their families, learn how to manage the illnesses, and learn how to assist the older person in managing the diseases.

chronic rather than acute situations because of the frequency of chronic problems in older adults.

• The differences between nursing care for acute and chronic medical conditions.
• The effect of the normal changes of aging on medical symptoms. These symptoms are discussed in terms of the specific effect that aging has on a health problem.
• Application of the concept of gerotranscendence to common medical illnesses of older people.

Five body systems have been selected for discussion in this chapter. The changes in these systems are commonly found with older adults in any setting. Frequently seen medical conditions are included as examples of the disorders that affect each system. Often these conditions do not occur alone. For example, two or more cardiac problems may be present at the same time, and arthritis often occurs with other chronic conditions.

ACUTE VERSUS CHRONIC CONDITIONS

Acute medical problems develop rapidly. The person experiencing an acute problem notices symptoms for a few minutes to less than a month. The acute symptoms may be caused by some previous chronic condition, such as congestive heart failure (CHF), or by a change in body function that is related to aging. For example, changes in kidney function could induce acute renal failure. An acute problem may also develop from an infection.

Research has shown that poor health does not have to be an inevitable consequence of aging. Older adults who practice healthy behaviors, take advantage of clinical preventive services, and continue to engage with family and friends are more likely to remain healthy, live independently, and incur fewer health-related costs. Important components to keeping older adults healthy are preventing chronic diseases and reducing associated complications.

A chronic disease is one that lasts 3 months or more. Chronic diseases cannot be prevented by vaccination but can be controlled with appropriate medication. Many chronic diseases can be prevented with healthy lifestyle intervention. Chronic diseases tend to become more common with age.

About 80% of older adults have one chronic condition, and 50% have at least two. Chronic conditions commonly found in elderly individuals include: cardiovascular disease (including hypertension), arthritis, diabetes, kidney disease, and mental health issues.

There are numerous ways to distinguish between acute and chronic medical conditions. Acute conditions may be thought of as requiring more immediate and often more sophisticated or technical levels of treatment. The goal with an acute condition is to cure the problem.

This woman has adapted to severe rheumatoid arthritis. She is unable to walk or straighten out her hands or legs, yet she lives a full and satisfying life.

Chronic conditions develop over time and often are not noticed by the person with the problem until major deficits manifest. These conditions tend to require more help from the informal system of caregiving, specifically from the family or a home-health nurse. Often an older adult develops a partnership with members of the informal system to gain more control over the chronic disease. Cure is not the goal with chronic conditions. From a nursing standpoint, the goal is to provide care that is helpful in managing chronic diseases. This care should be focused on assisting the older adult to function at the highest possible level in the physical, social, psychological, and spiritual arenas of life. Achievement of this goal should provide a higher quality of life for the individual and decreased morbidity (disability). An alternative goal is to work with an individual to enable him or her to die with dignity; this is a realistic goal that needs to be acknowledged when working with people who have chronic, debilitating diseases. Chapter 11, which focuses on end-of-life care in the elderly person, can assist you in understanding this goal.

Nursing care requires observation of the patient's physical functioning, which makes this one of your responsibilities. In the acute phase of illness, it is essential that the nurse note responses to medical treatments such as medications or surgery. New signs and symptoms may arise because of such treatments. All changes must be reported because the new symptoms may be critical in determining whether to continue treatment, or they may indicate complications from the medical interventions.

Nursing care for people with chronic diseases also requires the nurse to observe the person's physical functioning. In addition, it is important to have the observations of informal caregivers. The most critical information comes from the chronically ill person's observation of personal symptoms and overall condition. For treatment to be most effective, the person must be tuned in to the body's responses to treatment or to changes in total body function.

Various stressors may exacerbate a chronic but stable disease in the short-term and in the long-term. Such stressors include uncertainty about the future, such as relocation or transition stress; starting a new treatment; or the development of an acute condition. For example, a person with emphysema may develop pneumonia, and although antibiotics may cure the acute condition, the antibiotics may cause a flare-up of the previously controlled chronic emphysema.

Many nurses and other health-care workers have difficulty working with people with chronic conditions. There is a tendency to look for time lines, to place limits on how long the condition may last, or to predict when it might get worse. It is crucial for you, the licensed practical nurse (LPN), to recognize that each patient is an individual and to know that each chronic condition has its own pattern. Some conditions, such as cancer, may get progressively worse. For a patient with a cerebrovascular accident (CVA), the recovery and return of ability depend on the part of the body affected. There is no accurate prediction or measure of recovery because of variable factors that differ from person to person. Other conditions may not change over months or years. This situation can be seen with multiple sclerosis, in which a person goes through a period of remission or absence of symptoms that lasts for a prolonged period of time.

A person with a chronic health problem, such as hypertension, may have to learn to cope with a disease in which there are no visible signs or symptoms of pathology. Some people may not realize the disease is even present. Medications for hypertension often have side effects that cause people to stop taking their drugs. Other people stop taking their medication for hypertension when they feel good or believe the condition has been cured. This creates a very dangerous situation for the person. It can also occur with physical and emotional conditions and is something that the knowledgeable nurse frequently assesses and works to deter. Chronic diseases require long-term, treatments.

Working with people with chronic conditions can be a challenge for the nurse. It is common for people with chronic diseases to become discouraged. This type of nursing care calls on your creativity to assist the older person to conserve time and energy to participate in activities that have meaning for the individual. Fatigue should be prevented, and ways must be found to help the chronically ill person learn to cope with loss and change. Use of a self-care model in providing nursing care can help patients maintain their remaining capabilities. The nurse, patient, and family form the team that is needed to encourage self-care. A crucial part of the team's function is

FOCUSED LEARNING CHART

Understanding the differences between acute and chronic diseases

Older adults have both acute and chronic diseases

Acute	Chronic
Develop rapidly	Exist for at least 6 months
Need immediate care	80% of community living older adults have at least one chronic disease
Often, more sophisticated care	Develop over time until major deficits are manifest
Goal is to cure the problem	Require assistance from informal caregivers (family, friends)
In older adults, the acute disease treatment may exacerbate one or more chronic diseases	The goal is management, not cure

maintaining good communication. This begins with an understanding of the past history of the older person. One part of that past history comes from a review of systems.

REVIEW OF SYSTEMS

To determine pathology and functional ability, a review of systems is used as part of the history and physical examination. This review covers all of the body systems in an orderly fashion. One purpose of the review of systems is to uncover symptoms that may be associated with the current health problem.

Another goal is to identify chronic conditions that may have persisted for years and to learn how the person has managed those conditions over time. The review of systems also is a method of gathering data that can help in deciding on the

appropriate type of treatment for each individual. For example, some medications may be inappropriate if the person has problems with falling.

HEALTHY PEOPLE 2020
Objectives

Increase the proportion of older adults with one or more chronic health conditions who report confidence in managing their conditions.

Reduce the rate of emergency department visits resulting from falls among older adults.

Reduce the proportion of older adults who have moderate to severe functional limitations.

Increase the proportion of older adults with reduced physical or cognitive function who engage in light, moderate, or vigorous leisure-time physical activities.

http://www.healthypeople.gov/2020/topicsobjectives2020/objectiveslist.aspx?topicId=31

The review of systems is especially useful for an older adult because:

- Older people frequently have nonspecific, atypical symptoms. The review helps to identify possible causes for present problems. It is a method of defining the usual and unusual for the individual.
- Changes of aging may affect two or more body systems simultaneously. The review can help to show how an interaction between systems occurs.
- Older people often have a complex history. The review can help to tie the past into the present problem.

For the review of systems, each system and the usual questions asked are listed. Any positive response to a question is followed by other questions to determine the extent or duration of the problem and treatment, if any. It is desirable to have information about treatments used in the past and the effectiveness of those treatments. Treatments include medications bought over- the-counter (OTC) in addition to those prescribed by a health-care provider.

Pulmonary System

- History of frequent colds or upper respiratory infections?
- Cough? Productive or nonproductive of sputum?
- Appearance of sputum (not saliva)?
- Dyspnea, with exertion, changing position (orthopnea), or during the night (paroxysmal nocturnal dyspnea)?
- Immunization history (pneumococcal vaccine [Pneumovax, shingles vaccination (Zostavax)] and influenza)?
- Exposure to anyone with tuberculosis and knowledge about the purified protein derivative (PPD) test for tuberculosis?

Cardiovascular System

- History of hypertension?
- History of murmurs, irregular heartbeat, or palpitations?
- Fainting or falls, especially when changing position?
- Chest pain (at rest or after exercising) or presence of edema?
- Easy bruising? Varicose veins? Anemia? Blood clots (if so, where)?

Gastrointestinal System

- Food and fluid intake: Typical 24-hour food intake? Number and size of glasses of water and other fluids? Who prepares the meals? Any food intolerances? Likes and dislikes? Vitamins taken? Use of alcohol or tobacco?
- Stomach or abdominal discomfort before or after meals?
- Problems with bowels and frequency of use of laxatives (what types)? Fecal incontinence, presence of hemorrhoids (any bleeding, pain, itching)?
- Nausea or vomiting (under what conditions)?

Musculoskeletal System

- Pain, stiffness, or discomfort in joints (when and in what situations)?
- Pain or cramping in muscles (when and in what situations)?
- Weakness of arms or legs? Swelling in joints? History of broken bones or other injuries to muscles or bones?
- Ability to walk? Distance traveled before stopping and reason for stopping?
- Use of assistive devices such as cane or walker (if so, under what circumstances)?
- Type of daily exercise or activity?

Genitourinary System

- Difficulty holding urine and under what conditions?
- Burning, pain, or bleeding on urination?
- Sense of fullness in bladder even after urinating?

Women

- Number of pregnancies? Any problems?
- Symptoms associated with menopause?
- Vaginal drainage? Itching? Burning?
- If sexually active, any pain or discomfort?

Men

- Nocturia? Dribbling after urinating or difficulty starting to urinate? Change in urine stream?
- If sexually active, any problems?

Neurological System

- Falls or fainting with or without dizziness? Steady or unsteady gait?
- Periods of amnesia or forgetfulness?
- Inability to hold onto objects?
- History of stroke or seizures?

- Difficulty with vision or hearing? Ask to describe.
- Loss of feeling or numbness in legs or arms?
- Headaches?

Endocrine System

- History of increased thirst, hunger, or urination?
- Dry skin, loss or thinning of hair?
- Intolerance to heat or cold?

QSEN

COMPETENCY: Patient-Centered Care (Knowledge, Skills, Attitudes)

Meeting Individual Patient Needs

Ruby Hines is a 76-year-old widow who has just been released from the hospital after falling at home. After careful observation and assessment, it has been determined that she does not have any broken bones and has been released to her home with the supervision of her family who lives nearby. She lives alone in her own home and has a daughter who lives two houses away. She has several nieces and nephews who live in close proximity. She also has members of her church who check in with her frequently for any needs.

She has a 10-year history of type 2 diabetes and hypertension. She is on sliding scale insulin, which she administers after checking her blood sugar four times a day. Although she had bilateral cataract surgery 3 years ago, she has difficulty seeing the lines on her insulin syringe when she draws up the sliding scale insulin. The risk of improper dosing is always present if a second person is not there to verify correct amounts. Because Ruby has fallen twice in the past 4 months, the family is considering moving her to another place where she can be more closely monitored.

Patient-centered care means recognizing the patient's needs and preferences while being provided compassionate and coordinated care.

1. How can you support Ruby as she considers her options for staying at home or moving to an assisted living facility?
2. Describe Ruby's need for active involvement of her care.
3. How can you balance family concerns with honoring Ruby's wishes to remain in her home?

This review of systems provides only a baseline of information. As a physical examination is performed, the patient frequently remembers other symptoms or events to be added to the history. Often, the first contact with any patient does not provide all the information that may contribute to an understanding of the patient's health problems. The person may believe that symptoms were not important at the time, or the symptoms may simply have been forgotten, so the review remains incomplete. Consequently, the review of systems is always left open for additional information that may help with the planning and the continuity of care.

CHRONIC ILLNESSES COMMONLY FOUND IN OLDER ADULTS

This section provides some background information about chronic conditions frequently found in older adults. The primary focus is on continuation of care rather than on immediate treatment and nursing care.

Cardiovascular Conditions

Coronary Artery Disease

The term *coronary artery disease* (CAD) indicates that the heart muscle is not receiving a blood supply adequate to meet its needs. CAD includes angina pectoris, myocardial ischemia and infarction, arrhythmias, CHF, valvular diseases, and hypertension. Examples of three of these conditions are discussed to show how some of the changes of aging may compound a person's ability to manage the condition. The first example includes angina and myocardial infarction (MI).

For some people, the first sign of CAD is a heart attack. The mortality rate for adults older than 70 years is about twice the rate for younger individuals. Cardiovascular disease is the leading cause of death and disability in older adults. For an older person, the symptoms of MI are often atypical. Instead of crushing chest pain, there may be dyspnea, dizziness, weakness, abrupt confusion, fatigue, and upper abdominal pain. Chest pain occurs even less often in a person older than 85 years.

Because of the atypical symptoms, the diagnosis of myocardial ischemia or MI may be difficult to make in older people. The electrocardiogram

(ECG) may not be as specific in diagnosing MI in older people as in younger people because of age-related changes such as ventricular hypertrophy. The cardiac enzymes phosphokinase (CPK), creatine kinase (CK), and troponin may not be elevated as much as in a younger person because of decreased muscle mass. Younger people usually have a more extensive MI, however, because of lack of collateral circulation. Nurses who work with older people need to be alert to the possibility of MI even when the usual signs do not appear.

Medical management for an older person is essentially the same as that for a younger person. Coronary artery bypass surgery has been shown to be effective in older adults. Decreasing risk factors such as diabetes, high cholesterol, obesity, smoking, and hypertension also helps decrease the risk of a heart attack (Carro & Kaski, 2011). One goal of medical care is to avoid complications. CHF, arrhythmias, thrombi and emboli, and extension of the infarction are common complications. These may be prevented by close monitoring during the acute phase after an MI. The use of beta blockers, lipid-lowering therapies, and aspirin helps to decrease mortality.

Some people restrict their activity after MI and become less capable of self-care. Decreased activity can lead to *deconditioning*. This deconditioning may compound aging changes in the musculoskeletal system, such as decreased muscle mass and decreased muscle strength. The ability to balance activity and rest to avoid incapacity requires a strong cooperative effort among the patient, family members, and health-care personnel. Referral to cardiac rehabilitation may help the person to identify individual abilities and limitations and avoid deconditioning. Older people are capable of recovery and may return to their usual lifestyles. Sometimes alterations in lifestyle may be necessary, however.

Congestive Heart Failure

Most patients with CHF are older than 60 years. CHF is defined as the inability of the heart to pump blood to meet the metabolic demands of the body. The common causes of CHF in older adults include hypertension, heart valve calcification, MI, CAD, cardiac hypertrophy, arrhythmias, thyroid disease, and anemia. An acute episode of CHF can be brought on by treatment for other conditions. Overaggressive intravenous fluid replacement (too much, too fast) and medications such as beta blockers are common causes of CHF. The symptoms of dyspnea and frequent nighttime wakening often lead to fatigue and decreased activity.

The goal of medical treatment is to reduce the workload on the heart and improve the ability of the heart to pump. Because patients with CHF have a weakened heart muscle, the pathology of CHF is decreased cardiac output. The use of drugs, such as digoxin, is a primary treatment. Digoxin, which is used to strengthen the force of the contraction of the heart, is most frequently used when atrial fibrillation occurs with CHF. Some older people have taken digoxin for many years. Periodic blood level evaluation of this drug is necessary to prevent toxicity and ensure that the drug is still needed. Other drugs include diuretics and drugs that increase dilation of the blood vessels, such as angiotensin-converting enzyme inhibitors (ACEIs). A side effect with these drugs is falling, which results from a decrease in blood pressure with change in position (orthopnea). Refer to Mrs. O. in the case study.

Nursing responsibility in chronic CHF includes monitoring the older person for:

• Presence of edema in feet, legs, sacral area, lungs, abdomen, and around the eyes. Look for increased fluid in any dependent parts and weight gain, especially when appetite is decreased. Often, people gain weight because of fluid retention but lose actual body weight. This type of weight gain and loss can lead to decreased endurance and increased workload on the heart. A weight record is helpful to monitor fluctuations daily to weekly, depending on severity or level of control of CHF.

• Blood pressure changes with change in position (postural hypotension). Blood pressure and pulse should be checked after 5 to 10 minutes of rest in a flat position, again within 1 minute of sitting, and again 1 minute after standing. Also ask the person whether dizziness occurs with these changes. A decrease of 20 mm Hg in blood pressure on changing position is significant. Patients need to be taught how to control balance before walking and how to use support equipment, such as a cane. The medication may need to be changed, or the patient may not be drinking sufficient fluid. Postural hypotension may result from a physiological change of aging in which the body does not respond to pressure changes. This is due to changes in pressure receptors in blood vessels. The cause of postural hypotension may be any or all three of the preceding possibilities.

- Maintaining a balance between rest and activity. This balance is crucial to prevent fatigue and accompanying inability in self-care. Most patients find that they benefit from a daily routine that allows for short periods of activity followed by rest. During the acute phase of CHF, activity should be minimal. An example is sitting in a chair for 30 minutes three times a day. As cardiac function improves, increased activity is possible. The activity level should be determined by the health-care provider and closely monitored by the nurse.
- Maintaining an adequate diet to prevent loss of lean body mass. The patient's appetite may be decreased, or fatigue may be so great that five instead of three meals a day are needed. The DASH (Dietary Approaches to Stop Hypertension) diet of 1500mg/day may be prescribed, although many people do well on a diet with no added salt and no foods that are high in salt (Centers for Disease Control and Prevention, 2011). Decreased sodium intake may make food unappetizing and can cause anorexia. Use of spices instead of salt (e.g., cinnamon, thyme, lemon) and commercial salt substitutes may improve the taste of some food.

Hypertension

A blood pressure below 120/80 mm Hg is considered normal. A blood pressure between 120/80 mm Hg and 139/89 mm Hg is a condition referred to as prehypertension (Mayo Clinic, 2015). A blood pressure greater than 140/90 mm Hg is regarded as hypertension (HTN) for any age group. HTN is the leading cause of death and morbidity in the United States. The prevalence of HTN increases with age, and about 70% of adults older than age 65 are affected. Men, African Americans, diabetic patients, and obese people tend to be at greater risk. Most research now supports the need to treat a systolic blood pressure greater than 140 mm Hg and diastolic blood pressure greater than 90 mm Hg. Several factors associated with aging may predispose an older person to HTN. Stiffening of the aorta, increased cardiac afterload (the force needed to pump blood from the ventricle), and increased peripheral vascular resistance may be present. Changes in the baroreceptor reflexes may be indicated by fluctuation of blood pressure during physical activity or emotional experiences. Other causes of HTN may include changes in the kidney and endocrine system secondary to aging.

Blood pressure measurement is one of the most important parts of the physical examination. Following are some guidelines for obtaining an accurate blood pressure reading in older adults:

- Allow the person to sit quietly for 3 to 5 minutes before taking a blood pressure reading. Older adults, especially when physically deconditioned, require more time to adjust to a baseline function even after a minor stress, such as walking into an examination area.
- Select the cuff size appropriate to the person: the regular adult cuff may be too large or too small. Use of a pediatric cuff for people with small arms and a large adult or leg cuff for obese people is essential for accuracy. The cuff should be about 20% larger than the diameter of the arm.
- An auscultatory gap is often found with older adults. To avoid an inaccurate systolic reading, palpate the brachial artery and inflate the cuff in increments of 10 mm Hg while palpating. When the pulse disappears, inflate the cuff another 20 to 30 mm Hg, and then listen for the sounds as you deflate the cuff. The first sound may be followed by a gap of 20 to 30 mm Hg before the sounds are again heard.
- If this is the first contact with the older adult, take readings on both arms to determine whether there are differences of more than 10 mm Hg. For example, if there is an arteriosclerotic plaque in the right subclavian artery, the blood pressure is lower in the right arm. The correct reading is then obtained from the left arm.
- Determination of orthostatic hypotension is needed, especially when monitoring the effect of antihypertensive drugs. (See previous note

Think Like a Nurse

When digoxin doses are too high, a common side effect is confusion. This is often mistaken for a progressive sign of aging. When there is a sudden change in personality or level of consciousness, what questions are pertinent to ask?

under Congestive Heart Failure regarding technique.)

- If you have difficulty hearing the last sound for diastolic pressure, take the reading of a muffled sound as diastolic pressure. Make a note of this in your recording. One technique that can facilitate the diastolic reading is to elevate the arm above heart level.

Another nursing-care technique for someone with HTN is monitoring medications to ensure the maintenance of regular doses. This monitoring also will tell you the person's willingness to continue taking the drugs. The usual reason for a person to discontinue the drug or alter the dosage schedule is the experience of unpleasant side effects. The specific side effect varies with the classification of drug. Examples of side effects that may cause the person to stop taking the drug include constipation, drowsiness, depression, cough, dizziness related to orthostatic hypotension, anorexia, and, in men, impotence. In addition, some people stop taking diuretic medications if frequent trips to the bathroom interfere with their sleep or their daily activities.

When a person has had a consistent systolic pressure reading of 150 mm Hg or greater and then has a normal reading (120/80 mm Hg), further checking may be required. The decrease may be caused by side effects of medication. It also could be an indication of a heart attack. The usual symptoms of MI may not be present, but the person would be more fatigued and have less strength or energy to do things.

Teaching good health habits related to diet, weight loss, and exercise is also a nursing function. Some people may be placed on dietary restrictions, such as no added salt, reduced cholesterol, or reduced calories. Severe restrictions usually are not needed, but basic teaching is needed to alert older adults and their families to factors that can help control blood pressure. If these measures are successful, medications may not be needed.

Efforts to reduce blood lipid levels in people older than 75 years of age are still considered questionable by some practitioners. Measure-ments of fasting cholesterol and high-density lipoprotein (HDL) are minimal laboratory tests to determine lipid levels. An older person may have more difficulty than a younger person in changing a lifetime pattern of eating. Use of a food diary may help

with this change. Periodic contacts with nursing staff should check not only adherence to the diet, but also the person's reaction to the changes that have occurred. Emotional support provided in this way increases compliance with difficult dietary changes.

The use of regular exercise in controlling blood pressure is just as important for older people as it is for younger people. The health-care provider may prescribe aerobic exercise, especially walking, as an adjunct to control blood pressure and weight. Regular exercise may be just as beneficial as medication for some people. When people do not exercise regularly, they tend to start too fast. Instructions should be given for a minimum of 5 minutes of warm-up and stretching and a gradual increase in the amount of time spent in aerobic walking. Usually, the older adult can start with 10 minutes of aerobic walking two to three times a week. The time and frequency of aerobic activity can gradually be increased by 5 to 10 minutes each week. The person should be taught how to take a pulse to ensure that the pulse does not go beyond that person's maximum limit during the peak workout time. The maximum is based on resting heart rate and age. A cool-down period of at least 5 minutes after exercise also is needed.

Peripheral Vascular Disease

The maintenance of good vascular supply to the extremities is crucial for older people. When blood vessels are affected by arteriosclerosis and aging changes, the nutrition of tissues is impaired. Arteries and veins may be involved at the same time. A depleted oxygen supply results with retention of waste products in the body.

Think Like a Nurse

A common side effect when an angiotensin-converting enzyme inhibitor is used to treat hypertension is a nonproductive cough.

- If your patient presents with a sudden cough that was not precipitated by other cold symptoms, what interventions can you undertake?
- What important questions about the history of the cough can you ask?
- What physical assessment can you perform?

Critically Examine the Following:

Read the following patient care situation. Ponder how you would resolve the situation. Make some notes regarding what you decide, and be prepared to share your thinking in class.

Mrs. P. is your new home-health patient. She has been admitted and assessed by the registered nurse (RN), and your first visit is scheduled for this afternoon. Some of the things you think are significant from the RN's notes are that Mrs. P. is a 72-year-old, morbidly obese woman who underwent right total knee surgery 9 days ago (3 days hospital; 6 days nursing home). She lives alone. Her home is on one level. She requires oxygen hours a day because of right-sided heart failure with pulmonary HTN. She has been on antidepressants for most of her life; she finds them effective. Her HTN is managed with medication. The knee replacement was done because of severe degenerative osteoarthritis. A second total knee replacement is planned within the next 3 months. She has joint pain in shoulders and hips. She admits to being deconditioned because of chronic joint pain.

The RN has asked you to evaluate Mrs. P. and outline a plan to counteract her deconditioned state so that her next knee surgery and her recovery from it will be easier. This requires some very creative critical thinking. Give yourself some time to consider this problem; ask others what they think would be effective; and think of Mrs. P. as a real person who needs your help and knowledge.

Evidence of decreased vascular function is indicated by skin ulcers resulting from venous stasis. Venous stasis is marked by changes in the skin, such as thinning and dryness or overgrowth of epidermis. A permanent brown discoloration may appear because of small hemorrhages (petechiae). Any slight trauma to the area can break the skin and begin an ulceration. Prompt treatment is needed to avoid infection. Even when an ulcer is healed, the area is always at risk for further breakdown. Concern about the condition may cause the person to limit activity. Functional problems—for example, limited ability to ambulate—may result.

Prevention of further trauma and interference with blood supply is the guide for nursing intervention.

Neurological Conditions

Stroke

The fourth leading cause of death for older adults is stroke. The term "brain attack" has been advocated to raise awareness of the need for rapid emergency treatment. A stroke can occur when there is limited or no blood flow to a part of the brain; it is a medical emergency and can cause permanent neurological damage and even death. Strokes happen despite increasing emphasis on prevention. Risk factors include old age, high blood pressure, previous stroke or transient ischemic attack (TIA), diabetes, high cholesterol, tobacco smoking, and atrial fibrillation (American Heart Association, 2014). High blood pressure is the most important modifiable risk factor of stroke. Stroke is a leading cause of serious long-term disability.

About 60% of people who survive must cope with some disability and physical impairment. Such coping may involve sensory or motor abilities, memory, or language and other communication skills.

Strokes can be classified by type. Ischemic strokes, the most common type of stroke, occur when the blood supply to a part of the brain is suddenly interrupted. These are generally caused by a clot in the blood vessel. Hemorrhagic strokes

PATIENT EDUCATION

Teaching for Peripheral Vascular Disease

Keep legs elevated when sitting.

Avoid constricting clothing such as nylon stockings.

Avoid extreme temperature changes.

Keep legs uncrossed when sitting.

Use cotton socks and properly fitting shoes.

Report any break in skin as soon as possible.

Avoid applying tape or salves to the area.

occur when there is bleeding into the brain tissue or cranial vault. This can occur with brain trauma, aneurysms (weakening and bulging of a blood vessel), or uncontrolled HTN. Depending on the location of the stroke, there can be right- or left-sided weakness. If the stroke occurs in the right hemisphere of the brain, the left side is generally affected. If the stroke occurs in the left hemisphere, the right side is affected.

After the patient has been stabilized, usually in the hospital, planning for discharge and follow-up care is needed. Rehabilitation should begin as soon as possible, preferably in the hospital. Such an early beginning helps prevent the development of some of the physical complications of a stroke. Two common complications are contractures and skin breakdown. Continued care aids in regaining prestroke abilities, providing emotional support, and maintaining physiological defense mechanisms, such as resistance to infections.

Classification of stroke on the basis of the involved hemisphere is important because it points to the type of nursing care required. The goals for care and the way the nurse interacts with the patient are particularly affected. Frequently, a patient with a right hemisphere stroke exhibits the following characteristics:

- Left visual neglect: inability to recognize that there are objects on the left side of the visual field
- Difficulty with recognizing faces
- Poor awareness of deficits caused by stroke
- Impulsivity
- Disorientation to place and time
- Impaired attention or memory
- Monotone and flat affect
- Difficulty with organization and problem solving
- Difficulty with social aspects of language (e.g., poor turn-taking skills, providing too much information)
- Difficulty with retrieving words
- Weakness or paralysis on the left side of the body

A patient with a left hemisphere stroke tends to have more visible disabilities, such as:

- Extreme cautiousness
- Difficulty with speaking
- Inability to express self verbally
- Inability to write words

- Inability to understand written words
- Weakness or paralysis on the right side of the body

Physical, occupational, and speech therapies should be included as part of the interdisciplinary team plan of care. Fatigue may require scheduled rest times, but a limit should be placed on the length of time allowed for rest.

Other losses also occur that are independent of the hemisphere involved. Neglect of one side of the body may first be exhibited in failure to eat food placed on one side of the tray or by failure to turn toward a visitor. Homonymous hemianopsia (loss of vision in the left or right visual field) (Fig. 15.1) or bitemporal hemianopsia (loss of the peripheral or temporal area of vision) may cause each of these symptoms. Therapy is to teach the person consciously to look at a "total picture" of self and surroundings.

Prevention of complications is a major component of post stroke care. After a stroke, a person is frequently at risk for infections (respiratory and urinary), falls, malnutrition, repeated strokes, and deconditioning secondary to lack of activity. Prevention of complications includes all of the following:

- At a minimum, administering immunizations for pneumonia, influenza, shingles, and tetanus
- Keeping a routine for urination
- Monitoring fluid and food intake
- Monitoring medications
- Maintaining mobility and independence at optimal levels

Think Like a Nurse

Patients who have had a right-sided stroke are a challenge for you, the LPN, and the family. As the nurse, you have to help the patient and family cope with many frustrations. A major one is conflict between the patient and caregivers that may result from the patient's denial of disability or from impulsive behavior (acting without thinking). The patient may be unaware of the effect of this behavior, and the family must be constantly alert to the potential for injury to self or others. This type of behavior may persist throughout the remainder of the person's life. What are ways the LPN can assist the patient and family deal with these changes?

Homonymous hemianopsia

FIGURE 15.1 Homonymous hemianopsia results in the patient ignoring the entire side of the body that he or she cannot see because of the stroke.

Older people tend to drink inadequate amounts of fluid. Teaching the older adult and family members ways to ensure consumption of 1500 to 2000 mL of water per day is useful. Some people fill a quart bottle with water every morning and drink from that throughout the day, periodically refilling it. When encouraging fluids, however, be sure the person does not have difficulty swallowing. People with swallowing difficulties after a stroke frequently have more difficulty with fluids than they do with swallowing solids. Thicker liquids may be tolerated better than thin liquids.

The person's appetite may be affected by an inability to use a knife and fork. Occupational therapy should help with instruction on new ways for self-feeding. Meal plans may need to be altered to help the person lose weight or control sodium or cholesterol levels. Medications often are used to control HTN, cardiac arrhythmias, and blood clotting disorders. When a person begins to feel better, it is common to believe some medications are no longer needed. Compliance with medications must be frequently assessed. Accurate determination of blood pressure in the home or physician's office is essential. Listening to the apical heartbeat instead of relying on radial pulse is advisable. Laboratory work to follow prothrombin time and international normalized ratio (PT/INR) is critical (see Chapter 22). Following a set schedule to maintain a balance between rest and activity helps to minimize fatigue and to promote activity. Many older people who live at home may need continued follow-up after discharge from the hospital or nursing home. Home health care is important for the older adult to maintain optimal health.

Parkinson's Disease

Parkinson's disease (PD) is found more often in men than women. The condition can begin as early as the mid-40s, but it usually appears between 60 and 80 years of age. This is a chronic, progressive disease that is marked by slow movement, rigidity, unstable posture, and tremors at rest. There are some known causes for Parkinson-like symptoms, but the cause of PD is unknown.

The primary treatment for PD is medication. This condition also requires active involvement of the patient affected by the disease and the family. Education of the patient and family should be a primary objective for every nurse. Important information to be taught includes the following:

• Defining the disease and its problems
• Side effects and individual reactions to medications
• Methods to promote independence and activity while providing for safety

Some people with PD become very depressed and withdraw from social contacts. The person with PD can help to prevent depression by identifying times when fatigue occurs. The beneficial effect of medication may "wear off" close to the time for the next dose. Activity planned around these times of fatigue and decreased drug effect would help to maintain physical and social function.

As the disease progresses, the person is at risk for several complications. Infections, gastrointestinal problems, and injury from falls are most common. Respiratory infections occur when swallowing is affected. Aspiration of food and fluids can lead to pneumonia and malnutrition.

Urinary tract infections may result from urinary retention and from inadequate fluid intake. Eye infections may result from seborrhea (a dandruff-like skin problem).

Constipation is a common gastrointestinal problem resulting from a lack of bulk-type foods and fluids. Problems swallowing can lead to anorexia. Nausea and anorexia are common side effects of the medications. Consumption of semisolid foods or those with the consistency of pudding and foods with a high water content, such as fruits, may help.

A person with PD tends to be physically unstable. Many falls can be prevented by the use of a cane or walker. Safety devices should be installed in the home, such as handholds in the bathroom and banisters in the stairway. Floor coverings and furniture should enable a barrier-free route for walking. Shoes that fit well, are lightweight, support the foot, and do not cause either slipping or too much friction are needed.

The goal is to maintain the person's function for as long as possible. A secondary goal is to support the family as they help to manage the daily activities of the elderly person. Coping with the changes that usually occur is difficult for most families. Referral to support groups and helping with problem-solving are two important nursing functions.

Sensory Losses

Many adults find that visual and hearing losses begin around 50 years of age. The eyeball changes shape for most people so that they become farsighted and require glasses for near vision, such as when reading. This aging change is referred to as *presbyopia*. Changes in the shape of the lens and a yellow discoloration may alter the person's ability to focus and to distinguish colors.

Three common pathological visual conditions experienced by older people include cataracts, glaucoma, and macular degeneration. Clouding of the lens, resulting in cataracts, is the most common pathological visual condition. Blurred vision and difficulty with nighttime driving may be the first clues of cataract formation. Outpatient surgery to remove the cloudy lens and replace it with an artificial lens is a common and safe treatment. Other eye conditions require more adjustment, however.

Glaucoma is one of the leading causes of blindness and results from increased pressure in the eye that damages the optic nerve. Central vision is usually retained, but peripheral vision is lost. People speak of having "tunnel vision." This condition is generally controlled with medications instilled in the eye daily. All people older than 40 years of age should have a yearly examination for increased intraocular pressure (>22 mm Hg).

Macular degeneration destroys the point of maximum sight—the macula. Blindness does not result, but the person loses central vision. Peripheral vision is retained around that central blind spot. Increased magnification helps many people. Some people learn to adjust head positions to use peripheral vision. Use of zinc and vitamin A, C, and E supplements has been effective for some people in reducing the progression of macular degeneration.

Hearing loss increases with aging and is noted more among men than women. This condition may be due to an aging change called *presbycusis* that occurs without previous injury or other known

These women reside in a nursing home and have multiple chronic diseases. With the holistic care they receive in the nursing home, they are safe and satisfied with their lives.

cause. Hearing difficulties have social and emotional consequences because communication with others suffers. Many people tend to talk more loudly to individuals who are hard of hearing. Speaking loudly results in sounds becoming more muddled, so that comprehension is worse. Some people are helped by the use of hearing aids, whereas others cannot be helped in this way because of the type or extent of hearing loss. Adjustment to a hearing aid may be difficult because of lack of finger dexterity. The inability to tune out distracting noises also may discourage individuals from using the aid.

People with visual or hearing loss should be informed about available services. Centers for the visually impaired in large cities can provide materials to assist people with using their remaining vision. Often, people can be taught ways to compensate for the loss. Audio amplifiers are available for hearing-impaired individuals. These devices can provide greater amplification and are especially useful in open-room areas.

Following are general guidelines for nurses working with visually impaired or hearing-impaired older adults:

- Face the person before beginning to speak. Avoid sitting in front of a window or light so there will not be any glare. Glare reduces the ability of a person to read lips.
- Speak clearly and slowly so that words are distinct.
- Try not to exaggerate your speaking voice.
- If possible, use a low pitch when speaking.
- Touch the person to indicate where you are.
- Identify yourself by name and explain why you are there.
- Keep the patient's glasses and hearing aid clean.
- Refer to local, state, or national resources for assistance (e.g., centers for the visually impaired, audiologists, Lions Club for help with glasses).

Pulmonary System

Chronic Obstructive Pulmonary Disease

Chronic obstructive pulmonary disease (COPD) is a condition resulting from exposure to irritants, most commonly cigarette smoke. Other irritants include breathing in of chemical fumes, dust, air pollution, and second-hand smoke. Chronic bronchitis, asthma, and emphysema are included in this very broad category. COPD is the third leading cause of death for people older than 65 years. The primary signs and symptoms are cough and shortness of breath. The lungs become hyperinflated, and the diaphragm flattens. The person must use abdominal and intercostal muscles (accessory muscles) to breathe. Use of these muscles requires more energy than use of the diaphragm.

Some older adults who develop a barrel chest appear to have developed COPD. This appearance may be due to increased residual volume of air because of destruction of the alveolar walls. In this condition, there is less lung surface for diffusion of gases. Alternatively, the person may have a severe kyphosis (rounding) of the chest. This condition should not be confused with COPD.

Different forms of COPD have distinct symptoms; however, the end result for all forms is chronic lung disease that has a strong negative impact on physiological and emotional function. Often, there is one event, usually an infection, that causes the person to recognize the chronic nature of the condition. There is no typical pattern to the disease process except that COPD is progressive, and serious complications do occur, especially repeated infections. Hypoxemia may result with any form of COPD.

The adjustments that a person with COPD has to make in lifestyle, habits, and work can be overwhelming. Prevention of complications is the primary goal of long-term care. Each person (and family member or significant other, when available) needs to have knowledge about the disease process and how to aid in self-care. Teaching self-care includes the following:

- Ways to prevent infections with balanced diet, balanced rest and activity, avoidance of situations in which spread of infection may occur, and use of influenza and pneumococcal immunizations
- How to avoid triggers that cause flare-up of symptoms
- How to recognize signs and symptoms of infection, such as increased cough, change in sputum, and decreased tolerance for activity
- Instruction in medication, including the use of oxygen, the purpose of each medication, and side effects to be expected
- How to keep track of the medication schedule and medications to avoid, such as cough suppressants

Evidence-Based Practce

Wayne, P.M., Walsh, J.N., Taylor-Pilae, R.E., Wells, R.E., Papp, K.V., Donovan, N.J., & Yeh, G.Y. (2014). Effect of tai chi on cognitive performance in older adults: Systematic review and meta-analysis. Journal of the American Geriatrics Society, 62(1), 25-29.

Keeping active, both physically and mentally, has been demonstrated to slow down age-related cognitive decline in healthy older adults. One way older adults can engage their minds and bodies is through tai chi. Tai chi is an exercise that physically incorporates mild aerobic and agility training. It also incorporates choreographed movement patterns that can help with speed in processing new information and assist in memory recall.

Questions

1. What are other ways that older adults can increase their physical activity?
2. What are ways that older adults can increase their memory?
3. How can increasing light to moderate physical activity affect older adults' memory?

- Explaining the need for adequate hydration (2000 mL/day unless other conditions, such as heart disease, rule this out)
- How to distinguish between anxiety and airway obstruction, and measures to control both
- How to develop a support group or how to locate one

Musculoskeletal System

Osteoarthritis and Degenerative Joint Disease

Osteoarthritis is the major chronic condition reported by older adults. The incidence of arthritis increases with aging. There are more than 100 types of arthritis. Destruction of the joint cartilage occurs, often followed by overproduction of tissue at the joint margins. The result is a visible enlargement of the joint, especially in the knees and fingers. The cause of the most common form, degenerative joint disease or primary osteoarthritis, is unknown. Inflammation of the joint usually does not occur. Primary arthritis is permanent and progressive. It

also can fluctuate or vary in intensity, however. Secondary osteoarthritis develops from a combination of physical stress on joints and a medical problem such as diabetes or inflammation. Gout and rheumatoid arthritis are examples of this form.

A patient with degenerative joint disease usually reports joint stiffness in the morning with limitation of motion and muscle aches, cramps, or spasms. The extent of these symptoms varies from person to person. Some people have very little joint pain or stiffness. Others may experience joint pain most of the day. There is no specific treatment.

The goals for treatment may include the following:

- Control of pain with nonsteroidal medications, such as ibuprofen
- Steroid injection into the affected joint
- Weight loss if the person is overweight
- Maintain activity
- Cope with physical and lifestyle changes
- Joint replacement

To reach these goals, it is usually helpful for the person to understand the nature of the condition and to avoid the use of ineffective treatments. It also is important to learn to identify events or activities that increase and decrease pain to promote self-care.

Another crucial aspect of care is to teach the older adult to use medications to prevent pain rather than to control pain after it has started, that is, take pain medication before activity or on a routine basis. Meal planning is another challenge. Meals should meet but not exceed caloric needs. (This can be a problem for people with low income, minimal sources of emotional support, or lack of energy or motivation to change eating habits.) The nurse should teach the patient and family to plan activities around the time of day when the person feels best and there is less pain.

A physical therapist can teach the proper use of moist heat, physical therapy exercises, and equipment (e.g., a walker) to decrease pain or stress on joints. A walker or other equipment may need to be examined to ensure that it is appropriate for the person's needs. The nurse should focus on teaching the older adult self-expression to maintain self-esteem, decrease depression, and promote social interaction. Referral to an arthritis support group and use of teaching materials from such a group may be helpful to older persons and their families.

Osteoporosis

Osteoporosis is the most common bone disease in the older adult. Osteoporosis is a disease in which bones become fragile and are more likely to fracture. Usually, the bone loses density, which is determined by the amount of calcium and minerals in the bone. Caucasian women are at the greatest risk. Asian women and women who have small, thin frames are at higher risk. Men and women of all ethnic groups can develop osteoporosis. Women experience more rapid bone loss in their 50s than men do. A decrease in estrogen in women at the time of menopause and a decrease in testosterone men are leading causes of bone loss in the older adult (see Box 15.1 for other risk factors). By the late 60s, men and women lose bone mass at the same rate. The older adult may be unaware that he or she has osteoporosis until minimal trauma results in a fracture.

A major goal when working with someone with osteoporosis is to maintain safety. Injury resulting from a fall, especially a hip fracture, is one of the most frequent consequences. The resulting loss of mobility and restriction of activity create emotional problems and place the person at risk for other physical problems, such as skin breakdown and constipation. In addition, treatment is long and costly.

A major nursing responsibility is to teach the person and family to identify hazards in the home and community. Simple techniques that can be used to help maintain safety are the use of grab bars by the toilet in the tub or shower and the use of a tub chair for bathing. The house should be carefully examined for safety hazards such as "trippers" (e.g., scatter rugs, electric cords, uneven pavement, and pets). The person should be taught to maintain postural balance by rising slowly and avoiding sudden movement. Another area in which teaching is beneficial is the identification of risk factors—for example, limiting use of caffeine sources to one a day. Limiting the use of tobacco and alcohol may help decrease the progression of osteoporosis. Increasing the consumption of sources of calcium, such as fortified low-fat milk, yogurt, and cottage cheese, also increases the intake of vitamin D.

Metabolic and Endocrine Diseases

Type 2 Diabetes

Type 2 diabetes is becoming an epidemic. Diabetes is a condition in which the body does not properly process food for use as energy. Most of the food we eat is turned into glucose, or sugar, that our bodies can use for energy. The pancreas is an organ, located by the stomach, that makes a hormone called insulin. Insulin is necessary to help glucose get into the cells of our bodies to be used for energy. When an individual has diabetes, the body either does not make enough insulin or cannot use its own insulin as well as it should. This causes glucose to build up in the blood. This is why many people refer to diabetes as "sugar diabetes."

Type 2 diabetes is becoming more prevalent in the United States. The CDC estimates that by the year 2050, one in three Americans will have type 2 diabetes if current trends continue. Currently one in nine adult Americans has diabetes.

If an individual has prediabetes, his or her glucose is higher than normal, but not high enough to be considered diabetes. When a person is diagnosed with prediabetes, it alerts the individual that he or she is at risk for developing type 2 diabetes (see Box 15.2). Research shows that people with prediabetes can greatly reduce the chance they will develop type 2 diabetes by losing weight and increasing their activity level.

Individuals diagnosed with prediabetes also are at higher risk for heart disease, stroke, and eye disease. Diabetes can cause serious health complications including heart disease, blindness, kidney failure, and the loss of feet or legs. Diabetes is the seventh leading cause of death in the United States.

BOX 15.1 RISK FACTORS FOR OSTEOPOROSIS

Positive family history for osteoporosis

Inactivity or immobility

Low calcium and vitamin D intake

Smoking

High intake of alcohol

High intake of caffeine

Long-term use of corticosteroids or anticonvulsant drugs

Low body weight

Weight loss surgery

Disease conditions: autoimmune disorders, diabetes, leukemia, hyperparathyroidism

BOX 15.2   RISK FACTORS FOR TYPE 2 DIABETES

Age 45 years or older

Prediabetes diagnosis

Overweight

Family history of type 2 diabetes

Physically active fewer than three times
   per week

History of having given birth to a baby who
   weighed more than 9 pounds

History of gestational diabetes

Certain ethnic groups (African American,
   Hispanic/Latino, American Indian)

Think Like a Nurse

The symptoms of diabetes in the elderly can be masked, making the disease more difficult to diagnose. Warning signs such as increased thirst, frequent urination, and vision problems may be overlooked because of the common effects of aging on the body. Changes such as fatigue, weakness, mental confusion, incontinence, and other health complications related to diabetes are more often the presenting symptoms. In addition, it is not unusual for the older person to have high cholesterol levels along with elevated glucose levels.

   What questions can be asked to determine changes in symptoms

Older adults with chronic illnesses can live reasonably normal lives if they are willing to attend to the details of managing their disease. This woman was able to attend her granddaughter's college graduation because of her determination to live well with diabetes.

There is no cure for type 2 diabetes, but it usually can be controlled with diet alone. When the person is overweight, a reduced caloric intake coupled with regular exercise is recommended. Oral hypoglycemic drugs may be used if control is not achieved with diet and exercise. Some older adults may need insulin when adequate blood glucose level control is not achieved.

The types of complications associated with diabetes mellitus, such as skin lesions and renal and neurological problems, also may be typical of aging. Teaching about skin care, protection of the feet, periodic eye examination, dental care, and recognition of infections is critical in maintaining proper control of diabetes. The nurse also needs to teach older adults with type 2 diabetes how to follow a regular schedule involving medication, diet, exercise, and blood glucose monitoring.

Hypothyroidism

Hypothyroidism is common especially among older women. The presence of a low thyroid level is often overlooked because of the similarity between the symptoms of hypothyroidism and characteristics of aging. Symptoms of hypothyroidism, which are thought to be typical among older adults, are fatigue, memory loss, slowing of thought processes, dry skin, intolerance to cold, constipation, and thinning of hair. Symptoms can occur slowly over time.

Health-care providers can order blood tests to determine whether thyroid hormone levels are abnormal. Caregivers often attribute behavioral changes in an older person only to aging. Even small deficits of thyroxine or small increases in thyroid-stimulating hormone can result in slowed reactions. This should be a clear safety alert for every nurse.

Although hypothyroidism is common among older women, the symptoms often are ignored because they are confused with characteristics of aging. People must be taught how to recognize signs and symptoms of overmedication or under-medication for this disease. It is especially important to monitor respiratory and cardiac function. People usually begin to notice improved function within a few days of starting treatment.

GEROTRANSCENDENCE

Each of the diseases discussed in this chapter requires a great deal of commitment and courage to manage and live with successfully. The people who are most likely to commit to self-management are people who have embraced the concept of gerotranscendence. Most individuals, however, do not understand the concept. Gerotranscendence is something that comes from within after living a life that successfully follows Erikson's developmental stages. A person who has gone through Erikson's stages has managed life well and with successful human interaction. Such individuals have loved and been loved, have avoided despair despite life's tragedies, and have been industrious and successful. Consequently, such people are ready for the losses of old age and the inevitability of death. Many psychologists say that the family and friends who can talk about death openly are the ones who are very close to each other. This comfort with oneself and with the inevitability of death is one aspect of gerotranscendence.

An older adult who has succeeded in Erikson's developmental plan can accept death because of a life well lived. The individual generally can continue living with singular or multiple acute and chronic diseases because there are few regrets in his or her life. Such people accept illness and work to manage it; they also accept the inevitability of death and plan for it.

Consider a 68-year-old woman with multiple serious chronic diseases. Within the last 3 months, she has been diagnosed with an aggressive cancer that has spread. She is undergoing chemotherapy and will also have radiation. She has purchased a burial plot, picked out and had a head stone put into place, and written her obituary. She is affluent and is now working on her will to update it. She made a list of items that she wants to go to friends and each of her nieces and nephews. With those things done, she now plays with and makes plans to do things with her three grandchildren that include her only child and her husband. She has achieved gerotranscendence as she accepts her illnesses and the fact she will eventually die, and she has moved on to enjoy her life.

The way for older adults to achieve gerotranscendence is to have support from caring nurses like you throughout their lives. The way for you to achieve it later in your life is to be aware of Erikson's theory and apply it for yourself and to teach it to people who come into your life. It is worth the effort.

CONCLUSION

Although all of the conditions in this chapter have been discussed separately, you probably have noted that there are similarities in approaches that can be used. Involvement of the patient has been stressed throughout. The need for exercise, high-quality meals with lowered caloric intake, and prevention of complications are three common themes. The following case study serves as an example of thinking out a unified approach to the care of a person with chronic conditions.

CASE STUDY SOLUTION

1. You should consider the desired effect of her digoxin and any OTC drugs she may be taking. Consider the possible side effects of each, and whether there are any interactions among the medications. In addition, consider how frequently blood pressure needs to be checked (probably every 1 to 2 weeks after a medication is started; consider the use of a home-health nurse to monitor this or use of a senior center if there is one where blood pressure monitoring can be done). Check for edema, especially in the lower extremities, sacral area, and lungs. The area of edema depends on whether heart failure is right-sided or left-sided: Right-sided failure results in edema in the lower extremities, sacral area, and abdomen; left-sided failure results in fluid in the lungs. In each case, the location of edema is related to where the backup of pressure occurs. Monitoring also should include: keeping a diary of food eaten and looking at salt content and quantity of food and fluids. Even after a person has been on medications for some time, reviews of diet, activity, ability to take medications as prescribed, and ability to pay for the medications (to avoid skipping doses) are needed. One critical factor to monitor is weight. People with CHF may have increases in weight because of fluid retention and not because of an increase in lean body mass. They may look healthy because of that weight, but fluid accumulation decreases their ability to function by putting more stress on the heart; cardiac output available for daily activities and endurance is decreased.

2. You should discuss the effect of gradual loss of vision with possible development of cataracts. How does this affect a person's ability to take medications as ordered, to shop, to use transportation, to use the telephone, and to feel safe, especially at night? When the person also is hampered by osteoarthritis, a vicious circle may develop. Chronic pain may limit activity, which creates more stiffness and decreased range of motion. As a result, the person needs to exert more energy to do even simple housekeeping and can lead to a more sedentary lifestyle—so the cycle continues. When these limitations are superimposed on the chronic conditions of HTN and CHF, the person may gradually lose not only the ability but also the desire for self-care. These psychosocial losses are added to the physiological losses, and the need for assistance with activities of daily living is increased. You also might want to discuss the differences between acute and chronic pain and the effect of chronic pain on daily activities, perception of self-care abilities, involvement in social activities, and the effect that complaints about this type of pain have on social interaction.

3. One could make some assumptions that would need to be checked out about involvement with family. The case history indicates that Mrs. O. has been able to be self-sufficient, and that she has some support from family members. Family tends to be the first line of assistance for older people, and only if family help is unavailable do they rely on community support or formal and governmental agencies. The history of the individual is usually a good indication of what that person will do as an older adult, provided that there is some support when problems occur. Apparently, Mrs. O. has good cognitive ability and is capable of learning. Teaching and helping her to establish a program of monitoring herself (such as weight, food intake, type of food, shopping for inexpensive food) and teaching her ways to simplify housekeeping, conserve energy, and develop a daily schedule to do energy-requiring activities when she has the most energy could be very effective. Involvement of the patient in developing this program of care is essential. Allow the patient to be part of the decision-making process.

4. Look at community resources in her area. Investigate the county agencies on aging, home-health agencies, nutrition programs, transportation resources, and availability of neighbors or friends as well as family. What help is available to assist with visual problems? Is a program available to help with control of arthritic pain, such as water aerobics? Is physical therapy available? Talk to or visit some of these resources to determine if they would help Mrs. O.

REVIEW QUESTIONS

1. Chronic health conditions differ from acute conditions in which of the following ways?
   1. Chronic conditions begin at an earlier age.
   2. Acute conditions tend to take time developing.
   3. Chronic conditions require active work by patient or family.
   4. Acute conditions occur briefly and resolve quickly.

2. A review of systems helps the nurse identify which of the following?
   1. Possible interaction among health-care problems
   2. Whether the person has been taking care of his or her health properly
   3. How much the patient can remember about past health history
   4. To whom the patient should be referred based on a system need

3. When a person has a right-sided stroke one way to ensure the patient's continued attention to both sides of the body is to do which of the following?
   1. Observe for equal length of both arms.
   2. Observe the condition of the skin and mucous membranes on the affected side.
   3. Continue to teach the patient to strengthen the unaffected side and to avoid overuse of the affected extremities.
   4. Continue to approach the patient from the unaffected side to encourage communication.

4. A major concern with older adults who have chronic conditions such as osteoarthritis is lack of activity. Which of the following is an unwanted result of decreased activity?
   1. Diarrhea
   2. Poor hygiene
   3. Loss of sense of touch
   4. Deconditioning

5. An older person with a chronic condition such as HTN may not take prescribed medications routinely. The main reason for this is which of the following?
   1. Inability to remember a medication schedule
   2. Lack of symptoms that indicate blood pressure is high
   3. Fear of becoming dependent on the medication
   4. Undesired side effects of the medications

REFERENCES

American Heart Association (2014). Executive summary: Heart disease and stroke statistics—2014 update. *Circulation, 129*(3), 399-410.

Carro, A., & Kaski, J.C. (2011). Myocardial infarction in the elderly. *Aging and Disease, 2*(1), 116-137.

Centers for Disease Control and Prevention (2011). Prevalence of hypertension and controlled hypertension. www.cdc.gov/mmwr/preview/mmwrhtml/su6001a21.htm?s_cid=su6001a21_w

Centers for Disease Control and Prevention. (2014a). Chronic disease prevention and health promotion. www.cdc.gov/chronicdisease/overview/index.htm

Centers for Disease Control and Prevention. (2014b). Healthy aging. http://www.cdc.gov/aging/index.html

Centers for Disease Control and Prevention. (2014c). National vital statistics reports: Deaths final data for 2010.

Healthy People. (2014). Older adults. http://www.healthypeople.gov/2020/topicsobjectives2020/objectiveslist.aspx?topicId=31

Mayo Clinic. (2015). Prehypertension. http://mayoclinic.org/diseaseconditions/prehypertension/basics/definition/con-20026271

WEB RESOURCES

American Diabetes Association: www.diabetes.org

American Heart Association: www.heart.org

Centers for Disease Control and Prevention: www.cdc.gov

Physiological Assessment

16

KATHLEEN R. CULLITON

CONCEPT

Assessment

LEARNING OUTCOMES

1. Describe two unique aspects of physiological assessment for older adults.

2. Describe at least three normal aging changes for each body system.

3. List two tools that are commonly used to evaluate functional status.

4. Discuss the importance of nutrition to the physiological well-being of the older adult.

5. Describe at least two important components to include in a home assessment.

CASE STUDY

Miss S. is an 85-year-old woman who has been admitted to the medical unit where you work. She has been there for 2 days while being treated for heart failure (HF). You are assigned her care for the next 12 hours. In a report, you are told Miss S. is uncooperative and incontinent. Miss S. is responding well to her medication regimen for the HF and will be discharged tomorrow.

Discussion

1. What is your priority in terms of assessing Miss S. today?

2. How will you meet the requirements of the priority assessment items?

3. What other points of concern should you address in your assessment?

4. How will you do that?

 ## INTRODUCTION

Health assessment is a holistic look at a patient's data, including the patient's physical, psychological, social, cultural, spiritual, and environmental information. Nurses involved in health assessment are not just simply collecting information about problems; the assessment must include identification of strengths, assets, potential risks, and potential areas of growth.

This chapter provides you with the opportunity to learn how to do a holistic assessment. Holistic assessments go beyond the physical assessment and include all aspects of the older person's life. The ability to perform a holistic assessment requires a high level of thinking and a sophisticated ability to process information. This is your chance to learn and then to do something significant for the older adults in your care. This chapter outlines the parts of a physical, functional, discharge, and wellness assessment. The interrelationship between physical health, psychological well-being, and safety (Fig. 16.1) is highlighted. You, as the licensed practical nurse (LPN), need to be prepared to make a complete and thorough holistic assessment of the older patient in an effort to improve the person's overall health and happiness.

FIGURE 16.1 Interrelationship of physical health, psychosocial well-being, and safety.

techniques used to conduct a total examination. This assessment outline assists you, however, in completing a head-to-toe physical examination of an older adult. It is important to remember to report any abnormal findings to the registered nurse (RN) or the physician.

 ## PHYSICAL ASSESSMENT

The techniques for physical examination included in this chapter are not all-inclusive of the

 ## HISTORY

When taking a history on any system, there is information you need to have for an accurate

⏱ Priority Setting

It is impossible to say that learning how to assess one body system over another is the priority for this chapter. You simply need to learn it all! In the process of learning how to do a head-to-toe assessment, there is a simple list of priorities, however. Here is my list:

1. Learn how to auscultate and palpate so that you can trust what you hear and feel. The only way to do this is to practice. Do it over and over and over again. It can take more than 50 practice assessments before one can trust what one is hearing or feeling.
2. After you have mastered the basic skills, you need to focus on the body one system at a time. Do heart assessments until you are really good. Blending the health history and integrated physical assessment allows nurses to identify patient problems and assets more accurately. This is part of the Nursing Process.

This woman smokes a pack of cigarettes a day and seldom leaves her house. Based on this information, what other questions should you ask her about her health as you take her history?

record of the person's overall health. You need to know the person's:

- Exercise plan
- Eating patterns, including recent weight loss or gain
- Consumption of alcoholic beverages, caffeine, and water
- Sleep patterns
- Smoking habits, or lack of them
- Stress management techniques
- Sexual activity
- Medication record, including prescription and over-the-counter medications

For Miss S., taking her medications appropriately is a serious matter. Any information about Miss S. and her use or misuse of the medications ordered to manage her heart failure (HF) must be reported to the RN immediately.

After you have obtained the previously listed holistic information, you need to take a history and do an examination of the person's physiological systems. The following information serves as a guide (Dillon, 2007). If you identify aspects of the assessment or history that you do not understand or know how to do, discuss your concerns

in class or privately with the faculty person. I am sure you have been taught how to do a history and physical examination on middle-aged adults. What you are learning in this chapter is not extremely different, yet it includes the aspects of a history and physical examination that relate to people who are growing older. It is important that you learn to adapt from one age group to another as you work in nursing.

The following information is presented in a very didactic manner. That is for ease and efficiency in your study of the material. Read this material and master it! A nurse who can do an excellent history and assessment of a specialized group of people, such as older adults, is very desirable as an employee. Even more important is that you will have the skills and knowledge to "pick up" on a subtle symptom, such as "painless" heart attacks, infections without a fever, or increased white blood count (WBC), all of which many older adults have. Subtle symptoms are important to know because they may save a life.

The material in this chapter is divided into three basic skills for doing an assessment: history, inspection, and palpation (Wilkinson, Treas, Barnett, & Smith, 2016).

REVIEW OF SYSTEMS

Head, Neck, and Face
History
Evaluate the older adult's medical history for head injury, increased level of stress, thyroid dysfunction, neck injury, or infection.

QSEN

COMPETENCY: Quality Improvement (Knowledge, Skills, Attitudes)

Improving Patient Care

At an interdisciplinary team (IDT) meeting, Dr. K. complained that the nurses were calling him at crazy times with inappropriate requests. Before the nurse manager could respond, the pharmacist exclaimed that he was also getting unnecessary calls. When the nurse manager approached the physician and pharmacist for clarification, it seemed that the nurses were concerned about the well-being of a resident but were unable to communicate data to support their concerns. They would say things like, "the resident is acting funny" or "I don't know why but I have a funny feeling about how Mr. U. is doing."

The nurse manager called the nursing management team together to discuss this problem and possible solutions. The group decided the following:

1. They decided to change the reporting process. To help the nurses organize their thoughts and get all of the information they needed before they made a call, the group adopted Identification, Situation, Background, Assessment, and Recommendation (I-SBAR) as the reporting tool.
2. The nursing staff had a mandatory orientation and training on the use of I-SBAR. Online and printed worksheets were distributed to nurses as part of the training.
3. The staff used the I-SBAR for 2 weeks. At the end of 2 weeks, the nursing management team distributed a questionnaire asking the staff and other members of the IDT if there were any changes noted with the use of I-SBAR.

After the 2-week period, four of the nurses asked the management team to help them with physical assessment. They knew when a resident was agitated or anxious but felt ill equipped to perform an appropriate assessment. The nurse managers worked at the bedside with the nurses to help with not only assessment skills but also diagnostic reasoning.

If a resident was short of breath or having difficulty breathing the nurses, were taught the following: not just to take the resident's respiratory rate but to assess lung sounds; note when the difficulty breathing occurred (with activity or at rest); ask the resident whether he or she had any other symptoms; check capillary refill, oxygen saturation, pulse rate and rhythm, and blood pressure; and ask the resident whether he or she had ever had a similar problem and what were those circumstances.

This is an excellent example of how a change in process can definitely improve the practice of the staff and ultimately the care for a resident. It demonstrates the knowledge, skills, and attitude associated with quality improvement. The nursing management team demonstrated a commitment to quality care by looking at process and process improvement rather than simply pointing a finger at nurses who were not performing good assessments.

1. Why do you think the nurses came forward and asked for assistance with bedside assessments?
2. Can you identify a problem in your work setting that needs a process change to improve care?

Physical Examination

The assessment of the head and neck is the same for older adults as for younger people.

INSPECTION

Observe the older individual's head position. Note the size, shape, symmetry, and proportion of the head. If it appears abnormally large or small, measure the circumference or distance around the head. Evaluate hair distribution, pattern of baldness, and dryness of the scalp. Note if lice are found in the hair. The presence of lice demands immediate intervention. Assess the face for color, symmetry, and distribution of facial hair. Evaluate facial muscles by having the older adult demonstrate different facial expressions: raise eyebrows, close eyes, puff out cheeks, smile, show teeth, and frown. Note any wrinkles or dryness of the skin. Note the size of the neck. The trachea should be aligned with the midline of the suprasternal notch. Observe for symmetry of the neck muscles. Note venous distention, involuntary muscle tension, or swelling in the neck. Assess the active range of motion (ROM) of the neck by having the older adult tilt the head backward, forward, from side to side, and in a circular motion. ROM of the neck should be completed without limitation or pain.

PALPATION

Palpate the alignment of the trachea. Palpate the cervical muscles, and note any tenderness. Palpate the carotid pulses one at a time. What does the pulse feel like? Is it bounding? Weak? Or does it have a vibration-type movement? As the older adult moves the neck, palpate over the spinal area for crepitus. Crepitus is a slight grating sensation that occurs when you palpate, and it is not normal.

Abnormal findings include edema of the face (especially around eyes), involuntary facial movements (tic, tremor, droop), lack of symmetry, unusual size and contour, and tenderness.

Nose and Sinuses

History

Ask the older adult to describe any problems with the nose or sinuses. Note that epistaxis (nosebleed) is more common in older adults than in younger adults.

Physical Examination
INSPECTION

Observe the size, shape, and color of the nose. Note any flaring of the nostrils during breathing and any nasal drainage. Ask the older person to tilt the head so you can examine the nasal cavity for swelling, drainage, polyps, and bleeding. The nasal mucosa should be moist and dark pink. Frequently, men have an increased amount of nasal hair. Assess the movement of air through each nostril by occluding the nostril not being examined and asking the older adult to inhale and exhale through the nose. Assess the older adult's ability to smell by asking the person to identify different common smells (almond, vanilla, cinnamon, coffee). It is abnormal for the smell to be perceived differently in each nostril.

PALPATION

Palpate the nose for tenderness or masses. Abnormal findings include swelling of mucosa, bleeding, discharge, perforation, polyps, and deviation of nasal septum. It is uncommon to find nasal blockage, infection, crusting, and dryness.

Eyes

History

The nurse needs to discuss the following: vision changes, pain, excessive tearing or discharge, diplopia, infection, and cataracts. Ask whether the person wears glasses. When are the glasses worn? When was the last ophthalmic examination?

Physical Examination
INSPECTION

Assess the external eye and visual acuity. Examine the eyes for position and alignment. Note the symmetry of the eyebrows, eyelashes, pupils, and irises. Changes in the appearance of the eyelids can be due to systemic diseases such as hyperthyroidism, myasthenia gravis, or palsy. The eyes should be evaluated for redness, swelling, and discharge. Pupils should be equal in size unless they have been unequal throughout life or have become unequal as a result of surgery or trauma. They may react more slowly to light than they did in the person's youth. Normally, the pupils are black, equal in size, round, and smooth. If the older adult has cataracts, the pupils may appear cloudy.

Before testing visual acuity, you, as the nurse, need to make sure that adequate light is available. If the older adult wears glasses, the lenses should be checked for cleanliness and alignment because those two factors can affect visual acuity. The line of the bifocals may cause double vision if the glasses are misaligned. Evaluate distant vision with a Snellen's eye chart. Test each eye separately, with and without glasses. After testing separately, test the eyes together with and without glasses. Any person with 20/40 vision or less should be referred to a physician or nurse practitioner. To test near vision, use a newspaper or other conventional reading material; measure the distance from the face to the reading material. Have an alternate plan if the person cannot read. A possibility is to have the person look at an artistic picture and describe the details to you.

Ears

History

The nurse needs to help determine the effect of hearing loss on the older person's life. Does the older adult use any corrective devices, such as amplifiers or hearing aids? The following are some questions that can be used to elicit a history: Have you experienced pain from your ears? Have you had dizziness? In what situations? How long did it last? What relieved the dizziness? Have you had any discharge from your ears? What color? What consistency? Did it have an odor? Have you experienced a sudden or rapid change in your hearing? What were you doing when it occurred? Does it come and go?

Physical Examination

INSPECTION

Observe the older individual in conversation. Does the person lean forward or cup a hand to the ear to hear? Is a loud speaking voice used? Does the person request repetition of what has been said? If hearing loss is identified, speak to the person in a normal tone of voice and speak toward the better ear, if there is one. Assess the ear for size, shape, symmetry, redness, inflammation, swelling, discharge, and lesions.

PALPATION

The surface of the skin of the ear should have a smooth texture. Palpate around the ear and ask the older adult whether any pain or tenderness is present.

Mouth and Throat

History

The first aspect of history taking related to the mouth is to establish whether the older adult has any dental complaints. The following questions can be used to elicit a history.

Do you have any pain or discomfort? Are any of your teeth especially sensitive to hot or cold temperatures? Have you noticed any swelling in your mouth or throat? Do you have any difficulty chewing or swallowing? How does food taste? Is your mouth dry?

Do your dentures fit properly? Do you have any sores or lesions in your mouth or throat? How often do you brush your teeth, dentures, or tongue? Do you use dental floss? If so, how often? When was your last dental examination? What was the result? Do you clean your dentures at night in a cleaning solution?

Physical Examination

INSPECTION AND PALPATION

Inspection and palpation are used concurrently during the oral cavity examination. Use a gloved hand and a gauze pad to perform this part of the examination. If the older adult wears dentures, remove them before starting the examination. Evaluate the fit of the dentures to the gums or alveolar surfaces and the dentures themselves. Dentures are considered to fit improperly if there is inflammation and ulceration of the palate, mucosa, and alveolar ridges. Examine the dentures for cracks, missing pieces, and rough edges. Dentures should be stable and remain securely fixed during chewing. Underlying tissues should be pink and adhere tightly to the bone. There should not be food, debris, or excessive denture adhesive on the inside of the denture. If the older adult does not have dentures, examine the teeth. Note the number and position of teeth. Are they in good repair, or can you see cavities and broken teeth?

The gums should be pink, moist, and smooth. Inspect for signs of inflammation and lesions. The hard palate should be pale. The soft palate should be pink. Inspect for inflammation, lesions, pallor, and any purulent drainage or a white coating on the tongue. The uvula should be midline and red. It should move up as the older adult says "Ah." Tonsils, if present, should be small, pink, and symmetrical. Check the gag reflex with a tongue blade. The top and bottom of the tongue should be examined. A smooth, painful tongue may indicate vitamin B_{12} deficiency. The tongue and mucous membranes should be pink, moist, and free of swelling and lesions. The tongue should relax on the floor of the mouth. Varicose veins on bottom surfaces of the tongue are common. Ask the older adult to stick out the tongue to examine it. While you hold it out with a piece of gauze, inspect all sides of the tongue and the floor of the mouth. Report any white, scaly patches. The lips should be moist, smooth, and pink. Check the corners of the mouth for cracks. These cracks are a prime spot for *Candida* (yeast) infections.

Neurological System

History

Does the older adult have any problems with headaches? Shaking or trembling? Confusion or memory loss? In assessing the neurological system, the nurse also should ask if the older adult has experienced seizures. Is there an existing seizure disorder? What type of treatment has been received? What were the circumstances occurring before, during, and after the seizure?

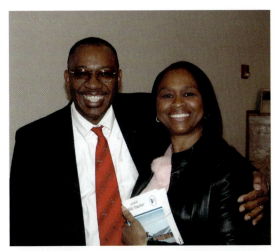

When taking a history on an older adult, it generally is helpful to obtain information from the family as well as the individual being assessed. In many older people, long-term memory may be based on facts that have been altered to "make the story better."

Physical Examination
INSPECTION

Examine the older adult's level of orientation. Is the person alert, lethargic, or nonresponsive? Oriented to place, time, and person? As the older adult answers questions, observe the face for symmetry of movement when smiling, talking, grimacing, or frowning. Evaluate the older adult's appearance throughout the examination. Is the person dressed appropriately? Is the person wearing multiple layers of clothing? If so, are they appropriate for the weather outdoors? Is there body odor? Does the person appear well groomed? Is the older adult's behavior appropriate? Evaluate the strength and symmetry of the older adult's upper and lower extremities. This is commonly done by asking the person to squeeze your hands. Ask the person to walk across the room and observe the gait for symmetry, balance, and coordination during ambulation. Note any weakness.

Peripheral Vascular System
History

Following are key history questions related to peripheral vascular functioning: Do you have diabetes? Do you wear garters or girdles? Do you wear ankle-, knee-, or thigh-high hosiery? When you take off your hosiery, is there an indentation in your leg that does not go away for several minutes? Do your shoes fit tightly? Do you have pain in your calves after walking? Do you ever experience pains, aches, numbness, or tingling in your calves, feet, buttocks, or legs? Are there any activities that you cannot do because of pains and aches in your extremities? What aggravates your pain? What relieves the pain? Does walking or climbing stairs cause pain? Do you ever notice change in the color of your extremities—red, blue, or pale? Have you noticed any hair loss over any part of your legs? Does your family have a history of problems with the legs? Do you sit for long periods with your legs crossed? Do you experience swelling of your legs at the end of the day? Does swelling return to normal in the morning?

Physical Examination

The physical examination of the peripheral vascular system includes inspection, palpation, and auscultation. The nurse should always compare one side of the body with the other when using these assessment methods.

INSPECTION

Skin color should be evaluated with the older adult lying down. Inspect the upper and lower extremities. Venous insufficiency is indicated if the legs are cyanotic when they are dependent (hanging down) or when petechiae or broken pigmentation is present on the skin over the legs. Chronic venous insufficiency is common in elderly people. If the legs become pale when they are elevated and turn dark red when they dangle, arterial insufficiency is indicated. The signs of chronic venous insufficiency are distended tortuous veins, hair loss, hyperpigmentation, cool or normal skin temperature, and pretibial edema or pedal edema that is worse during the day but improves at night when the older adult lies down to sleep. The signs of chronic arterial insufficiency include thin, shiny, atrophic skin; hair loss over feet and toes; thick and rigid toenails; and cool skin.

Edema of the legs and feet should be noted. The nurse may choose to record the width of the edematous area by using a measuring tape. When measuring the legs to assess edema, be sure to measure at the same place on each leg. If you wish to monitor changes in edema, lightly mark the location on the leg you are measuring with a felt-tipped marker and measure in the same place each day. Stasis ulcers are rare with varicose veins, but they commonly occur with deep vein insufficiency. Venous stasis ulcers are located on the sides of the ankles. Arterial ulcers may involve toes or places where the skin has been bumped or bruised.

PALPATION

Check the skin temperature of the older adult's arms and legs by using the back of your hand. Increased temperature can be caused by a localized response to inflammation. Cool temperature indicates decreased blood flow. Peripheral pulses should be evaluated by using the pads of the index and middle fingers. The pulse is evaluated for rate, rhythm, amplitude, and symmetry. Normal vessels feel smooth and resilient. In most older adults, increased resistance to compression may be palpated because of rigid and tortuous artery walls. The nurse should practice palpating the pulses of a young person and an older person to be able to differentiate the changes associated with aging. Pulses should be evaluated one at a time (carotid, brachial, radial, femoral, popliteal, and dorsalis pedis). They should be regular, strong, and equal bilaterally. Lack of symmetry between extremities indicates possible impaired circulation. If you have difficulty finding a pulse, feel throughout the area where it is expected to be and vary the pressure of your finger. Be sure you are not feeling your own pulse. The rate you feel should be different from your own heart rate. If you had difficulty finding a pulse, you can mark its location with a felt-tipped pen after it is found.

Cardiac System

History

Older adults should be asked questions for assessment of cardiac disease risk factors, including smoking and exercise: Do you have any problems with dyspnea (shortness of breath)? Does your shortness of breath increase with activity (i.e., dyspnea on exertion)? Do you have chest pain? When does it occur? What are you doing when it occurs? Is the chest pain relieved by rest?

Physical Examination

INSPECTION

A cardiac physical examination procedure is the same for older and younger persons. The older adult should be evaluated while lying down, sitting up, and standing. Observe the neck and chest to detect any visible pulsations, lifts, or heaves. The heartbeat is usually not visible, but it may be if the individual is emaciated. It is abnormal to observe the heart beating on the chest wall of an older adult who is obese or of normal weight. Note any cough, shortness of breath, venous or abdominal distention, or cyanosis of mucous membranes and nailbeds. The legs, ankles, and feet should be observed for edema.

PALPATION

Feel the front of the chest over the heart for any thrills, heaves, or lifts. A thrill is a palpable vibration. A lift or heave is a pulsation that is more forceful than anticipated. There should be minimal changes in the pulse when the older adult changes positions between lying, sitting, and standing. Press on the nailbeds and observe for the return of a pink color; this is called capillary refill and should occur quickly. It is abnormal for a refill to take longer than 2 seconds. Skin temperature should be palpated for unusual coolness or heat. The blood pressure should be checked using the orthostatic technique that you learned in Chapter 15. Orthostatic hypotension is a common problem with older adults.

AUSCULTATION

Older adults have more rapid and less distinct heartbeats. Many older persons live normal, everyday lives with chronic atrial fibrillation. Any irregularity of the heartbeat noted while listening to the heart should be reported to the RN or physician. Infrequent extra beats (ectopic) are fairly common. Another common abnormal finding is a heart murmur. A heart murmur is caused by thickened and rigid heart valves and decreased strength of myocardial contractions. It sounds like a hum or click and results from turbulent or backward flow of blood through the heart. If detected, it should be reported.

Respiratory System

History

Questions that are used to assess an older adult's respiratory status include the following: Do you have any difficulty breathing? Do you get short of breath with exercise or exertion? Do you have a cough? Is your cough dry or productive? What color and consistency is the mucus that you cough up? Is there any blood in the mucus?

Dyspnea or difficulty breathing is not a part of normal aging. It is often related to HF, pneumonia, anemia, and other lung diseases. It is present in only one-half of older persons with pneumonia. The first signs of pneumonia often include a nonspecific deterioration in health, such as slight cough, altered mental status, and tachycardia.

Ask the older adult if there is any history of lung disease. If so, what effect does it have on activities of daily living (ADLs)? Is oxygen used? Ask questions to determine if the older adult is

FOCUSED LEARNING CHART

Assessment of Cardiac Risk Factors

Risk	Management
Advancing age	Understand medications
Being male	Smoking cessation
Women after menopause	Appropriate exercise plan
Obesity	Manage obesity
Elevated blood glucose levels (diabetes mellitus)	Decreased sodium intake
Elevated blood lipids (hyperlipidemia)	Low-fat diet
Elevated blood pressure (hypertension)	No constricting clothing
Sedentary lifestyle	
Smoking	

using oxygen safely in the home. Other questions that can be used to elicit history of lung disease are as follows: Do you live in an area that has air pollution? Have you or any member of your family ever had tuberculosis? What is the date of your last chest x-ray study? Have you had the pneumonia vaccine (Pneumovax)? If so, when did you receive it? Have you had an influenza shot this year? Have you received one within the last year? Have you had a tuberculosis skin test? When?

Physical Examination
INSPECTION

In the older adult population, barrel chest, slight use of intercostal muscles, and slightly prolonged respirations may occur normally. If these signs and symptoms occur suddenly, they should be considered abnormal. The respiratory rate for normal older adults is 12 to 24 respirations per minute. A rate of 24 or greater is considered tachypnea. Observe for the use of accessory muscles and nasal flaring. A rate of less than 12 respirations per minute is considered bradypnea. Overt signs of the lower oxygen levels resulting from bradypnea include decreased consciousness, confusion, and lethargy. The character of respirations also should be evaluated. A normal respiratory rate is even and unlabored. The older adult's skin, lips, and nail color should be inspected for cyanosis and pallor. Posture while sitting and standing should be noted. Posture affects the ability to breathe.

PALPATION

The anterior and posterior chest should be palpated for masses and tenderness of the ribs. The tracheal area should be palpated for any deviation.

AUSCULTATION

An older adult can become dizzy from hyperventilation if asked to take deep breaths for a long time. Allow the person periods of normal breathing between deep breaths. Listen fully to inspiration and expiration. Softer vesicular sounds and diminished breath sounds in the bases of the lungs are normal. Listen for abnormal (adventitious) sounds. These sounds are superimposed on the normal breath sounds. Crackles are often heard when the older adult has HF or pulmonary edema. Crackles result from air passing through moisture and sound like hair being rubbed between the fingers. Scattered crackles in dependent lung segments of some older adults should not be mistaken for bronchitis or HF. If the crackles disappear after coughing, they are not pathological. If they are present after coughing, pathology may be present. Wheezes are a whistling noise caused by air passing through a narrowed airway. This happens with bronchospasm and swelling of the bronchioles. It is commonly heard in chronic obstructive pulmonary disease and in older adults with asthma. Pleural friction rub is due to inflammation between the membranes lining the chest cavity. It sounds like leather rubbing together.

Gastrointestinal System

History

In taking a gastrointestinal (GI) history, the nurse needs to focus on nutritional status, bowel habits, and medications. Ask the older adult or family member to give a 24-hour recall of the older person's diet. Evaluate the reported intake for nutritional balance. Is it full of fatty foods? Is it low in fiber? Does it have a high starch content? Calculate the amount of fluids the older adult drinks in a 24-hour period. The older adult needs 2,000 to 3,000 mL of fluids per day. Continue with more health history questions: How do you tolerate eating and drinking? Do you have problems with swallowing? Do you have the sensation that food is stuck in your throat? What is your bowel routine? Do you have abdominal pain? Do you use laxatives? Have you used laxatives in the past? How long did you use them? What kind of laxatives? How often were they used? Have you experienced any recent injury or infection?

Physical Examination
INSPECTION

Inspect the skin of the abdomen and note any lesions caused by rubbing of belts or corsets over the years. Check for fungal rashes in skin folds of adults who are obese or incapacitated. Does the abdomen look rigid? If so, refer the individual to the RN or physician. Abdominal rigidity can indicate bowel obstruction.

FOCUSED LEARNING CHART

Adventitious (abnormal) breath sounds

	Crackles	Wheezes	Plural friction rub
Pathology:	HF or pulmonary edema	COPD Asthma	Inflammation between membranes lining chest cavity
Caused by:	Air passing through moisture	Air passing through narrowed airway	Inflammation
Sounds like:	Hair being rubbed through fingers	Whistling noise	Leather rubbing together
Report to RN if:	Coughing does not relieve crackles	Present	Present (is very painful)

AUSCULTATION

Listen to the abdomen with your stethoscope. Mentally divide the abdomen into quadrants that intersect through the umbilicus. Auscultate each quadrant until you hear bowel sounds, or if there are no bowel sounds, listen continuously for 5 minutes. Bowel sounds are decreased in the older adult because of decreased gastric motility that accompanies normal aging. While the history was being taken, did the older adult complain of pain in the abdomen? Ask the older adult to point to the area of pain. Right lower quadrant pain may indicate appendicitis. Left lower quadrant pain may indicate diverticulitis. Tenderness at the base of the xiphoid process may indicate stomach pain, hiatal hernia, or referred pain from the aorta. Palpation provides further information.

PALPATION

Relaxation of the abdominal muscles enhances palpation. If the older adult is obese, palpation may be difficult. If you palpate a mass in the abdomen, it could indicate diverticulitis, fecal impaction, mesenteric thrombosis, or cancer.

Integumentary System

History

History taking is the most important aspect of the skin assessment. The most common skin complaints are pain, pruritus (itching), paresthesia (numbness), and dermatitis. The nurse needs to find out as much as possible about any skin problem mentioned. Questions to ask include the following: Do you have any skin problems? What kind? How were they treated? Are you allergic to any drugs or environmental allergens? What are they? How long have you had the allergy? Have you been exposed to an infectious disease? What is your history of sun exposure? What is your skin care regimen? Evaluate all medications that the older adult is taking. Anything that can cause an allergic reaction, no matter how long the product has been used, should be discussed. Common allergens are soaps and topical medications.

Physical Examination

INSPECTION

Look at the older person's skin in a well-lit room. Skin folds should be evaluated for dampness, irritation, and fissures. Common skin folds are under the breasts and inguinal areas. Observe the scalp, behind the ears, the fingernails and toenails, genitalia, buttocks, and face. How clean is the older adult's skin? Is there an odor present? Assess skin color for variations that are not uniform and have changed since the previous examination. Note any pallor, jaundice, cyanosis, erythema, petechiae, and ecchymosis. Older adults with deeply pigmented skin tones should be evaluated for changes in color such as duskiness, graying, and blackish areas. Jaundice in a person of color should be evaluated on the hard palate and the soles of the hands and feet. Check pressure points over bony prominences, especially on individuals who are debilitated or immobilized. Pay particular attention to the areas over the scapulae, back of the head, earlobes, hips, heels, coccyx, and elbows.

The Braden scale is a common assessment tool used to evaluate the risk of pressure ulcer formation. This is a helpful assessment to complete on every older individual who enters a health-care setting. It provides baseline information on the older person's risk for pressure ulcer formation. Individuals at high risk should have preventive measures implemented from the start. The Braden scale (Fig. 16.2) also can be used for periodic assessment of the older person. If the older adult's risk for pressure ulcer development increases over time, new and more aggressive interventions for prevention should be implemented.

Evaluate the skin for lesions. Some lesions are normal. Table 16.1 describes normal and abnormal skin lesions. Note the consistency of the lesions. If there has been a change in color, consistency, edges, or growth, the lesion may have changed from normal to abnormal.

PALPATION

Check the skin for turgor. Gently pinch the skin on the forehead or anterior chest to see how quickly it returns to place. Poor turgor may be a normal aging change. It also could indicate dehydration or malnutrition or both. Palpate skin texture and note the temperature. Notice if the skin has become rough, dry, or coarse. Normally, the skin is smooth with some dryness. Check the skin temperature with the back of your hand. During this evaluation, note the symmetry of temperature and texture.

PATIENT EDUCATION

Patients should be taught to observe for any new skin lesions on their bodies or changes in existing lesions. This information should be shared with either their nurse or primary care physician.

Braden Scale
FOR PREDICTING PRESSURE SORE RISK

Patient's Name _____ Evaluator's Name _____ Date of Assessment

	1	2	3	4			
SENSORY PERCEPTION Ability to respond meaningfully to pressure-related discomfort	**1. Completely Limited:** Unresponsive to painful stimuli (does not moan, flinch, or grasp), due to diminished level of consciousness or sedation. OR Limited ability to feel pain over most of body surface.	**2. Very Limited:** Responds only to painful stimuli. Cannot communicate discomfort except by moaning or restlessness. OR Has a sensory impairment which limits the ability to feel pain or discomfort over ½ of body.	**3. Slightly Limited:** Responds to verbal commands, but cannot always communicate discomfort or need to be turned. OR Has some sensory impairment that limits ability to feel pain or discomfort in 1 or 2 extremities.	**4. No Impairment:** Responds to verbal commands. Has no sensory deficit that would limit ability to feel or voice pain or discomfort.			
MOISTURE Degree to which skin is exposed to moisture	**1. Constantly Moist:** Skin is kept moist almost constantly by perspiration, urine, and so on. Dampness is detected every time patient is moved or turned.	**2. Very Moist:** Skin is often but not always moist. Linen must be changed at least once a shift.	**3. Occasionally Moist:** Skin is occasionally moist, requiring an extra linen change approximately once a day.	**4. Rarely Moist:** Skin is usually dry, linen requires changing only at routine intervals.			
ACTIVITY Degree of physical activity	**1. Bedfast:** Confined to bed.	**2. Chairfast:** Ability to walk severely limited or nonexistent. Cannot bear own weight and/or must be assisted into chair or wheelchair.	**3. Walks Occasionally:** Walks occasionally during day, but for very short distances, with or without assistance. Spends majority of each shift in bed or chair.	**4. Walks Frequently:** Walks outside the room at least twice a day and inside room at least once every 2 hours during walking hours.			

FIGURE 16.2 Braden scale for predicting pressure sore risk. (From Braden, B. J. & Bergstrom, N. [1992]. Pressure reduction. In G. Bulechek & J. McCloskey [eds.], *Nursing Interventions* [2nd ed., p. 63]. Philadelphia, PA: W. B. Saunders, with permission.)

	1	2	3	4
MOBILITY Ability to change and control body position	**1. Completely Immobile:** Does not make even slight changes in body or extremity position without assistance.	**2. Very Limited:** Makes occasional slight changes in body or extremity position but unable to make frequent or significant changes independently.	**3. Slightly Limited:** Makes frequent though slight changes in body or extremity position independently.	**4. No Limitations:** Makes major and frequent changes in position without assistance.
NUTRITION *Usual* food intake pattern	**1. Very Poor:** Never eats a complete meal. Rarely eats more than ½ of any food offered. Eats 2 servings or less of protein (meat or dairy products) per day. Takes fluids poorly. Does not take a liquid dietary supplement. OR Is NPO and/or maintained on clear liquids or IVs for more than 5 days.	**2. Probably Inadequate:** Rarely eats a complete meal and generally eats only about ½ of any food offered. Protein intake includes only 3 servings of meat or dairy products per day. Occasionally will tkae a dietary supplement. OR Receives less than optimum amount of liquid diet or tube feeding.	**3. Adequate:** Eats over ½ of most meals. Eats a total of 4 servings of protein (meat, dairy products) each day. Occasionally will refuse a meal, but will usually take a supplement if offered. OR Is on tube feeding or TPN regimen, which probably meets most of nutritional needs.	**4. Excellent:** Eats most of every meal. Never refuses a meal. Usually eats a total of 4 or more servings of meat and dairy products. Occasionally eats between meals. Does not require supplementation.
FRICTION AND SHEAR	**1. Problem:** Requires moderate to maximum assistance in moving. Complete lifting without sliding against sheets is impossible. Frequently slides down in bed or chair, requiring frequent repositioning with maximum assistance. Spasticity, contractures, or agitation leads to almost constant friction.	**2. Potential Problem:** Moves feebly or requires minimum assistance. During a move, skin probably slides to some extent against sheets, chair, restraints, or other devices. Maintains relatively good position in chair or bed most of the time but occasionally slides down.	**3. No Apparent Problem:** Moves in bed and in chair independently and has sufficient muscle strength to lift up completely during move. Maintains good position in bed or chair at all times.	

FIGURE 16.2 (Continued)

TABLE 16.1   NORMAL AND ABNORMAL SKIN LESIONS

NORMAL SKIN LESIONS	
Lesion	**Description**
Seborrheic keratosis	Raised; vary in size; tan to black; appear warty or greasy; frequently appear on trunk
Senile purpura	Vivid purple patch; well demarcated; eventually fades
Senile lentigines	Brown; irregularly shaped patches; age or liver spots; occur most frequently on back of hands, forearms, and face
Cherry angioma	Bright; ruby red elevated area; frequently found on trunk; common; insignificant; increase in size and number with age
Sebaceous hyperplasia	Yellowish, flat, solid elevations with central depression; looks like a small doughnut; common on face, forehead, and nose; more common in men
ABNORMAL SKIN LESIONS	
Senile or actinic keratosis	Precancerous; superficial patch covered by a persistent scale; common on sun-exposed areas
Squamous cell carcinoma	Firm, red-brown nodule; may arise from senile keratosis; common on sun-exposed areas and in fair-skinned individuals
Basal cell epithelioma	Starts as pearly colored solid elevation on face or ear; ulcerates leaving a crater with an elevated border and depressed center
Malignant melanoma	Brown-black lesion; may have flecks of red, white, or blue irregular border, irregular surface; arise from moles or appear as new pigmented, irregular lesion
Lentigo maligna melanoma	Less aggressive form of malignant melanoma specific to elderly adults; arise from lentigines that enlarge laterally

From McGovern, M., & Kuhn, J. K. (1992). Skin assessment of the elderly client. *Journal of Gerontological Nursing,* 18(8), 40–41, with permission.

Musculoskeletal System

History

The most common musculoskeletal complaints are related to the joints. Complaints include pain, stiffness, redness, limitation in movement, and joint deformity. If the older person complains of pain, determine where the pain originates and where it radiates. The most common soft tissue problem is pain in and around the shoulder joint. If the older adult has a sudden onset of low back pain, report it to the RN or physician. This pain could indicate a compression fracture of the spine.

Physical Examination

INSPECTION

If possible, observe the older adult while the person is participating in ADLs and instrumental activities of daily living (IADLs). (See Functional

Assessment section in this chapter.) Doing so allows the nurse to assess ROM, muscle mass, and level of independence in self-care. Some decline in ROM is expected. There is a general rigidity of the lower extremities.

Observe the older adult's ability to walk. Have the person ambulate a specified distance to determine endurance. It is normal for older men to have a slight anterior-flexion of the upper body while the arms and knees are slightly flexed. Note the kind of shoes worn by the older adult. Intervention is necessary if the person has an unstable gait yet wears high-heeled shoes. Have the older adult transfer in and out of the bed and chair, on and off the commode, and from the commode to the bathtub. Observe for symmetry of movement. Determine if the person needs assistance. Some older people may be independently mobile with the use of a wheelchair. Assess their ability to maneuver the wheelchair in the environment. Check the older adult's feet for lesions and deformity because these can interfere with gait and mobility. As with physical examination of all of the systems, report all abnormal findings of the musculoskeletal system to the RN or physician.

Reproductive System

History: Female Patient

Although questions about sexual functioning and the reproductive organs may be uncomfortable for the nurse and the older adult, it is important to ask them. Ask the older woman if she knows about breast self-examination (Fig. 16.3). If not, education on the subject is needed. Do not be surprised

BREAST SELF-EXAMINATION

1 OBSERVE FOR SYMMETRY, LUMPS, DIMPLING, NIPPLE RETRACTION, OR FAILURE OF NIPPLE ERECTION

4 GENTLY SQUEEZE NIPPLE AND OBSERVE FOR SECRETION AND NIPPLE ERECTION AFTER EACH NIPPLE IS GENTLY STIMULATED

5 WHILE LEANING FORWARD, OBSERVE BREASTS AS THEY ARE REFLECTED IN MIRROR TO DETECT IRREGULARITY, RETRACTED AREAS AND NIPPLE RETRACTION ESPECIALLY ON ONE SIDE ONLY

3 FEEL FOR NODES, IRREGULARITY, AND TENDERNESS BOTH IN BREASTS AND AXILLARY AREAS

FIGURE 16.3 Breast self-examination. (From Venes, D. [ed.]. [2009]. *Taber's Cyclopedic Medical Dictionary* [21st ed., p. 310]. Philadelphia, PA: F. A. Davis, with permission.)

if the older woman is familiar with breast self-examination and does it regularly. Many older women are more compliant than younger women in performing this examination. Inquire about symptoms of breast cancer. Does the person have any pain, nipple discharge, lumps, skin discoloration, or change in breast shape? Is there any family history of breast cancer or other cancerous conditions? Determine if the older woman has used estrogen or other medications that affect the breasts, such as digitalis, thyroid drugs, and antihypertensives. Has the older woman ever had an abnormal Papanicolaou (Pap) smear? If so, was she treated? Did she receive any medications for menopausal symptoms? Has there been any unusual bleeding since menopause?

Some common physical complaints that older women experience with intercourse include vaginal dryness, pain, and limited mobility from arthritis. These complaints should be addressed, and ways to deal with them should be suggested. Lubricants and using different positions during intercourse, such as the side-lying position, can help the older woman manage these concerns. Note the discussion in Chapter 14 on sexually transmitted diseases.

History: Male Patient

The older man should be evaluated for symptoms of benign prostatic hyperplasia. Is there any change in the urinary stream? Any dribbling of urine? A sense that the bladder is not completely empty after urinating? Is there urinary frequency? Urgency? Burning during urination? Does the older man experience nocturia? How often? Review his medications and note whether he takes diuretics or an anticholinergic that might worsen benign prostatic hyperplasia. Does he realize the importance of checking his breasts periodically? Although male breast cancer is rare, it is possible for older men to develop breast cancer.

Physical Examination

INSPECTION

During the examination process, you should inspect the external genitalia on older male and female patients. Assess for skin or mucous membrane lesions, rashes, discoloration, hair loss, inflammation, discharge, asymmetry, and circumcision.

Urinary System

History

In gathering information about the urinary tract, the nurse needs to discover the chief complaint and the nature and extent of the older adult's underlying problem. The most common complaints are urgency to void, leakage when changing position, pain on urination, frequency of urination, voiding small amounts, and incontinence caused by coughing, sneezing, and laughing. The subject of urinary incontinence frequently causes the older adult to feel embarrassed. Incontinence may cause the older person to withdraw from usual social contact for fear of having an accident. It is also a major risk factor for pressure ulcer formation and urinary tract infections. Despite the difficulties and embarrassment that may be associated with discussing incontinence, it is a serious problem that can have multiple untoward effects.

If the older adult reports any complaints related to the urinary tract, determine the person's normal urinary and bowel habits before the symptoms began. Assess the past medical history for childbirths, previous surgeries involving the lower abdomen and pelvic floor, renal disease, and bladder cancer. Evaluate the older adult's medications. Diuretics and antiparkinsonian drugs can affect the urinary system. Periods of prolonged rest or immobility can cause urinary stasis. Urine that is allowed to pool in the bladder creates a favorable environment for the development of infection. To empty the bladder fully, it is important for the older adult to be able to use the sitting-with-legs-dependent position. Full bladder emptying may not be possible on a bedpan. Decreased fluid intake results in low urine volume and infrequent urination. This situation can create pooling of the urine and increase the risk for infection. It also can lead to dehydration, elevated blood glucose levels, and electrolyte imbalance. These conditions may manifest in the older adult through alterations in mental status.

Physical Examination

INSPECTION

Assess urine amount and color for the presence of any sediment.

PALPATION

Palpate the abdomen for distention of the bladder and signs of pelvic discomfort or masses.

 ## FUNCTIONAL ASSESSMENT

For an older adult, a functional assessment is as important as a physical assessment. Very often, the older person demonstrates changes in function as the first or only sign indicating the onset of illness. Although the older person has many chronic illnesses, these typically are not problematic until function is affected.

Functional assessment encompasses a holistic approach to evaluating the older adult that includes physical, cognitive, and social function. Physical function comprises the individual's current health status in addition to how well the person performs ADLs and IADLs. Cognitive function includes the individual's memory, judgment, and thinking abilities. Cognitive function is discussed in Chapters 19 and is not included in this section on functional assessment. Social function involves a psychosocial approach to determine how the individual interacts with the environment and with others.

Functional assessment involves evaluating the older adult to determine what the person can do (strengths) and cannot do (deficits). What the health-care team members see as a deficit may not correlate with what the older adult views as a problem. The older adult's true abilities, as assessed by the nurse, and the older adult's perception of these abilities must be considered.

Functional assessment assists in setting realistic goals. Cure as a goal is inappropriate for an older individual with chronic, irreversible conditions. The goal for such a patient would be to maximize functional strengths and compensate for deficits to achieve and maintain optimal independence in function.

In almost any health-care setting, the nurse is the health-care professional who spends the most time with the older adult. The nurse has many opportunities to observe the client's physical functioning. A decline in functional ability may represent a change in an underlying chronic disease or the onset of a new acute illness. Monitoring functional status helps track improvements and setbacks. It also indicates when additional services are needed. Use of a formal tool to evaluate functional status allows the nurse to validate, monitor, and communicate clearly clinical impressions to other members of the interdisciplinary health-care team.

Activities of Daily Living

The Katz ADL scale is widely used to assess ADLs. It is a well-rounded tool that is appropriate for use in most settings, including home, hospital, and nursing home. ADLs are the activities performed in taking care of oneself. The following areas are considered ADLs: bathing, dressing, toileting, feeding, ambulating or transferring, and continence. Direct observation is the most valid indicator in assessing ADLs. Watch the older adult perform ADLs and check for abnormal body movements. Rate the older adult on each of the ADL items of the Katz scale. Using the scale supplies specific information on how the older adult performs in each of the ADL areas, and the composite score can give you and other members of the interdisciplinary health-care team an overall view of the person's level of ability. The score also gives an objective means to monitor progress over time. Goals in each of the ADL areas can be set on the basis of scores on the scale.

If you were assigned to assess this man on admission to the nursing home where you work, what observations could you make even before talking to him? His left arm is hanging without good positioning or apparent control. Does this man have a muscle or enervation problem in the arm, or has he possibly had a left-sided stroke? He is in a wheelchair. Why?

Think Like a Nurse

You are caring for a patient on home-care services. The family states that the person is losing weight. What assessments can you do to identify the problem?

Instrumental Activities of Daily Living

IADLs include the ability to use the telephone, cook, shop, do laundry, manage finances, take medications, and prepare meals. These activities are needed to support independent living. Lawton's scale for IADLs is used widely (Fig. 16.4).

If possible, observe the older adult while he or she is performing IADLs. Look for abnormal body movements such as tremors or twitching, for lack

---

Instrumental Activities of Daily Living (IADL) Scale

Self-Rated Version Extracted from the Multilevel Assessment Instrument (MAI)

1. Can you use the telephone:
   without help, — 3
   with some help, or — 2
   are you completely unable to use the telephone? — 1

2. Can you get to places out of walking distance:
   without help, — 3
   with some help, or — 2
   are you completely unable to travel unless special arrangements are made? — 1

3. Can you go shopping for groceries:
   without help, — 3
   with some help, or — 2
   are you completely unable to do any shopping? — 1

4. Can you prepare your own meals:
   without help, — 3
   with some help, or — 2
   are you completely unable to prepare any meals? — 1

5. Can you do your own housework:
   without help, — 3
   with some help, or — 2
   are you completely unable to do any housework? — 1

6. Can you do your own handyman work:
   without help, — 3
   with some help, or — 2
   are you completely unable to do any handyman work? — 1

7. Can you do your own laundry:
   without help, — 3
   with some help, or — 2
   are you completely unable to do any laundry at all? — 1

8a. Do you take medicines or use any medications?
   (If yes, answer Question 8b) Yes — 1
   (If no, answer Question 8c) No — 2

8b. Do you take your own medicine:
   without help (in the right doses at the right time), — 3
   with some help (take medicine if someone prepares it for you and/or reminds you to take it), or — 2
   (are you/would you be) completely unable to take your own medicine? — 1

8c. If you had to take medicine, can you do it:
   without help (in the right doses at the right time), — 3
   with some help (take medicine if someone prepares it for you and/or reminds you to take it), or — 2
   (are you/would you be) completely unable to take your own medicine? — 1

9. Can you manage your own money:
   without help, — 3
   with some help, or — 2
   are you completely unable to handle money? — 1

SOURCE: Lawton MP, Brody EM. Assessment of older people: self maintaining and instrumental activities of daily living. *Gerontologist.* 1969;9:179–185. Reprinted with permission.
For additional information on administration and scoring refer to the following references:
1. Lawton MP. Scales to measure competence in everyday activities. *Psychopharm Bull.* 1988;24(4):609–614.
2. Lawton MP, Moss M, Fulcomer M, et al. A research and service-oriented Multilevel Assessment Instrument. *J Gerontol.* 1982;37:91–99.

FIGURE 16.4 Instrumental Activities of Daily Living Scale. (From Lawton, M. P., & Brody, E. M. [1969]. Assessment of older people: Self maintaining and instrumental activities of daily living. *Gerontologist* 9, 179–185. Copyright © The Gerontological Society of America, with permission.)

Evidence-Based Practice

Hoogerduijn, J.G., Schuurmans, M.J, Korevaar, J.C., Buurman, B.M., & de Rooij, S.E. (2010). Identification of older hospitalised patients at risk for functional decline. Journal of Clinical Nursing, 19, 1219-1225.

The researchers' goal was to identify a tool that was sensitive to predict functional decline in older adults. The study population consisted of 177 adults older than age 65 years in an acute care hospital. The Katz functional assessment tool established a functional baseline for each participant. Data collection included administration of three older adult assessment instruments to each participant. The three tools (instruments) used were the Identification of Seniors at Risk (ISAR), the Care Complexity Prediction Instrument (COMPRI), and the Hospital Admission Risk Profile (HARP). All of the participants were assessed again after hospitalization. Researchers defined post-hospitalization functional decline as a drop of at least one point on the Katz functional assessment. To summarize their findings, the authors reported that the ISAR was the tool with the closest assessment that predicted functional decline. The COMPRI was somewhat predictive, but the HARP was not predictive. The authors suggested that continued study of the validity of tools and instruments used to assess older adults is very important to accuracy and application of assessment data.

Questions

1. What functional assessment tools do you use in your care setting or the setting where you have clinical experiences?
2. Is the information gathered used to predict functional decline in your patients?

of balance, or for poor vision. In addition to checking the person's ability to complete the IADL, it is important to assess the older adult with regard to safety. The older person may be able to cook a meal, but if the burner is left on, a serious safety concern exists.

In completing an IADL assessment, the nurse often must rely on reports from the older adult or family members. Keep in mind that individuals tend to overrate their abilities, and family members tend to underrate them.

Tools for assessing ADLs and IADLs are used to measure the older person's ability to do self-care and home-care tasks. They can be used to help identify needed services and to monitor the progress or deterioration of the older individual.

Social Function

Social function is how the older adult interacts with self, the environment, and others. It is the degree to which a person functions as a member of the community. Cultural and socioeconomic background and the older adult's environment define and limit social activities and relationships. Self-concept affects the older adult's ability to perform self-care activities. Psychological interventions may be

necessary to enhance the older person's self-esteem before achieving independent functioning.

 ## DOCUMENTATION OF THE ASSESSMENT DATA

It is challenging to have spent a long time collecting data only to find that when you sit down to document the assessment, words do not come.

Just like in the beginning of the chapter, when practicing was discussed, documentation also requires practice.

Electronic health records are helpful because the programming gives you options for documentation in the form of pop-up cues.

The Resident Assessment Instrument (RAI) discussed in Chapter 4 has very scripted documentation. When assessment data is entered into the RAI form, the program generates a plan of care, goals, and evaluation parameters.

 ## CONCLUSION

This chapter contains a great deal of information about performing a holistic physical assessment and a functional assessment. To be an effective gerontological nurse, you need to be very good at both of these skills. There is a great deal of information in this chapter. The only way you will learn it is to go over it several times, practice asking the questions, and practice the skills. Have the courage to use the skills (even with a cheat sheet) whenever you go to your student clinical assignments. This is not a chapter to read and then move on to the next one. This is the one you need to internalize through rereading and practice. Best wishes!

CASE STUDY SOLUTIONS

In doing a holistic assessment, it is important that you determine the underlying cause of the "little" problems as well as the big ones. The big problem for Miss S. is the management of her HF. According to the report, that is going well. You need to verify that her medical treatment is still managing her symptoms. Heart failure is the priority concern because it is life-threatening and the reason she was admitted to the hospital. How will you assess Miss S related to the HF? Following are some suggestions:

1. Assess for edema by checking her ankles, abdomen, lumbosacral area, and hands for swelling, and listen to her lungs for adventitious breath sounds.

2. Is she able to perform ADLs without dyspnea?

3. Does she understand her medication administration?

Now let's consider her incontinence and lack of cooperation. Some nurses would not be concerned about these items, but because you are committed to holistic nursing care, these concerns are important to you. One idea should come to your mind right away. Assume Miss S. is on furosemide (Lasix) for the HF. Lasix is associated with increased urination. At age 85, this probably is a major inconvenience for this person. Has she cut down on her fluid intake to decrease the stress urination and incontinence, which has resulted in an electrolyte imbalance and confusion? This is what I would investigate as I did my assessment. It will be a very serious problem if it is not resolved before Miss S. goes home.

REVIEW QUESTIONS

1. The following are normal aging changes except:
   1. Presbyopia, presbycusis
   2. Presbyopia, urinary incontinence
   3. Kyphosis, ptosis
   4. Osteoporosis, arteriosclerosis

2. Activities of daily living include:
   1. Shopping
   2. Managing finances
   3. Bathing
   4. Using the telephone

3. A common tool used for evaluating ADLs is:
   1. Lawton's scale
   2. The mini-mental status examination
   3. The Katz scale
   4. 1 and 3

4. A common symptom of myocardial infarction in an older adult is:
   1. Chest pain
   2. Lethargy
   3. Confusion
   4. 2 and 3

5. An important health problem that the nurse should help the older adult prevent is:
   1. Fecal impaction
   2. Dehydration
   3. Malnutrition
   4. All of the above

REFERENCES

Dillon, P.M. (2007). *Nursing health assessment: A critical thinking, case studies approach* (2nd ed.). Philadelphia, PA: F.A. Davis.

Wilkinson, J.M., Treas, L.S., Barnett, K.L., & Smith, M.H. (2016) *Fundamentals of nursing: Theory, concepts, and applications* (3rd ed.). Philadelphia, PA: F.A. Davis.

WEB RESOURCES

Hartford Institute for Geriatric Nurses Assessment Series: http://consultgerirn.org/resources

Common Clinical Problems: Physiological

17

TAMARA DAHLKEMPER

CONCEPTS

Mobility

Safety

Tissue Integrity

LEARNING OUTCOMES

1. Describe how the nurse can assist in maintaining mobility for the older adult at risk for impaired mobility.

2. Define two categories of risk factors for falls in older people.

3. Identify two categories of incontinence.

4. Explain how prompted voiding and habit training schedules can be used by the nurse for prevention or reversal of incontinence.

5. Identify the mechanical and physiological risk factors for pressure ulcers.

6. Discuss the problems pertaining to adequate food intake in older people.

7. Describe two sleep disorders common to older adults.

8. Define iatrogenesis, and list common iatrogenic problems experienced by older persons.

CASE STUDY

Mrs. S. is an 84-year-old widow who was admitted to the hospital after a right-hemisphere cerebrovascular accident (CVA). Her medical history includes hypertension, atrial fibrillation, and bilateral total hip replacements because of degenerative joint disease. Before the CVA and this hospitalization, she was living in her own apartment, where she was social and able to meet her own needs except for shopping and heavy housecleaning. Her family did those things for her. When admitted to the hospital, she was found to have left-sided weakness and some speech problems, although she could be understood.

The family is planning to admit her to the nursing home; they do not know if she will be able to return to her apartment, but they are hopeful that she will be able to go to an assisted-living apartment. The report given to the nursing home from the hospital includes the following facts:

- During her hospitalization, she became incontinent. A Foley catheter was placed to control the urinary incontinence, but she subsequently developed a urinary tract infection, so the catheter was removed.

- She developed aspiration pneumonia, which the physician assumed was due to aspirating food because of a swallowing deficit from her stroke. Her diet was changed to puree, and she has had no further episodes of aspiration, although she is taking only about 30% of her diet.

- She has started physical therapy and has progressed from the parallel bars to short distances with a walker. She does not own a walker, so she has not walked on the unit; she has only walked in the therapy department.

- Mrs. S. has not spoken much during her hospitalization, although she follows simple directions. The nurse thinks that she "might be a little confused at times."

- The family is very concerned that if she falls, she may damage the hip replacements, and they have requested that she be restrained.

Discussion

Examine the list of facts in the case study for iatrogenic problems. How would you prevent such problems? How would you deal with them?

 ## INTRODUCTION

With aging, every body system undergoes some changes. These changes, although they do not result in illness or disease, cause health problems that are more prevalent in older people. As you learned in Chapter 15, most people who are older than 65 years of age have multiple chronic diseases. As a result of normal aging changes combined with underlying chronic diseases, the older person has less physical reserve than a younger person has to respond to the increased demand of an illness. With diminished physical reserve, the older adult is less capable of adapting to physical stressors and is at increased risk for clinical problems such as immobility, falls, incontinence, pressure ulcers, and alterations in nutrition and sleep. This chapter reviews the clinical problems that are common to older adults. In addition, effective management approaches, based on nursing diagnoses, are discussed.

 ## ALTERATION IN MOBILITY

The process of aging, combined with the presence of chronic illness, places the older adult at risk for developing an alteration in mobility status. Immobility is a major medical disability for elderly adults and one that is frequently overlooked by health-care providers. Immobility often leads to numerous complications for older people in long-term care facilities, people in the hospital, and people in the community. Nursing care is essential to maintaining and improving an older adult's ability to be mobile.

Musculoskeletal System

Normal aging changes that occur in the musculoskeletal system increase the risk of developing problems related to mobility. The bones of an older person are less dense and more brittle owing to changes in the formation of bone at the cellular level. As a result, older adults are likely to develop osteoporosis and subsequently be at risk for bone fractures.

With a fracture, mobility is restricted still further. Mechanical stresses, such as walking and standing, tend to stimulate the process of bone formation. When the body is immobilized, there is bone dissolution. This process is called *disuse osteoporosis*, and it makes the bones of the older person still more brittle.

Generalized muscle weakness is also a normal aging process. There is a noticeable decrease in muscle strength with aging. The antigravity muscles are most affected by this change so that standing up can be a difficult movement. In time, if muscles are not used, walking, balancing, and turning become severely impaired. At complete rest, muscle strength can decline at a rate of 20% to 30% in a 7- to 9-day period (Strax et al., 2004). *The loss of muscle mass is not only a symptom of generalized deterioration, but it is also a factor in the risk of falling.*

The mobility of the joints is affected by the length and composition of the muscle fibers. When there is immobility, the muscles that bridge the

joint shorten. With decreased muscle length and thickening of the joint cartilage (which is the connective tissue that surrounds the movable surfaces of the joint), the joints become stiff, which seriously impacts the ability of the person to move.

Osteoarthritis, or degenerative joint disease, occurs in 33.6% of people age 65 years and older (CDC, n.d.). It is marked by deterioration of the cartilage and formulation of new bone at the joint surfaces. With aging, the cartilage is less elastic, thicker, and more easily stretched. As a result, the joint is stiff, and there is decreased range of motion

Evidence-Based Practice

Park, J., & McCaffrey, R. (2012). Chair yoga: Benefits for community dwelling older adults with osteoarthritis. Journal of Gerontological Nursing, 38(5), 12-25.

Yoga is known as an effective treatment for osteoarthritis. However, traditional yoga may be difficult for individuals with decreased balance or the concern of falling. This study looked at the possible effects of chair yoga on pain and stiffness, physical function, and depressive symptoms for older adults with osteoarthritis. The study sample included seven older adults with the average age range of 71 to 81 years who had a diagnosis of osteoarthritis. These participants attended an 8-week chair yoga class with 45-minute biweekly sessions. The results showed a statistically significant improvement in stiffness and physical function. Although there was some improvement in pain symptoms, the changes were not statistically significant. These results were the same for depressive symptoms. Although the sample size was small, the study does support chair yoga as beneficial for improving stiffness and physical function for older adults with osteoarthritis. The authors of the study suggest incorporating yoga as a complementary alternative medicine treatment for providing holistic care to older adults.

Question

Although this study focused on community-dwelling older adults, what is the feasibility of using chair yoga as a form of exercise in an assisted living or long-term care facility?

Priority Setting

The priority for this chapter is easy to identify. After you understand the content of this chapter, you need to assist every older adult to whom you give care to achieve his or her maximum physical ability. Keep that thought in mind and do not stray from it. By doing so, you will enhance the lives of all of the older people in your care.

(ROM) of the joint. Over time, an older adult can lose the ability to mobilize efficiently as a result of stiffness in the joints. As joints are immobilized, contractures (a permanent contraction of the muscles that bridge the joint) can develop and limit mobilization further.

Cardiovascular System

Many of the changes in the cardiovascular system that accompany aging are closely related to inactivity. Similarly, these aging changes can be exacerbated, or become more severe, when there are prolonged periods of immobility.

Oxygen consumption and cardiac output are known to decrease with aging and may vary among older adults. This change is evident from the fact that the pulse rate of an older person does not increase in response to exercise as efficiently as in younger people. After physical exertion, the pulse takes longer to return to a normal level. The inefficient cardiac response to activity causes activity intolerance, but most older adults learn to adjust to the changes.

Respiratory System

As is true of all of the body systems, aging changes to the respiratory system put the older person at risk for complications when immobility is present. Normal anatomical changes in the aging body compromise lung function. Increased rigidity of the rib cage, kyphosis, and osteoporosis reduce the compliance of the chest wall, making it more difficult to inflate the lungs fully. The reduced compliance of the chest wall makes it more challenging for the older adult to maintain activity, and it increases the potential for complications caused by immobility. The lungs of most older adults have diminished vital capacity (the amount of air that can be expelled from the lungs after inspiration). Other changes include less efficient gas exchange by the alveoli and less stretchability of the lung tissue. The result is impaired ventilation and decreased blood supply to the lungs. Such changes not only may hinder the older person's ability to move, but, more importantly, they also place the older person at increased risk for developing atelectasis and pneumonia when immobilized.

Response to Illness

Chronic health problems may cause older people to restrict their movement. Poor eyesight may cause someone of any age to avoid activity because of fear of falling over an obstacle. Pain in

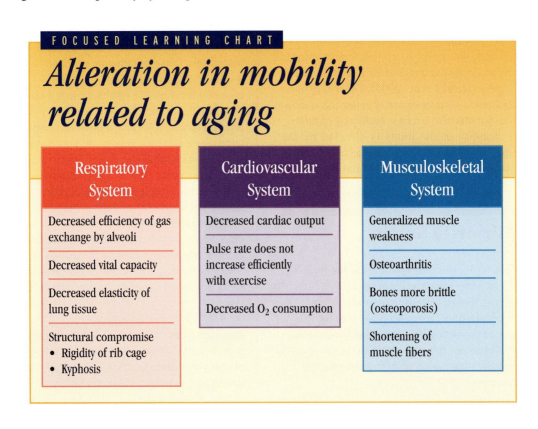

FOCUSED LEARNING CHART

Alteration in mobility related to aging

Respiratory System	Cardiovascular System	Musculoskeletal System
Decreased efficiency of gas exchange by alveoli	Decreased cardiac output	Generalized muscle weakness
Decreased vital capacity	Pulse rate does not increase efficiently with exercise	Osteoarthritis
Decreased elasticity of lung tissue	Decreased O_2 consumption	Bones more brittle (osteoporosis)
Structural compromise • Rigidity of rib cage • Kyphosis		Shortening of muscle fibers

the joints owing to arthritis or pain in the lower extremities owing to impaired circulation generally limits ambulation and causes older adults to become sedentary. Shortness of breath or angina secondary to chronic cardiovascular disease also may cause the individual to avoid activity.

Acute health problems can lead to immobility. The onset of an acute illness, whether or not it requires hospitalization, may lead to confinement in bed. Often, well-meaning family members and health-care providers encourage immobility. Bedrest often is ordered during hospitalization for an acute illness. In contrast to a younger person, an older adult who is on bedrest deteriorates rapidly and may develop irreversible complications. Although rest can promote healing, immobility promotes deterioration. Prolonged immobility is detrimental to the physical and mental health of a person of any age. When immobilized, the older person can develop complications such as contractures, pneumonia, thrombophlebitis, pressure ulcers, incontinence, constipation, dehydration, loss of appetite, and psychological problems related to sensory deprivation and depression. Although Mrs. S. had a stroke, it is important to keep her mobile to prevent further complications.

 ## NURSING IMPLICATIONS

Nurses as well as the older people to whom they give care need to be aware that promoting physical activity not only prevents complications, but also slows the rate of the aging process. In the hospital setting, the time for enforced bedrest needs to be limited as much as possible. As soon as it is medically safe to do so, the nurse needs to ensure that the patient is up and out of bed. If orders for bedrest are in effect, it is the nurse's responsibility to inquire whether such orders can be changed. Even transferring the person from a supine to a sitting position has beneficial effects. While on bedrest, older adults can be taught isometric and active ROM exercises. If the person is incapable of performing these exercises independently, the nurse must assist the patient in meeting this need through passive ROM exercises.

As soon as it is medically indicated, the older patient should be ambulated with assistance. This intervention is as important to the patient's health as receiving the proper medication or a dressing change. Nursing staff should support physical therapy services by ensuring that appropriate sturdy footwear, eyeglasses, and any assistive devices such as canes or walkers are available. Because of reimbursement issues, hospital stays are becoming shorter. As soon as the person is physiologically able, attempts to restore functional ability should begin.

As in the hospital setting, promoting functional mobility is central to the care of the older person at home or in a nursing home. The nursing home environment offers different possibilities for fostering mobility. In contrast to the hospital setting, where the presence of an acute state may impede the nurse's attempts to restore function, the nursing home environment allows the nurse to monitor and promote mobility over an extended period. All residents should be considered for assisted walking unless the underlying chronic illness absolutely precludes such an activity. An older person who does not walk deteriorates even further and eventually loses all ability to walk. Family members and other caregivers for the older adult who lives at home need to be taught the importance of mobility.

Critically Examine the Following

Although immobility is a prevalent health problem, it often is not addressed in the care of the older adult. Identifying immobility as a patient-care problem and intervening to prevent it are central to nursing care of older persons. In addressing mobility needs, the licensed practical nurse (LPN) may prevent complications and shorten the length of time that the older person is in the hospital or rehabilitation facility. Often nurses do not like to disturb patients when they are asleep or have visitors in order to ambulate their patients or have them participate in physical therapy. After reading this chapter, what are your thoughts on the importance of ambulating patients? Will you modify your care related to the importance of mobility for your patients?

POTENTIAL FOR INJURY FROM FALLS

As with alteration in mobility, the potential for falls is closely related to many of the bodily changes that occur with aging. The aging of the musculoskeletal system, which may cause deterioration in mobility, also may increase the older person's risk for falling. One-third of adults who are older than 65 years living in the community fall each year (CDC, 2013). As an individual gets older, the risk of being injured in a fall increases. Falls can lead to mild or severe injuries and are the leading cause of injury death in older adults (National Safety Council, n.d.). The presence of chronic illness accompanying the aging process places all older adults at increased risk for falls.

When an older person falls, the person often becomes fearful of falling again. The older adult may limit activities and become more withdrawn and dependent on others, less mobile, and more at risk for future falls. Caregivers also may place restrictions

This woman has severe physical limitations, but she can get around because she is in the right type of wheelchair for her needs. Her chair does allow her some physical activity.

on the older person's mobility to prevent another fall. At home, the family may admonish the older person to restrict activities so that a fall does not occur again. In the health-care setting, restraints should never be used to prevent the risk of another fall. These options do not promote health for the person.

Factors that predispose to falling are typically divided into two categories: intrinsic and extrinsic. Intrinsic factors include factors inherent to the individual, such as normal aging changes, deficiencies in health status, changes in mental status, immobility, and changes in functional ability. Extrinsic factors refer to environmental conditions, which may include poor lighting, slippery floors, inappropriate or poorly placed furnishings, and inadequate footwear. Falls among older adults often stem from the presence of intrinsic factors that hinder the older person's ability to manage the environment or from environmental conditions (extrinsic factors).

Intrinsic Factors

Age-related changes in posture, balance, gait, and vision predispose an older person to falls. Postural changes are common in older people and are due to a decline in strength and flexibility. In older adults, the head tends to be carried forward, the shoulders may be rounded, and the upper back may have a slight curvature, or kyphosis. Changes in posture and spinal alignment can affect balance and increase the risk of falls.

Posture and Balance

The body's ability to maintain its coordination in a standing position and to react to prevent a fall depends on coordination among the musculoskeletal system, the neurological system, and the visual system. Postural sway occurs when one or more of these three systems are not functioning at an optimal level. Balance problems are associated with postural sway, which can cause falls. Prolonged bedrest, aging changes, medications, and the presence of some chronic diseases are contributors to postural sway.

Postural reflexes play a role in fall prevention by responding to disturbances in balance during standing or walking. With aging, these reflexes become slower; older people are less able to "catch" themselves when they trip or begin to fall. Inactivity may result in a slower response to disturbances in balance.

Gait

With aging, the gross motor movements necessary for maintaining posture and gait, or walking, are altered. The gait of older people often is marked by decreased speed and step height; small, hesitant steps; diminished arm swing; and stooped posture. These changes are almost universal in people older than 80 years. The alterations in speed of movement and maintenance of upright posture adversely affect balance and often lead to a higher incidence of falls by older adults.

Vision

All older people experience changes in vision as part of the normal aging process. With aging, there is a decline in visual acuity, peripheral vision, depth perception, night vision, and tolerance for glare. The loss of vision that accompanies aging is a risk factor for falls because there is a decreased ability to focus on objects at a distance and to judge distances correctly. The result is that an older person may miss a step or trip over a curb. The decline in peripheral vision may cause an individual to trip over objects at the edge of the visual field. Visual deficits can compound a gait disability because vision is necessary to maintain stability while walking.

These normal, age-related changes in posture, gait, and vision, when compounded by the presence of an underlying chronic or acute illness, make falls the leading cause of death from injury in people older than 65 years. Because of the presence of these intrinsic factors, many older people are less capable of coping with the extrinsic factors that may be in the environment.

Extrinsic Factors

Most falls affecting older adults result from environmental factors. Such factors include clutter in the halls, inadequate lighting or glare, and unsafe furniture or equipment in the person's immediate area. Attempting to function in an area that is not designed to accommodate the aging person's needs can diminish the older person's confidence. The individual may begin to fear falling and may eventually become more sedentary. Such behavior leads to an eventual loss of function and an increased need to depend on others for activities of daily living.

Nursing Implications

It is important for nurses to understand the role that intrinsic and extrinsic factors play in falls. The individual's ability to maneuver safely in the immediate environment is best monitored by the nurse. In the home and the institutional setting, most falls occur in the bedroom and the bathroom. It is important to assess the older person walking about the bedroom, getting into and out of bed, and getting on and off the toilet. Only by assessing the individual's ability to manage these daily activities in his or her own environment can you, the nurse, begin to anticipate needs and take steps to prevent a fall before it occurs.

Having assessed the older person's safety, the nurse, along with members of the interdisciplinary health-care team (IDT), should plan care according to the observed need. The nurse may observe that the older person cannot safely get on and off the toilet independently and may advise the individual not to attempt this maneuver unassisted. If the person is not cognitively intact, you may use a toileting schedule to discourage the individual from attempting self-toileting when you, the LPN, or other caregivers are not present to assist. If the

---

BOX 17.1   MEDICAL CONDITIONS ASSOCIATED WITH FALLS

Alcohol use

Arrhythmias

Delirium

Dementia

Depression

Diabetes mellitus

Muscle weakness

Orthostatic hypotension

Osteoarthritis

Parkinson's disease

Polypharmacy: more than four medications

Recent hospitalization

Sleep disorders

Visual and hearing impairment

From Moylan, K.C., & Binder, E.F. (2007) Falls in older adults: risk assessment, management and prevention. *American Journal of Medicine,* 120(6), 493-497.

older person cannot safely ambulate alone, the IDT may decide that physical therapy is indicated or that a program of daily assisted ambulation should be initiated.

Older adults who cannot safely stand or walk unassisted, but who may still attempt these actions, should not be left alone for extended periods. One idea is to bring the person out of the room so that staff members can observe the older adult and in that way keep the individual safe. When someone who is not safe is left alone, mobility alarms would help the staff know when the individual is getting up unassisted. Mobility alarms can be attached to the bed and wheelchair. All members of the IDT need to remember to remove clutter and to maintain clear walking paths for older people, to adjust lighting to provide an optimal environment, and to wipe up spills from the floor as soon as they occur or are noticed.

ALTERATION IN ELIMINATION

Urinary Incontinence

Urinary incontinence, a problem that affects millions of Americans, is defined as an involuntary loss of urine that is sufficient to be a problem. It is a problem most often seen in the elderly in general, with an increase in incidence in nursing home residents (Adelmann, 2004). The cost of caring for individuals with urinary incontinence can be expensive.

Even greater than the economic cost are the psychological and social costs to the individual who is incontinent of urine. Incontinence is seen as a major reason older adults are placed in nursing homes. People who are incontinent may feel embarrassed and socially isolated. They may withdraw from participation in social activities and become depressed. Incontinence is associated with the development of other health problems, such as skin breakdown, and urinary tract infections. Identifying the presence of urinary incontinence should be part of the nursing assessment.

Age-Related Changes Affecting Incontinence

Although incontinence is more prevalent in older people, it is not a normal aspect of aging. There are, however, numerous age-related changes that make the older person susceptible to developing incontinence. In older adults, the bladder capacity diminishes to about half that of younger adults. The diminished ability of the kidneys to concentrate urine makes urinary frequency and nocturia (excessive urination at night) common problems for the older person. In addition, many older people experience sudden and unexpected contractions of the detrusor muscle (the smooth muscle that makes up the outside wall of the bladder), which cause an urgent need to void. Changes in the central and autonomic nervous systems of the older person cause a decreased ability to contract the external sphincter of the bladder, which exacerbates urinary urgency further. Many postmenopausal women experience thinning and weakening of the muscles of the pelvic floor because of estrogen loss. In men, an enlarged prostate, often associated with aging, may lead to urinary retention, irritability of the detrusor muscle, and bladder spasms.

The urinary urgency that many older people experience often leads to incontinence in an institutional setting. When an older adult cannot go to the toilet independently or as often as needed, incontinence is likely to result. This situation is exacerbated further by the immobility that results from being ill or from needing medical interventions, such as intravenous therapy.

Think Like a Nurse

You have been asked to present the educational section at the next staff meeting. Your nurse manager has requested that you develop a teaching plan for your colleagues regarding the importance of mobility in older adults. You have been asked to discuss two former patients who had mobility problems. As part of your lesson plan, write out the reasons an older person should be mobile. Identify ways mobility can be done successfully with the following patients:

1. An 87-year-old man with a fractured hip. He is deconditioned (a word from a previous chapter; do you remember it?), yet insists he can walk "by himself."
2. A 72-year-old woman who is "pleasantly confused" while recovering from a fractured femur. She is experiencing a great deal of pain and thinks you are her son.

Address both patients' ambulation plans.

At age 83, this woman is incontinent. Many older adults admitted to nursing homes are placed there because their family members cannot manage the problems associated with incontinence. This woman wears disposable briefs, and the staff members keep her clean and free of urine odor.

Types of Incontinence

For the nurse to intervene in the management of incontinence, it is important to understand the underlying causes of incontinence.

Acute Incontinence

Acute or transient incontinence is incontinence that occurs because of the presence of a treatable medical condition, and it often resolves when the underlying illness is treated. The following mnemonic highlights the possible causes of acute incontinence:

D: Delirium
R: Restricted mobility
I: Infection, inflammation, impaction
P: Pharmaceutical, polyuria, psychological

Delirium is an acute confusional state that is brought on by an acute illness and that disrupts the physiological homeostasis in the older person. In a delirious state, the person is unaware of the need to void, and the person does not have the capability to get to the toilet.

Restricted mobility, as already discussed, is a common cause of incontinence in elderly people. Individuals who are experiencing pain may be less likely to attend to urinary urges to avoid an increase in pain sensation. Individuals with physical limitations, such as Mrs. S., are also at risk for incontinence.

Urinary tract infections cause frequency, urgency, and painful urination. This condition can lead to increased bladder contractions and incontinence. Many residents in long-term care have bacteria in their urine, a condition that is asymptomatic and does not require treatment. When bacteriuria is accompanied by urinary incontinence, however, the person should be treated, and the effect of the treatment on the incontinence should be noted. Fecal impaction may obstruct the bladder outlet and may cause overflow urinary incontinence.

Many medications can cause urinary incontinence. Following is a list of drug groups that adversely affect an older person's ability to maintain continence:

- Sedatives/hypnotics
- Antipsychotics
- Narcotics
- Anticholinergics
- Diuretics
- Caffeine

Endocrine disorders that lead to hyperglycemia or hypercalcemia may cause urinary incontinence. Psychological causes that have been associated with urinary incontinence include depression and confusional states.

NURSING IMPLICATIONS

Most instances of bladder incontinence are transient and often reversible. In most cases, acute or transient incontinence can be resolved with treatment of the underlying illness or with discontinuation of a causative medication. Incontinence should never be accepted without first

PATIENT EDUCATION

Patients and family members should be taught that infrequent urinary incontinence that is not bothersome can lead to more frequent urinary incontinence and should be evaluated by their primary provider.

ascertaining that the older person has been assessed for underlying conditions and that treatment has been initiated.

Chronic Incontinence

There are four types of persistent or chronic incontinence. Incontinence is considered to be persistent if it continues after reversible causes have been ruled out or treated. In addition, persistent or chronic incontinence usually has a gradual onset, worsens over time, and occurs when there is a failure either to empty or to store urine. The four types of persistent or chronic incontinence are as follows:

Urge incontinence is the most common form of incontinence in older adults. In this type of incontinence, the individual feels the urge to go but does not have enough time to get to the toilet before the urine is released.

Stress incontinence occurs when a small amount of urine is released after there is a sudden increase in intra-abdominal pressure caused by coughing, sneezing, laughing, or lifting. This type of incontinence results when the bladder outlet sphincter is incompetent or weak. Stress incontinence is more common in women and is often a result of poor pelvic muscle tone and a shorter urethra.

Overflow incontinence is caused by impaired bladder emptying and overdistention of the bladder. When the bladder is not emptied sufficiently, the resident experiences frequent dribbling of urine.

Functional incontinence results when the individual is unable or unwilling to attend to toileting needs. In this situation, the bladder and urethra function normally, but cognitive, physical, psychological, or environmental impairments make it difficult for the older person to get to the toilet. Inaccessible toilets, unavailable caregivers, depression, and inability to find the toilet all are possible causes of functional incontinence. Mrs. S. is experiencing this type of incontinence and will need to be assisted to the toilet on a regular schedule.

NURSING IMPLICATIONS

Treatment of urinary incontinence is based on the underlying cause. Medication intervention may be used to treat infection or stop abnormal bladder muscle contractions and tighten sphincter muscles. Surgical intervention is used to correct anatomical anomalies and remove obstructions. Behavioral interventions require that the health-care professional provide education and positive reinforcement to the older adult and family members. Behavioral interventions sometimes may be used in combination with medical or surgical interventions.

BEHAVIORAL INTERVENTIONS

Behavioral interventions, which are most often provided by nursing personnel, include the following:

- Bladder training (retraining)
- Habit training (timed voiding)
- Prompted voiding
- Pelvic muscle exercises

These techniques are most helpful with stress and urge incontinence.

Bladder retraining is used to restore the normal pattern of voiding by inhibiting or stimulating voiding. The goal is to lengthen the time between voidings. This is best done by instructing and assisting the individual to learn to suppress the urge to void in an attempt to increase the amount of urine the bladder can hold. This technique is used with individuals who are capable of understanding and remembering the instructions. Most bladder-retraining schedules begin with a schedule of toileting every 2 hours and gradually increase the amount of time between voidings to every 3 to 4 hours while awake.

Prompted voiding is different from bladder training in that the goal is not to increase bladder capacity, but rather to teach the incontinent person to be aware of toileting needs and to request assistance from the caregiver. In this technique, the person is asked to try to use the toilet at regular intervals and is praised for maintaining continence and using the toilet. The schedule that is followed usually involves toileting on awakening, after meals, at bedtime, and, if awake, at night. More voiding times can be added if the individual's voiding schedule indicates a need. This intervention works well with moderately confused people.

Habit training works best with cognitively impaired or confused people and requires the caregiver to take the patient to the toilet at regular intervals. The toileting schedule may be every 2 to 4 hours, or the caregiver may toilet the individual on awakening, after meals, midmorning and midafternoon, at bedtime, and at night, if awake.

Pelvic floor muscle exercises, also known as Kegel's exercises, are used to alleviate stress incontinence. The goal of such exercises is to strengthen the pelvic floor muscles. Patients who are taught Kegel's exercises must be cognitively intact and willing to participate in this exercise regimen. The exercise consists of the person contracting the pelvic floor muscles and holding them for 3 to 4 seconds and then relaxing the muscle. This should be done 15 times in succession at least three times per day, increasing to 10-second contractions each time. Once the person has met the increased seconds per contraction, a schedule of 10-second contractions and releases per day can be maintained.

In dealing with incontinence, nurses play a key role in education and treatment. Incontinence is not a normal part of aging but is more prevalent in elderly people. Many forms of incontinence are reversible, and all attempts should be made to assess, treat, and resolve incontinence when it is present.

Constipation

Bowel functioning and the avoidance of constipation are common concerns for older adults. Many older people were raised during a time when anything but a daily bowel movement was considered abnormal. The concern regarding this problem is appropriate because numerous age-related changes in the gastrointestinal system make constipation more likely.

It is probable that an older person has an extended gastrointestinal transit time as a result of slower peristalsis. More water is removed from the stool when it is in the colon for longer periods. The stool becomes harder and more difficult to pass. Immobility, decreased exercise, and a lack of fiber and water in the diet are common problems in older people, and these factors tend to exacerbate the tendency to become constipated. Certain drugs also may lead to constipation, including the following:

- Antacids containing aluminum and calcium
- Anticholinergics
- Iron supplements
- Laxatives (when abused)
- Narcotics
- Some antidepressants
- Diuretics
- Calcium channel blockers
- Anticonvulsants
- Antispasmodics

Immobility is particularly problematic in the maintenance of regular bowel movements. Muscular atrophy, which is a loss of tone in the muscles of the intestine, and generalized weakness of the muscles necessary for the expulsive mechanism of evacuation occur during periods of immobilization. The overuse of laxatives also causes a loss of muscle tone in the bowel.

Immobility not only affects the physiological functioning of the gastrointestinal system, but it also prevents the individual from interacting efficiently with the environment to meet the needs of the body. Factors such as strange environments, disruption of the usual elimination patterns, being forced to defecate in an unnatural position in unnatural surroundings (as occurs with the use of a bedpan), and suppressing the urge to defecate because of the inability to get to the toilet inhibit normal defecation.

Nursing Interventions

Nursing interventions aimed at prevention of constipation should be focused on establishing a regular pattern of bowel elimination that is not associated with straining or discomfort. It is important for the older person's overall health to attempt to correct constipation without resorting to the use of laxatives. These interventions should include increasing physical activity, increasing water intake, increasing dietary fiber, and establishing a regular bowel routine. Regular exercise stimulates motility in the gut.

The older adult should be encouraged to drink 1,500 to 2,000 mL of fluids daily unless this is contraindicated by other health problems. Dietary fiber also plays an important role in the avoidance of constipation. Fiber holds water, making the stool softer and bulkier, which speeds the passage of stool through the intestine. It can be difficult to increase fiber in the diet of the older person because of lifelong dietary preferences and poor dentition. It may be helpful to consult a dietitian.

Assisting the patient to develop a regular bowel routine is an essential part of bowel maintenance and one in which the nurses play a pivotal role. In facilitating regular bowel routines, the nurse must assess how much, if any, assistance the person requires in getting safely to the toilet. The use of bedpans should be avoided whenever possible, but when they are used, the patient should be in an upright position unless this position is contraindicated. The nurse also needs to ensure that regular toileting times are maintained and that privacy is provided during toileting time.

ALTERATION IN SKIN INTEGRITY: PRESSURE ULCERS

A pressure ulcer is defined as any lesion caused by unrelieved pressure that results in damage to the underlying tissue. Pressure ulcers are an extremely serious health problem that can lead to pain, extended hospital stays, and further complications from infection. In hospitals, the pressure ulcer rate has been estimated to be 10% to 18%, in nursing homes 2.3% to 28%, and in home care 0% to 29% (National Pressure Ulcer Advisory Panel, 2014). Older persons are particularly at risk, especially if they have multiple health problems. Approximately 60,000 deaths per year are associated with pressure ulcers (Agency for Healthcare Research and Quality, n.d.). The development of pressure ulcers has been associated with the quality of health care and may signal overall poor care by the health-care system. Because pressure ulcers are, for the most part, preventable, maintaining adequate skin integrity is a quality-of-care issue for all nurses. Even more important than knowing the various treatment modalities is knowing how pressure ulcers develop. You need to become an expert in prevention techniques.

Risk Factors

Mechanical Risk Factors

Four mechanical factors that contribute to the development of pressure ulcers are pressure, shearing, friction, and moisture.

- *Pressure* ulcers usually occur over bony prominences such as sacrum, ischium, trochanters, heels, elbows, and the back of the head, where normal tissue is squeezed between the internal pressure of the bone and an external source of pressure or friction, such as the chair or the bed. External pressure that lasts long enough and is sufficient enough to decrease blood flow results in inadequate oxygenation and nutrition to the area and the subsequent development of a pressure ulcer. Immobility is the most important risk factor in the development of pressure ulcers. Pressure of high intensity that is left unchecked for more than 2 hours can result in irreversible tissue damage.
- *Shearing* occurs when the head of the bed is elevated more than 30 degrees and the person slides toward the foot of the bed. In this situation, the skin over the sacrum does not move, whereas the subcutaneous tissue and gluteal vessels are stretched. Rupture of the blood vessels results. Subcutaneous fat, which lacks the ability to stretch, is particularly vulnerable to injury from shearing forces. Sores that develop on the sacrum, heels, and anterior tibial region are most probably a result of shearing. When shearing and pressure are both present, the amount of pressure necessary to cause tissue damage is half the amount that causes tissue damage when shearing is not present.
- *Friction* occurs when the skin is moved across the sheets, such as when the person is being pulled up rather than lifted up in the bed. The result of this motion is damage to the epidermis, which can lead to ulceration or a break in the skin. *Moisture* caused by perspiration or incontinence can increase the friction between the surface and the skin. Moisture also can cause maceration (softening of the skin), which weakens the skin and increases the risk of infection. In the presence of moisture resulting from urinary or fecal incontinence, the risk of pressure ulcer development on the sacrum and buttocks increases fivefold. Incontinence is a strong predictor of skin breakdown.

Physiological Risk Factors

In addition to mechanical forces, there are factors that are inherent to the individual that increase the risk of skin breakdown. Examples include aging skin, immobility, and malnutrition.

- *Aging skin* increases the likelihood of developing pressure ulcers because it is less resistant to the mechanical forces that can damage the skin. With advancing age, there is a decrease in the thickness of the cell layers of the epidermis, a flattening in the epidermal-dermal interface, and a loss of subcutaneous tissue. These changes cause impaired wound healing and decreased thermoregulation, causing the skin to become more fragile.
- *Immobility,* combined with the age-related changes of the skin, greatly increases the risk of pressure ulcer formation. Normally, spontaneous body movements that occur during sleep and throughout the day protect the skin from pressure. Many situations prevent the body from spontaneous movement, however, including physical disability, loss of sensation, presence of pain, or use of sedating drugs or anesthesia.

- *Malnutrition* is another physiological factor that can lead to pressure ulcer formation. Deficiencies in zinc, iron, vitamin C, and protein adversely affect the health of the skin. The more severe the malnutrition, the more severe the pressure ulcer. In older adults who have experienced weight loss or who are underweight, it is important to check the albumin level of the blood. A serum albumin level less than 3.5 g/dL indicates that nutritional intervention is necessary to prevent skin breakdown. Malnutrition and the subsequent weight loss lead to loss of muscle mass and subcutaneous tissue. This diminishes the body's protective padding and increases the pressure over the bony prominences.

Staging

Pressure ulcers are graded according to the degree of tissue damage. The staging of a pressure ulcer dictates the type of treatment to be implemented. Staging provides a means of describing an ulcer that allows for the ulcer to be monitored over time. Commonly used staging criteria are presented in the following list:

Stage I: Nonblanchable erythema of intact skin. (The skin is reddened, even in the absence of direct pressure.)

Stage II: Partial-thickness skin loss involving epidermis or dermis. The ulcer is superficial and manifests clinically as an abrasion, blister, or shallow crater.

Stage III: Full-thickness skin loss involving damage to or necrosis of subcutaneous tissue that may extend down to, but not through, the underlying fascia (fibrous membrane covering the muscles). The ulcer manifests clinically as a deep crater with or without undermining of adjacent tissue.

Stage IV: Full-thickness skin loss with extensive destruction, tissue necrosis, or damage to muscle, bone, or supporting structures (e.g., tendon or joint capsule). Undermining and sinus tracts also may be associated with stage IV pressure ulcers.

Prevention

Assessment of risk is a vital first step in prevention of pressure ulcers. If a person is found to be at risk for developing pressure ulcers, interventions to prevent skin breakdown can be initiated before an ulcer develops. Numerous assessment tools are available. Review the Braden Scale presented in Chapter 16.

Assessment should be done using the following criteria:

Acute care: Assess on admission and every 24 hours or sooner if the patient's condition changes.

Long term: Assess on admission and weekly for 4 weeks. Then assess every quarter or as the resident's condition changes.

Home care: Assess on admission and on every nurse visit.

When an older adult is found to be at risk for alteration in skin integrity, preventive measures should be aimed at reducing pressure on bony prominences, preventing shear or friction, keeping skin clean and dry, and providing adequate nutrition and hydration. To reduce pressure, the person should be repositioned at least

---

QSEN

COMPETENCY: Quality Improvement
(Knowledge, Skill)

Promote Quality Outcomes for Patients

Providing quality care and ensuring positive outcomes for patients should be a priority for all nurses. Knowing how to find information by reading research articles and national guidelines regarding appropriate outcomes for the patient population you serve is a skill that is important in providing care to your patients. Taking that information and working with the health-care team to identify gaps between local and best practices and then helping to develop the processes to adopt best practices in your facility will improve outcomes for your patients. The Agency for Healthcare Research and Quality has developed a toolkit for preventing pressure ulcers in hospital settings. The toolkit can be found at http://www.ahrq.gov/professionals/systems/long-term-care/resources/pressure-ulcers/pressureulcertoolkit/putoolkit.pdf

1. How can the information in the tool kit be used to prevent pressure ulcers and improve patient outcomes in your patient population?
2. How will you share the information with the rest of the health-care team to involve them in preventing pressure ulcers in your facility?

every 2 hours. This regular repositioning decreases the amount of time that pressure is exerted on any one body part. The appearance of reddened areas indicates that more frequent turning or other interventions may be indicated. When placing an older adult on either side, a wedge should be placed behind the person to prevent the person from lying directly on the trochanter (which is the bony prominence located below the neck of the femur).

Although at one time it was common practice to massage reddened areas over bony prominences, this is no longer the practice. Massage may exert pressure on the area and may cause further breakdown of the small capillaries. In some cases, it may be necessary to use pressure-relieving devices, such as air-filled, water-filled, or gel-filled chair pads or mattresses, and foam heel protectors and mattresses. The use of egg-crate mattresses, although common, does not provide sufficient pressure relief to prevent pressure ulcers. Walking programs and passive and active ROM exercises not only improve muscle strength and joint flexibility but also are important in the prevention of skin breakdown.

PATIENT EDUCATION

You are a home-health nurse for a 79-year-old woman who is cared for by her husband with drop-in visits from three daughters. Sarah, the patient, is home bound because of general fatigue and postoperative total hip replacement. She can ambulate with a cane but is fearful and will not leave the house except on rare occasions. She says she is happy to be at home with her husband and not to have the arthritic hip pain. The problem is she is either in bed or a recliner chair most of the day and night. Her husband lifts her to and from the chair and bed when Sarah is "too tired to move herself."

You have noticed that Sarah's buttocks are reddened, as are her heels. Focus on a teaching plan for this couple. What do they need to know about pressure ulcers? What is the best way for you to share the hazards of immobility with Sarah? What can you do to prevent the stage I pressure ulcers from developing into something worse?

To reduce friction, persons should be lifted and not pulled when repositioned. The use of a lift sheet or a turn sheet is essential to distribute the person's weight evenly and avoid undue friction and stress on the skin. Shear can be reduced by decreasing the amount of time and frequency that the person's head is elevated above 30 degrees while in the bed. When out of bed and in a chair, the person should be repositioned at least every hour, and long-term sitting should be discouraged. While in the chair, the individual needs to be examined for appropriate posture and alignment because an inappropriate sitting posture can lead to pressure ulcers and increased shearing forces.

Although skin should be kept clean and dry to prevent pressure ulcers, older adults do not need to be bathed daily. Excessive bathing and rubbing can be drying and damaging to the skin. Using a mild cleansing agent that does not promote dryness and patting the skin dry are essentials of good skin care for the older person.

Treatment

Treating pressure ulcers is expensive and can extend the recovery and rehabilitation time. The treatment of pressure ulcers is extremely individualized, and it requires a team approach. Any suspicion of a pressure ulcer should be reported immediately to the RN so early treatment can begin. Nursing care is aimed at maintaining skin integrity by preventing irritation to the skin from friction and moisture. Providing adequate nutrition and good hygiene are also important to assist with the healing process.

ALTERED NUTRITIONAL STATUS

Adequate nutrition is essential to the maintenance of health, prevention of disease, treatment of chronic illness, and recovery from acute illness. When the body is inadequately nourished, the individual is more likely to develop an illness and is less able to recover from illness. Caloric or protein malnutrition is a concern for older people.

To be adequately nourished, the body must have a sufficient intake of carbohydrates, fats, proteins, vitamins, minerals, and water. Difficulty obtaining appropriate nutrition can be a result of lack of knowledge about good nutrition, inadequate income or means of obtaining the appropriate foods, lack of socialization (which may lead to disinterest or overindulgence in food), or housing that is inadequate for storing and preparing nutritionally sound meals. The older person's diet is often lacking in calcium, vitamin C, riboflavin, niacin, and iron. A deficiency of any essential nutrient can cause changes to the body that, if left unchecked, can lead to illness. Chapter 8 covers additional information on nutrition of older adults.

Risk Factors

Anorexia (loss of appetite) is a major cause of inadequate nutritional intake in older people. Poor dentition, poorly fitting dentures, or lack of dentures may make it difficult for the individual to chew, and a soft or puree diet may be unappetizing. Not only may diminished mobility make it difficult for the older person to obtain and prepare food, but a sedentary lifestyle also may lead to a decreased appetite. Polypharmacy, a common situation with elderly patients, can adversely affect appetite by altering taste sensation, impairing cognition and mood, or interfering with the absorption of nutrients. Other causes of anorexia in older adults may include the increased incidence of chronic illness, social isolation, depression, and unappetizing institutional foods.

Changes in the metabolism of older people translate into changes in nutritional requirements of the body. With aging, there is a decreased metabolic rate, and the body requires fewer calories for maintenance. Decreased mobility and the loss of muscle mass associated with aging also suggest that older people may need to decrease their caloric consumption. Older adults use more energy, however, than younger people to do the same activities. If the individual is active, there may be a need to increase the caloric intake. With aging, the body does not metabolize protein as efficiently, so older people may need more protein in their diet.

Maintaining adequate nutrition in older persons who have a disease process poses a particular challenge to the nurse. People with advanced dementia may have weight loss even when there is an adequate intake of nutritional requirements. It is suspected that this weight loss may be due in part to the increased use of antibiotics in a population that tends to have a higher rate of infection. Neuroleptics, another commonly used class of drugs in demented patients, also may cause a loss of appetite. It has been postulated that there may

be a disturbance in the metabolism of patients with advanced Alzheimer's disease, and this, too, may account for the unexplained weight loss in these patients. The term "failure to thrive" has been used to describe another entity associated with weight loss. Failure to thrive occurs when some elderly nursing home residents experience a gradual decline in physical and cognitive functioning associated with weight loss, withdrawing from food, withdrawing from human contact, and exhibiting signs of depression.

A significant problem for many older adults who have had a stroke or generalized weakness is aspiration, the inhalation of solids or liquids into the upper respiratory tract. This is a critical problem because of the serious consequences of an aspiration. It can cause pneumonia or death by choking. The symptoms of aspiration include a sudden severe cough or cyanosis while eating or drinking, voice changes, and increased respiratory rate after eating or drinking. The possibility of aspiration is increased with dysphagia (difficulty swallowing) and gastroesophageal reflux problems.

Assessment

Assessing the nutritional status of the older person can be a difficult task for the nurse. The recommended dietary allowance (RDA) that is established by the National Academy of Science Research Council is one way of monitoring how well an individual is meeting nutritional requirements. The RDA does not consider the specific needs of the population older than 65 years of age, however. Additional nutrients that may be needed as a result of infection or chronic illness are not addressed by the RDA.

Complicating the assessment for malnutrition further are the changes of the aging body itself. Many physical manifestations of malnutrition are similar to changes that are associated with aging. These changes include dry, thin hair; dry, flaky skin; sunken eyes; dry oral mucosa; weight loss; and muscle weakness. Using skinfold measures to estimate percentage of body fat may not yield accurate information because mean body mass (muscle tissue) decreases with age. Probably the most reliable indicator of adequate nutritional intake is a normal serum albumin level (3.5 to 5.5 g/dL). Monitoring an individual's weight over time is also an appropriate means of recognizing alteration in nutritional status.

Nursing Implications

To reestablish adequate nutritional intake, healthcare providers should strive to maintain oral feedings, possibly with appropriate modifications. The diet may need to be made more palatable with foods that have different textures and flavors. Providing the individual's food favorites whenever possible is also a good approach. Family members can be asked to provide favorite foods for the older person. Ensuring that the older person has dentures if needed and that they fit well and providing a diet that is appropriate for the person's dental status are imperative.

Everyone responds well to meals that are served in an attractive manner and in an environment that is relaxed and pleasant. Nursing staff should strive for this kind of atmosphere during mealtime by not raising their voices and trying to keep noisy dietary carts out of the eating area. Eyeglasses help the resident to see the food on the tray, and hearing aids allow the resident to socialize with tablemates during mealtime. It is important that the nurse ensure that the individual has whatever assistive devices are needed to make the eating experience a more pleasant one.

If the person's nutritional status does not improve despite these efforts, the nurse needs to consider other interventions. It may be necessary to offer more assistance with meals. The individual may need to be fed or have containers opened, or he or she may just need ongoing gentle encouragement throughout the meal to continue eating. Often, gently touching the arm or shoulder while encouraging feeding helps the older adult to attend to the task of eating. Touch is a caring behavior that indicates value and respect for the person being touched. Older people often are not touched or hugged frequently and generally respond positively to the act of being touched. A nutritional supplement also may be needed.

The dietitian should assist in deciding what, if any, supplements are needed. Liquid dietary supplements are best offered between meals so that the supplement is not substituted for the meal itself. The supplement can provide a large percentage of the RDA requirements but does not completely meet all dietary requirements.

Tube feedings and parenteral feedings can be used when all other attempts at oral feedings have failed. These methods have numerous complications, however. Striving to maintain adequate oral intake should be the goal of all nursing personnel.

This father and son have lived together since the father's discharge from a nursing home. He was admitted for falling and for generalized weakness; he was malnourished. The son enjoys cooking and caters to his father's wishes, which has improved the older man's health remarkably. Now, the two of them go to the nursing home to visit the father's friends.

Adequate nutrition affects every aspect of the individual's health and well-being.

SLEEP PATTERN DISTURBANCES

Older people often complain of not getting enough sleep or not feeling well rested after sleeping. Sleep disturbances increase with age. It is estimated that sleep pattern disturbances affect half of people older than 65 years who live at home and two-thirds of older people living in institutions.

Normal Sleep Patterns

A review of normal sleep patterns is necessary to understand the changes in sleep patterns that tend to occur with aging. There are five stages to normal sleep. Refer to Chapter 10 if you need to review this material.

Age-Related Changes in Sleep Patterns

In the course of aging, people tend to sleep less than 8 hours per night. Older people have an impaired capacity to maintain sleep; sleep tends to be marked by more frequent and prolonged awakenings during the night. In addition, stage IV and REM sleep diminish. In extreme old age, changes in cerebral blood flow and organic brain syndrome also are associated with a shortening of the REM stage of sleep.

The sleep patterns of older people can be disturbed by factors such as needing to void frequently during the night (nocturia) and changes in vision and hearing that cause incorrect perceptions of their immediate environment. These changes can lead to ineffective sleep or sleep deprivation. Sleep deprivation is marked by fatigue, tiredness, eye problems, muscle tremor, muscle weakness, diminished coordination and attention span, apathy, and depression.

Sleep Disorders

In addition to age-related changes in sleep patterns, some sleep disorders are common to older adults. Sleep apnea, a medical condition in which breathing stops for 10 seconds or longer numerous times throughout the night, is more common in older people. There are two types of sleep apnea. Central sleep apnea is caused by a defect in the central nervous system that effects the diaphragm; obstructive sleep apnea is caused by an obstruction in the upper airway that impedes airflow. Untreated sleep apnea is associated with cognitive decline, cardiac disease, stroke, and decreased quality of life. Death can result because of the effect on the cardiovascular and respiratory systems. The affected person complains of excessive daytime sleepiness and constant interruption of sleep. Cessation of breathing for 10 or more seconds, followed by very loud snoring or choking, is the primary objective symptom of sleep apnea.

Night-shift personnel are often the first people to discover the symptoms of sleep apnea when a patient or resident is admitted to the hospital or nursing home. The treatment for sleep apnea is usually weight reduction, continuous positive airway pressure (CPAP), oxygen, and occasionally surgery. CPAP is a technique that forces air down the nose, through the throat, and into the lungs; it is used during sleep for persons who have been diagnosed with sleep apnea.

Sundown Syndrome

Sundown syndrome is another disorder that affects many older people. Sundown syndrome is defined as the appearance or exacerbation of symptoms of confusion associated with the late afternoon or evening hours. This syndrome is marked by behaviors such as agitation, restlessness, confusion, wandering, and screaming that occur usually in the evening hours (sundown). Little is known about this disorder, which is a tremendous management problem for caregivers. Risk factors for sundown syndrome seem to be impaired mental status, dehydration, being awakened frequently during the night for nursing care, and recent relocation either to a new room or to the institution.

Nursing Interventions

Sleeping medications, tranquilizers, and sedatives are commonly used to promote sleep but should be avoided at all costs in older persons. Sedatives and barbiturates that depress the central nervous system may lead to other problems by depressing vital body functions, lowering basal metabolic rate, decreasing blood pressure, and causing mental confusion. Sleeping medications decrease spontaneous body movements that may lead to skin breakdown. Most of the medications used to promote sleep are not efficiently metabolized by the aging body, and the person may experience a hangover effect the next day. In addition, these drugs tend to cause blurred vision, dry mouth, and urinary retention. Because it is known that an elderly person cannot sleep as long as a younger person can, it is unreasonable to put an individual to bed at 8 p.m. and expect that person to stay in bed until 7 a.m. the next day.

There is much the nurse can do to promote sleep without resorting to the use of medications. Meeting the individual's comfort needs by offering back rubs or snacks such as warm milk, assisting with toileting needs, providing socks or an extra blanket to increase body temperature (which may be diminished in an older person), repositioning, and alleviating pain are just a few of the nursing interventions that may reduce insomnia. If these interventions do not promote sleep, it is prudent to allow the older person to come out of the bed and perhaps sit for a while in a comfortable chair near the nurses' station. This may reassure the individual of the surroundings and prevent attempts to get out of bed unassisted, perhaps risking a fall. During the daytime, increased physical activity may promote sleep.

IATROGENESIS

Iatrogenic disorders can be defined as disorders that a person acquires as a result of receiving treatment by a physician, nurse, or other member of the IDT. Iatrogenesis also can occur if the person does not receive treatment when it is indicated or receives incorrect treatment. An older person often presents with numerous chronic conditions that require complex interventions, numerous medications, and increased exposure to the health-care system; this puts older adults at increased risk of experiencing untoward effects of medical treatment. Iatrogenic disorders include the disorders previously discussed in this chapter: immobility, falls, incontinence, malnutrition, pressure ulcers, and disturbances in the sleep-wake cycle.

Common causes of iatrogenesis in the hospital are misuse or overuse of drugs, prolonged immobilization, nosocomial (hospital- acquired) infections, and malnutrition and dehydration secondary to preparation for diagnostic tests. In the nursing home, common iatrogenic disorders include immobilization, adverse drug reactions, falls, pressure ulcers, and nosocomial infections.

Iatrogenic disorders often cause a vicious circle in which one disorder quickly leads to another. Consider the older person who is admitted to the hospital for abdominal discomfort. This person is unable to sleep and is prescribed a sleeping pill. Having taken this medication, the person is groggy when getting out of bed and sustains a fall. The staff, not wanting the patient to be hurt again, assigns a volunteer to sit with the person to remind him or her not to get up. The older person is now unable to get up and suffers from some of the adverse sequelae of immobility, such as incontinence, disorientation, and pressure ulcer formation. In time, the person's muscles become deconditioned, and the next time the patient is assisted out of bed, there is another fall, the person sustains a hip fracture, and the cycle continues. One can see what a high price is paid for the effects of negative medical and nursing interventions.

CONCLUSION

The health-care needs of older adults are multiple and complex. Health-care providers often are not educated in the normal aging process or in the older person's response to illness and health-care interventions. As a result, the layperson and the health-care provider may believe that there is little that can be done to improve the health status of older adults. Not only is this not true, but also this attitude can lead to a self-fulfilling prophecy in which older people are expected to be ill and to experience functional decline. Assessment and interventions aimed at correcting the illness, promoting function, and averting a subsequent decline may not be initiated, and the older person is likely to become more ill and more dependent on others.

LPNs can and should play a pivotal role in ensuring that the health-care needs of older persons are being met. They also need to be aware of the problems that besiege the older person as a result of medical interventions. Iatrogenesis can be prevented. Many of the clinical problems that the older person faces in health and in illness can be averted or alleviated with nursing interventions that are focused on improving and maintaining wellness and promoting function.

CASE STUDY SOLUTION

In this case study, there are numerous potential iatrogenic problems that the nursing staff should address. The report from the hospital notes that Mrs. S. had a Foley catheter inserted because she was incontinent. The question the nurse should be asking here is, "Why is Mrs. S. incontinent?" True, the incontinence can be a result of damage from the stroke, but until attempts are made to take the patient to the bathroom, one cannot be certain. It may be that Mrs. S., having had a stroke that affected her speech, could not tell the staff that she needed to go. She may have to go to the bathroom as soon as the urge presents itself. A prompted voiding schedule would be helpful in beginning to assess whether this incontinence is reversible. A Foley catheter should not be the first intervention used in the presence of incontinence. In this case, the use of the catheter prolonged the hospitalization by causing a urinary tract infection.

Another possible iatrogenic problem may be aspiration pneumonia. In a person who has had a stroke and who has difficulty talking, one should consider the possibility of a swallowing deficit. A patient such as Mrs. S. should never be left alone to eat. In addition, the nursing staff should be assessing her during mealtime for any difficulty swallowing. If a difficulty is noted, a speech and swallowing consultation is warranted. When the diet was changed to puree, Mrs. S. apparently had no further problems with swallowing but had a decreased nutritional intake. The nurse needs to assess the person to understand why the diet is not being taken. There may be many reasons. The patient may not like her diet, she may still be having difficulty swallowing and is afraid of choking again, or she may be depressed and without an appetite.

It is a positive step that Mrs. S. has been started on physical therapy and is walking, but there is more that the nursing and physical therapy staffs can do to promote functional ambulation. Walking does not have to be done just in the therapy department. The therapist needs to lend a walker to Mrs. S. or to instruct the family to buy one for her so that ambulation can be done on the nursing unit. Therapy takes place for only about 1 hour a day. Walking the person on the unit augments therapy, improves the person's gait, helps her to regain her confidence in her functional ability, and prevents the negative effects of immobility.

The nurse reports that Mrs. S. might be confused; however, there is little evidence here to support that conclusion or to suggest that confusion should be expected. From the report, Mrs. S. was not confused before her hospitalization. If she is confused, it may be related to the urinary tract infection, the pneumonia, the relocation to the hospital, or the depression from the stroke. The possibility of confusion should not deter the nurse in any way from pursuing a plan of care that focuses on promoting the highest level of functional ability for this patient.

The family requests that Mrs. S. be restrained to prevent injury to her hip replacements. Instead of a restraint, the staff needs to consider ways of preventing a fall so that the family will understand that a restraint is not needed. Possible interventions to prevent a fall might include helping Mrs. S. to understand her limitations, toileting her at regular intervals, promoting lower extremity strengthening through exercise, keeping her out of her room and within sight of the staff, and perhaps using an alarm if she is unpredictable in her attempts to get up. Honoring the family's request for a restraint may serve only to cause contractures, skin breakdown, a worsening of her urinary incontinence, depression, and general deconditioning related to immobility. The family needs to be educated to the dangers of using restraints. The use of restraints would not promote a positive outcome for this patient.

REVIEW QUESTIONS

1. An example of an intrinsic risk factor for falls in the older person is:
   1. The use of diuretics
   2. Weakened muscles in the lower extremities
   3. Glaring lights in the hallway
   4. The use of a cane

2. To promote mobility in the older adult, the nurse would:
   1. Turn the patient every 2 hours
   2. Encourage the patient to cough and take deep breaths
   3. Ask the family to bring in the patient's walker from home
   4. Assume that the physical therapist is helping the patient to walk

3. The best way to promote urinary continence in the older person is to:
   1. Stop giving the diuretic because it causes the patient to have urinary urgency
   2. Obtain a urine specimen for culture and sensitivity
   3. Offer the bedpan every 2 hours
   4. Assist the patient to the toilet in the morning, after meals, and at bedtime

4. When seeing a reddened area on the patient's coccyx, the nurse would do all but one of the following interventions:
   1. Turn the patient every 2 hours
   2. Ask the physician to order a medication to treat the skin
   3. Help the patient to the toilet more frequently
   4. Measure how much of the diet the patient is taking every day

5. Which of the following is not an example of an iatrogenic disorder?
   1. Falling because of dizziness after receiving medication for pain relief
   2. Depression because of a stroke
   3. Incontinence because the patient could not find the bathroom
   4. Loss of weight because the patient cannot chew the food that is provided

REFERENCES

Adelmann, P.K. (2004). Prevalence and detection of urinary incontinence among older Medicaid recipients. *Journal of Health Care for the Poor and Underserved,* 15(1), 99-112.

Agency for Healthcare Research and Quality (n.d.). Preventing pressure ulcers in hospitals. www.ahrq.gov/professionals/systems/long-term-care/resources/pressure-ulcers/pressureulcertoolkit/putoolkit.pdf

Centers for Disease Control and Prevention (n.d.). Osteoarthritis. www.cdc.gov/arthritis/basics/osteoarthritis.htm

National Institute on Aging (2014). NIH, PCORI announce major award to prevent falls injuries in older people. https://www.nia.nih.gov/newsroom/2014/06/nih-pcori-announce-major-award-prevent-falls-injuries-older-people

National Pressure Ulcer Advisory Panel (2014). Elimination, sleep, skin, and foot care. In: Toughy, T.A., & Jett, K. *Ebersole & Hess' toward healthy aging: Human needs and nursing response.* (8th ed). St. Louis, MO: Elsevier.

National Safety Council (n.d.). Slip, trip and fall protection for older adults. www.nsc.org/safety_home/HomeandRecreationalSafety/Falls/Pages/OlderAdultFalls.aspx

Strax, T.E., Gonzalez, P., & Cuccurullo, S. (2004). Effects of extended bed rest—Immobilization and inactivity. In: Cuccurullo, S. (ed.). *Physical medicine and rehabilitation board review.* New York, NY: Demos Medical Publishing.

WEB RESOURCES

National Pressure Ulcer Advisory Panel: http://www.npuap.org/

Pressure Ulcer Guidelines: http://www.guideline.gov/content.aspx?id=34754

Psychological Assessment

TAMARA DAHLKEMPER

LEARNING OUTCOMES

1. Identify three cognitive functions.

2. Use a standardized examination to screen for cognitive functioning.

3. Identify four uses of psychological assessments.

4. Describe the impact of depression on the mental status score.

18

CONCEPTS

Assessment

Cognition

CASE STUDY

Ms. F. is 81 years old and in general good health. At age 78, she decided to move into an assisted living facility. Her family became concerned for her safety and noted some minor problems with memory, a decline in her energy level, and an inability to take care of herself. She was placed on a unit with other residents who functioned independently. A few months after admission, some of the residents began to remark to the staff that Ms. F. was ignoring some of their efforts to engage her in conversation. She started retreating to her room a little more. She seemed more withdrawn in general. She favored a chair off to herself rather than an available seat in a group of other residents.

Discussion

1. Based on this information, what is the first step you will take to identify the change in Ms. F.'s behavior?

2. What are the next steps you will take?

 ## INTRODUCTION

Psychological assessments are essential tools in identifying the mental health of older adults in all health-care settings. Such assessments provide the basis for determining the psychological illness or wellness of a person as well as determining how much of a return to normal an individual can expect to achieve. Psychological assessments are important in any health-care setting, but especially when the focus is restorative care.

Restorative care, in its truest application, requires a body-mind-spirit connection. Relate this concept to Jean Watson's theory of caring—the two theories are conceptually the same, and it is hoped that they are beginning to have meaning for you in your practice. Nurses practicing within this framework are concerned with the physical indications that a person is declining, such as falling, incontinence, and immobility. Even though behavioral or psychological indicators have received less prominence in terms of restorative care, they are equally important. Some examples of psychological indicators are failure to eat and a decline in functional level, such as severe memory loss or confusion without a physiological basis.

Although one can expect a certain amount of decline in older people who have vascular and central nervous system disease, it is important to identify the psychological areas of decline and recognize when interventions are essential. Maintenance of mental health and cognitive functioning is as important to restorative care as the maintenance of physiological processes. Nurses working with elderly people need to understand basic concepts of mental health and cognitive function so that they can participate in the care of the older adult more effectively. Assessment tools provide a brief, methodical approach to noting changes commonly found in individuals with cerebrovascular diseases, delirium, and dementia disorders.

 ## MENTAL HEALTH

Over the years, clinicians in the field of mental health have tried to diagnose symptoms, traits, and patterns of behavior that identify disease. The view that identification and treatment of disease result in optimum health is known as the medical model. The simplest definition of mental health would be the absence of identifiable disease. Most people have short-term or long-term psychological disorders at intervals throughout their lives; examples include grief over the death of someone close, post-traumatic stress disorder, or an eating disorder. A more comprehensive approach to mental health is to define the traits of the mentally healthy personality.

Practitioners use terms that have been formulated by theorists to describe and discuss psychological problems. Words such as *id, ego,* and

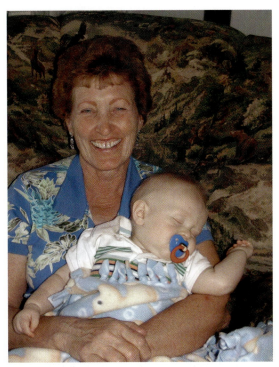

Review the four characteristics of mental health, and then look at this woman's face. You would need to interview her to determine whether or not it is true, but she does have the appearance of someone with purpose and meaning in her life.

Priority Setting

The most important priority you can set when assessing older adults psychologically is to be able to do an effective assessment very, very well. You can't fake an assessment and assume it will do any good for the person who is ill. Pick one of the assessments in this chapter and learn it well. Read about it in professional journals, talk to experts about how they perform the assessment, and look for a mentor. The mentor could be an experienced nurse or nurse practitioner. Let your mentor know that you want to be expert at doing the MMSE, for example. Perhaps your mentor will talk to you about the things that he or she does, or perhaps your mentor will take you along as he or she does assessments. You cannot assess people unless you have developed the expert skill required to do an excellent assessment. So, get busy! Pick one tool and stick with it until you are really, really good.

superego are used by therapists who base their practice on Freud's theory. *Enmeshment* is a term used by some family therapists to describe interactions among family members that keep them dependent on each other. A therapist practicing within a Gestalt framework may focus on the feeling experiences of an individual.

The current trend is to identify wellness in mental health. Although it is difficult to define wellness, some characteristics have been des-cribed by psychologists, nurses, and physicians and are included in the following list:

- A clear meaning and purpose in life
- A strong reality orientation
- An ability to cope creatively with life's situations
- A capability for open, creative relationships

Notice how these statements complement the concept of gerotranscendence? If an individual has achieved gerotranscendence, that person has increased personal life satisfaction, made a redefinition of self and relationships with others, and become open to new and creative possibilities. Gerotranscendence is psychological well-being.

Mental health is not a product of good nurturing or of a life of positive experiences. There are individuals who function well in life—for example, they maintain a satisfying job and career, have a family, and make a contribution to their community—despite poor nurturing and environmental handicaps. Most views of mental health now embody a continuum of health and illness. This continuum is dynamic rather than static. Many situations have an impact on the functioning of an individual, including the following:

- The death of someone close
- Unemployment
- The birth of a child
- Relocation

Any individual, if sufficiently stressed, can show some signs of impairment. One concept refers to the continuum of functioning as a scale of the differences in people. Individuals who are higher on this scale require more stressors to impair their functioning than individuals who are lower on this scale, and they choose a life course based on thought and conviction rather than on impulse; they also show an ability to stand by a belief that is different from that of their peer group.

It is important for nurses working in gerontology to identify and promote positive mental health traits. Nurses can reinforce healthy traits and interactions in older persons. This is nursing care being given in the nursing model (Watson's theory) rather than the medical model. Because it is nursing model care, it is caring and holistic, which are strong traits of the profession of nursing and characteristics that you want to work to develop as a licensed practical nurse (LPN).

Cognition

Cognition is a mental activity concerned with processing information. It refers to a broad range of mental behaviors, including awareness, thinking, reasoning, and judgment. This process is very complex and involves many abilities or functions. Because it cannot be directly observed, many psychologists define cognition in terms of cognitive functions. The cognitive functions can be conceptualized in numerous ways and can be defined as perceiving, thinking, remembering, communicating, orienting, calculating, and problem-solving (Desai et al., 2010).

Memory

Generally, the more active people have been, the better their overall memory is as they age. A dysfunction in memory occurs in almost all of the cognitive disorders common in older adults. Psychologists generally refer to two categories of memory: short-term memory (STM) and long-term memory (LTM). The time interval for measuring STM is seconds, whereas for LTM it is minutes and beyond. Many elderly persons demonstrate excellent long-term recall, although this recall may be rooted more in a belief than in fact; this is the nature of LTM. It means that the stories older persons tell of their childhood or young adulthood are stories based on their belief systems rather than on what actually happened. This skill may be enchanting to staff and can be used effectively as a tool for reminiscence to strengthen a person's self-esteem.

Memory functions are extremely important to a person's ability to think. A deficit in STM means that a person is unable to recall some of today's events. An older adult with severe impairment of STM experiences the routine of each day as a new experience. Such a person is trapped in an endless cycle of requesting basic information about the environment from strangers, such as "Where is my room?" or "When do we eat?"

Memory impairment limits the ability of a person to form a new idea or relate one fact with another. It is nearly impossible for memory-impaired individuals to organize new information into categories. A place where one can put something (a pair of glasses) for safe keeping may change several times a day. This makes a never-ending search for an important item an everyday event.

Screening for memory impairment is the most important part of any assessment for an elderly patient. The loss of STM is the first symptom of Alzheimer's disease. A stroke also may impair memory function, but in this case, the type and extent of impairment depend on the location of the damage in the brain. Other STM deficits may be due to depression. Individuals with depression are inattentive to their environment. They often are preoccupied or self-absorbed. A decline in STM is an important finding on assessment and should prompt further investigation. The family of Ms. F. from the case study was concerned about her memory loss. This issue should be assessed further to determine whether it is an initial sign of a more severe problem.

Perception

Psychologists believe that all behavior depends on how one sees oneself, the situation one is in, and the interaction between the two. Behavior changes as individuals become aware of details in their surroundings. Learning, problem-solving, remembering, and forgetting all are part of one's awareness of the environment. Effective communication with an older person depends on the nurse's ability to understand the perceptual world of that person. With such an understanding, the most bizarre behavior often becomes comprehensible.

The first phase of forming a perception is the ability to use the five senses to collect information about the environment. Frequently, older adults have impairments in the sense organs. In Chapter 2, you learned about the deficits in vision, hearing, touch, taste, and smell that may occur in older persons.

There is an emotional or feeling component to perception as well. Individuals take in information

Memory function

Assessing memory function is the most important assessment when working with cognitively impaired adults.

In general, the more active people have been, the better their memory is as they age.

Long-term Memory (LTM)

Measured in minutes and beyond

Rooted in belief rather than fact

Short-term Memory (STM)

Measured in seconds

Unable to recall daily events: "Where is my room?"

Without STM, a person is limited in forming new ideas or relating one fact to another

Loss of STM is symptomatic of Alzheimer's disease, cerebral vascular accident, and/or depression

---

from the environment and form opinions about such information. Perceptions are normally evaluated against past experiences. An older adult may compare a meal eaten within the institutional setting with recollections of meals eaten with the person's own family. These recollections of past experiences are a part of forming perceptions.

Perceptual distortions also are known as hallucinations and delusional thinking. Although both may indicate a psychiatric illness in younger individuals, perceptual distortions are common in illnesses with dementia. Impaired memory and a natural distrust of a strange environment exaggerate this tendency in an institutionalized older person.

Orientation

Orientation refers to a person's awareness of self in the context of a particular time and place. Tests for orientation determine whether the persons being tested know their names, where they are, and the approximate time of day. Sometimes the expression "oriented times three" is used to indicate that an individual's orientation to time, place, and person is correct. Assessment of orientation is covered on every mental status examination. This is important information because a disturbance in orientation is one of the most frequent symptoms of brain disease. Awareness of time and place requires that individuals know where they are and can remember it. In this way, individuals keep in touch with ongoing history. Orientation depends on a person's ability to link each minute with the previous minute. Disorientation with respect to time is the first major confusion to occur as a result of dementia. Loss of a sense of place is likely to follow. Finally, the person loses the ability to recognize other people and, eventually, cannot remember who he or she is.

Think Like a Nurse

You are caring for an 81-year-old woman who was just admitted to the medical unit where you work. The charge nurse asked you to do something about the woman because she is screaming, "Don't hurt me! Don't hurt me!" and thrashing out at the staff. Because you are experienced in gerontological nursing, you assess the woman to determine the problem rather than restrain or confine her because her behavior is inconvenient. Think in terms of first-stage dementia and list three reasons why this woman would legitimately be fearful. Then, list what you can do about it. The first clue is in the section you just read on perception. The next clue is that the woman was just admitted and might be experiencing transitional stress. You think of a third reason and list all three with an appropriate intervention. Be prepared to share your thinking in class.

Thinking

Every area of the brain is involved in the mental operation of thinking. The ancient Greeks believed there were "higher" levels and "lower" levels of thinking, a distinction that is still relevant. Higher level thinking includes the ability to form concepts and think in an abstract manner. Asking a person to interpret a proverb tests the person's ability to think abstractly. If a person interprets the proverb "a stitch in time saves nine" in a way that conveys that prompt attention to a problem prevents trouble in the future, the person's ability to think abstractly is considered intact. A concrete interpretation adheres closely to the exact meaning of the phrase. Concrete thinking is a "lower" mental ability. Someone with concrete thinking may answer the question about the proverb with something like, "If I make nine stitches, the cloth will hold."

Thinking processes have a hierarchical order. The lower mental abilities are more enduring and less affected by brain injuries and disease processes. The higher levels of thinking tend to be more fragile. At first glance, interpreting proverbs may seem a bit removed from a person's ability to function in the real world. The use of good judgment, the ability to think abstractly, and the capacity to reason are higher level abilities, however, that indicate the difference between independent and supervised living. To some extent, these abilities can be determined by proverb interpretation. In general, tests for abstract thinking are not included as part of the short tests of mental function.

Communicating

The only vehicle for assessing thinking processes in an individual is communication. People understand human thought when it is reflected in language. It is important to assess language problems because they are common in cerebrovascular and dementia disorders. Assessment of communication patterns, word order, and the general sense of a sentence provides a window into the dementia process. This is especially true with a person who has experienced a stroke. Sometimes persons who have had a stroke have severe problems with communication. Small connecting words such as "if," "and," and "but" are missing. There are also several types of aphasia that impair an individual's ability to communicate.

Calculating

Calculating is a cognitive function that must be assessed carefully in terms of the person's intelligence and educational level. Poor performance may indicate dementia or delirium, anxiety, or depression. Serial 7s is one test that can determine a person's ability to calculate. The person is asked to

Critically Examine the Following

Whenever you are asked to complete this type of exercise, you are asked to think on a higher level. Has it seemed that way to you? Think back to your reactions in doing the critical thinking assignments. Did you avoid doing some? Were you irritated or upset at any of the assignments? Did you enjoy the challenge of doing them? Were you bored with them or saw them as not being a challenge? Take some time and consider your reactions to these assignments. Consider how you felt when certain items were discussed in class. Did you benefit from the thinking of your classmates? Were your ideas and thinking valued by others? Take the time to write your reactions regarding the higher level thinking experiences. Be prepared to share them in class.

subtract 7 from 100 and then to subtract 7 from that remainder, continuing five times. A nurse interviewed a moderately to severely impaired patient with Alzheimer's disease. Although the patient was completely disoriented with regard to time and place and could not recall the names of three objects seconds after they were told to him, he performed magnificently with the serial 7 calculations. In seconds, he completed the operation and then turned to the nurse, announcing proudly that mathematics was always his favorite subject. This is an example of why you should assess all components of cognitive function.

Problem-Solving

Problem-solving skills are essential to an individual's ability to function in any environment. Even people with dementia can exhibit aspects of problem-solving ability. Individuals in the early stages of Alzheimer's disease frequently make lists. Lists are coping devices that enable the recall of event sequences. When asked questions of orientation, some elders search for familiar cues in the environment. Examples of this behavior include the patient who was asked the date, spied a newspaper, and then winked and, smiling broadly, gave the correct answer. Another patient called to a nursing assistant passing by the door. When the nursing assistant entered the room, the patient asked him for the date and promptly relayed this information to the nurse interviewer.

An individual's environment is filled with a multitude of clues that facilitate orientation, aid a failing memory, and maintain a stable perceptual field. Use of these clues enables older adults to maintain communication with nurses, other patients, and family members. Because a patient's environment is rich with problem-solving clues, room changes and unit changes should be made infrequently and only after the most careful thought.

ASSESSMENT TOOLS AND HOW TO USE THEM

Mental status examinations are the most frequently used psychological assessments. Mental status assessment includes probing of the cognitive functions and level of consciousness (LOC). In selecting a tool, it is important to remember that examinations with brief instruments are generally better tolerated by an elderly person.

This man is a deacon in his church. This responsibility requires that he communicate, calculate, and problem solve. He also needs a good memory to do his job well. Interviewing people about their activities gives you important information for a psychological assessment.

A short examination is much less tiring for an older person to sit through than a lengthy one. No brief instrument is a perfect detector of cognitive impairment, however.

Screening tools initially may seem intimidating or cumbersome to use in clinical practice. Most tools are short and can be easily committed to memory after using them a few times. The following tests are commonly used and easy to learn and administer: Pfeiffer's Short Portable Mental Status Questionnaire (SPMSQ) (Pfeiffer, 1975), Folstein's Mini-Mental Status Exam (MMSE) (Folstein, Folstein, & McHugh, 1975), and the Mini-Cog. These scales are compared in Table 18.1 and are listed with a brief description in Box 18.1.

An important factor to consider in the scoring of all tests is that the educational level of the person being tested influences test results. An older adult with a lack of a formal education can score several points lower than an older person with greater deficits but more education. Some mental status tests have a method of scoring to correct for education.

TABLE 18.1   MENTAL STATUS EXAMINATIONS

	SPMSQ	MMSE	MINI-COG
Level of consciousness (LOC)		X	
Cognitive functions			
Remembering	X	X	X
Communicating			X
Problem-solving			X
Perceiving			
Thinking			
Orienting	X	X	
Calculating	X	X	
Corrects for education and culture	X		X
Number of questions	10	30	
Time required (minutes)	5	10	3

Modified from Gurland, B. J. (1987). The assessment of cognitive function in the elderly. *Clinical Geriatric Medicine, 3,* 53–63; and Waszynski, C. M. (2012). The Confusion Assessment Method (CAM) retrieved from http://consultgerirn.org/uploads/File/trythis/try_this_13.pdf.

SPMSQ = Short Portable Mental Status Questionnaire; MMSE = Mini-Mental Status Exam;

There are important reasons for an LPN to gain skills in using assessment tools. A standardized test allows you, as the caregiver, to collect pertinent information in a short time. The collection of this information is organized and methodical. The initial test establishes a baseline and allows for comparison of changes over time.

Memory

Assessing memory function is the most important assessment in working with cognitively impaired older adults. There are three steps in the memory process. Each step needs accurate assessment. The steps are reception (encoding), storage (retention), and retrieval (recall). Folstein's MMSE tests memory by asking the older adult to repeat three words after the nurse three times—for example, apple, ball, and lamp. The number of trials it takes for the older person to recall the three items is noted. Immediate repetition enables the nurse to determine whether the person has heard the three words correctly. After the older adult repeats the words accurately, the nurse requests that the person remember them. In 5 minutes, the nurse asks again for the older adult to recall the three words.

Orientation

All short mental status examinations include questions about orientation. Time orientation is tested by asking for the date (day, month, year, and day of the week) and the time of day. Because older adults often become quite skilled in using clues from the environment, it is important to remove newspapers or calendars that may help them find the answer. An older adult can sometimes have an accurate sense of time passing yet may not remember the exact date. The nurse may ask questions such as "How long has it been since you last saw me?" or "What was your last meal?"

Assessment of orientation in place generally begins with questions about the name or location of the place in which the person is being examined. You, as the LPN, need to determine whether patients know the kind of place they are in—a nursing home or hospital. Short mental status examinations ask questions about the state, county, or country of residence. Many people with moderate to severe dementia are unable to recall places. It may be more functional to question an older adult regarding the location of the bedroom or the dining room, for example, "Can you tell me where your room is?"

Assessing Delirium

Nurses sometimes have a difficult time recognizing delirium and ofter refer to it as confusion. Sudden onset is the most significant feature described by experts. Older individuals may develop

BOX 18.1 BRIEF DESCRIPTION OF COMMON SCREENING TOOLS

The MMSE was developed by Folstein to be used with medical and psychiatric patients. Scores in the range of 9 to 12 indicate a high likelihood of dementia. Scores of 25 and higher are considered normal.

The *SPMSQ* was developed by Pfeiffer. This test is a little quicker to administer than Folstein's MMSE. Questions of orientation and memory are addressed, and there is one question concerning calculation. LOC is not assessed. An advantage over the MMSE is that there are specific directions for scoring this test to correct for education and race. A test score of 8 to 10 indicates severe intellectual impairment; 5 to 7, moderate impairment; 3 to 4, mild impairment; 0 to 2, intact status.

The Mini-Cog is a tool that can be used quickly to identify cognitive impairment and is best used to identify individuals needing more thorough evaluation. The first part of the test asks a patient to remember three common objects and then repeat those objects a few minutes later. The second part of the test asks a patient to draw all 12 numbers on a clock and place the hands at ten minutes after 11:00. The clock must be drawn within 3 minutes. A correct response is all numbers drawn in the appropriate spot on the clock and the hands at the appropriate time. Refusal to draw the clock is scored as abnormal.

---

a delirium gradually, however, over the course of 2 or 3 days. A nursing home resident was being assessed for delirium by the nurse. The resident, who was talking about snakes in her bed, suddenly stopped and turned to the nurse. "Your hands are very chapped," she said. "You should use gloves to do your housework. I always did." Then the resident returned to her delirious state.

Another feature of delirium is disorientation. One person may be mistaken for another. Sometimes an older adult imagines being at home or in another location. Other cognitive functions may become impaired. There also may be a disturbance

in the sleep cycle. Many delirious elders are awake all night and then sleep during the day. A common tool used to assess for delirium is the Confusion Assessment Method. Once delirium is identified, the person should be reassessed every shift to assess if the person is still experiencing delirium. (Waszynski & Petrovic, 2008). Assessment findings should be combined with results from the physical assessment and nursing observations.

Assessing Depression

Although research indicates that depression is no more prevalent in older people than it is in younger people, its manifestation is different and difficult to identify. It is important for you, as the nurse, to gain skills in the assessment of depression because of your focus on the quality of life for all people.

There is a heavy emotional cost to depression that ultimately affects the immune system, which can lead to physical illnesses and infections. Depression predicts the onset of disability almost as powerfully as disability predicts depression. Older individuals who are depressed are in a high-risk category for institutionalization because they are less motivated to care for their personal hygiene and nutrition. This lack of self-care increases their vulnerability to disease. In addition, depressed individuals are frequently withdrawn and socially isolated, and so they have weak support systems. The path to a nursing home for these individuals is apt to be very short and direct. It is possible that Ms. F. has depression and if diagnosed earlier and appropriately treated, she may have delayed admission to assisted living.

Some people older than 65 years of age are beginning to face some significant losses: economic, vocational, family supports, and friendships. Physical disabilities are frequently viewed as the beginning of the end. "If you have your health, you have everything," one grandmother reports. The loss of health signals a life of dependency for most older adults. Generally, the most impressive feature of depression is an unpleasant mood. To psychiatrists, the term clinical depression refers to a cluster of specific symptoms. These symptoms are clearly defined in a diagnostic manual called the *Diagnostic and Statistical Manual of Mental Disorders* (DSM).

Depression may be chronic or acute, and the symptoms may vary in intensity. Severe depression is thought to impair cognitive functioning at any age. Memory seems to be the function most influenced by a depressed mood, but there are many ways that memory can be affected. Information committed to memory when a person is depressed is likely to be biased. Other clinicians focus on the ability or lack of ability of older adults to attend to their environment as the indicator of a depression.

An assessment tool used to identify depression in older adults is the Geriatric Depression Scale, Short Form. This tool consists of 15 questions and can be used with patients who are physically ill or have mild to moderate dementia.

Evidence-Based Practice

Waszynski, C.M., & Petrovic, K. (2008). Nurses' evaluation of the Confusion Assessment Method: a pilot study. Journal of Gerontological Nursing, 34(4), 49-56.

The purpose of this study was to examine nurses' evaluation of the usefulness of using the Confusion Assessment Method (CAM) to identify delirium in hospitalized adults in a major metropolitan hospital. The study also assessed the nurses' willingness to evaluate patients' cognitive status beyond the standard orientation of person, place, and time. The study was conducted on 2 units in an 850-bed hospital; a total of 223 patients were assessed using the CAM. The study identified delirium in 18.4% of all patients studied. An interesting result is that 5 of the 25 patients age 40 to 49 years demonstrated "substantial incidence of delirium."

At the end of the study, nurses were asked to evaluate the usefulness of the assessment tool. Of the nurses who participated in the study, 98% agreed that using the CAM was beneficial in identifying delirium in their patients, and many agreed that the tool should be used on each shift to assess the cognitive status of their patients.

Questions

1. As an LPN working in a long-term care facility or home care, how could you incorporate the CAM into your nursing assessments?
2. How would use of this tool change the way in which you would provide care to your patients?

PATIENT EDUCATION

When using tools to assess older adults, it is important to educate them on why the tool is used. The nurse should explain to the older adult that it is an objective method to identify potential problems that may need to be addressed to improve their well-being and their nursing care.

WHEN TO ASSESS

Many hospitals and nursing homes use some sort of standard mental status examination to screen for gross impairments on admission. This is an excellent practice. Although some initial confusion, agitation, or depression is often seen in older adults who are newly admitted because of transitional stress, this practice, if consistently done, helps staff to get a baseline of the person's overall cognitive function. The assessment can be repeated if the older adult exhibits acute changes in behavior, mental status, or functional level—for example, if there is a decline in activities of daily living (ADLs). Although screening tools are not diagnostic—that is, they do not point out the exact nature of the problem—they do show, in a factual way, specific areas that have changed.

Validity and Reliability of Assessment Scales

Whenever a questionnaire is used in any clinical setting, psychologists are concerned about two questions: validity and reliability. Is the test question a valid question? For example, does the question really measure memory, or orientation, or thinking? Validity is determined by the agreement reached by a panel of individuals who are experts in the content of the particular test questions used. The more experts that are involved in designing the process, the greater the validity of the test questions. Reliability is concerned with consistency. Would two nurses, each asking the same person the same questions, get the answers? When the answer to this question is "yes," the test questions are reliable. All standard mental status questionnaires considered in this chapter are valid and reliable instruments. They have been used by a variety of experts for many years with consistent results. Because rating scales are designed to collect standard information about older persons in a methodical way, nurses should review the methods of using the rating scales together. This practice ensures that information is gathered in the same way. One nurse can interview an older adult while another nurse observes. Then they can reverse roles and compare the answers they received. Some experts recommend continuing this technique with 10 patients or until 80% of the ratings are the same.

ASSESSMENT TECHNIQUES

Older adults generally remain cooperative unless they perceive the questions asked as challenging their mental competence. Catastrophic reactions such as screaming or leaving the room angry can be precipitated when a person is pushed to perform beyond the person's competency. An older adult's refusal to answer questions should be accepted. This information in itself is significant. Older persons, aware of their cognitive impairments, may become defensive when their vulnerabilities are exposed. Attention to the following factors promotes the success of the psychological assessment.

Timing

The timing of an interview is an important factor in determining success. Regular staff members, especially nursing assistants in the nursing home setting, are especially skilled in knowing the best time to interview a resident. Allowing an older person to select a time may be the most effective way to gain cooperation.

Privacy

Privacy is very important. Questions that to caregivers may seem routine are often considered deeply revealing and very personal to older persons. All interviews should be conducted in the person's room or in a location that ensures confidentiality. When assessing Ms. F, it is important that you do the assessment in a private room with no family members present.

Elimination of Interruptions

Interruptions undermine the importance of psychological assessments. They negatively affect a person's attention span, and they distract the nurse from focusing on the person being interviewed. Some interruptions are beyond your control as the nurse and occur regardless of the precautions taken. Reasonable efforts should be made to eliminate as many interruptions as possible because they have an impact on the reliability and validity of the assessment.

Positive Introduction of the Assessment

Introducing the psychological assessment in a positive and respectful manner is useful. Describing

---

QSEN

COMPETENCY: Evidence-Based Practice
(Knowledge, Skills, Attitudes)

Incorporating Assessment Tools in Your Practice

As a nurse, it is important for you to recognize the importance of using assessment tools to guide your nursing care. Assessment tools can be used to identify changes in a person's ability from one period to another. They can also be used as a means of communication among health-care workers. Communicating specific information about the patient is important in providing patient-centered care. In the case of cognitive status, a tool can be used to identify changes in that person's cognitive abilities from shift to shift, and changes in the care plan specific to that patient can then be made. Potential safety concerns can also be identified. A nurse needs to become competent in using assessment tools to ensure reliability in the information that is gathered. Practicing using the tools on several patients is the best way to become proficient in using the tools.

 Point of Interest

As an LPN, you should develop polished skills with using assessment tools. Learn to use them well, practice on people many times, and then be prepared to share your skill and knowledge with the interdisciplinary team. This will make you a strong, positive asset to the place where you work.

This nurse is performing a cognitive assessment on an elderly patient.

the test as "a lot of silly questions" may prompt the response that "If they are so silly, why should I answer them?" Let the older adult know that the information gained from this assessment will help the nurses in planning and providing care.

WHAT TO DO WITH THE ASSESSMENT INFORMATION

All information obtained from the older person must be used on the individual's behalf. This information should be dated and appear in an accessible place on the chart with a notation that this document must remain on the chart. Assessment information generally is not updated unless a person exhibits a behavioral problem or has a marked decline in functional level.

Applications in Clinical Practice

In the hospital or nursing home, psychological assessments may be used as one of the factors determining the unit assignment of a new resident on admission. They contribute to the identification of the person's strengths and potentials. When used in conjunction with the person's ability to perform ADLs, psychological assessments may point out the need for psychiatric evaluation. When a person's mental functioning seems much lower than the score of a psychological assessment might indicate, a mental illness is suspected.

Psychological assessments can be used as a basis for care planning. This assessment is especially important when an older adult's social graces lead staff members to conclude that the person is functioning at a higher level than is the case. Many individuals with dementia learn strategies to cover for losses in cognition. They may rely on list making, props in the environment, and social cues from others. Staff members sometimes can make excessive demands on older persons if they are unaware of cognitive deficits.

Psychological assessments can allow a broad determination of the effects of an intervention. For example, a person with sadness, who wishes to die, may be treated with an antidepressant. Effective treatment may enhance the abilities of depressed older persons to attend to their environment, improving memory and perception. On the mental status examination, such people may achieve higher scores in the area of recall. This information is useful to a consultant when a more extensive evaluation is considered necessary. It is helpful to be able to tell a consultant that an older adult has dropped 4 points on Folstein's MMSE because the examination was conducted 6 months earlier. It also is useful to note the specific area of decline—for instance, the area of decline is in orientation to time and place or in immediate recall.

Older adults vary greatly in symptom severity and the rate of progression. Although older persons in the later stages of dementia present similarly regardless of disease process, the initial symptoms may clearly indicate one disease over another. The initial symptom of Alzheimer's disease is the gradual progressive decline in the ability to learn new information. The most significant early symptom of Pick's disease is a change in personality. This is an important distinction.

Symptoms of dementia are a moving target that must be tracked. The tracking is done by frequent, well-recorded assessments. If an assessment tool has been used to establish a baseline in the early stages of the disease process, it may contribute to the diagnostic process.

Observations of a person's behavior and functional status are subjective and often inconsistently reported. It is difficult to get a clear idea of decline or progression over time without objective

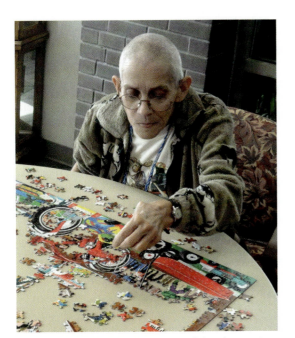

Working a puzzle helps this man with his depression.

Assessments help establish a person's baseline functioning. They can be used to establish a diagnosis, plan care, and evaluate treatment efforts. Psychological assessments also enable the nurse to define problem areas in a more specific manner to consultants. Older adults cooperate well with assessments if the nurse is sensitive to timing, respects the person's privacy, limits interruptions, and presents the assessment tool in a positive manner.

 ## CONCLUSION

Many institutionalized elderly people are well aware of their declining abilities. These losses have a dynamic impact on their self-concept. A life once vital and central to a young family now does not seem worth the effort to maintain. A lowered self-concept and diminished self-esteem complete the picture of physical decline. The process can become circular without the intervention of a caring and knowledgeable staff.

The performance level of most individuals improves in a supportive environment. Recognition and reinforcement of cognitive skills and abilities and of attributes of mental health can positively affect restorative care efforts. Nurses who consistently identify strengths in a factual way are instrumental in improving the quality of life for older adults in their care.

measures. Psychological assessments and other assessment tools provide the means for collecting factual information about older adults.

Brief mental status examinations universally identify assessments of memory and orientation as the two features that provide the most information about an individual's cognitive functions.

CASE STUDY SOLUTIONS

1. The first step you should take is to talk to Ms. F. in a private setting to discuss the noted change in behavior. You want to hear directly from her what she is thinking and feeling. She may just feel the need to spend more time alone, or there may be some issues with the other residents that need to be resolved.

2. Complete a physical assessment to make sure she is not experiencing a physical condition that needs to be managed, such as pain. Also check to see when she had her last hearing examination in case she is having troubles hearing, thereby limiting her ability to participate in conversation. You will also want to complete the Geriatric Depression Scale to see whether she is experiencing some depression. The results of these assessments need to be reported to the registered nurse.

REVIEW QUESTIONS

1. A common tool used to assess delirium in older adults is:
   1. Mini-Cog
   2. Geriatric Depression Scale
   3. MMSE
   4. CAM

2. The nurse practitioner of a unit annually conducts an MMSE on all the residents. She informs you that Mrs. H.'s score in the area of orientation has dropped 2 points from last year. You suspect that the drop is due to:
   1. Delirium
   2. Arthritis
   3. Progression of dementia
   4. Depression

3. The activities department has alerted you to the fact that recently Mr. J. has not been interested in attending programs sponsored by their department. This morning, he complained to you that he believes that he is having problems with his memory. He did not eat breakfast and only picked at his lunch. He denies feeling depressed. You conduct an MMSE. There is a change in score from the admission MMSE conducted 3 months ago. His immediate recall of three objects on Folstein's MMSE has declined. You suspect:
   1. Delirium
   2. Progression of dementia
   3. A urinary tract infection
   4. Depression

4. Mrs. C. does not come out of her room for breakfast. The night shift staff members report that she was up all night and that she has a fever. You go to Mrs. C. to determine whether you can assist her. She seems to be asleep. When you touch her arm, she opens her eyes. She does not quite recognize you, her favorite nurse. She believes that it is bedtime and her main concern is that her husband (who has been dead for 20 years) is late coming home from work. When you leave the room, she returns to "sleep." Yesterday her MMSE score was 30/30. You know immediately that she is:
   1. Depressed
   2. Having a massive stroke
   3. Delirious
   4. Confused, owing to dementia

5. Important considerations when conducting psychological assessments are:
   1. Timing
   2. Privacy and elimination of interruptions
   3. Positive introduction of the assessment
   4. All of the above

REFERENCES

Desai, A.K., Grossberg , G.T., & Chibnall, J.T. (2010). Healthy brain aging: A road map. *Clinical Geriatric Medicine, 26*, 1-16.

Folstein, M.F., Folstein, S.E., & McHugh, P.R. (1975). Mini-mental status: A practice method for grading the cognitive state of patients for the clinician. *Journal of Psychiatric Research*, 12, 189.

Pfeiffer, E. (1975). A short portable mental status questionnaire for the assessment of organic brain deficit in elderly patients. *Journal of American Geriatrics Society*, 23, 433.

Waszynski, C.M., & Petrovic, K. (2008). Nurses' evaluation of the confusion assessment method: A pilot study. *Journal of Gerontological Nursing,* 34(4), 49-56.

WEB RESOURCES

Confusion Assessment Method (CAM): http://consultgerirn.org/uploads/File/trythis/try_this_13.pdf

Geriatric Depression Scale: http://consultgerirn.org/uploads/File/trythis/try_this_4.pdf

Mini-Cog: http://consultgerirn.org/uploads/File/trythis/try_this_3.pdf

Mini Mental State Exam (MMSE): http://www.mountsinai.on.ca/care/psych/on-call-resources/on-call-resources/mmse.pdf

Common Clinical Problems: Psychological

19

TAMARA DAHLKEMPER

LEARNING OUTCOMES

1. Recognize three behaviors that may signal the presence of a psychological problem in an older adult.

2. Explain how to use nursing interventions for older adults with common psychological problems.

3. Describe how to manage difficult behaviors of older adults.

4. Compare reality orientation, reminiscence, remotivation, resocialization, and validation techniques.

5. Select important information about psychological medications to include in teaching.

CONCEPTS

Cognition

Mood and Affect

Stress and Coping

CASE STUDY

Mr. A. is an 80-year-old retired farmer. He lived with his wife on the farm until 1 year ago, when he became too ill for his wife to manage his care alone. At that time, he became a resident of a nursing home in a nearby town. He has been forgetful for several years and now wanders the halls looking for his pickup truck. During the winter, he walked away from the nursing home and wandered for several hours. This resulted in frostbite on several fingers and toes. He becomes agitated when he is told that he cannot go back to his home. What actions can be taken to assist Mr. A.?

 ## INTRODUCTION

Psychological problems are disturbances in mental or emotional health that occur as a result of external or internal stimuli. These problems are usually assessed by examining thought patterns, behaviors, and emotions. Because psychological difficulties are not as obvious as some physical problems that can be diagnosed by laboratory tests, it may be difficult to diagnose and treat older adults with these problems correctly.

Almost any psychological problem that can occur with other age groups also can occur with older adults. It is estimated that approximately 20% of the adult population age 55 years and older have some type of mental health illness. The most common include anxiety, cognitive impairments, and depression (Centers for Disease Control, n.d.). A few common psychological problems found in clinical situations are described in this chapter. A glossary of terms used in this chapter is presented in Box 19.1.

GENERAL GUIDELINES FOR COMMUNICATING WITH OLDER ADULTS

It is helpful to review some basic principles for good communication, particularly as they relate to communicating with an older person with a psychological disorder. It is important to practice the skills outlined throughout this chapter to develop your own style for working in an individualized way with each person in your care.

Forming Relationships With People Who Have Psychological Problems

Generally, relationships have three stages. During each stage, there are concepts with which you should be familiar. At the beginning of a relationship, people sometimes are uncomfortable. After all, they are sick, and you are new to them. As time goes on and trust is established, people enter a stage of the relationship that allows for more open communication that can be therapeutic in its purpose. The last stage of a relationship involves termination or saying goodbye. Problems in relationship-building can be prevented by understanding these normal stages.

Beginning a Relationship

People who have psychological problems may not be easy to get to know initially. They may have had problems starting relationships all of their lives, and forming a relationship with a new nurse might be difficult. Some people with mental illnesses have trouble trusting others and find it difficult to trust a new nurse or a new roommate in a hospital or long-term care facility. There are some things that can be done to help make the beginning of a relationship more comfortable.

If the person with a psychological problem does not talk or becomes upset at first, do not take it personally. The person may be feeling uncomfortable and unsure of how you will react. You, as the nurse, can be creative in dealing with problems such as this and need to respond in a natural way. Some approaches to consider are using humor to diffuse tension or finding an interest of the person's, such as fly tying or crocheting, and asking him or her about it.

Important points to keep in mind are the need to establish trust and not to reject the person. You may need to say to the individual, "It seems like you'd rather not talk right now. I'll come back in an hour and sit here (or at the desk, or at a table) just in case you want to talk to me then."

BOX 19.1 GLOSSARY OF PSYCHOLOGICAL TERMS

Anxiety: Generalized unpleasant feeling of apprehension.

Behavior modification: Treatment method of changing behavior.

Bipolar affective disorder: Psychological disease involving mood swings from mania to depression.

Delirium: Sudden, reversible state of confusion.

Delusion: False, fixed idea or belief.

Disorientation: State of not knowing what day or time it is, or not knowing where one is.

Hallucination: False sensory impression, often seeing or hearing something that is not there.

Illusion: Misperception of a real event or object.

Neurolinguistic programming: A way of communicating using neurological, behavioral, and speech patterns.

Neurotransmitter: A chemical in the brain that carries electrical impulses to neurons.

Paranoia: A way of thinking that systematically interprets others as being intentionally harmful.

Phobia: Exaggerated fear of a particular object or group of objects.

Schizophrenia: Psychological disease involving severe thought and perception disturbances.

Sensory deprivation: Condition of decreased stimulation that can cause hallucinations, illusions, and disorientation.

Social support: Emotional and physical assistance given by loved ones.

Somatization: Extreme preoccupation with physical problems.

 Priority Setting

When working with any person with psychological problems, the absolute priority is *safety*. As a licensed nurse, you are responsible for the safety of each person who is ill as well as the employees and visitors.

1. Some people with mental illness can hurt themselves. The most serious injury that can occur is suicide. The attempt at suicide can result in major injuries such as cuts at the wrist and falls. You must protect such people against their own self-destructive behavior. Suicidal people must be on a "suicide watch," which refers to additional staff caring for them in a smaller and more confined space. With the proper treatment—mainly medication—suicidal people recover, and their underlying condition, depression, is managed.
2. Some people with mental illness try to hurt others. It is their effort at gaining control of their out-of-control lives. Such people could start a physical fight with someone much weaker than themselves, be verbally abusive, or go to extremes to hurt others.

Because you are licensed, you are responsible for what happens on the unit. Be ever diligent; listen to the certified nursing assistants as they work closely with the patients; get to know the patients and develop a relationship of trust with them; then do your best to provide an environment of safety.

Developing a Relationship

Once you have developed a trusting relationship with an older adult, you are ready to be an instrument in the work of healing for a person with psychological problems. With the development of trust, the older person is able to share with you emotions such as fear and anger and the symptoms of more serious illnesses such as delusions or hallucinations. Your responsibility is to listen and guide the discussion.

If the older person has a serious disease, most of the verbal therapy is done in group or private sessions with a psychologist. Your responsibility is to listen, be genuine, and report anything unusual to the registered nurse (RN).

Ending a Relationship

Nurses begin and end relationships with many people every day. Sometimes this happens in small ways, such as taking a weekend off or going away for a conference or vacation. Sometimes it is more permanent, such as discharging a person to another facility or to the home, changing jobs, or saying goodbye to a person who is dying. During this phase of a relationship, people generally try to avoid the termination process. This often is exhibited when the patient ignores you and other staff members or acts out.

If a nurse is going away for a short time, the older adult may start demanding more attention by ringing the call light more frequently, becoming angry or irritated by small things, or not responding or talking. To prevent this from happening, it is best if the person knows as soon as possible when to expect the separation. Provide opportunities for the older adult to talk about it openly with you. If a permanent separation is approaching, some kind of formal farewell, such as a goodbye party, might be helpful. Taking pictures with patients and staff also can help ease the difficulty of a separation. If an older person is being discharged home, do not always assume it is a joyous occasion. Sometimes the situation at home is worse than being in the nursing home or hospital. Even if a person is looking forward to going home, mixed feelings may exist about having to adjust to another new situation. Remember the difficulty of transitional stress.

It is not unusual for a patient who is ready to go home suddenly to become worse. If this happens, it may be a clue to you that the person is having problems with ending his or her present relationships. If you, as the nurse, talk about this openly by sharing feelings, such as "Things just aren't going to be the same around here without you, Mr. M.," the person may be more willing to discuss personal feelings.

Verbal Communication

Communication skills described in general nursing books also can be used successfully with older adults. Some skills are important to emphasize when working with elderly people who have psychological problems. The following discussion includes validation techniques, which are especially useful with disoriented individuals. Validation therapy is discussed in more detail later in the chapter.

Open Questions

Verbal communication can be helpful by using open questions instead of closed questions. A closed question is a question that can be answered with a simple "yes" or "no." An open question tends to encourage the person to talk more. Open questions are asked using such words as "who," "what," "where," "when," and "how." "Why" questions usually are not helpful, especially with someone who is disoriented. Some people with psychological problems may be unable to answer a "why" question logically or rationally. If a resident in a nursing home says she is looking for her mother, you may validate her by asking open questions, such as "What did your mother look like?" "What did you like to talk about with your mother?" "What did you and your mother do together?" If you were to ask, "Why do you want your mother?" the resident likely would be unable to tell you.

Giving Instructions

When giving directions, it is best to do so slowly, one step at a time. Individuals who are disoriented may be unable to perform any self-care activities unless they are prompted by very simple cues. Telling someone who is disoriented to brush his or her teeth may not get any results. If you tell the person to pick up the toothbrush, then pick up the toothpaste, then put the toothpaste on the brush, then put the brush in the mouth, and then brush up and down, the person may be able to do more than you originally thought.

Guided Choices

Some people may not respond to open questions as well as they do to guided choices. When asked, "What would you like to do today?" someone with a psychological problem may not know how to respond. When given a choice between two activities, with choices given one at a time, however, the person may be able to make a choice. An example of guided choices is: "Would you like to go to singing time today, or would you rather go for a walk outside?"

Empathy and Genuineness

When a nurse shows the desire to understand someone, it promotes more meaningful communication. Empathy can be expressed by maintaining eye contact, using a caring tone of voice, listening closely to what someone says, and making statements such as "This must be difficult for you," or "It sounds like you are having a rough time right now."

The opposite of empathy is patronizing a person. Using a tone of voice as if talking to a child is an example of being patronizing. This type of communication keeps the nurse from using empathy and is not helpful in communicating with older adults. Referring to an older person as "honey" or "dearie" is also patronizing and a hindrance to effective communication. Another example of patronizing behavior is referring to an older person in a report to another nurse as a "real cutie" or a "sweetheart."

It is important that the nurse be genuine when showing empathy. Being genuine means that nurses must truly represent themselves. Finding things you sincerely want to say to a person is more important than saying the right thing from a book.

Listening

Listening to someone includes listening to feelings, words, and behaviors. Sometimes people with emotional problems may forget or confuse the facts or use words that do not make sense. When this happens, it is especially important to listen to feelings instead of trying to get the facts straight. If a resident is incomprehensible but is speaking loudly and has tearful eyes, you might respond by saying, "This is extremely frustrating for you."

Another aspect of listening is to ensure the older adult can hear you. A review of the basic principles may help you. Start by placing yourself directly in front of the person. Stand so that there is not a bright light (e.g., a window on a sunny day) behind you so the person can read your lips as well as listen to you. Speak in a normal tone; do not shout even if the person cannot hear you. If you suspect the person is having difficulty hearing you, move closer to the person. Ask permission to move close to one of the person's ears and repeat what you were saying, in a normal tone. If the person seems comfortable with touch, place your hand on a shoulder and express nonverbal acceptance and caring with touch. Remember to smile and do not act rushed even if you are. You may find other successful methods for promoting the older adult's way of listening. If so, use them and share them with others.

Values and Culture

There are many different motivations for behavior during a conversation. Two that can enhance or

Do you recognize the cultural background of this man by looking at him? It is important to gather information quickly on cultures unfamiliar to you so that you can give caring, holistic health care.

interfere with effective communication are the values and culture of the nurse and the older adult. What one person sees as normal may be seen as unacceptable or offensive by a person who has different values or comes from a different cultural background. For example, a nurse who has been educated to value touch as a way of communicating concern and an older adult who perceives touch without permission as an invasion of privacy would have problems with the communication process.

Nurses know that older adults, as with other age groups, come from a wide variety of backgrounds. A Hispanic resident may stand very close while talking to staff members. A staff member who is unaware of this cultural difference may interpret such behavior as being intrusive. An older Japanese person who values modesty may have difficulty talking openly about bowel and bladder problems. Some Native Americans want their shaman, or medicine man, to perform a sacred "sing" to help them heal. This ritual involves music, dance, and numerous family members and friends. To have meaningful communication with older adults, all caregivers need to understand and respect the various differences that can occur because of personal values and cultural behaviors. Review Chapter 9 if you feel you need more information on cultural awareness.

Being patient also is very important. Some nurses have to be available to the older person to whom they are assigned for several days before seeing a positive response. When the results do come and the nurse is able to communicate successfully with the older person, it is a very rewarding experience.

Nonverbal Communication

Psychologists say that nonverbal communication, such as tears or the inability to smile, is the most honest communication a person can make. To be an effective listener, you need to watch and listen to what is being said. Using direct eye contact and a caring tone of voice can help the communication process. Positioning the body at eye level also helps.

Touch

Touching is an important part of communicating with people. Many older people miss human contact and enjoy being touched. A person with psychological problems, however, may become frightened, withdrawn, or agitated if touched. When the nurse touches someone who has an emotional problem, it is a good idea to ask the person first if it would be all right. Saying "Would it be okay if I gave you a hug?" might be a way of asking for permission. Carefully note the response of the person to the question and the actual touch. Some people who are very withdrawn may respond only to touch.

Touch can be used to stimulate sensory memories as well. Different people respond to touch in different ways. Table 19.1 lists common responses to touch. A person who talks about his mother or says "Ma, ma, ma" repeatedly may respond well to stroking on the upper cheek. This stimulates the rooting reflex and can bring back memories of a loving mother. Stroking the upper arm from the shoulder to the elbow is perceived by many people as a universal symbol of friendship. It feels comforting and safe to have someone touch in that way. If a patient is agitated, you can try stroking his or her upper arm while you talk quietly and gently to the patient.

Matching and Mirroring

Research has determined that it helps the communication process if a person can match or mirror another's behavior. Mirroring is doing exactly what the person is doing as if the person were looking into a mirror. Matching is using the same pattern or intensity of tone the person is using. This technique must be done in a respectful way and not as a way of making fun of the individual. If the nurse feels uncomfortable doing this, it is not genuine and does not help communication.

Matching and mirroring are nonverbal ways of helping someone know that you hear what he or she is saying. Matching of emotions can be done by labeling the emotion out loud and using the same intensity used by the older person. Mrs. C. may pound her fist on the arm of her wheelchair and say, "I hate them, I hate them, I hate them." Using matching and mirroring, the nurse would pound on the table with the same rhythm she is using and say, "You're angry, you're angry, you're angry," using the same intensity of emotion.

Universal Symbols

A universal symbol is an object in the present that represents something important from the past. Sometimes these symbols increase in importance for people who develop disorientation as they grow older. The symbol can be something that has meaning to the older person, such as a reminder of

TABLE 19.1 COMMON RESPONSES OF DISORIENTED OLDER ADULTS TO TOUCH

Remind Client of	Touch Technique
Mother	Palm of hand in a light circular motion on the upper cheek
Father	Fingertips, in a circular motion, medium pressure, on the back of the head
Spouse/lover	Hand under the earlobe, curving along the chin, with both hands, a soft stroking motion downward along the jaw
Child	Cupped fingers on the back of the neck, with both hands, in a small circular motion
Brother or sister or good friend	Full hand on the shoulders and upper back by the shoulder blades; use full pressure in a rubbing movement
Animals or pets	Fingertips on the inside of the calf

From Feil, N. (1989). *Validation: The Feil Method.* Cleveland, OH: Edward Feil Productions, pp. 47–48, with permission.

a hobby or life's work, or it can be a different type of symbol. Some typical symbols are listed in Table 19.2. An apron can be made with a large pocket in the front that can contain significant symbols. A farmer may touch farm tools placed in the pocket of an apron and by doing this revive a memory of a time in life he enjoyed. As the farmer touches the tools, the nurse can encourage communication using these symbols of his previous life. Think about Mr. A in the case study. Is this a technique that might work to help Mr. A?

Problem Behaviors

If a person with a psychological problem begins to display any unusual behaviors, it may be due to numerous different causes. Recent changes in relationships may contribute to increased wandering, shouting, and aggressive or withdrawn behaviors. These behaviors are common after a room or roommate change or when the person is becoming accustomed to new staff members.

 Point of Interest

In all likelihood, you will not eagerly want to use the touch techniques just described. This is a test of courage of sorts. These touch techniques have a powerful impact on people with dementia. You need to have the courage to step into the situation and give the techniques a try. What if you use the rooting reflex touch on a resident and the person reacts loudly and with fear or anger? Don't walk away and say that technique never works. Instead, critically examine what has happened and consider what the mother of the older person did to cause such a strongly negative reaction so many years later. You have learned something important about the person by using this technique: The mother was not a positive influence in the older person's life, and the issues surrounding the mother may need to be resolved for the older adult.

TABLE 19.2 UNIVERSAL SYMBOLS AND WHAT THEY CAN MEAN

Symbol	Possible Meaning
Jewelry, clothing	Worth, identity
Shoe	Container, womb, male or female sex symbol
Purse	Female sex symbol, vagina, identity
Cane or fist	Penis, potency, power
Soft furniture	Safety, mother, home
Hard furniture	Father, God
Napkin, tissue	Earth, belonging, baby
Flat object	Identity
Food	Love, mother
Drink from a glass	Male power, potency
Any receptacle	Womb
Picking the nose	Sexual pleasure
Playing with feces	Early childhood pleasures

From Feil, N. (1989). *Validation: The Feil Method*. Cleveland, OH: Edward Feil Productions, p. 73, with permission.

These behavioral changes also may indicate that a medication change needs close monitoring or that symptoms of the person's illness are becoming more acute.

When you are caring for a person who is exhibiting difficult behavior, you need to take special precautions. Be alert to any situation that would place you, the older adult, or other patients in danger. Report anything suspicious to the RN, and stay calm.

All persons with psychological problems do not act in a dangerous way. Some sit quietly and never talk or move. This person needs your attention and expertise as well. Talk gently and kindly to the person. Sit with this quiet individual even if there is no conversation. Touch the person if it seems acceptable. All of these simple acts indicate acceptance of the person and are important for healing.

What should you do if an older adult is "yelling" at you? First, do not respond with anger. Stay calm. Be empathetic and kind. Listen to what is being said to identify what the problem really is. Get help if you need it. Be alert to what is going on throughout the unit and with the individuals in your care.

Some older adults with psychological disorders have hallucinations, delusions, and illusions. These are symptoms of serious mental illness. People exhibiting these symptoms may think that they are Jesus Christ, or they may see bugs crawling all over their arms, or they may think you are a princess and want to wait on you. When dealing with such problems, the first rule is to stay calm. The next most important thing is to tell the truth. Do not play into the symptom by saying, "Yes, I am Princess Laura," or something of that nature. Be caring, honest, and genuine with the person. If you feel uncomfortable or in danger, get help; this is never a wrong response.

 AGITATION

Agitation can occur as a result of physiological or psychological problems. Some people become agitated because of physical causes that result in delirium. Common psychological problems that can cause agitation are the manic phase of bipolar affective disorder, stress or anxiety, flashbacks from traumatic experiences, reactions following abuse, or dementia. When people become agitated, they also may become violent. Such violence can be directed toward themselves or others. Preventing agitation and managing it when it occurs can be accomplished by following a few simple principles, as follows:

• Watch for signs of agitation. Some people show signs of increasing irritability before a severe problem occurs. Others may have sudden, explosive outbursts. Notice if someone is talking very loudly, pacing more or faster, or making threatening comments to staff or others. Before an actual outburst occurs, try to keep the person talking to you by using some of the communication skills discussed in this chapter. With many people who are agitated, simply matching their breathing patterns or tone of voice is calming. With most people who are agitated, it is best to step back about 4 to 6 feet while talking with them. With disoriented elderly people, the reverse may be true, especially if a sensory deficit is present. It may be more calming to move closer to maintain sustained eye contact and touch. This movement must be done cautiously to protect your own safety and that of others. If there is the possibility that other patients or visitors may be harmed, move them out of the way.
• If a person becomes physically aggressive, it is important to remember that the thumb is the weakest point of the hand. If a person has a

hold on you, the way to remove yourself is by rotating away from the thumb of the person's hand. Most psychiatric facilities provide training sessions that allow you to practice dealing with these behaviors in a way that minimizes harm to yourself and protects the agitated person.

Dealing With Psychological Problems Caused by Stress

This section provides some general guidelines for dealing with older adults with psychological problems who are experiencing stressful situations. Making an extra effort to assign the same staff members to an older person in the hospital and in the nursing home may help to prevent emotional distress. A hospitalized patient may be assigned six different nurses during a 3-day stay. The sheer number of names to remember is difficult, but it is especially challenging for an older adult with emotional problems.

In addition to the "normal" stress of being admitted to a hospital or nursing home, an older

Reminiscence is an excellent tool to use to strengthen an older person's self-esteem.

person with psychological problems has to deal with whatever illness caused the admission and the symptoms of the psychological illness. An example is a person who has hallucinations. Hallucinations are real to the person experiencing them, and they add a tremendous level of confusion to the daily life of the person. Hallucinations interfere with one's ability to perceive information accurately. The nurse's instructions or even a greeting may be misinterpreted; medications may look like spiders; walls and doorways may keep moving. The approach to such problems includes keeping the same caregiver with the patient throughout his or her stay. The nurse will begin to understand the behaviors of the older adult and be able to work within the limitations of the mental illness of the person.

It also helps when an older person's familiar belongings can be kept in the room; this promotes self-worth and helps to prevent disorientation. Small objects and pictures can be placed near the older person during a hospitalization to prevent the disorientation that can accompany stressful changes during an illness. Playing taped music of familiar songs generally is better than television viewing in preventing sensory overload. These are just a few examples of simple nursing interventions that can be used to prevent psychological problems caused by stress in older adults.

Violent Behavior

If older adults start to act violently, the nurse must remember to protect these individuals from their own behavior at all times. The nurse needs to call for help and, as a member of a team, decide what the intervention should be. Do not raise your voice; stay calm. These are the basic rules for handling someone who is violent.

Some violent behavior can be life-threatening. If you are in that type of situation, slowly gather any endangered patients and take them to safety. There is no formula for what to do in every possible situation. Simply stay calm and safeguard the patients and yourself.

Sexual Acting Out

Acting out feelings of anxiety may take many forms. Sometimes older adults with dementia lose social controls and express sexual feelings openly. Some people, such as individuals in the early stages of Alzheimer's disease, have an increased desire for sexual activity. People with other types of psychological problems, such as bipolar affective disorder, show sexual feelings in ways that are socially inappropriate. Dealing with these behaviors is almost always difficult, no matter how experienced the nurse is. Always consider if the acting out is an expression of the need for affection and touch. Notice any factors that seem to trigger the behavior to intervene before the behavior occurs.

SPECIALIZED COMMUNICATING SKILLS

The hallmark of nursing care for persons with psychological problems is the ability to communicate effectively. In addition to the skills just described in this chapter, there are other communication skills that can be used to make it easier to talk to older people with psychological problems. Some standard communication skills and concepts from the Validation Method (Feil and Klerk-Rubin, 2014) are described in this section.

The Validation Method, a communication approach for relating to disoriented older adults, helps disoriented persons express themselves. Sometimes communication with someone who is disoriented is blocked by the listener's need to have the disoriented person think or talk in a "logical" way. When the listener is able to put aside the need to communicate in a normal way, it becomes possible to communicate in other, more effective ways. The listener becomes able to understand and validate the disoriented person's experiences.

Preferred Sense Words

All people relate to their surroundings through their senses. Most people respond more through one sense than through others. How a person talks can give an idea of that person's preferred sense. If Mrs. J. says, "I see what you mean. Look at this," she probably is a person who responds best to sight or visual words. Some people respond best to hearing or auditory words, and others respond best to words about feelings or movement (kinesthetic words). Table 19.3 lists commonly used visual, auditory, and kinesthetic words. The nurse can use the person's preferred sense to establish rapport. If an older adult says, "No one listens to me anymore," a response such as "What would you like for me to listen to, Mr. J.?" would

receive a better response than "What would you like me to see, Mr. J.?"

Vague Pronouns

If a person is unable to fill in the details with enough facts to be understood, try using vague or ambiguous pronouns to help foster communication. Sometimes people refer to all women as "she" and all men as "he." If the nurse becomes too concerned about accurate details, the opportunity to communicate may be lost. Instead of worrying about the facts, such as who "he" or "she" is, try to focus on the feelings. If an older person says, "She's all alone. She can't stay there," you can respond, "You're worried about her. She's important to you." That type of sensitive response generally elicits more communication.

Speaking Slowly

Many people who have emotional problems have slowed thought processes. When this problem is combined with normal aging changes, it is very important for the nurse to use slightly slower speech and wait a little longer for the person to respond. Asking questions one at a time, instead of running several questions together, can also make it easier to talk to an older person with an emotional problem.

Asking the Extreme

When someone who is disoriented is upset about something he or she thinks happened, ask questions about the extremes of the situation. What is the worst? What is the best? Imagine the opposite. When is it better? When does it not happen? Suppose every night an elderly woman thinks some men are coming to attack her. The nurse might ask, "When do they usually come? When are they not there? What helps you feel safe? What doesn't help you very much?" Often by looking at the extreme of a situation, the person can recognize what is happening in the "here and now."

GRIEVING AND DEPRESSION

Surviving losses is part of the aging process. An older person may lose relationships with people through death, retirement, or relocation, or he or she may lose the ability to maintain contacts with friends and family because of physical problems. An older adult also may experience the loss of valued social roles, a home, financial security, vision,

TABLE 19.3   COMMONLY USED PREFERRED SENSE WORDS

Visual	Auditory	Kinesthetic
See	Listen	Feel
View	Hear	Grasp
Picture	Sound	Move
Look	Loud	Touch

hearing, or other body functions. The loss of a loved one is one of the most powerful losses a person can experience.

Dealing With Grief

It is helpful to keep in mind the stages of the grieving process—denial, anger, bargaining, depression, and acceptance—when dealing with losses (see Chapter 11). These stages do not always occur with every person. Some people who experience losses may become angry but not go through the other stages. As a nurse, it is important to accept each person's response to grief and not have a preconceived idea of how a person should respond.

If an older adult is grieving over the loss of a job, the nurse can help him or her to talk about the grief by asking open-ended questions, such as "What did you do at your former job?" "When did you start working there?" "How did you get started working there?" Asking open-ended questions about feelings also can help another to express grief. Sometimes it can be uncomfortable to hear a person talk about negative emotions such as anger and sadness. Encouraging someone to express feelings and allowing expressions of anger or crying can help that person deal with feelings effectively. Saying something like, "How did you feel about that?" or "What upset you the most about that?" can encourage someone to talk about feelings. Telling someone who is sad and grieving "Don't cry now, it will be all right" only gives false reassurance and tells the person to keep such powerful emotions inside. If emotions are not expressed, they tend to be expressed later in dysfunctional ways, such as extreme anger, agitation, or withdrawal. Mr. A. is grieving the loss of his farm and home. Because he is unable to verbalize his feelings, he is expressing his feelings by showing signs of agitation.

Depression

Depression in later life is usually triggered by a life event such as illness, placement in a nursing home, or loss of a loved one (see Table 19.4). It can also be a relapse of depression earlier in life. Approximately 25% of older adults experiencing one or more chronic illnesses are depressed. These chronic illnesses include heart disease, stroke, cancer, arthritis, Alzheimer's disease, and Parkinson's disease. Depression also occurs in 50% of older adults living in long-term care facilities (Geriatric

TABLE 19.4 RISK FACTORS FOR DEPRESSION

Medications

Grieving

Loneliness

Alcohol and substance abuse

Changes in environment

Previous episodes of depression

Lowe socioeconomic status

Loss of independence

Loss of functional status

Chronic medical illness or disability

Mental Health Foundation, 2014). Although depression in older adults is underdiagnosed, it is the most treatable psychological disorder.

When the effects of the losses of aging are combined with the effects of physical risk factors, it is clear why many elderly people are depressed. The good news is that most people who have depression can be helped by antidepressants and psychotherapy. Antidepressants that are used to treat depression are generally effective.

Tricyclic antidepressants were widely prescribed in the past and are still effective for many people. Major problems with using tricyclic antidepressants are anticholinergic side effects such as constipation, urinary retention, hypotension, and tachycardia.

With the advent of serotonin-selective reuptake inhibitors such as citalopram (Celexa), fluoxetine (Prozac), paroxetine (Paxil), and sertraline (Zoloft), safer treatment options are available for people who have depression. Another antidepressant used very effectively with many elderly people is bupropion (Wellbutrin), but it is contraindicated in individuals with seizure disorders (Tabloski, 2007).

Medications are an important part of treating depression but are most successful when used in conjunction with other types of therapy. Psychotherapy with a therapist educated to work with older adults can help the person develop coping skills for dealing with depression.

Along with psychotherapy and antidepressants, older adults should maintain good health habits. as this can have a positive impact on mood. Older adults should be encouraged to participate in regular physical activity and maintain a nutritional diet. For older adults with physical limitations, it may be difficult to participate in regular activity. Likewise, older adults with physical limitations or financial issues may find it difficult to provide a nutritious diet. The nurse should assess an older adult's needs and provide opportunities for some form of activity and a healthy diet for the older adults in their care.

Refer to Chapter 18 for information on assessing for depression.

Depression and Confusion in the Elderly Person

Assessing someone who is depressed is complicated by factors that occur as a result of normal aging. Chapter 18 describes how to assess someone with depression and how to use standard measures of depression. Some of the behaviors seen in people with depression may be very similar to behaviors seen with other problems that are common in older people. Individuals who are depressed may not care about their surroundings and begin to be disoriented and confused as they draw inward. It can be very difficult to know whether the mental slowing and memory loss attributed to depression are actually caused by the depression or represent changes commonly found in the early stages of dementia. Many elderly people who have depression are thought to have dementia and are not treated for their depression (see Table 19.5).

Depression and Suicide

Assessing for the risk of suicide is essential for someone who is depressed. The suicide rate among older adults is high. It may not seem likely that an older person would have thoughts about suicide, but it happens too frequently. If an older person says something like "I just don't want to live anymore," the tendency may be to discount the person and say, "Oh, you don't mean that," or "You'll feel better tomorrow, you're just having a bad day." If a person expresses a wish to die, makes funeral plans, has a major change in life, or begins to give away cherished possessions, these can be signs that the person may be planning suicide.

Asking people whether they are having thoughts about killing themselves is not "putting the thought into their heads." Many people are relieved to talk to someone about suicide if asked in a calm, matter-of-fact manner. Finding out whether the person has a plan and what it is are essential pieces of information. If a homebound older adult describes a hoard of potassium supplements or cardiac medications that are readily available, and if the person's conversation indicates a plan to take the medication after the nurse leaves, the situation requires immediate action. Persons who say they do not want to live but have not thought about how they would end their lives are at a much lower risk for an immediate suicide attempt than persons who have a plan. Many incidents of so-called noncompliance with medications are actually intentional attempts to overdose. If an older adult is having thoughts about suicide,

TABLE 19.5   DIFFERENCES AMONG DELIRIUM, DEMENTIA, AND DEPRESSION

	Delirium	Dementia	Depression
Onset	Rapid	Slow	Rapid
Duration	Short	Long	Short or long
Night symptoms worsen	May worsen	Frequently worsen	Usually do not
Cognitive functions	Variable	Stable	Variable
Physical causes	Common	None	Possible
Recent changes	Common	None or minimal	Common
Suicidal ideation	Rare	Rare	Common
Low self-esteem	Rare	Rare	Common
History of psychiatric symptoms	Not usually	Rare	Common
Mood	Labile	Labile	Depressed
Behavior	Labile	Labile	Slowed thought and motor processes

Critically Examine the Following

Many people believe that depression is not an actual illness and that the depressed person just needs to deal with it and get on with life. What are your thoughts about individuals who suffer from depression? Do you have anyone in your life who has depression? How has it impacted their life and those around them? After learning about depression, have you changed your views?

listen carefully, intervene immediately if necessary, and refer the person for treatment.

Failure to Thrive

The term *failure to thrive* is most often applied to young children who do not grow and develop as expected. Some elders who are depressed also may have a failure to thrive or a giving-up complex. This may be the case when the older person no longer makes an effort to continue with life, such as by refusing to eat, refusing medications, or choosing to resist or refuse treatment for health problems. If there is not an intervention that involves the interdisciplinary team and the family, the older adult may die in this situation.

 ### DELIRIUM AND DEMENTIA

Because depression can cause some confusion and disorientation, it can be difficult to determine whether the older person has a problem with delirium, dementia, or depression (see Table 19.5). Many factors influence a person's ability to think clearly.

Emotional stress and change can cause anyone to have difficulty remembering scheduled appointments or to be distracted easily from activities of daily living, such as turning off the burner when cooking. Sometimes physical factors such as illness, insufficient oxygen, or high or low blood glucose levels may cause a person to show signs of confusion. A person who has a problem with disorientation can be found in any setting. When a person becomes disoriented, the caregivers may become resigned to the problem and consider this to be a normal part of the aging process. That is not a correct assumption. Clarification of the differences between delirium and dementia can provide guidance for effective intervention in both situations.

Delirium

Delirium refers to a situation in which an older person has a rapid change in behavior and thinking ability. Mental status changes that occur with this acute problem usually affect an individual's ability to recall where he or she is, what day or time it is, or even the individual's own name. Delirium may cause agitation or rapidly changing moods. Someone who is delirious commonly has an anxious facial expression. Short-term memory may or may not be intact. With delirium, the older adult pays little attention to surroundings or may respond slowly to new surroundings.

A person with delirium usually talks in a rambling way that does not make sense. The individual may have difficulty staying awake, or the individual could have increased activity and be awake all the time. Sensory and perceptual disorders, such as hallucinations and delusions, may be present. A person with delirium may perceive that a nurse holding a syringe has a knife or that a baby is crying when no baby is there. Changes in thought content and process also may be present. Fixed ideas or beliefs as well as disjointed or flighty thoughts may be evident.

Delirium can result from various physiological causes and can be reversed. Malnutrition, electrolyte imbalance, infection, change in blood glucose, hypoxia, drug reactions, pain, sensory deficit, and dehydration are common causes of delirium. Delirium can also result from excessive environmental noise, unfamiliar surroundings or people, use of restraints, and excessive bedrest. It is important to determine what is causing the delirium because the sooner the problem can be treated, the sooner the delirium resolves. Refer to Chapter 18 for information on assessing for delirium.

When an older adult has a period of delirium, it can be very upsetting for the family and nursing staff. Explaining what is happening to all involved can help reduce stress and make it easier for everyone to handle the problem behaviors that occur.

Think Like a Nurse

A 75-year-old man who has just had surgery develops delirium, is agitated, and tries to pull out his nasogastric tube. How will you respond to this situation?

PATIENT EDUCATION

An important part of providing patient education is also educating family members. When an individual is experiencing delirium it can be stressful for family members who may not understand why their loved one is behaving in such a manner. The nurse should inform the family that the behavior is temporary and once the underlying reason for the delirium is addressed, the behavior will stop.

Family members should be encouraged to maintain a quiet environment and limit the number of visitors during an episode of delirium. The goal is to provide a stress-free environment for the older adult.

Dementia

The symptom of dementia is usually defined as the loss of intellectual abilities to the extent that it interferes with normal activities of daily living. Dementia is characterized by problems with cognitive ability, personality changes, memory impairment, decreased intellectual functioning, and changed judgment and mood.

Dementia usually occurs gradually, over months or years, and is the result of deterioration of the brain. Neurological diseases such as Pick's disease or Huntington's disease can cause this damage, or the damage can be the result of vascular problems such as multi-infarct dementia. Advanced AIDS also has an associated dementia. The most common type of dementia is associated with Alzheimer's disease (AD). It is estimated that in the future dementia will outweigh heart disease and cancer as a major health problem. This estimate is based on the growing number of elderly people in the population and the strong correlation between aging and AD.

Because dementia is such a significant concern, new approaches to dealing with this problem are being examined. Validation therapy is a way of communicating with people who have dementia (Feil and Klerk-Rubin, 2014). Validation means respecting the feelings of the person and confirming that, from the individual's perspective, the experience is true.

The Validation Method is being used in many countries for people who are disoriented to decrease stress, to promote self-esteem and communication, to reduce use of chemical and physical

Evidence-Based Practice

Dong, X., Simon, M.A., Wilson, R.S., Mendes de Leon, C.F., Rajan, B., & Evans, D.A. (2010). Decline in cognitive function and risk of elder self-neglect: Finding from the Chicago Health Aging Project. Journal of the American Geriatrics Society, 58, 2292-2299.

This study examined the association between decline in cognitive function and risk of elder self-neglect in older adults living in the community. The sample consisted of 1,017 older adults reported to social service agencies for suspected elder self-neglect from 1993 to 2005. Elder self-neglect is defined as the behavior of an elder person that threatens his or her own health and safety. Self-neglect usually manifests as the person's inability or refusal to provide housing, food, water, personal hygiene, clothing, and basic safety. The study showed an association between the decline in cognitive function and a greater risk in self-neglect; however, the association was small, and the researchers suggest that further research is needed. One potential area of research should address the possibility that elder self-neglect may be the cause of cognitive decline.

1. What assessment tool or tools will you use to assess for a decrease in cognitive function?
2. When working with older adults in the community, how will you assess for potential self-neglect?

restraint, and to make it possible to sustain independent living for a longer time.

A brief introduction to the Validation Method follows. More information on communication strategies is given later in this chapter.

Stages of Disorientation

Naomi Feil (2014) has described four stages of disorientation that occur with people who are "old-old" (older than 80 years of age). Disorientation is a term used by Feil to describe symptoms associated with late-onset Alzheimer's disease. These changes occur in people who have had fairly normal lives until they reach their 80s, when they begin to show signs of disorientation. The stages are malorientation, time confusion, repetitive motion, and vegetation.

MALORIENTATION

Malorientation is the first stage of disorientation. People who are maloriented may initially appear as if nothing is wrong with them. These people may be oriented as to where they are and who the president of the United States is, but they are beginning to forget information important for maintaining normal activities of daily living. They may try to cover up their memory loss by making up excuses. They do not like to be around people who are disoriented because they are threatened by their own memory loss. They deny their feelings and blame other people for their problems.

People who are maloriented respond best to open questions about facts, not feelings. It is important to hold on to acceptable social roles and rules for people who are maloriented. Encouraging someone who has been a teacher to lead the Pledge of Allegiance may be a way of helping maintain dignity and promote self-esteem. Often, the technique of using commonly preferred sense words assists this person to relate to the caregiver. It is best to listen to a maloriented person until you identify what the person's preferred sense is and then address the person with words that represent that sense. For example, someone who often says, "Oh, yes, I see what you mean," probably is a visual person and may respond to visual words better than to other choices (see Table 19.3).

TIME CONFUSION

As people become more disoriented, they withdraw more from the real world and retreat into their own inner world. During this stage, people lose a sense of real time and respond to an inner sense of time.

A person may think about his or her mother (who is dead) and because past time has fused with present time talk about her as if she was present. Because the nurse feels a need to orient the time-confused person, he or she might say something like, "Your mother is dead; you can't go to see her." This only agitates and distresses the individual, who has no real need to stay in a painful present reality. Using the validation approach, the nurse would move close, use touch, and say, "You miss your mother. What color eyes did she have? Blue or brown?" This is an effort to stimulate pleasant thoughts and memories for the person. There are several different methods of touching a person with dementia that are designed to evoke feelings about a loved one. See Table 19.1 to review common forms of touch.

REPETITIVE MOTION

If people with dementia continue to retreat from present reality, they may enter the stage of repetitive motion. During this stage, movements or sounds are repeated constantly. Usually, speech is limited to single-syllable words, and eye contact is made only after someone touches and talks to the person. The use of touch with these people is very important. Individuals with repetitive motion are often ignored emotionally, with caregivers providing physical care only. Validation techniques of sustained eye contact, stroking, and touching can help reach people in this stage of disorientation and prevent the final stage, which is that of vegetation. When persons are in the repetitive motion stage, they often communicate through universal symbols. These people use objects to represent thoughts. A common example is carefully folding and holding or caressing a napkin, which could represent a baby. Other examples are given in Table 19.2.

VEGETATION

The final stage of disorientation and withdrawal is vegetation. In this stage, very little movement or sound is noted. Eye contact is very rare. Using touch and familiar music can help reach a person in this stage.

Alzheimer's Disease

Alzheimer's disease is an irreversible, progressive brain disease. It involves parts of the brain that control thought, memory, and language and can profoundly affect a person's ability to carry out daily activities. In most people with Alzheimer's disease, symptoms first appear after age 60 and the risk increases with age. Alzheimer's disease is the most common cause of dementia among the elderly. As many as 5 million Americans suffer from Alzheimer's disease (National Institute on Aging, n.d.). Although younger people may develop Alzheimer's disease, it is much less common. Nearly half of those age 85 and older may have the disease. It is important to note, however, that Alzheimer's disease is not a normal part of the aging process.

Plaques and protein tangles that develop in the brain are two of the main features of Alzheimer's disease that are responsible for the changes in cognitive abilities. There probably is not one single cause of the disease, but several factors that can affect each person differently. Age is the most important known risk factor for Alzheimer's disease. Family history is another risk factor. Scientists are also researching the role that high blood pressure,

FOCUSED LEARNING CHART

Stages of disorientation in persons with dementia

Malorientation	Time Confusion	Repetitive Motion	Vegetation
1st Stage	2nd Stage	3rd Stage	4th Stage
Appear normal	Ambulatory, but confused	Generally non-ambulatory	Bedridden
Forgetful regarding day-to-day information	Withdrawn from real world and retreat to own inner world	Retreat from present reality	Vegetative state
Make excuses to cover up memory loss	Respond to inner sense of time (childhood, newly married)	Use objects to represent thoughts; make sounds, not words, or just single-syllable words	No words or eye contact and very little movement
Ask open questions about facts, not feelings; use commonly preferred sense words (Table 19.3)		Use touch (Table 19.1) and universal symbols (Table 19.2)	Use touch and familiar music to comfort

increased levels of cholesterol, and blood glucose play in developing Alzheimer's disease.

Lack of communication between the neurons may cause inappropriate or demanding behavior. For example, a patient may not understand the need for appropriate toileting needs. They may not remember the steps on how to undress in order to bathe. Often times, the elderly adult with AD may become combative or uncooperative. The anger can be a mask for his confusion and anxiety. A person with AD may constantly follow his spouse or caregiver around and fret when the person is out of sight. The world can be strange and terrifying to a person who cannot remember the past or predict the future. Having a trusted and familiar caregiver close by may be the only thing that provides security and peace of mind. Having a set routine also helps the person with AD cope with the uncertainty. Many patients with AD do not like to be in unfamiliar environments and will often refuse to leave the comforts of their home or room. Understanding of the person with AD and his or her frustrations with the loss of control of behavior and physical abilities is very important.

Although medication and brain exercises can help manage symptoms in some people, currently there is no cure for this devastating disease. Researchers are continuing to examine the evidence for physical, mental, and social activities as protective factors against Alzheimer's disease.

PARANOIA

Some people with emotional problems fear that other people are trying to hurt them. Such paranoid ideas are an indication of problems the person may have with trusting others. This paranoia can occur with several forms of dementia, Parkinson's disease, or other psychological disorders. Paranoia is an early symptom of Alzheimer's disease. People who are paranoid often seem very convincing and logical. Developing trust is the priority with someone who is paranoid. Being consistent and reliable in all that you do with the person can be the best way to develop trust. Do not make promises you cannot keep. If you say you will do something, following up with the paranoid person is especially important. It is also important to identify potential stressful situations and alleviate the situation when possible to decrease anxiety. It is particularly important to avoid putting medicines in food or drink without the paranoid person's knowledge.

 ## DEVELOPMENTAL DISABILITIES

Historically, people who had developmental disabilities did not live to an old age. With advances in health care, more individuals who have developmental disabilities, such as Down's syndrome, are living longer. There is evidence that as individuals with Down's syndrome grow older, they are at high risk of developing Alzheimer's disease.

Individuals with developmental disabilities may have some of the problem behaviors that have been identified in this chapter. Principles for setting limits on behavior include the following:

• Recognize the person's feelings and encourage expression of them.
• State the limit clearly.
• Point out ways that behavior can be expressed within the limits and what is outside the limits.
• Allow the person to express anger at having limits placed on him or her.

SUBSTANCE ABUSE

Health care workers who are working with people who have chemical dependency problems recognize that there are a growing number of older adults with substance abuse problems. Because many older people are treated for a wide variety of physical problems, sometimes they receive prescription drugs from several different sources. The availability of prescription drugs contributes to the problem of drug abuse among older persons.

Alcoholism is another problem for many elderly adults. Many of the same reasons that people use substances to self-medicate (e.g., depression, losses, loneliness) in other stages of life are even more of a problem for elderly people. Because many

memory lapses found with substance abuse are similar to the memory lapses in the early stages of dementia, substance abuse may not be discovered until it is advanced. Sometimes families have difficulty confronting older family members about substance abuse problems. The denial of a problem, which is characteristic of most substance abuse problems, is especially difficult to deal with when working with older adults. This situation creates a problem with the treatment process. If a substance abuse problem is suspected, it is best to contact trained professionals to assist with interventions.

 ## GROUPS FOR THE ELDERLY

Many older adults with psychological problems can benefit from group interactions. Some types of group therapy that have been used successfully with older persons are discussed next.

Reminiscence

Based on memories of similar events or experiences, many older adults form bonds in groups. Stimulating memories of childhood or early adulthood can serve to improve feelings of self-worth and provide an opportunity to review their lives. Memories may stimulate laughter and happiness or other emotions and serve as a way of coping with present circumstances. Groups can be conducted around an important event, such as Pearl Harbor Day. Common, shared experiences, such as early school days, can be recalled to promote socialization and provide mental stimulation. Reminiscence also can be used individually as a means of helping people process any unfinished business in their lives.

A very structured form of reminiscence is the life review process. This process provides an opportunity for evaluation and integration of life experiences. People in more advanced stages of disorientation are unable to benefit from this type of therapy.

Remotivation

To improve interest in and quality of life, remotivation techniques can be used. The emphasis with remotivation is the use of real objects to stimulate senses and provide new motivation in life and the surrounding world. Pictures, plants, animals, or sounds can be used to encourage group interaction. Because Mr. A. was a farmer, he may benefit from a group garden. Holidays, birthdays, or hobbies can be used to focus on participating in the here and now. The focus is on factual information as opposed to exploration of feelings. These groups work best with people who have depression or early stages of disorientation.

Resocialization

Encouraging residents to assume social roles can stimulate feelings of increased self-esteem. The focus for this group is on social roles and not on problem-solving. Discussion may occur about previous social gatherings and how people behaved during these events. The emphasis is on the present and on the discussion of factual information.

Many older adults with psychological problems can benefit from group interactions. Group members are assigned roles, such as the greeter, or to serve each other refreshments. Feelings are not the focus of resocialization groups, which can be helpful for mildly disoriented individuals.

Reality Orientation

The goal of reality orientation is to help residents become oriented to present reality. Constant reminders about the present—that is, where they are and what day it is—are given. Current events on the television or in the newspaper can be used as topics to stimulate discussions. The season of the year, holidays, and the weather are other topics to promote orientation to reality. These groups are focused on keeping people oriented to present reality and are not usually very effective with people who have more than mild disorientation.

Validation

Validation groups combine some of the other types of techniques with group problem-solving and a focus on support. Members are assigned roles, sing familiar songs, serve each other refreshments, and reminisce about the past. Movement is encouraged during group activities. The group is presented with a problem to solve. Resolving losses and expressing feelings are emphasized. Validation groups are most effective for people who have moderate disorientation.

 ## PSYCHOTROPIC MEDICATIONS

As with all medications, adaptation is necessary when using psychotropic medications with an older adult. Teaching the older person and his or her family about the reason for the medication, side effects, toxic effects, and what to do if a dose is missed are very important when psychotropic drugs are used.

Many psychotropic drugs require time—sometimes several weeks—before a therapeutic effect is achieved. This waiting period may be longer for some older people. Older people may show more signs of toxicity at lower-than-usual doses because their ability to excrete the drug is impaired, resulting in a buildup of the drug in the bloodstream. Older people could also be more difficult to treat because of side effects that occur secondary to the difference in distribution and excretion of drugs in the aging body.

This group of older adults is being led in a resocialization group. Many older adults with psychological problems benefit from group interaction.

Psychotropic medications work in the brain in various ways. Most medications work by helping to change the level of neurotransmitters or chemicals in the brain. It is hoped that reestablishing a more normal balance will help the person have fewer psychological problems. Because these drugs work on the brain, it is important to use them only for psychological problems and not just because the resident has behaviors that irritate other people. Before any drugs are used to sedate a person with problem behaviors, all other types of nursing interventions must be used along with documentation of the interventions.

Because of physical health problems, some medications used to treat mental health problems may be contraindicated or may require careful administration in the older patient.

A common side effect of many psychotropic drugs is constipation. When combined with normal aging changes, the constipation resulting from psychotropic medications can become a problem for the elderly person.

Orthostatic hypotension results from many psychotropic drugs. Simple teaching techniques can help manage some of the postural blood pressure changes; however, these changes often are severe enough to require that the medication be discontinued.

PHYSICAL AND MENTAL HEALTH

Because there is such a strong relationship between physical and mental health, many professionals believe that all diseases have physical and emotional aspects. Some older people grew up in a time when it was frowned on to admit that mental illness existed, but it was more socially acceptable to have a physical problem. One grandmother described a time early in her marriage when she became so upset with her husband that she became "sick" and took to her bed for a week.

This expression of emotional problems through physical complaints is called somatization. If a stressful situation is encountered, the person who uses somatization may develop a backache, headache, or stomach ache to avoid dealing with problems. This does not mean the ache is "all in the head," but it may mean that the person finds it easier or more acceptable to have a physical pain than an emotional one. For someone who has done this for 80 or 90 years of life, it may be difficult or impossible to change this way of coping. The nurse can help the patient learn to meet needs more directly by encouraging the person to talk about feelings openly.

PATIENT RIGHTS AND LEGAL RESPONSIBILITIES

The current standard of care in nursing homes and in mental health centers is that the older person has the right to the least restrictive form of treatment. Federal and state regulating agencies have specific regulations protecting these rights. In most states, treatment can be administered involuntarily only if a danger exists to the individual or to others. The length of time allowed for this type of treatment varies from state to state but is usually only a few days. If a longer treatment schedule is required and the older person is unwilling to consent, an application for guardianship may be made; the person's rights to make personal decisions are taken away and assigned to a guardian. This procedure may be necessary for people with some types of mental illness, including dementia.

When agitated behaviors become severe, the nurse has to make a decision about how to handle the problem. Points that must be considered are the patient's right to the least restrictive treatment environment and the legal issues related to the use of chemical and physical restraints. If an older adult has an episode in which increased symptoms of bipolar affective disorder or schizophrenia are exhibited, an antipsychotic drug is likely to be more effective than it would be for someone with dementia or delirium. Before giving a chemical restraint, it is necessary to try talking to the person as well as using behavioral interventions. When all else fails, physical restraints may be necessary on rare occasions. If using physical restraints, remember the following safety precautions:

1. Use the least restrictive device.
2. Check on the person often.
3. Remove the restraints every 2 hours for a brief period.

CONCLUSION

The care of elderly people in all arenas of nursing is an opportunity to practice the art of nursing at its highest level. The skills and understanding that are needed to give meaningful care to the elderly patient with psychological problems are complex, and they require a personal and professional commitment to the needs of people as they age.

CASE STUDY SOLUTION

Working with the entire nursing staff, a plan is developed for using validation therapy with Mr. A. When he asks about his truck or home, the staff ask him questions such as, "What color is your truck?" "What did you do with your truck?" "Where did you go?" "With whom?" Coveralls with a front pocket are obtained, and a small hammer and screwdriver are placed in his pocket. His toolbox is brought into his room. The staff has put him in charge of a small garden outside the nursing home. Individual sessions of validation are scheduled 20 minutes a day, three times a week, by the activities staff.

Over a 6-week period, the staff notices that Mr. A. spends quiet, productive time in the garden area. He carries his toolbox with him most of the time but does not use its contents. He no longer leaves the building except to work in his garden. He is still forgetful.

REVIEW QUESTIONS

1. The best intervention for an elderly resident of a nursing home who has paranoia is:
   1. To encourage him to lead a large group singing
   2. To plan one-on-one activities with staff and other residents
   3. To invite the resident to sit on the residents' council of the nursing home
   4. To have the resident join a weekly bingo group

2. An elderly homebound person taking medication for a psychological problem needs to know which of the following?
   1. If dizziness occurs, notify the nurse.
   2. It may take several weeks to get the desired effect.
   3. Report any changes in vision.
   4. All of the above.

3. Validation techniques are best described as:
   1. A way of helping someone resolve past experiences
   2. Helping someone find new meaning in growing older
   3. A reminder of a painful present reality
   4. Bringing someone from the past into the present world

4. A hospitalized older adult shows signs of depression. The best intervention is which of the following?
   1. Ignore the person's feelings because they are a normal part of aging.
   2. Tell the person to cheer up because things are not so bad.
   3. Do not allow the person to talk about being sad because that makes it worse.
   4. Encourage the person to discuss feelings openly because it helps to talk about problems.

5. When teaching older adults or their families about the use of psychotropic drugs, one of the most important concepts to teach is:
   1. The meaning of the different colors of the medications
   2. The stress psychotropic drugs put on the kidneys
   3. To anticipate the chronic light-headedness that most people experience
   4. Not to expect the full effect of the drug for several weeks

REFERENCES

Centers for Disease Control and Prevention. (n.d.). The state of mental health and aging in America. http://www.cdc.gov/aging/pdf/mental_health.pdf.

Feil, N., & de Klerk-Rubin, V. (2014). *The validation breakthrough: simple techniques for communicating with people with Alzheimer's and other dementias*. (3rd ed.). Baltimore, MD: Health Professions Press, Inc.

Geriatric Mental Health Foundation (2014). Late life depression: A fact sheet. http://www.gmhfonline.org/gmhf/consumer/factsheets/depression_factsheet.html

National Institute on Aging. (n.d.). About Alzheimer's disease: Alzheimer's basics. http://www.nia.nih.gov/alzheimers/topics/alzheimers-basics#what

Tabloski, P.A. (2007). *Clinical handbook for gerontological nursing*. Upper Saddle River, NJ: Pearson Prentice-Hall.

WEB RESOURCES

Geriatric Mental Health Foundation: http://www.gmhfonline.org

Validation Training Institute, Inc.: http://vfvalidation.org

Rehabilitation and Restorative Care

20

KATHLEEN R. CULLITON

LEARNING OUTCOMES

1. Define the concepts of rehabilitation and restorative nursing in a holistic framework.

2. Identify the clinical implications of restorative care in walking programs, continence training, and feeding and self-help programs.

CONCEPTS

Care Coordination

Functional Ability

CASE STUDY

At age 60, Mr. A. suffered a severe, incapacitating stroke. He is able to communicate verbally and with gestures, but he is unable to move his right arm and his right leg is very weak. Mrs. A is very upset because Mr. A is sleeping all of the time and refusing to work with the physical and occupational therapists.

Mr. A. and his wife had planned to retire in 5 years and travel. The stroke has created major questions for Mr. and Mrs. A. regarding current employment, living arrangement, financial stability, and retirement plans.

Discussion

As the LPN working with the interdisciplinary team, what are the care focus priorities for Mr. and Mrs. A?

 ## INTRODUCTION

Nurses strive to promote the health of older adults. Generally, nursing care involves assisting older persons in overcoming the symptoms of an acute health problem or the worsening of a chronic condition. Nurses use medications, treatments, and referrals to help the individual overcome physical, psychological, social, and spiritual illness. In the acute-care setting, nurses assist older adults through the crisis of illness and discharge them back into the community to their homes or a supportive living environment. The goal of nursing care is to assist older adults back to the highest level of health possible and to allow them to live in their homes or whatever environment provides them with optimal safety (Chen, 2010). Assessment of their general health and ability to meet their personal needs are considerations during the discharge process. Sometimes older adults are no longer physically or emotionally able to return safely to their homes. You, as the licensed practical nurse (LPN), play a significant role for older adults who need restorative care.

This chapter presents an overview of gerontological nursing concepts based on rehabilitative and restorative care. Rehabilitative and restorative nursing care surpasses the traditional custodial approach that prevailed in the care of older adults before the initiation of the 1990 Omnibus Budget Reconciliation Act (OBRA) regulations. Data collection for residents in nursing homes is done on the minimum data set (MDS) (see Chapter 4) and emphasizes restorative care of older adults as a major priority of care.

As people age, they experience increased incidence of chronic disease processes such as hypertension, diabetes mellitus, and heart failure; these processes can lead to disabilities such as mobility issues, paralysis, and activity intolerance. With the elderly population increasing, nurses are called on to provide rehabilitative and restorative care to older people in health-care facilities and community settings.

 ## UNDERSTANDING REHABILITATION AND RESTORATIVE CONCEPTS

Rehabilitation is the process of teaching and training individuals to achieve their highest level of independent function (Benjamin, Edwards, Ploeg, & Legault, 2014). People are most familiar with rehabilitation programs for spinal cord injuries. For older adults, rehabilitation often is prescribed for paralysis after a stroke or deformity from rheumatoid arthritis and after joint replacement surgery for severe degenerative joint disease. Rehabilitative care is a multidisciplinary care model. Physical therapists, occupational therapists, speech therapists, dietitians, respiratory therapists, recreation therapists, social workers, psychologists, nurses, and rehabilitation physicians all are

⏱ Priority Setting

When dealing with rehabilitation and restorative care, there are three priorities for you:

1. Get to know the person admitted to the unit and the person's family and significant others. To make the rehabilitation and restorative program meaningful for the person receiving treatment, you need to know the person's personal goals and dreams. Because people are not brought to a rehabilitation and restorative care unit in a life-and-death crisis, you have time to meet this priority. Take the time to identify the person's goals and share them with the rest of the IDT team.

2. Use your knowledge and skills as a nurse to prevent disabling consequences (i.e., foot-drop, contractures, pressure ulcers, depression) while carrying out rehabilitative and restorative programs.

3. It is assumed that you will carefully follow all physicians' orders. The third priority goes beyond doing what is legally and morally required of you, such as following orders. It is to support the people in your care as they go through the challenges of a rehabilitative or restoration program. It is difficult and demanding. Your support can make a significant difference in the outcome for each individual.

BOX 20.1   DEFINING REHABILITATIVE AND RESTORATIVE CARE

Rehabilitation: Processes of teaching and training individuals to achieve their highest level of independent function.

Restorative care: Assisting patients who have reached their highest level of function through rehabilitation to maintain that level of function over time.

members of rehabilitation care teams. The priority for Mr. A. and his wife is to get them networked with the interdisciplinary team (IDT). In an IDT meeting, Mr. and Mrs. A. are participants in a clinical conference in which the rehabilitative team reviews Mr. A.'s case and allows him to make informed decisions on how to proceed with the goal of discharge.

Rehabilitation is initiated after an extensive assessment of an individual's physical, emotional, spiritual, and functional assets and liabilities. To develop a rehabilitative plan, assessment information and the resources available to assist the individual are reviewed. Often, an individual does not need all available services. The team is restructured to include the necessary health-care team members. This team works with individuals and their families to develop rehabilitative goals and to decide the best way to work toward the goals. Mr. A. has a significant physical disability to his right arm and leg. The nurses, physical therapists, and occupational therapist will evaluate not only the right-sided weakness but also how the weakness affects Mr. A.'s ability to perform activities of daily living (ADLs), walk, climb stairs, and manage instrumental ADLs (IADLs).

Selecting a short-term or long-term living environment is one of the first choices that a rehabilitation team must make. Every care environment has the potential to be a place for rehabilitation. Limiting factors often are insufficient family support, environmental safety, insurance reimbursement, and access to the rehabilitation team. An older adult with a total hip replacement may want to go home, but home has an upstairs bathroom, and there is no one available to prepare meals. These factors present a problem. A man may be recovering well from knee surgery and wants to have intensive inpatient therapy, but his insurance company does not approve the cost. An elderly woman may want to go to her rural community hospital for rehabilitation after a stroke, but the services she needs are unavailable in that community. The rehabilitation team works to help the person access support services and find the most appropriate environment for the rehabilitation process.

Restorative nursing care is related to rehabilitation. It has the same goal—to assist older people with reaching their highest functional ability. The major difference is the intense involvement of the entire health-care team. Because of the direct involvement of therapists and other health-care professionals, rehabilitation is an expensive service. Restorative care is initiated after an older person has reached the rehabilitative goal or has not shown any further improvement. The whole health-care team is involved in designing restorative care plans but is not directly involved in the implementation. An older person who is in a rehabilitation program after a stroke would have the benefit of a physical therapist to learn exercise, safe walking, and transferring techniques. The older adult continues to need assistance with exercises and walking, but a nurse or a nursing assistant encourages the person to do as much as possible independently and assists him or her only if necessary.

Rehabilitation provides individuals with intensive short-term strengthening and retraining, whereas restorative care continues the process over time. Older adults often have a major health crisis and go through intensive therapy and training only to move to an environment where everything is done for them, and the benefits of the therapy are lost. Examples of restorative programs are ambulation, personal care, feeding, and toileting. The challenge for the nursing team is to continue to promote high levels of independent function. It is faster to transfer a person into a wheelchair and push the person to the dining room for breakfast, but that is not promoting independence. Promoting independence in care and use of adaptive equipment can encourage Mr. and Mrs. A. to work with the IDT to meet short- and long-term rehabilitation goals.

This same concept of needing to hurry is associated with high incidences of incontinence. It is often perceived as faster to change an older adult's briefs and bedclothes than to anticipate the need for voiding and walking the person to the bathroom. With rehabilitative and restorative nursing care, "faster" is not the goal.

The same principle applies to eating and personal care. Have you ever watched someone struggle to put a shirt on a paralyzed arm? Watching that struggle is uncomfortable because nurses know they could help that person get the shirt on faster and without as much stress and strain. It is very difficult to watch someone try to eat independently when they have a disability and to see the stress and frustration that can occur. Yet that older person deserves the right to feel the satisfaction of accomplishing a task or meeting a personal goal.

The concepts of rehabilitation and restorative care are crucial to promoting an older adult's optimal level of function. The focus of rehabilitative and restorative care is to maximize the abilities and functions of older adults to ensure the highest level of independence and quality of life. Rehabilitation and restorative care are not isolated treatments with limited application. They embody a broad set of principles to incorporate into every facet of nursing care in all settings.

Within the context of the IDT effort and after clinical conferences with the team to determine what plan is to be designed, LPNs, working cooperatively with the registered nurse (RN), prepare the goals and the nursing care plan. In this capacity, the LPN's role becomes one of practitioner, educator, counselor, case manager, researcher, and consultant.

NURSING ROLES

Bedside Caregiver

As caregivers, LPNs provide direct care to older adults until the skills necessary for self-care have been developed by the individual. Nurses need to give older adults positive reinforcement, encouragement, hope, and an opportunity to develop and use their physical and social skills.

Educator

When serving in the role of educator, nurses provide older people and their families with information related to the disability and its treatment and management. Included in the education plan should be health measures to obtain and retain function and to prevent further disability. Effective outcomes are more likely to occur when older adults and their families are included in the process of determining the goals of rehabilitation and restoration of function and treatment. It is important for older adults and the family or other caregivers to recognize that they are responsible for the decisions made and actions that result from those decisions. That is a predominant principle of rehabilitative and restorative care.

Counselor

As counselors, nurses assist elderly people with describing, analyzing, and responding to the current situation that makes rehabilitation or restorative care necessary. Counseling is the process of helping people solve and cope effectively with their problems. Counseling disabled people and their families is an ongoing process that requires supportive behaviors from the entire IDT. LPNs, after establishing trust and rapport with the older adult and the family, need to focus on assisting them in dealing with their grief over the losses imposed by the older person's current disability. The opportunity to express personal feelings assists the elderly person in developing coping skills related to the event of trauma that made rehabilitation and restorative therapy necessary. The LPN should counsel disabled elderly persons and their families to respond to the feelings of loss, frustration, and anger that they generally feel. It is important to express and deal with such feelings as a family.

Advocate

When assuming the role of advocate, LPNs use their influence and power as health-care professionals to bring about necessary changes for the older person and the family's well-being. That advocacy allows the rehabilitation and restorative care to have maximum effect. The LPN's interventions aid the older adult and the family members in obtaining necessary community-based services; the community-based services assist older disabled adults in maintaining their status as fully functioning, independent individuals within the constraints of the limitations imposed by the disability. Such interventions may include the use of assistive or adaptive devices such as crutches, a walker, a plate guard, and a padded spoon.

Case Manager

Generally, an RN is the case manager for disabled persons. In some situations, the LPN is asked to serve in that role. The case manager role places the LPN as a central figure working with the total health-care team throughout the entire episode of illness. The major focus for a case manager is to resolve actual problems and prevent potential problems for the aging person. The treatment plan, once agreed on by the IDT, is under the supervision of the licensed nurses (RNs and LPNs) working in conjunction with each older adult and family. When the plan is agreed on, a contract is entered into by the individual, family members, and nurse. This contract allows the plan to be implemented with clear communication with each person involved. This management may take place

This LPN is meeting with the IDT to plan care for the residents in her care.

in a hospital or nursing home and continue into the community where home-based care is provided.

Researcher

Many LPNs work in conjunction with RNs and a qualified nurse researcher to gather data on the rehabilitation and restorative care of older adults. Many questions remain unanswered regarding rehabilitative and restorative care of older adults in numerous areas. Each area provides a rich arena for research. Some research interests are the following:

- Management of behavioral symptoms
- Feelings about placing disabled family members outside the home and into an institution for care on a permanent basis
- Barriers that prevent the use of respite and day-care services
- Accurate measures of caregiver burden
- Effective coping strategies used by caregivers
- Types of educational and support programs needed to assist caregivers
- Services needed to individualize care at different stages of an illness or injury

 Point of Interest

Refer back to the chapter on end-of-life issues (Chapter 11). Review Kübler-Ross's five stages of grief. The older adult and the family will be going through these stages related to the physiological, emotional, or functional loss they are experiencing.

All of these clinical questions need to be raised when older individuals experience a traumatic episode and require nursing care. The nurse is responsible for raising questions regarding the specific needs of the older individuals and seeking systematic answers through research. A research approach helps build a body of knowledge regarding rehabilitation and restorative care.

GOALS OF REHABILITATION AND RESTORATIVE CARE

A goal is defined as a written statement of desired behavioral outcomes from which steps or strategies may be designed to achieve that desired end. Goals provide direction. They are the measuring tool for an effective plan of care. For example, "I will buy a car today" is a statement of the desired outcome. A defined series of steps needs to be taken before the accomplishment of that goal. Some of the steps are establishing a means to pay for the car, deciding what type of car to buy, finding out the selling price of cars at various car dealers, checking on insurance, and buying the car.

From the time of injury or disability, the efforts of all health-care professionals involved in care of the older adult are to be focused on the ultimate goal: the highest level of personal independence possible within the limitations imposed by the injury. In setting goals, LPNs assess the older person to determine what assets of mind, body, and spirit are present that would aid in the accomplishment of the goal. For instance, can the person ambulate sufficiently to make trips to the bathroom, dining room, and physical therapy department? The LPN might ask the following questions:

- Is the person able to communicate needs verbally?
- Can the person feed himself or herself?
- What are the goals of the older adult?

The information derived from the assessment is important in determining realistic and achievable goals for each individual. For lifelong quality of living, the components of a successful rehabilitation and restorative program must include the following goals, which should be individualized toward increasing the function and performance of the individual:

- Independence and self-care
- Mobility

- Involvement in activities—social, civic, family, church, and recreation
- Fulfillment of life's goals
- Holistic approach to living with a disability

You must be knowledgeable in evaluating the current holistic status of the older adult. For older adults, major changes in three areas are crucial to the success of a rehabilitation and restorative care program. Changes must be noted in physical, functional, and psychological status. Each of these areas can greatly affect the ability of the older adult to carry out the goals identified in the plan of care.

Physical Changes Affecting Restorative Care

Numerous physical changes may be present when an older adult sustains an injury or trauma necessitating rehabilitation. Existing health problems must be considered in planning rehabilitative and restorative care, as follows:

- Musculoskeletal changes secondary to old fractures, osteoporosis, arthritis, osteoarthritis, muscular dystrophy, or loss of strength in arms and legs can create mobility difficulties. Such situations can occur because of muscle atrophy, decreased bone mass, loss of subcutaneous fat, and decreased flexibility of the joints and limbs.
- Cardiovascular changes secondary to diminished cardiac output, irregular heart rate, and increased blood pressure readings can result in diminished circulation that does not bring sufficient oxygen to the body. Such conditions often cause a lack of activity because of fatigue. Cardiac changes may be the result of thickening of heart valves, thickening of blood vessels, or delayed response to stress.
- Respiratory changes related to diminished respiratory rates can create ventilation challenges for the older person and may be caused by long-standing asthma, obstructive lung disease, emphysema, tuberculosis, upper respiratory illnesses, limited rib cage expansion, atrophy of respiratory muscles, decreased arterial oxygen tension, decreased vital capacity, and diminished cough.
- Renal and digestive tract changes create elimination difficulties that may impair the proper

FOCUSED LEARNING CHART

Holistic functional assessment

Psychological	Physiological	Sociological
Memory	ADLs	Interaction with others
Judgment	IADLs	Family support
Thinking ability	Current health status	Involvement in the community

implementation of a restorative program. These changes may include decreased peristalsis of the intestinal tract that results in constipation or diarrhea, decreased intestinal enzyme levels that reduce the ability to digest foods properly, diminished glomerular filtration in the kidney, and decreased bladder capacity resulting in incontinence or retention of residual urine. The last-mentioned may create edematous lower limbs that make it difficult for the older person to ambulate comfortably.

- Consciousness and mental status changes may result in short-term memory loss, slower thought processing, and decreased pain threshold (Galik, Resnick, & Pretzer-Aboff, 2009).
- Perceptual changes may be exhibited by loss of visual acuity, diminished hearing, decreased sense of taste, lower sensitivity to touch, and decreased proprioception (spatial sensitivity or awareness of where things are in the available space).

Functional Changes Affecting Rehabilitative and Restorative Care

Changes in function in older adults may result from the impact of social and environmental situations (Resnick, Gruber-Baldini, Galik, Pretzner-Aboff, Russ, Hebel & Zimmerman, 2009) and can include the following:

- Inability to negotiate stairs in the home
- Functional implications of acute or chronic disease processes

Think Like a Nurse

When LPNs are asked to be involved in research, they are asked to gather data for the principal investigator. This is an opportunity you should take. You will learn from the principal investigator, will be able to spend time with older adults while gathering data, and will have pride in the finished research project.

- Physical factors, such as limited range of motion (ROM), strength, and endurance
- Inability to consume sufficient nutrients to maintain optimal health
- Inability to cook food, clean a home, or complete the laundry and other crucial chores

These functional changes need to be assessed by a nurse so that realistic goals can be established.

Psychological Changes Affecting Rehabilitative and Restorative Care

The psychological status of an older adult is a crucial component of any rehabilitation and restorative care program. When the older person possesses psychological well-being, there is a strong motivation to work toward the highest possible level of function. When older people feel needed and wanted by family, friends, and associates, they generally possess self-esteem and a positive self-image—two critical factors in developing a high degree of motivation to proceed with the restorative care program. Mr. A. is obviously

PATIENT EDUCATION

The nurse should teach patients and family members the importance of self-care as it relates to rehabilitative and restorative care. Patients should be instructed to do as much of their care as possible. Although doing most of their care by themselves may be difficult and even painful at times, it is critical to meeting their goals.

having difficulty coping with the disability and the rehabilitation program. Often a psychologist or psychotherapist is part of the IDT. The mental health specialist can help Mr. A. develop positive coping skills and motivation for rehabilitation.

DEVELOPING GOALS FOR REHABILITATIVE AND RESTORATIVE CARE

When developing goals for rehabilitative and restorative care, LPNs need to complete a full nursing assessment under the guidance of the RN. The nursing assessment should include a database with the following elements:

• Nursing history that includes the older adult's past medical conditions, psychological impairments, hospitalizations, and previous injuries (see Chapter 16)
• Physical assessment of all bodily systems (see Chapter 16)
• Functional assessment to check for functional ability and mobility (see Chapter 16)
• Mental status and psychological parameters that may be present, such as depression or anxiety (see Chapter 18)
• A spiritual assessment to determine any spiritual needs or deficits that may be a deterrent to good rehabilitation progress

Following the assessment, the LPN and RN work together as a team to analyze the data and prioritize rehabilitative and restorative goals for the older person. The following principles of holistic nursing care should be the guidelines for identifying goals:

• When the older adult enters the hospital or nursing facility, rehabilitation must begin immediately.
• Proper body alignment is to be maintained at all times.
• Pressure ulcers are to be prevented on all body parts.
• Rehabilitation is to be implemented concurrently with the illness, whether chronic or acute, temporary or permanent, or disabling or nondisabling.

Evidence-Based Practice

Poynter, L., Kwan, J., Saver, A.A., & Vassallo, M. (2011). Does cognitive impairment affect rehabilitation outcome? Journal of the American Geriatrics Society, 59(11), 2108-2111.

Over a two-and-one-half-year period, 241 older adults (all were older than 70 years old) admitted to 2 rehabilitation units were administered a Mini Mental Status Examination (MMSE) to categorize their cognitive function. At admission, week 2, week 6, and discharge, each participant's functional ability was measured using the Barthel daily activities of living score. The study found that all of the participants had an increase in function through the study period. An interesting finding was that participants with lower cognitive function continued to improve in ADL function through the whole 6-week period of rehabilitation. Participants with high cognitive function progressed in ADL function in the early period of rehabilitation.

Questions

1. What does this imply for care planning for residents of an Alzheimer unit?
2. How could this affect care standards and insurance reimbursement for long-term care?
3. How do the results of this study affect your approach to ADL function and confused older adults?
4. How could this study influence how you assign unlicensed assistive personnel to approach ADL care with older adults?

- All joints must be kept free through proper exercise and ROM.
- Convalescence is a gradual process and may extend over a considerable period of time for the older person.
- Nurses must understand the person's self-concept and feelings of dependency and isolation, if they exist.
- The time period for rehabilitation depends on the person's psychological acceptance of the condition and his or her physical condition.
- People born with disabilities usually have less difficulty accepting their condition than persons who acquire disabilities later in life.
- More severe emotional reactions are produced when accidents are traumatic.
- Loss and its meaning vary with every person.
- Any personality problems that may be exhibited are generally the result of the person's personality characteristics before disability.
- The usual initial reactions to physical injury are shock, fear, disbelief, and anxiety.
- Periods of grief occur when loss of any physical ability is experienced.
- Depression, anger, and denial may be present.
- Values are examined and limitations are put in perspective over time.
- Time is essential for acceptance.
- The family needs emotional support and comfort during the acute phase of the trauma or illness.
- All information should be given to the family and older adult, including information about resources for rehabilitation services and economic assistance.
- The nurse or social worker should be familiar with community agencies that can help.

IMPLEMENTATION OF GOALS IN REHABILITATIVE AND RESTORATIVE CARE

Goal 1: Maintenance of Joint Function

The implementation of planned care for older people requires that a holistic approach be adopted. The major concern in implementing care is the prevention of deformities through passive exer-cises that keep joints movable, promote venous return and lymphatic flow, and help prevent excessive demineralization of bones. This goal and care depend on the physician's orders that identify the extent of the exercise program to be implemented. By means of a thorough assessment of the physical condition of the older adult and the specific illness and prognosis for recovery, nurses assume responsibility for the passive exercise program. Such a program may include ROM activities in which each joint is put through the normal activities of which it is capable — supine, prone, lateral, medial, anterior, and posterior positions. This approach maintains the wellness capability of the joints and reduces the complications of contractures, strictures, and limitation of activity. By implementing passive ROM, nurses assist the injured person to resume independence of function and perform at optimal levels.

Goal 2: Active Exercise

Active exercise is designed to improve function and performance. It entails transferring from bed to chair, ambulating with assistive devices, using crutches properly, knowing how to maneuver the wheelchair, using hand-eye coordination, and using assistive devices that promote independent living in a normal manner. In each of these activities, nurses, in the role of teachers, help motivate the person to be as active in personal care as possible. Always follow the physician's orders for active exercise. A physical therapist is an excellent resource for these activities as well.

Goal 3: Bladder Continence

In some situations, it is necessary for the LPN to initiate bladder-training programs. Achievement of continence avoids the use of indwelling catheters. Bladder training aids in reducing the chance for urinary tract infections and increases self-esteem. Retraining is based on the development of clear patterns of communication between staff, the older adult, and the family regarding the schedule for toileting (usually every 2 hours). It is necessary for the bladder to be emptied at set times throughout the day. Limiting fluids after 6:00 p.m. so that the bladder can retain urine throughout the night is another strategy. Periodic catheterization may be employed sometimes to develop reflex emptying when the sensation for voiding is diminished or absent.

Goal 4: Bowel Continence

In addition to bladder training, it is important to employ bowel-training techniques if they are needed. Bowel training requires the establishment

BOX 20.2 SPIRITUAL ASSESSMENT

You are working with the RN to do a holistic assessment on an 80-year-old victim of a motor vehicle accident. Sister Agnes, a Catholic nun, was walking to prayers when she was hit by a speeding car. She has multiple fractures that will keep her in bed for days. She is in pain, and the RN is working to resolve her discomfort. You are working with the RN to complete the spiritual assessment.

Spirituality discussions make some people uncomfortable. If that is true for you, please work on your skills in this area to overcome such feelings. When considering this discussion with Sister Agnes, you already know two significant things about her that will influence your interview. First, because she is a nun, you can feel reassured that she is a spiritual person and will welcome the discussion. The second thing you know is counterproductive to the first. She is in pain and will not feel like having a lengthy discussion. What two questions could you ask Sister Agnes that would give you the basic information you need without causing her undue distress?

Thoughtfully write your questions and come to class prepared to share them. Below are two sample questions that may help you shape your questions for this activity.

1. Do you believe in a higher power or God? Note: For a Muslim, the higher power would be Allah; for an agnostic, it would simply be a higher power. For Sister Agnes, her response probably would be that she believes in God.
2. What can I do for you or with you, while you are here, to assist you in meeting your spiritual needs? Note: Some people may want you to pray with them, others may want religious artifacts in the room, and others may want a visit from their spiritual leader. Other people will want nothing.

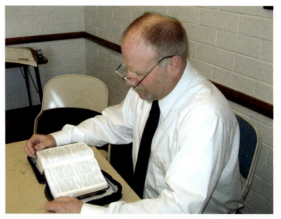

A holistic assessment includes asking about the older adult's spirituality. Religion has a significant role in the lives of most older people. You need to know about their spiritual needs and strive to meet them. This man takes great comfort in reading his scriptures. To do so, the scriptures need to be easily accessible, there should be good lighting, and he needs his glasses.

of a routine for emptying the bowel daily. This occurs most normally in the morning approximately 20 minutes after breakfast. The intake of breakfast stimulates the duodenocolic reflex, which assists in bowel elimination. A diet consisting of whole-grain breads, cereals, fresh fruits, whole bran, and increased fluid intake is helpful in providing the bulk and fluid needed for effective bowel training. This approach also reduces the complication of constipation in the older adult. If constipation does occur, it may be necessary to provide medication to soften the stool and allow the bowel contents to move into the lower colon area for elimination. It also is helpful in bowel-training programs to request that the older adult use the toilet instead of the bedpan to facilitate bowel elimination. This is

QSEN

COMPETENCY: Patient-Centered Care (Knowledge, Skills, Attitude)

Meeting the Individual Needs of Patients

You work in a long-term care rehabilitation facility. Recently, the adult children of a patient have come to the nurse manager to make a complaint.

Every time one of the children comes to visit their mother, she is holding hands and talking in a quiet and intimate manner with a male resident. The children want the time together stopped. The nurse manager has asked you to look into the situation. When you ask the resident about her male friend she shares that she has never met such a kind man. She shares, "We were both very lonely. No one gets excited about rehabilitation for knee and hip replacement but we may have never met if we did not have surgery." You report your findings back to the charge nurse, and she schedules a care conference with the interdisciplinary team (IDT), the resident, and the resident's children.

During the care conference the children become emotional and challenge the resident's behavior as "childish" and disrespectful of their father who passed away 6 years ago. The resident becomes tearful. The RN and social worker use therapeutic communication techniques to diffuse the emotionally charged challenges of the children and encourage the resident to discuss her feelings about the situation and her feelings about the fellow resident. The geriatrician goes on to explain the seriousness of loneliness and discusses with the children the therapeutic value of friendships, touch, and intimacy.

Think about it: The focus of team work and collaboration is positive outcomes for the resident. Through education about and demonstration of respect for the resident and her expression of affection to a fellow resident, the team is attempting to educate the children about the resident's rights and the positive benefits to expressing affection.

Patient-centered care really describes the behavior of the nurse, by going to the resident and asking her direct questions about the children's concerns, along with advocating for her in the IDT meetings.

Is there additional information you need to gather? If so, what is it? How important is sexual expression for older adults? Is it being expressed appropriately in this situation? Please carefully ponder your response and be prepared to share your thinking in class.

not always possible. Rectal suppositories are useful when initiating a bowel-training program. Enemas are rarely used as part of a bowel-training program.

Goal 5: Appropriate Sexual Expression

When implementing a holistic plan of care, the LPN must be aware of the older adult's intimacy needs. This means building in time during the rehabilitation and restorative care process for partners to have privacy. It also can include offering the sense of touch by holding hands with the elderly adult in appropriate ways and, when given permission, for squeezing the shoulder or forearm with a firm but gentle touch.

Goal 6: Psychosocial and Spiritual Well-Being

It is crucial to include interventions that address the psychosocial and spiritual needs of older adults. Communicating, increasing self-concept and self-esteem, treating the person with dignity and respect, and meeting spiritual needs are essential to holistic nursing care. Examples could include uninterrupted time to pray, arrangements for visits from the local clergy, and allowing religious artifacts in the room.

In implementing rehabilitation and restorative care, nurses follow the plan of care outlined by the IDT. Such information comes from the database (MDS) of information collected during the admission assessment and periodically throughout the course of the care. The nurse must be alert to changes that need to be made in the plan of care as the older person improves, stays the same, or declines in physical abilities.

Final Thought About Implementing Goals

The implementation of care measures should focus on the older adult's previous coping skills. It is important that older adults become partners in the care regimen by sharing knowledge and adaptability. The goals are established by the older person, the family, and the nurse as a member of the IDT based on the assessment data. When the goal is stated in specific, measurable terms, evaluation of the progress and outcome of care are easily measured.

The terms of the goal are to be put in the framework of self-care and self-responsibility.

 ASSESSMENT OF GOALS

Goals are assessed at intervals—sometimes daily, sometimes weekly, sometimes monthly—depending on the goal to be accomplished. When the goals have been stated in observable, measurable terms, the assessment of their achievement is relatively easy. In the course of the disease or traumatic injury, in-depth documentation is extremely important for noting the progress of the person. A systematic approach to fulfill all the stated goals assures the patient, family, and health-care team that a holistic approach has been incorporated into the older adult's care. This approach reassures the older adult and the nurse that custodial care will be avoided and that rehabilitation and restorative nursing from a holistic perspective is in place.

Goals Specific to Elderly Adults

Restorative nursing goals specific to older adults include the following:

- Improvement of function
- Delay of deterioration
- Accommodation to dysfunction
- Comfort in the dying process

Improvement of Function

Functionality is defined as the ability to continue to live one's preferred lifestyle without disruption. In other words, each older adult can live independently, do ADLs and IADLs, be mobile, and have self-care ability. To live independently suggests that there is no need for physical assistance or supervision from another person. Goal assessment on a daily or weekly basis is essential to good care.

To improve function, it is necessary to take into account the impact of the older person's social and environmental situation, the functional implications of acute or chronic disease proc-esses, and the physical factors that may influence function. By combining these factors, a picture of the capability of older adults to live and function should emerge for the health-care team.

ROM exercises are exercises performed on a regular basis to preserve the function of the joints and muscles. It is crucial that this maintenance function be performed correctly and on a schedule so that no deterioration of the physical status of the person occurs. The nurse, under the direction of the physical therapist, does this activity or instructs another health-care team member to carry out the activity correctly.

Improving the strength of the muscles necessitates that some resistance be exerted so that the muscle works hard to maintain or improve its function. Resistance is often accomplished through the use of weights or by pushing against an object to provide resistance. The actual testing of the muscle strength and endurance is done by the physical therapist, and a plan of exercise is identified. This plan must be carried out meticulously so that every muscle and its function are duly exercised, and strength and endurance are improved.

Mobility is identified in various stages, depending on the type of injury or disease present in the older adult. The progression is usually from bed mobility, through transfer activities, to wheelchair or ambulatory locomotion. Transfer includes getting from bed to a chair and back to bed, on and off a toilet, and in and out of a bathtub or car. These activities involve standing, sitting, pivoting, turning, or side-slide movement (sliding from bed to chair using a transfer board). To promote function in mobility involves locomotion or moving from one point to another. Older adults may need to use a wheelchair, so the ability to propel and maneuver the wheelchair is important. Wheelchair use involves the development of arm strength with the use of weights or other forms of strength building. Other assistive devices such as crutches, braces, and splints may be needed to assist in locomotion. To help the individual reach optimal function, instruction needs to be given in the best approaches to maintaining balance and endurance and in the use of devices to prevent falls.

When the goal is to improve function, there is a positive outcome orientation. For example, if the nursing diagnosis is stated:

- Body Image Disturbance: functional— self-esteem disturbance related to function limitations, role and lifestyle change.

Then the goal should be written:

- The older adult will verbalize positive statements about self.
- The older adult will identify and demonstrate appropriate strategies to deal with functional limitations.

Some of these strategies could be the ability to manipulate buttons and zippers, to tie shoelaces, and to put on underwear. If the older adult is unable to perform these functions, devices such as long-handled reachers, button hooks, and elastic shoelaces may allow the person to perform more independently.

In helping older people retain functional ability and avoid deterioration, it is important to be aware of the disease processes that may interfere with their ability to achieve independent living. Such limiting problems most often involve cardiorespiratory, neurological, or musculoskeletal systems. Many of these conditions may impose significant functional limitations on the person. All of these factors must be kept in mind when implementing goals for rehabilitative and restorative care for the elderly person. Dedication to the restorative care plan helps older people keep motivated and engage in the purposeful and varied activities that promote function and performance.

Delay of Deterioration

A primary goal of rehabilitative and restorative nursing is the delay of deterioration in all functional aspects. If bouts of depression are noted on admission and during the course of treatment, the RN should be notified and a psychiatric consultation requested if it is determined to be appropriate for the individual. Depression signals initial deterioration of motivation. Helping the person maintain a spirit of hopefulness is one way to assist in the delay of deterioration.

Another approach to ensure delay of deterioration is to ensure that the nursing care plan calls for exercise of all mobile bodily parts—legs, arms, fingers, toes, neck, hips, and knees. Move-ment of all of these joints is essential in the maintenance of a healthy state. No nurse should ever allow a contracture to occur. Use of pillows, a footboard to prevent footdrop, and resting splints for wrists and fingers aids in proper alignment of the body to maintain function and delay deterioration. Properly aligned and supported body parts assume their natural posture and position. Passive ROM exercises for all joints can delay deterioration to a great extent. Caution must be exercised, however. If care is not used in moving the joints, soft tissue injury can result from undue stretching of the muscles and joints; this could cause additional injury and slow the rate of recovery, or it could cause great pain when the person becomes active again.

Another priority concern is the prevention of pressure ulcers. Excellent skin care should be a daily part of nursing care for all persons. This is especially important for elderly people who have impaired nutritional status. Pressure ulcers may develop over any bony prominence and on the occiput, ear parts, sacrum, and greater trochanter. Special devices to cushion these parts need to be used as a preventive measure, such as special pillows, donuts, gauze dressings, and special mattresses (circulating water or air). Turning the person every 2 hours is the best preventive measure to ensure skin integrity. When turning the person, the support of limbs and back for good body alignment is essential to keep weakened muscles from further deterioration.

Cognitively impaired elderly persons are in need of individualized nursing care. These people need appropriate sensory stimulation to maintain their contact with the world. Putting the person in a position where others can be seen and the careful use of the radio and TV can help stimulate cognitive functions and lessen the possibility of further deterioration.

To delay deterioration, older adults should participate in out-of-bed activities as soon as they have achieved a medically stable condition. First, they should dangle their feet for several minutes to gain a sense of balance. When this activity is tolerated, the nurse should help the older adult to stand by the side of the bed with whatever assistive device is needed (e.g., a walker or cane). Finally, the person should be assisted to walk to a chair and sit with proper support for approximately 15 minutes at a time. You, as an LPN, are essential for providing the appropriate encouragement to the individual.

Accommodation to Dysfunction

The goal of helping elderly people accommodate to dysfunction requires a great deal of motivation on the part of the nurse. It is essential for the LPN to listen attentively and actively to the personal fears, hopes, thoughts, feelings, and values that are expressed by the person who is adjusting to the deficits left by an accident, injury, or stroke. Nurses should be aware that a rehabilitation program is primarily a learning and training process. Each person must have the ability to absorb new information on how to use personal potential and how to practice new skills. If a person has sustained an injury that created a footdrop gait, the individual must learn to accommodate walking by lifting the foot intentionally so that it remains flat as weight is shifted from one side of the body to the next. This action requires

This woman was admitted to the nursing home in a weakened condition. The first goal was to prevent her from deteriorating any further. As you can see, she now can be up in a wheelchair for short periods.

major concentration until the old adage "practice makes perfect" becomes second nature to the walker. The nurse's role is to encourage the person to keep working for the highest outcome possible.

Holistic wellness occurs for the older adult receiving restorative care when:

• The psychological self-image of the person incorporates personal limitations into a healthy and acceptable image.
• Social activities and interactions with friends and family continue to be a major part of the person's life.
• The person exhibits gerotranscendence by accepting the new lifestyle with joy, peace, and gratitude for the remaining strengths of his or her personhood.

These are the elements to be found when the goal of accommodation to dysfunction is achieved. As the grief and sense of loss diminish, older people adopt a healthier view so that life, once again, is worth living for them.

Comfort

Restorative nursing may include providing comfort measures and palliative care to elderly people.

Palliative care means providing the care requested by the older person in terms of advance directives and a living will. The individual's decisions must be honored by the nurse and family members. The older adult may have requested that no food or water be given after it has been determined that no benefits would be derived from such comfort measures. Life-sustaining technologies such as intravenous solutions or use of a respirator also may be terminated if no positive outcome is predicted. All of these wishes are to be followed using the Code of Ethics for Nurses.

Nurses are to be supportive of the advance directive wishes of terminally ill older adults and their family members. Nurses must be accountable to support advance directive decisions and facilitate implementation of the individual's wishes. All care decisions are to be carried out in a compassionate and caring manner. Nurses need to approach care of the dying older adult with reverence for body, mind, and spirit as the dying adult approaches end of life. The nurse should attend to the dying person with dignity and respect. Chapter 11 contains more information on end-of-life issues.

CLINICAL IMPLICATIONS OF REHABILITATIVE AND RESTORATIVE CARE

Using the framework of the restorative care principles and guidelines that were cited earlier in this chapter, four clinical rehabilitative programs for older adults are outlined:

• Walking programs
• Bladder and bowel continence training
• Feeding and self-feeding programs
• Self-care—ADL programs

Walking Programs

Mobility is crucial to optimal functioning for older people. To be mobile means that the individual enjoys the satisfaction of independence in living. Nurses play a key role in providing motivation for a walking program. Depending on the type of assistive device needed by the older adult to aid in gait control, the nurse follows the directions given by the RN, primary care provider, or physical therapist. Excellent foot care is critical to maintaining a walking program. Also, properly fitting shoes are important to establish proper posture while walking. Mr. A. may require referrals to community resources, home-care services, and durable medical supply companies to assist him in obtaining medical equipment for home use and even receiving nursing care in the home.

The older adult may need braces or crutches to walk. Leg and back braces are devices that are used to support body weight, limit involuntary movements, or prevent and correct deformities. Crutches are devices that may be necessary to help the person learn to walk again in a normal manner. Crutches may be used on a temporary or permanent basis, depending on the type of injury sustained during the trauma.

For successful crutch walking, it is important to strengthen the muscle groups used in this activity. This strengthening should begin as soon as the physician believes that the older adult has recovered sufficiently to consider walking. Strengthening exercises should be provided while the person is still confined to bed. These exercises include the muscles of the arms, shoulders, chest, and back. Before ambulation, the older adult should be taught how to move from the bed

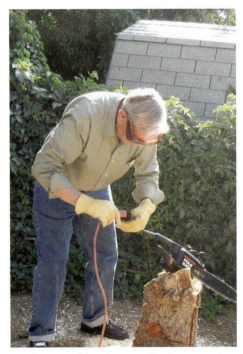

As people grow older, they need to keep moving. This 85-year-old man has spent most of his life working outdoors. He will never go to a gym because "they are for sissies!" He keeps busy with outdoor projects. They keep him moving, provide him with satisfaction, and a purpose in life.

to the chair and should be capable of performing this movement without assistance. Older people who need assistance to learn to stand, balance themselves, and ambulate again sometimes experience difficulty. Patience on the part of the nurse is an important quality.

Important points in crutch walking include correct measurements for crutches so that they have a proper fit. Crutches need to have heavy rubber tips to prevent the crutch from sliding. The crutches need to be moved in a rhythmic way that propels the person forward. Finally, crutches should have padding on the underarm piece so that weight is not placed on the radial nerve. The hand-hold on the crutches may have padding to reduce irritation there as well. The nurse should emphasize good posture for a person who is crutch walking: The head should be held high, and the pelvis should be kept over the feet for excellent balance. Crutch walking is best taught in several short lessons to reduce fatigue in the older adult. When ambulation begins, it is important to have an attendant in front and in back of the person to provide stability and to reduce anxiety about possible falls.

Several types of gaits may be used in crutch walking, depending on the type of injury and the physician's orders, as follows:

- *Four-point gait*: The person bears weight on both feet and has four-point contact with the floor (both crutches and both feet).
- *Two-point gait*: There are two points of contact with the floor (crutches only).
- *Swing-to gait*: Crutches are placed ahead of the person, and, with weight on the crutches, the body swings through to the crutches.
- *Three-point gait*: Partial weight-bearing is permitted.

As the older adult practices the walking program outlined earlier, the person should master sufficient ADLs to be independent. This independence includes being able to get up and down steps and in and out of cars. It is important for nurses to be very familiar with all assistive devices used in walking programs.

Walking programs also are initiated for elderly adults without assistive devices. Walking for the older adult is an excellent physical fitness activity. It provides cardiovascular fitness and aerobic exercise. Walking for 20 to 30 minutes, three times a week, has been supported by research as a way to maintain good physical fitness and conditioning. Walking should be a lifelong program to promote wellness and joy in living.

Continence Training

A second major clinical challenge is maintenance of bladder and bowel continence in a traumatized, disabled older adult. An older adult who is the recipient of good nursing care should not experience urinary or bowel incontinence. The use of an indwelling catheter is ineffective bladder management. Urinary infection can result within 24 hours of catheter insertion. Catheter insertion also lowers the self-esteem and self-concept of the person trying to regain control of a traumatized life.

Bladder retraining is generally successful when a regular time schedule is established for emptying the bladder. Retraining of the bladder takes patience on the part of the older adult and the nurse. A similar program for bowel training should be initiated soon after admission. As noted earlier, increasing the patient's fiber and fluid intake and a regular toileting regimen promotes bowel elimination on a regular schedule. If constipation does occur, stool softeners are the treatment of choice to resolve this problem. The use of enemas is not part of a retraining program. Enemas should be used only in an emergency.

Feeding and Self-Feeding Programs

The clinical challenge of maintaining nutrition adequate for tissue repair and health demands a high level of skill on the part of the LPN. In the early stages of rehabilitative and restorative nursing, the older adult may need to be fed through a nasogastric or enteral feeding tube. A specially formulated calorie-specific formula is administered through the feeding tube in either bolus feedings or continuous drip infusion.

As the older adult progresses in recovery, he or she may need to be placed on a feeding program in which manual assistance by the LPN or nursing assistant is needed until the person has sufficient strength for self-feeding. Older adults should be fed at regular mealtimes, and snacks should be provided. Promoting the older person to a self-feeding program is a definite sign of progress. Encouragement should be given by the nurse so that the older adult consumes sufficient calories to have adequate nutrition to meet the energy demands of rehabilitation.

Self-Promoting Behaviors and Activities of Daily Living

Independence in personal care is a challenge for older adults with disabilities that affect their ROM, mobility, strength, coordination, and dexterity. It is important that members of the nursing care team allow older adults to have time to perform aspects of their own care independently. Occupational therapists can provide assistive equipment that makes self-care easier. Built-up handles for toothbrushes and hairbrushes are easier for older adults to hold. A chair in the tub or shower may allow a weak individual to be able to bathe independently. Lowered sinks, counters, and mirrors might allow a wheelchair-bound person to sit up to the sink to wash and perform other personal care. Specially designed plastic devices with long handles to insert inside a person's socks and long-handled shoehorns allow older people who are unable to bend over to put on their own socks and shoes. Clothing with Velcro fasteners is easier to fasten and unfasten when dressing. Adjustments in the care environment and education of all of the personal care staff are essential to the success of self-care–ADL programs.

 ## CONCLUSION

This chapter provides an overview of the principles that govern rehabilitation and restorative nursing practices for LPNs who care for older adults in various settings. Through appreciation of the uniqueness of older adults and their special needs, rehabilitative and restorative nursing care can help them achieve optimal functioning to live life to the fullest.

CASE STUDY SOLUTION

1. Mr. A. needs assurance from the health professionals, nurses, and therapists that he will gain sufficient strength to walk with the aid of a walker and eventually to walk independently.

2. The LPN and Mr. A. contract to carry out the walking and exercise program on a daily basis to correct the footdrop problem.

3. By setting goals, Mr. A. perceives his condition in a more positive light and is encouraged by his progress.

4. The LPN also is concerned about Mr. A's despondency. She documents Mr. A.'s behavior and informs the RN about his psychological state. Together, the nurses talk with Mr. A. about his depression and seek his approval to obtain a psychiatric consultation. This problem is then referred to a mental health professional.

5. The LPN arranges for Mr. A. and his wife to become participants in a clinical conference in which the rehabilitative team reviews Mr. A.'s case and allows him to make informed decisions on how to proceed on discharge. This may include referral to various social agencies that could assist him in obtaining medical equipment for home use, receiving nursing care in the home if his wife feels unable to take care of Mr. A., and seeking Social Security and pension payments if Mr. A. believes he can no longer work.

6. Mr. A. is encouraged to eat nutritious meals so that his tissue can make repairs. He needs sufficient energy from his nutritional intake to do his exercises and walking program properly.

7. Activities are scheduled for him so that he can regain his social skills and interact with people without embarrassment and hesitation. Mr. A. was discharged from the hospital within 2 weeks of the incident, feeling that he was in charge of his life and that life was worth living. He also could see that the goals he and his wife had established for retirement could be accomplished. Mr. A. learned to live with his disability, and because of good nursing care, the quality of his life was not diminished.

REVIEW QUESTIONS

1. The aim of rehabilitation for older adults is to:
   1. Engage in limited ADLs
   2. Deny function and performance that existed before the incident
   3. Keep food and fluids at a level so that energy and strength are minimized
   4. Restore an individual to his or her former or best possible function and environmental status

2. Which of the following directives most closely coincides with the desired goals of a successful rehabilitation program?
   1. Keep physical changes at a minimum and promote self-esteem.
   2. Promote independence and self-care, along with mobility and a holistic approach to living with the disability.
   3. Promote involvement in limited activities and ROM exercises.
   4. Promote the fulfillment of the patient's life goals despite mobility problems.

3. Principles of rehabilitation include the most important step in nursing care, which is:
   1. Doing passive ROM
   2. Understanding the patient's self-concept and encouraging feelings of dependency
   3. Beginning rehabilitation immediately on the patient's admission
   4. Giving selective information to the family

4. Rehabilitation goals specific to older adults include:
   1. ROM exercises, transfer skills from bed to chair, dependency on enema usage
   2. Improvement of function, delay of deterioration, development of codependent behavior
   3. Accommodation to dysfunction, comfort in the dying process, accommodation to an indwelling catheter
   4. Delay of deterioration, improvement of function, accommodation to dysfunction, comfort in the dying process

5. In continence training for bladder control, the nurse should:
   1. Increase fluids, especially during the evening hours, and toilet the patient every 4 hours
   2. Restrict fluids during the nighttime hours and toilet the patient at his or her request
   3. Increase fluids during the daytime hours and toilet the patient every 1000 mL
   4. Increase fluids during the daytime hours and toilet the patient every 2 hours

REFERENCES

Benjamin, K., Edwards, N., Ploeg, J., & Legault, F. (2014). Barriers to physical activity and restorative care for residents in long-term care: A review of the literature. *Journal of Aging and Physical Activity,* 22, 154-165.

Chen, Y.M. (2010). Perceived barriers to physical activity among older adults residing in long-term care institutions. *Journal of Clinical Nursing,* 19, 432-439.

Galik, E. M., Resnick, B., & Pretzer-Aboff, I. (2009). "Knowing what makes them tick": Motivating cognitively impaired older adults to participate in restorative care. *International Journal of Nursing Practice,* 15, 48-55.

Resnick, B., Gruber-Baldini, A.L., Galik, E., Pretzer-Aboff, I., Russ, K., Hebel, J.R., & Zimmerman, S. (2009). Changing the philosophy of care in long-term care: Testing of the restorative care intervention. *Gerontologist,* 49(2), 175-184.

WEB RESOURCES

Association of Rehabilitation Nurses: www.rehabnurse.org/

National Rehabilitation Information Center: www.naric.com/

Pharmacology and Its Significance for Older Adults

21

KATHLEEN R. CULLITON

LEARNING OUTCOMES

1. Discuss how aging changes affect the pharmacodynamics and pharmacokinetics of medications.

2. Explain the impact of polypharmacy on safety for older adults.

3. List four ways a licensed nurse can support the physician in implementing Beers criteria.

4. Define the purpose of understanding chronopharmacology.

5. Develop a nursing care plan to synthesize interventions to assist older persons in maintaining proper pharmacotherapeutics.

CONCEPTS

Managing Care

Safety

CASE STUDY

Mr. W.'s neighbor called the home health-care agency where you work and requested that a home visit be made because Mr. W. seems to be getting thinner and thinner. The agency assigns you to go visit. You find Mr. W. sitting on the porch with his feet propped up and half asleep. Mr. W. is 74 years old and lives at home alone. He does fairly well on his own. He has difficulty seeing, but he can read soup can labels. He has arthritis in his hands and opens cans with an electric opener.

Mr. W.'s drug history includes

- Captopril, 25 mg oral twice a day for heart failure
- Carvedilol 25, mg oral twice a day for heart failure
- Furosemide, 20 mg oral every day for hypertension
- Ibuprofen, 600 mg oral three times daily for arthritis
- Simvastatin, 10 mg oral daily for hyperlipidemia
- Potassium chloride, 500 mg oral twice a day for potassium replacement

Mr. W. denies any use of street drugs and states that he "doesn't believe in that stuff." Mr. W. drinks a six-pack of beer each week and occasionally has a tomato juice and vodka before he goes to bed. When asked about other medications, he states that he uses Mylanta "several times a day, just one tablespoon full," and Ex-Lax every day for a bowel movement. He also takes a small blue-and-white capsule that his brother gave him because it helps his brother's arthritis. He takes that capsule "once or twice, maybe three or four times a week."

Mr. W. is currently complaining of weakness, dizziness, and occasional chest pains that he treats with Mylanta. His feet and hands seem to be swelling lately.

Discussion

1. What is the first step in your home visit?

2. What nursing diagnoses may apply to Mr. W. at this time?

3. While looking at his brother's blue-and-white capsule, you discover the name of the drug on the side. What is your best course of action regarding this "over-the-fence" drug?

4. What role does the Ex-Lax play in Mr. W.'s pharmacotherapeutics?

5. What referrals does the nurse need to make?

6. What should the nurse do to assist Mr. W. in becoming compliant?

 INTRODUCTION

One of the biggest advances in medical care has been the discovery and rediscovery of plants and chemical compounds that formulate drugs. Drugs are prescribed to manage and sometimes cure physical and mental illnesses. Ancient civilizations used various herbs and other plant and mineral substances to prevent and treat physical and mental problems. Many modern drugs used in Western medical practice have a long history of effectiveness in healing. Some medicines that are prescribed today were originally discovered and used by medical practitioners and healers from other cultures. Quality medical care and medications are responsible for increasing the life expectancy of large populations of people. A dilemma of Western medicine is the heavy dependence on the use of medications for managing and treating diseases. Many people do not consider a medical treatment complete unless they receive a prescription for a drug. This can be a serious issue for older adults. Mr. W. is taking six prescription medications for hypertension, hyperlipidemia, heart failure, and arthritis, all chronic diseases. Because these medications manage and do not cure diseases, Mr. W. may be taking these medications for the rest of his life.

This chapter examines issues related to drug use and older adults. Following are some basic terms related to drug use:

- *Pharmacology*—The study of medications.
- *Pharmacotherapeutics*—The use of medications to treat diseases. The benefit of a medication (desired effect) is weighed against the unwanted and dangerous effects (side effects) to measure the appropriate use of any medication.
- *Pharmacodynamics*—The effect of specific medications at the site of action. Pharmacokinetics, half-life, protein binding, disease processes, and aging affect pharmacodynamics.
- *Pharmacokinetics*—The study of how a medication moves into and through the body and how it is excreted from the body. The processes of absorption, distribution, metabolism, and excretion are affected by aging and diseases and influence the pharmacodynamics of any drug.
- *Half-life*—The time required for half the medication to be excreted or inactivated by the body.
- *Protein binding*—Binding properties of proteins. Proteins in the bloodstream are binding sites for many drugs. The portion of a drug that is bound to a protein is inactive (only a free drug is available to have a desired effect). Two drugs that are both highly protein-bound compete for protein-binding sites. This competition significantly increases the level of free drug in the bloodstream (drug molecules that were bound to the protein and have been released). The significant increase has an impact on the effects and adverse effects of the drug.
- *Adverse drug reactions (ADRs)*—Unwanted effects or side effects of a medication. ADRs are related to changes in pharmacokinetics, dosage amounts, timing of doses, and interactions of medications with other medications or foods (Hale, Griffin, Cartwright, Moulin, Alford & Fleming, 2008).

FACTORS AFFECTING PHARMACOTHERAPEUTICS FOR OLDER ADULTS

Sensory Changes

As individuals age, changes occur that can affect pharmacotherapeutics. Changes in vision, hearing, taste, and sensations all can affect the safe use of medication for older adults. Nurses need to be aware of the negative impact of sensory changes and adapt nursing care to ensure safe medication use.

Changes in Vision

Changes in vision can have a serious impact on the safe use of medications by older adults. As individuals age, they experience increased difficulty distinguishing colors, especially blue and green, because of the hardening and yellowing of the lens in their eyes. This yellowing often makes it difficult for older adults to differentiate shades of blue, purple, brown, and green, yet older people can see bright yellow, red, and black more clearly. Many older adults have difficulty distinguishing individual pills by color. When older adults are instructed to take the "pink pill in the morning and the blue one at night," they may make errors.

Reading small print is also a challenge for many older adults. Older people often have trouble reading the label on drug bottles because of the small print. Mr. W. can read a soup can label, which is a good indicator that his vision is good enough to read a medication label. Why is this an important assessment for Mr. W.?

Mr. W. needs to be able to see to read medication labels and to read and review medication schedules. Attaching a large-print tag to a bottle and having a magnifying glass by drug bottles can help an older person read the medication bottle label and avoid medication errors. Using a medication box or mediplanner is a good idea for many older individuals. Medication boxes are filled with the person's ordered medication. The box has a separate compartment for each time during the day that the older person has to take a medication. The box is usually filled for 1 week at a time, and the days of the week and times of medication doses are clearly marked in large, bold, raised initials and symbols. Family members and friends can be taught to assist the older person in preparing the medication box for a week at a time.

Sensitivity to glare is another visual challenge for aging eyes. Shiny surfaces such as plastic tape over medication labels can be difficult for older people to read. Portions of instructions written on paper that has been laminated may be missed or difficult to read because of reflecting glare. Labels for drug bottles should be printed on paper that is not shiny. Medication instructions should be in bold, large print on white or yellow paper to ensure they can be read.

Decreased Hearing Acuity

Hearing changes, such as presbycusis, increase the possibility that an older person may be unable to hear and understand instructions. Often, out of habit, older adults may nod their heads or state that they understand instructions even if they did not hear them all. Asking an older adult to repeat or demonstrate instructions is an excellent way to ensure that the instructions have been heard. Using large print instructions and following them when giving verbal instructions also helps older people. Many people with hearing difficulties develop lip-reading skills. Ensure that the older adult can see your mouth while you are giving instructions. Wearing lipstick if you are a woman and speaking slowly and intentionally, rather than louder, enhances an older person's ability to read lips. Throughout the time that you, the nurse, are giving verbal instructions, stop and ask older patients if they have any questions. Clarify information and have the older patient restate and demonstrate the teaching that is occurring.

Decreased Taste Acuity

With age, older adults experience changes in taste. It is most obvious in foods. A common complaint is that food is bland or has no taste. Changes in recognizing tastes and flavors result from changes in the taste buds and often in the sense of smell. The ability to differentiate medications by taste is inhibited, and the potential for unknowingly taking nonmedications or caustic poisons increases. Encourage older adults to throw away old prescription bottles and not to use them for storing household cleaning products and other poisons that may be mistaken for medications.

Changes in Touch and Dexterity

Older adults experience decreased touch sensitivity as they age. This decreased sensitivity can be worsened with decreased circulation and peripheral nerve deterioration in the hands and feet. Arthritic joint changes can combine with decreased touch to minimize strength, which can make it difficult to open modern packages. Childproof lids that require a person to push down and turn at the same time are very difficult for older people to open. Individual drug doses in plastic bubbles that require the plastic to be torn or the backing to be ripped off also are difficult to open. Pharmacists use alternative packaging for older adults if the older person requests it. Flip-top lids can replace the hard-to-twist childproof lids. Bubble-packed medications can be cut out of the packaging and placed in a pill bottle or a pill box.

Cognitive Changes

With increasing age and subsequent risk for disease, older adults may have changes in their thought patterns. It is important for the nurse to question what has caused the thought pattern changes. Are the causes pathological or drug-induced? Sometimes older adults have trouble remembering if they have taken their medications. Multiple drugs with varying dosages administered at different hours often create confusion.

The technical language that health-care professionals frequently use can be difficult for older people to understand, and they often are unwilling

---

QSEN

COMPETENCY: Safety (Knowledge)

Older Adult Issues That May Affect Safety of Medication Use

Visual changes
- Difficulty identifying colors (blue pill/green pill)
- Difficulty reading small print
- Sensitivity to glare on shiny surfaces of bottles.

Hearing changes
- Inability to hear instructions
- Not asking questions for clarification for fear of "looking dumb" when they have not heard instructions

Cognitive changes
- Trouble remembering if medications were taken
- Confusion with complex medication regimens
- Inability to remember correct medication for specific symptoms

to ask questions. Many older adults do not want to seem uninformed and state that they trust the physician or nurse to do what is right.

Challenges With Taking Medications Correctly

Often individuals do not follow their drug regimen correctly. This can be intentional or the result of poor understanding. If older adults do not understand how a drug works or do not like the effect of a drug, they may make mistakes in administering their medications. Common problems are taking doses at the wrong time and altering the dosage amounts.

Forgetting to take medications is a routine compliance issue. When giving older people medication instructions, ask them to describe a typical day. Instructing older adults to take a medication everyday before breakfast rather than instructing them to take the drug at 8:00 a.m. may encourage compliance, especially if they sleep until noon or are up at 5:00 a.m. Studies have shown that more medication doses are forgotten when a drug is dosed frequently during the day rather than once a day. Simplified dosing schedules that consider the older person's daily routine and the use of medications that are dosed only once a day can help the person be compliant in taking medications.

Drugs are taken for the chemical effect that they have on the body. Unwanted effects or side effects are common for many medications. Individuals often choose to alter the dosages or quit taking an ordered medication because of the side effects. One of the most common side effects that older adults complain of is upset stomach; this often is caused by the medication dissolving in the stomach and irritating the stomach lining. Stomach irritation can be lessened if the older adult takes the medication with food, so instruct the older adult to do so as long as the medication does not need to be taken on an empty stomach. If the medication needs to be taken on an empty stomach, encourage the person to drink at least 8 oz (1 cup) of water with the medication. Drinking water washes the medication through the stomach faster and, it is hoped, lessens stomach irritation. Encourage people to talk about the uncomfortable side effects of their medications. Often by simply changing the timing of a medication dosage (from morning to bedtime dosing), unwanted or bothersome side effects may decrease significantly.

Both of these women take medications daily. Because they are compliant and follow their drug regimen correctly, they are able to attend, for example, this cookout. They also spend time with their families and give a great deal of service to their community. They both agree that their health is improved because of the medications they take.

People commonly simply stop taking a medication. News in the media and advice from neighbors or friends may make older people uncomfortable with specific drugs or fearful of the drug's long-term effects on their bodies. Encourage older patients to discuss these concerns. Patients who are not accurately following prescribed drug regimens are reluctant to tell their physician. Not following orders could be interpreted as questioning the physician's skill and knowledge, and most older people do not want to be disrespectful. Many older adults manipulate drug routines to fit their beliefs about personal medication needs. Encourage an open dialogue about medications. Allow the expression of concerns or questions. Review magazines and newspapers that older people read to keep informed regarding potential questions and concerns they may have regarding their medications.

Polypharmacy and Chronic Health

A good rule to follow for pharmacotherapeutics in older people is "the smallest number of drugs should be prescribed at the lowest possible dose."

Older adults often have multiple chronic diseases. People with chronic health problems frequently have several drugs prescribed for each problem. The result for older patients often is multiple medications and a complex medication regimen. This complexity is compounded when the older individual has different physicians prescribing medications for each disease. Pharmacists are skilled at identifying potential drug interactions, but their effectiveness depends on awareness of the total medication regimen. If an older person uses more than one pharmacy, a pharmacist may not be aware of other drugs that the older adult is taking. Increased numbers of medications and varied dosing schedules can lead to mistakes in taking medications and serious drug interactions. For example, an older adult with Alzheimer's disease may have periods of anxiety and agitated behavior. An antianxiety medication may be prescribed to decrease the anxiety and agitated behavior. Antianxiety medication has a central nervous system sedating effect that can increase drowsiness and cause the older adult to be at risk for immobility and falls. Immobility can lead to joint pain and stiffness that may require pain medications. Pain medications can increase sedation and drowsiness and lead to an increased risk of falls. Using drugs to treat disease symptoms and using other drugs to treat the side effects of such drugs can lead to the severe adverse drug effects of polypharmacy. Simplification of drug regimens is an important step in avoiding adverse effects of polypharmacy.

Complex medication routines are not the only cause of polypharmacy. Many older individuals take multiple nonprescription medications, such as laxatives, herbs, vitamins, and other home remedies. These widely available, over-the-counter

(OTC) medications may interact or interfere with prescribed medications, leading to adverse drug reactions (ADRs).

Older adults are significantly more prone than younger adults to having undesirable drug reactions.

Evidence-Based Practice

Richardson, K., Ananou, A., Lafortune, L., Brayne, C., & Matthew, F.E. (2011). Variation over time in the association between polypharmacy and mortality in the older population. Drugs Aging, 28(7), 547-560.

This article examines the mortality of 12,423 individuals older than 65 years of age over time. The original data on medication use (both prescription and over the counter), health conditions, and disability were collected in 1991 through 1993. The study followed these participants from England and Wales for up to 18 years.

As the data were analyzed, there was a strong correlation between use of five or more medications and death in the short term, identified as the first 2 years. The association of multiple medications and death for women in the 2- to 18-year period was significant but was nonsignificant for men.

This was a surprising study. Through reading about medications and older adults, adverse drug reactions, multiple emergency room visits, falls, and other negative happenings are the result of polypharmacy. One may assume that increased mortality would also be associated with increased number of medications used.

These authors put forth the challenge that polypharmacy is not a simplistic problem. The types of medications and the disease processes being treated also need to be considered when examining drug use in older adults.

One of the explanations the authors discussed was the culture of medicine in the United Kingdom. The conservative prescriptive practice of United Kingdom physicians was discussed as a possible variable for decreased association of polypharmacy and mortality.

Question

Can you think of some ways that cultural practices may affect medication use and polypharmacy for older adults?

Point of Interest

It is becoming common for older adults to purchase medications from Mexico or Canada either by traveling there or through the Internet. Medications may not have the same strict manufacturing controls that are in place in the United States and the dosages of the medications may not be equivalent to those in the United States. This is an important point for discussion with older persons.

This potential increases in direct proportion to the number of medications being taken. Common ADR symptoms include changes in mood or behavior, restlessness, confusion, irritability, anxiety, insomnia, and hallucinations suggestive of mental deterioration. Many of these symptoms can be misidentified as confusion or dementia and the ADR may go unrecognized and untreated. More medications may be prescribed to treat the symptoms of ADRs, and the cycle of problems continues.

Financial Concerns

Medications are expensive. Sometimes financial concerns lead older adults to misuse prescription medications. Taking a medication every other day rather than every day and sharing medications with other seniors are common but dangerous practices.

The cost of physician office visits and getting prescriptions filled may be difficult for an older person to manage. Some chose never to get their prescriptions filled. Others save their prescriptions until they can get to the pharmacist with the

This is the man whose wife has rheumatoid arthritis. He feels concern over being able to pay for the medication necessary for her to move as little as she does. His commitment is to his wife, however, and the quality of her life. He says he always has made it work, and he will in the future as well.

Think Like a Nurse

Mr. and Mrs. Washburn spend 3 months in the winter in Texas, New Mexico, or Arizona and take regular trips into Mexico to purchase medications because they are much less expensive than in the United States. What are some concerns that you can share with the Washburns? Be sure to consider all possible concerns.

right amount of money (this may result in not taking the medications for a month or more). Some people choose OTC medications for relief of the same symptoms as the prescribed drug. Some people take the medications until the symptoms decrease and then put the rest away for "later."

 ## PHARMACOKINETICS

Physiological changes related to normal aging and various disease processes affect the pharmacokinetics of many medications. When an individual takes a medication, there are certain expected events that assist the medication in getting to the intended site of action or effect. Medications in pill form are usually formulated to break down in the stomach acid or the small intestine. The dissolved medication is absorbed in the same place. If the individual has had a part of the stomach removed or has a low concentration of stomach acid, the pill may not be dissolved enough to be absorbed as expected. A good blood supply is necessary for the distribution of medication. Diminished blood supply to or from an area of the body alters the effective distribution of the medication. The liver metabolizes most medications. Liver disease or changes in the blood circulation to the liver change the expected metabolism of a medication. Excretion is the last step in pharmacokinetics. The kidneys have a major role in the excretion of most medications. Kidney disease or decreased blood flow to the kidneys can seriously change the intended excretion of medications. A discussion of the specific pharmacokinetic concerns for older adults follows.

Decreased Absorption

The overall effect of aging changes in older adults is decreased absorption. A major complaint by many older individuals is change in gastrointestinal (GI) motility, with resulting diarrhea or constipation. Drugs are absorbed poorly if they travel through the intestines at a rapid rate. Chronic diarrhea and overuse of laxatives move a medication through the intestines at a rapid rate and decrease the time that the drug is in contact with the intestinal wall to be absorbed. Drugs also are absorbed poorly if the intestine is impacted with stool, as in constipation.

Changes in the GI tract probably interfere with normal absorption of medications. Older adults often have changes in the quality and quantity of digestive enzymes that are important for dissolving and transforming medications into a form that can be absorbed through the intestine. Gastric pH becomes less acidic, and there is an overall decrease in the number of absorbing cells in the intestinal mucosa. The smooth muscle tone and motor activity of the GI tract decline with advancing age. These changes, along with slowed intestinal motility, decreased intestinal blood flow, and slowed gastric emptying time, serve to decrease potential drug absorption further. Atherosclerotic changes reduce the flow of blood to the major organs, resulting in slower disintegration of solid dosage forms such as tablets. Because of the changes in GI motility, drugs that are manufactured for normal adult GI motility are not suited to the slower geriatric bowel. Some drugs may be absorbed in lesser amounts. For example, acidic drugs are ionized to a greater extent, resulting in decreased absorption. Acetylsalicylic acid (aspirin) is more ionized in older people because their secretion of stomach acid is decreased. Absorption of aspirin may be decreased in older adults. Some drugs may be absorbed in greater amounts. Drugs that are absorbed from the intestines are more thoroughly absorbed if they remain in contact with the intestinal wall for a longer time.

Distribution

Drug distribution is greatly altered in older persons. As people age, the body mass becomes leaner with decreased parenchymal tissue and increased fat content. Increased fat results in increased absorption of fat-soluble drugs, resulting in decreased activity and prolonged effects for such drugs. Examples of drugs showing this effect are hypnotics, sedatives, fat-soluble vitamins, and heparin.

Changes in the cardiovascular system of older people may result in delayed arrival of the medication at the target receptors, slow release of the drug from the storage tissue, and slowed excretion of the drug. Decreased blood flow to the specific target tissue may result in decreased drug distribution.

Older people may have decreased plasma protein concentrations related to chronic disease processes or decreased nutrition. Plasma protein level is an important factor directly impacting the amount of a protein available to bind with a drug and the amount of free drug (unbound to protein) available to provide the intended drug effect. Most drug dosages are set for people with normal plasma protein levels. If the older person has less plasma protein, more of the drug is free (i.e., unbound to the protein) and is free to act on the receptors and cause its effect. For example, warfarin (Coumadin) is 90% bound in the average adult. Its dosage is regulated because 90% of it is bound to protein and is unavailable to the person. If the person is elderly, has dementia, is eating less than 30% of meals, and has half the normal adult protein level, a normal dose of warfarin would be an overdose.

Some researchers believe that the number and nature of drug receptors in the body change with aging. A decreased or increased response to a normal dosage of medication could result.

Another factor that influences drug distribution is dehydration that may be related to limiting fluids or the inability to drink adequate fluids, treatments that include diuretics or other medications that increase fluid loss, or illness that causes fluid loss, such as vomiting and diarrhea. Dehydration can result in decreased serum volume, which would increase the concentration of a medication in the blood.

Metabolism

Older adults experience a decrease in the rates of overall metabolism, microsomal metabolism, and hepatic biotransformation of the drug and a decline in the body's ability to transform active drugs into inactive drugs. The overall effect of these changes is that the medication remains for a longer time in an active form in older people. Some drugs may remain in the body twice as long as in younger adults.

Excretion

The altered filtration and decreased plasma volume that occur with dehydration commonly found in older people change the excretion of medications. Age-related renal changes result in slower excretion of the drug. Slowed excretion keeps drugs in the body longer and can lead to drug toxicity. Decreased respiratory and vital capacity, with increased carbon dioxide retention, results in decreased excretion of drugs normally excreted by respiration, such as anesthetics. Decreased and changed excretion results in an overall increased pharmacological effect of medications in older people (Carlson & Pfadt, 2009).

The overall effect of aging changes in older adults is increased pharmacological effect. Although less medication is absorbed, it stays longer in the body and remains in the circulation for a longer time.

 ## PHARMACOLOGY PROBLEMS

Pharmacology in older adults is frequently identified as a "can of worms." Problems include misuse, overuse, underuse, erratic use, and contraindicated use of drugs. Misuse phenomena include incorrect dosing, sharing of medications between neighbors and friends, and use of the same medications for a variety of purposes. As an individual ages, the dosage requirements for most medications decrease. Many medications given in normal adult doses to older adults result in an overdose. Another aspect of misuse occurs when a drug is taken for a variety of symptoms. An older adult may reason, "Well, this pill works for my upset stomach; it will probably work for my diarrhea."

Overuse may result from the belief that if one pill works well, then two pills will work better. People may believe that if they feel better with a vitamin supplement, then two vitamin supplements would definitely improve their health. This behavior may lead to serious ADRs.

In underuse problems, the person takes less medication than prescribed to "save" pills or money if finances are a problem. Many older adults are on fixed and limited incomes, the cost of medication is high, and medication is sometimes too expensive for the person to afford. Erratic use frequently occurs with short-term memory loss or forgetfulness; for example, a person may forget to take medications for 1 or 2 days.

Contraindicated use can apply in numerous situations. Sometimes older adults receive several drugs from several physicians. They also may have the prescriptions filled at several pharmacies. The end result is that the older population is at a much greater risk for drug interactions, allergic reactions, and problems with polypharmacy (taking multiple medications).

Specific Drug Problems for Older Adults

If all medications were carefully monitored and taken properly, and if the dosage were regulated and accompanied with instructions, the older adult would still be at greater risk than a younger adult for drug-specific problems because of aging changes in drug absorption, metabolism, and excretion. If an older person was prescribed the proper dosage of digoxin, understood the medication regimen, and was in full compliance, the older person would still be at a higher risk for complications to develop. Older people simply experience more side effects and difficulties.

Table 21.1 identifies categories of drugs that may precipitate side effects and adverse effects in older persons. It is important that you, as the licensed practical nurse (LPN), be aware of the possibility of potential problems and monitor for them.

Another specific drug problem is the use of home remedies and OTC medications. Home remedies, antacids, laxatives, and alcohol frequently interfere with the proper functioning of medication. Use of home remedies and OTC medications frequently interferes with pharmacotherapeutics. Some home remedies have actual benefits, some have only psychological benefits, and some are detrimental. For example, the use of bicarbonate of soda for "acid stomach" is detrimental and may result in serious acid-base imbalance. The ingredients of the home remedy and

The problem of polypharmacy is a challenging one for older adults. This man has multiple chronic diseases. The medication prescribed for him from his three physicians adds up to 22 pills each morning and 12 at night. It worries him, and he wants help in organizing the medications. Where would you refer him if he were your neighbor or family member?

TABLE 21.1   SPECIFIC DRUG PROBLEMS OF ELDERLY PATIENTS

Effect	Drugs
Drugs that cause dry mouth	Analgesics, anticholinergics, antidiarrheals, antilipemics, antiemetics, antipsychotics, antiulcer medications, muscle relaxants, antihistamines, antiparkinsonian medications, antihypertensives
Drugs that promote gastroesophageal reflux	Anticholinergics, beta-blockers, diazepam, dopamine, theophylline
Drugs associated with ulcer formation	Adrenocorticotropic hormones, aspirin, indomethacin, iron, histamine, phenacetin, potassium
Drugs that alter absorption of nutrients	Colchicine, neomycin, cholestyramine, antacids, tricyclic antidepressants, sucralfate (Carafate)
Drugs that promote constipation	Aluminum-containing and calcium-containing antacids, narcotic analgesics, anticholinergics, diuretics, iron, tricyclic antidepressants
Drugs that may promote diarrhea	Analgesics, anti-inflammatory agents, antacids, antiulcer medications, antibiotics, antihypertensive medications, asthma drugs, cardiovascular drugs, diuretics, iron
Drugs that may promote hepatic damage	Acetaminophen (Tylenol), analgesics, anesthetics, antibiotics (especially penicillin and sulfa), antineoplastics, cardiovascular drugs, oral hypoglycemics, steroids
Drugs that may cause excessive depression	Antihistamines, antipsychotics, anxiolytics, cardiac glycosides, narcotics, sedatives/hypnotics
Drugs that may cause dysrhythmias	Antidepressants, cardiac glycosides, phenytoin
Drugs that may damage the kidneys	Aminoglycosides, antibiotics, colchicine
Drugs that may precipitate electrolyte imbalances	Corticosteroids, diuretics
Drugs that may precipitate blood dyscrasias	Antineoplastics, antipsychotics

OTC medications need to be evaluated. The LPN must evaluate the frequency of use and the possible interactions.

Antacid Abuse

Some older people consume large amounts of antacids. Physically, a decreased amount of gastric acid has been documented with aging; paradoxically, antacid use usually increases with age. The antacids may be used by the elderly person for symptoms of chest pain. Early angina attacks may be considered heartburn and treated with antacids. Other pathological processes also may be perceived

as heartburn. This behavior can result in lack of care for serious health problems. Many antacids are high in sodium content. Excessive use of antacids can increase the severity of cardiovascular and renal disease, exacerbate hypertension, and result in increased fluid load for the aged body. Antacids are notorious for altering the motility of the gut, with resulting diarrhea or constipation. Mr. W. is taking Mylanta (magnesium hydroxide and aluminum hydroxide), an antacid. Complaints of stomach and chest pain can be serious and need to be evaluated by Mr. W.'s physician. Because he is taking ibuprofen, a nonsteroidal antiinflammatory medication

(NSAID) and is regularly using alcohol, he is at risk for stomach irritation and potential gastric bleeding. Chest pain is always considered to be heart related unless heart problems are ruled out. Mr. W. has a history of heart disease and is currently being treated for heart failure, hyperlipidemia, and hypertension. All of these diagnoses place him at risk for angina or a possible myocardial infarction.

Laxative Abuse

Another class of drugs sometimes abused by older adults is laxatives. Laxatives may be taken once, twice, or more than three times a day. Some older people forget that they have had a bowel movement and take more laxatives to facilitate another bowel movement. Although there is no consistent alteration in frequency of bowel movements with advancing age, the ingestion of laxatives increases significantly.

Laxative abuse may result in damage to the intestinal mucosa. The ascending colon is often the site for this damage, and it may dilate and shorten, losing its typical muscular features, resulting in decreased absorption of other medications (and nutrients) that are administered orally. Laxatives also inhibit the absorption of medications from the intestine; this results in decreased levels of the available drug being absorbed, causing a decreased therapeutic effect. Laxatives also result in fluid and electrolyte imbalances that may exacerbate cardiovascular or renal problems. A person who is a frequent abuser of laxatives should be assisted in developing other bowel-training methods. Psychological intervention may be necessary. Mr. W. is taking Ex-Lax (sennoside) a stimulant laxative every day. Daily use can lead to laxative dependence, which means that the bowel (peristalsis) no longer responds to normal reflexes and stretching stimuli to move the bowels. Overuse of laxatives may cause Mr. W. to have diarrhea, excess fluid and electrolyte loss, and even a decrease in the gastrointestinal absorption of medications. Because the laxative is stimulating the bowel to empty, medications are also "speeding" through the small intestine and do not have adequate time in contact with the absorbing surface of the small intestine, so less medication is absorbed.

Alcohol Abuse

Alcohol abuse is a social health problem in some older people. It is the primary drug of abuse worldwide. Alcohol abuse interferes with pharmacotherapeutics and frequently results in altered nutritional status. This may be seen in decreased serum protein levels (as discussed earlier in this chapter), decreased protein binding, and resultant overdosing of older people. Acid-base balance and fluid and electrolyte levels are adversely affected by alcohol abuse. Changes in these two homeostatic mechanisms result in changes in the pharmacotherapeutic effects of the medication regimen (Rigler, 2000).

Alcohol impairs thinking, judgment, and psychomotor coordination, all of which may lead to decreased medication compliance. Alcohol increases or decreases the effects of several other drugs, and other drugs often increase or decrease the effects of alcohol. Alcohol is a central nervous system depressant that potentiates other central nervous system depressants, particularly barbiturates. When taken concurrently, these two drugs may result in central nervous system depression, coma, and death.

Alcohol has a vasodilating effect and consequently increases the hypotensive effects of most antihypertensive drugs. The effect of alcohol on oral anticoagulants varies. Alcohol intake decreases the effects of the anticoagulants until liver damage occurs, at which point the anticoagulant effects are increased.

Medication Administration Considerations

An evaluation of how older adults manage multiple medications and when they take their medications could reveal potential pharmacology problems. Beer's criteria and chronopharmacology address these concerns and can help you to provide suggestions for more effective medication administration.

Beers Criteria

Beers criteria (American Geriatrics Society, 2012) were originally developed in 1991 as a list of potentially inappropriate medications (PIM) for nursing home residents. The criteria were revised in 1997 and 2003. The latest revision, 2012, is divided into three separate groups:

1. Potentially inappropriate medications and classes to avoid in older adults
2. Potentially inappropriate medications and classes to avoid in older adults with certain diseases and syndromes that the drugs listed can exacerbate

3. Medications to be used with caution in older adults Because aging is associated with a progressive decline in physiological function (which refers to the absorption, distribution, and elimination of medication) and multiple diseases, such as hypertension, arthritis, and diabetes, there is a strong need for oral medications to be given with attention to the personal needs of the older adult. Beer's criteria presents a standardized and collaborative approach for medication reduction and simplification.

Fifty-three medications or medication categories were placed in the groups based on the evidence of drug related medication issues and research supported adverse drug events for older adults.

The use of Beers criteria is the responsibility of the physician because physicians are responsible for ordering medications. There are several things you can do, however, to promote and support these criteria that would result in better medication administration for your elderly patients.

As the LPN, you need to be aware of Beers criteria so that you can talk to older people and get the needed information, share that information with the registered nurse (RN), and ask about the possibility of a Beers criteria review of the elderly person's medications. In general, a medication review is suggested for any older person.

All older adults admitted to long-term care facilities have mandated physician, pharmacist, and nursing interdisciplinary team members involved in reviewing the medication treatment plan.

Because aging is associated with a progressive decline in physiological function (which refers to the absorption, distribution, and elimination of medication) and multiple diseases, such as hypertension, arthritis, and diabetes, there is a strong need for oral medications to be given with attention to the personal needs of the older adult. Beers criteria present a standardized and collaborative approach for medication reduction and simplification.

Promoting Safe Medication Use

Listed here are some very practical things that you, as an LPN, can do to encourage the safety of medication use and older adults.

1. *Remove or discard unnecessary or expired drugs to prevent confusion.* This can be done without a physician's order. If you are a home health nurse, go through all medications with the older person or family members. If you are in a hospital or nursing home and have someone with multiple medications, ask a family member to bring them all in to you. You or the pharmacist can go over the medication with the older person or a family member.

2. *Encourage the use of a single pharmacy to enhance regimen review and collaboration with the pharmacist.* This can be done without a physician's order. It is simply good common sense. When you review the medications at home or medications brought into the facility, you can note what pharmacies are used and make suggestions to the family as to how to get them all transferred to one pharmacy.

3. *Consider nonpharmacological alternatives.* This can be done without a physician's order. You can suggest elevation of swollen feet, meditation and deep breathing for a headache, or mild heat for arthritis. Any alternative that can decrease the amount of medication being taken is considered a positive action. Mr. W. was elevating his legs when the nurse went to his home to visit him. This promotes venous return and decreases peripheral edema that can be an uncomfortable side effect of heart failure.

Point of Interest

Remember, do not flush or place quantities of medication in the garbage. Instruct the older person or a family member to dispose of the medications at a drug disposal station. Call the city or county for information about drug take-back services in your community. The United States Drug Enforcement Administration sponsors National Prescription Drug Take-Back Days with local law enforcement groups. For more information check the Food and Drug Administration site http://www.fda.gov/ and search Safe Drug Disposal.

4. *Coordinate administration times with established sleep and activity patterns.* This can be done without a physician's order. Ask for a list of times the medications are taken, and compare that with nap, sleep, and meal times. What can be changed to make compliance easier for the person who takes the medication? Associating medication administration with meal time or nap and sleep times encourages compliance in taking the drugs. Talk to the person about compliance and offer advice if you have it.

Chronopharmacology

Circadian rhythm is the reaction to the rotation of the earth around its axis in 24 hours and around the sun in 365 days. We each have variations of our personal circadian rhythms. There are people who stay up late, and others who get up early. Some nurses love to work the night shift, and others spend an entire career trying to avoid night shifts. All of these things and many more behaviors are driven by our personal circadian rhythms.

The rhythms of the human body can impact the absorption, distribution, metabolism, elimination, and even the effect of some medications. The study of this phenomenon is called chronopharmacology. Research scientists have defined the major circadian rhythms in humans that impact the body's use of medications; they also recognize that diseases do not display characteristics that are consistent over a 24-hour period. For example, research indicates that most asthma attacks occur at night. What does that tell you about administering asthma medication? Other consistencies include allergic rhinitis symptoms, which are generally worse in the morning; gastric acid secretion, which peaks between 2:00 a.m. and 4:00 a.m.; and the incidence of gastric ulcers, which is greater in the winter. Another example is cardiac disease: Angina, myocardial infarction, and thrombolytic stroke generally occur in the first 4 hours after waking. What does this indicate to you regarding compliance with administering morning medications?

Scientists have managed the most difficult aspect of chronopharmacology by inventing necessary timing elements for the medications that you deliver to the people in your care. These elements include enteric coatings, time-release capsules, and specific administration times. Your responsibility is to deliver medications on time and in the form they were ordered. Do not cut an enteric-coated pill in half or open a capsule and give just part of it. The science of developing medications for specific timed release is sophisticated and well established, and it is one that you need to honor.

Every persons' circadian rhythms are well established and are an important factor to consider when administering medications. Honoring circadian rhythms results in more effective use of medication by the body. It also can reduce the amount of medication needed by the older person because it is given at the time the body needs it. Both factors have the potential of decreasing toxic effects and improving therapeutic impact.

NURSING CARE OF OLDER ADULTS RECEIVING MEDICATIONS

When managing care of older adults receiving medications, the nurse should follow the nursing process as taught in Chapter 3. The five-stage nursing process consists of assessment, diagnosis, planning, implementation, and evaluation.

Assessment

Before administration of medication, a thorough assessment of the older adult should be completed. A thorough health history is extremely important. Ask the person about past diseases, illness, or symptoms and how they were handled. Inquire about the person's current health status. The history must include past use of drugs, present use of drugs, prescribed drugs, OTC drugs, "over-the-fence" drugs, and street drugs. Specifically ask about use of laxatives and antacids. Assess the person's allergies. Did the allergic reaction cause the person to have difficulty breathing? Hives? Nausea? Vomiting?

Assess the older person's social support network and home environment. Is the person able to get prescriptions filled? Are family members or friends available to help with medication compliance? Assess cognitive skills. Is the person confused or disoriented? Is this problem transitory? Is the person capable of understanding any teaching that occurs? Is depression present?

Assess the older adult's sensory status. Is vision impaired? Is hearing impaired? Is the person strong enough to open pill bottles? Assess the individual's current understanding of therapies and

Critically Examine the Following:

You are doing clinical hours for school in a community setting in an economically deprived area of the city. There are predominately older adults with multiple chronic diseases being seen by the nurse practitioner (NP). You have been asked to review the laboratory work before the person is seen by the NP. You notice that approximately 50% of the older adults have a serum albumin below the norm (3.5 to 5.5). You are puzzled by this occurrence and begin interviewing the older persons in an attempt to identify what is causing the problem. Consider what you would be most likely to discover if this scenario were true, answer the questions listed, and bring your best thinking to class. Whatever you discover, describe what impact a serum albumin level below normal might have on a person's drug regimen.

1. Most likely causative factor:
2. Impact on drug regimen:

medication regimen. Does the person understand the drugs, dosage, side effects, or adverse effects of current medications?

Assess compliance. Does the person take medications at the proper time? For what reasons would the older adult miss a medication? Is there someone to provide transportation to the physician's office or the pharmacy?

A thorough physical examination must be performed. Watch the older adult for nutrition and fluid status. Is the person thin and emaciated? Is the person dehydrated? Is the person's serum protein level low? This finding may necessitate a reduction in some drug dosages. Is the person obese? If so, the person may require increased dosages of fat-soluble vitamins and medications.

Diagnosis

Many nursing diagnoses are applicable to the older adult receiving medication therapy. Applicable diagnoses include the following:

- Altered Health Maintenance related to insufficient teaching

- Ineffective Management of Therapeutic Regimen related to lack of motivation
- Noncompliance related to lack of financial resources
- Noncompliance related to inability to open bottles

Planning

To promote responsible medication habits in older adults, LPNs must help them become informed medication consumers. Because many older people remain in acute-care settings for only a limited time, discharge planning and teaching must begin on admission.

Before beginning any teaching session, some preparations are important. Choose an environment with good lighting and minimal environmental distractions. Ensure that the older adult who has glasses and hearing aids is wearing them. Prepare visual aids and reading materials with strong colors and large print.

Plan the teaching session to be only 15 to 20 minutes long. Speak clearly and slowly. Use a low-pitched voice (some older people have difficulty hearing a higher pitch). Always face the person when speaking.

Whenever possible, relate the learning to prior life experiences. For example, when teaching about a thyroid drug, help the patient identify personal health problems that occurred before seeking medical treatment and relate those symptoms to how the patient will feel if the medication dose is too low. Tie administration times for medications to the person's daily schedule. If the older person eats oatmeal every morning without fail, the morning dose of digoxin can be associated with the oatmeal breakfast.

Treat older adults as mature and capable people. Do not be patronizing in your teaching approach. Teach a family member, friend, or neighbor at the same time. Have the older person teach the other person and observe the integration of knowledge. Provide sufficient time for review, questions, and return demonstrations.

Consider the need for assistive devices. Medication boxes come in many styles with individual compartments for different days and times. Consider the need for nonchildproof caps. Medication containers can be color-coded and accompanied by a wall chart with the color coding system shown. Teach the person to turn bottles upside down after the medication is taken. Allow the older person to

PATIENT EDUCATION

When setting priorities for teaching medication administration to older adults, you must think holistically. Before you begin any medication administration instructions, sit and talk with the older person you are teaching. Can the person hear what you are saying? Can the person read? Does the person have the visual ability to identify colors to differentiate pills? Does the person have arthritic hands that make it difficult or impossible to open medication wrappings and bottles? What are the person's financial resources; can the person afford the medication ordered? Who else should be invited to the teaching session (e.g., spouse, children, other caregivers)? Have a family member bring in the proverbial "brown bag" of medication that the older adult has been taking so that you can ensure there is nothing at home that is contraindicated.

After you have determined the answers to the previous questions, you can plan your teaching session. When you teach, sit close so that the older person can see and hear you. Be organized and have a plan ready that meets the needs you assessed previously. Those of you with more clinical experience may be thinking "no one has time for such a demanding teaching session." This is where you learn *the priority* for medication administration. You must take the time to assess, plan, and teach all older adults about their medications and how to take them!

What good is the power of modern medications—many of them actually miracle drugs—if the person taking them does not do it properly? It does no good. Many older persons take multiple medications with diverse administration schedules, such as diuretics every other day and potassium twice each day. If that person is admitted to the emergency department because of a fall from low potassium and dehydration, what could be the cause? Yes, you're right. The older adult mixed up the instructions and was taking the diuretic twice a day and potassium once every other day. The fall could easily result in a fracture and a prolonged hospital stay after surgery to repair the break.

The priority with medication administration is to assess, plan, and teach the person about all pertinent aspects of the medications given.

be responsible for taking personal medication the last few days in the hospital. The nurse should monitor these actions and review any areas of knowledge deficit.

Encourage all older adults to carry a list of medications (including prescription and nonprescription drugs) at all times. Another family member should carry the same list. The older person should be encouraged to share the list with all physicians and pharmacists before receiving or filling any new prescriptions. Encourage all older adults to locate a pharmacy they like and fill all prescriptions there. On all admissions to the hospital, the nurse should review all medications and refer incompatibilities to the physician or pharmacist.

Implementation

In administering medications to older persons, several strategies are important. When administering medications by mouth, be aware of the medication form. Time-release capsules (e.g., many cold capsules) should not be opened or crushed and mixed with food. If the person is unable to swallow the capsule, contact the physician or pharmacist for a liquid form. Enteric-coated capsules should not be crushed or dissolved. Disruption of the enteric coating allows gastric acid to come into contact with the medication and inactivate it. Offer the most important medication first. Give the person enough fluid so that the medication reaches the stomach.

Parenteral injections should be given into the dorsogluteal or ventrogluteal sites. The deltoid muscle should be avoided because in most older people it has lost much of its mass. The vastus lateralis muscle should be avoided owing to its decreased muscle mass and decreased circulation. Avoid injections into edematous areas that have decreased circulation.

Intravenous therapy needs to be closely monitored in older people because many older adults are in a slightly dehydrated state. Fluid overload is especially critical in a person who may have underlying cardiac and renal disease that would be exacerbated by excess fluid.

Some older people experience visual changes with changes in a medication regimen. Recommend that the person not change prescription eyewear until the medication regimen is established.

Evaluation

Evaluation, the final step in the nursing process, is critical in administering medication for older

Point of Interest

You are admitting an older person to the medical unit for chest pain, shortness of breath, and edema, and neither the older person nor the family member can recall the medications the older person is taking. A solution to this problem that is easy for the family is the "brown-bag" solution. Ask the family member to go home and put all medications the older person is taking into a brown bag and bring them to you. Be sure the family member brings prescription, OTC, and natural remedies. Assure the family member that all medications will be returned. This will give you the opportunity to make an accurate list of medications being taken by the older adult. It also gives you the opportunity to point out outdated medications that should be discarded.

The outcome of a successful medication plan can be evaluated by the following criteria:

- The older adult's ability to solve problems related to polypharmacy
- Communication of adverse reactions
- Adherence to regimen

adults. Evaluate the person's learning curve by doing a return demonstration teaching session. Ask questions about situations the older adult may encounter in the home setting. Allow the person to ask questions of you.

Evaluation of compliance is based primarily on personal and family report. Ask the older adult if medications are being taken, and then clarify how and when the medications are being consumed. Ask about the occurrence of side effects. If expected side effects do not occur, the nurse should question whether or not the medication is being taken. Blood levels (if available for a given medication) should be evaluated to determine whether the levels are commensurate with the person's report. Monitor the older adult's laboratory results to determine kidney and liver function. Ask for a personal evaluation of how the new medication is working. Does it help? What concerns does the person have?

 CONCLUSION

Pharmacotherapy for older adults is complex. The nursing care of the older adult must include attention to the details of the medication regimen. The LPN needs to be familiar with the aging changes that affect pharmacotherapeutics, including pharmacokinetic changes, sensory changes, psychological changes, problems of polypharmacy, chronic health changes, and financial changes. It is important that the nurse understand the drugs likely to be misused and be aware of specific drugs that are frequently misused by elderly patients: antacids, laxatives, alcohol, and home remedies.

The nurse needs to be able to implement the nursing process on behalf of older adults to assist them to develop into well-informed medication consumers. The ability to teach regarding medication administration and evaluate the impact of medications on the older person is a crucial skill for you to have.

CASE STUDY SOLUTION

1. Introduce yourself, explain why you have come, and begin a complete assessment. The history, drug history, and physical assessment need to be complete. View Mr. W.'s environment. Ask about support services, friends, family, and neighbors. Explore nutritional status and assess what food is available for Mr. W. Assess eyesight. Can he read drug labels? Assess compliance. Does he know when and how to take the medications?

2. Knowledge deficit related to medication regimen
   Noncompliance related to lack of understanding
   Ineffective management of therapeutic regimen
   Sensory deficit related to diminished visual acuity

3. Although the blue-and-white pill is a non-narcotic analgesic and nonsteroidal anti-inflammatory drug, it has not been prescribed for Mr. W. Identify his feelings about the medication. Does it seem to help his arthritis? Does he have side effects with the drug? Explain to the patient why it is important not to use this drug unless it is prescribed by the physician. Identify interactions of the drug with other prescribed medications (decreases the effectiveness of diuretics and antihypertensive therapy, increases gastric irritation, increases serum levels and risk of toxicity from digoxin). Stress the importance of not taking drugs unless his physician prescribes them. Offer to make an appointment for him to see his physician and ask for a prescription for a medication to relieve arthritis pain.

4. Ex-Lax facilitates movement through the gut, decreasing absorption of all the other medications; it probably contributes to fluid and electrolyte imbalance.

5. Refer to the physician for evaluation of chest pain (if this resembles cardiac angina, consider emergency referral) and to social services for necessary social support. Call on family members for assistance with medications and transportation, and suggest Meals-on-Wheels.

6. Set up a scheduling plan. Draw a calendar with medications depicted. Teach Mr. W. to take medications at specific times each day. Encourage discontinuance of Ex-Lax, Mylanta, and the blue-and-white pill. Build on the knowledge that he already has. Relate medications to events in Mr. W.'s lifestyle. If he seems unable to manage medications on his own, ask the physician for a referral for home-health nurses to administer medications as needed.

REVIEW QUESTIONS

1. Considering the pharmacokinetics in the older person, which of the following statements is true?
   1. Overall absorption is decreased.
   2. Overall distribution is enhanced.
   3. There is an increase in receptors with aging.
   4. Excretion is facilitated, resulting in a shorter duration of drug action.

2. Which of the following factors would be the strongest in influencing compliance in an older person on a fixed income?
   1. Dietary habits
   2. Cost of filling prescriptions
   3. Body fat-to-lean muscle weight ratio
   4. Family support

3. When working with the interdiscplinary team to simplify a resident's medication regimen, the LPN should:
   1. Discontinue all multiple medications.
   2. Review all oral medications with the person who is ill and the family, and try to unify the prescriptions to one pharmacy.
   3. Make a note to the physician with all of the high-risk medications the ill person is taking on it.
   4. Ignore the oral medications except to give them as they are ordered.

4. Chronopharmacology relates to:
   1. What time people wake up in the morning
   2. The science of time-release and enteric-coated medications
   3. The correlation between one's circadian rhythm and medication effectiveness
   4. The correlation between one's circadian rhythm and injection effectiveness

5. Mrs. M., age 82, lives at home alone. Her daughter visits once a day and helps her bathe. Mrs. M. cooks her own meals and works in her home and yard. Which of the following factors could place Mrs. M. at risk of making a medication error?
   1. Multiple medications
   2. Visual changes
   3. Different schedules for different drugs
   4. All of the above

6. Mrs. M.'s daughter reports that she seems to take laxatives two or three times per day. What effect would laxative abuse have on the other medications Mrs. M. is taking?
   1. Increased absorption owing to clearance of the GI tract
   2. Increased absorption owing to facilitation of medication through the GI tract
   3. Decreased absorption owing to increased gut motility
   4. Decreased distribution owing to increased fluid consumption

7. Mrs. M. seems to have difficulty remembering whether or not she has taken her pills. Which of the following would be helpful to her?
   1. Medication pill boxes with compartments
   2. Turning the bottles upside down
   3. Color coding the medications with a check-off list
   4. All of the above

REFERENCES

American Geriatrics Society (2012). Updated Beers criteria for potentially inappropriate medication use in older adults. *Journal of the American Geriatrics Society,* 60(4), 616-631.

Carlson, D.S., & Pfadt, E. (2009). *Clinical coach for effective nursing care for older adults*. Philadelphia, PA: F.A. Davis.

Hale, L., Griffin, A., Cartwright, O., Moulin. J., Afford, S., & Flemming, R. (2008). Potentially inappropriate medication use in hospitalized older adults: A DUE using the full Beers criteria. *Formulary, 43*(9), 326.

Rigler, S. K. (2000). Alcoholism in the elderly. http://www. aafp.org/afp/2000/0315/p1710.html

WEB RESOURCES

Beers Criteria: http://www.americangeriatrics.org/files/documents/beers/2012AGSBeersCriteriaCitations.pdf

Reducing adverse drug events: http://consultgerirn.org/topics/medication/want_to_know_more

Laboratory Values and Older Adults

22

DEBORAH JUDD

DEBORAH JUDD

LEARNING OUTCOMES

1. Identify laboratory tests that are important indicators of health and disease in elderly patients.

2. Apply an understanding of laboratory tests to the health of elderly persons.

3. Identify at least three reference resources for understanding laboratory values.

4. Identify medications that have an influence on laboratory tests for elderly patients.

5. Describe nursing actions appropriate for abnormal laboratory values.

6. List and describe the rationale for laboratory tests related to social and lifestyle choices.

CONCEPTS

Assessment

Managing Care

Clinical Decision Making

CASE STUDY

Mr. K. is an 85-year-old resident of a small, independent group home where he has been caring for himself but sharing provided meals with the other residents. He underwent a transurethral resection of the prostate 4 years ago for benign prostatic hyperplasia. He has been treated for a heart irregularity and congestive heart failure in the past. Today he is being admitted to your intermediate care facility by his daughter because of several recent falls. Mr. K. reports that he has been nauseated and has not been eating well for the past few days. He also complains of wetting before reaching the restroom and blames this on his slow movement because of severe degenerative arthritis of his joints. Medications include the following:

- Furosemide (Lasix) 40 mg in the morning
- Digoxin 0.125 mg in the morning
- Ibuprofen (Motrin) 600 mg twice a day
- Acetaminophen (Tylenol) 500 mg every 4 hours as needed

   On physical assessment, you find the following:
- Height 5 feet 10 inches
- Weight 135 lb
- Blood pressure sitting 120/70 mm Hg and pulse irregular at 80/min
- Blood pressure standing 90/60 mm Hg and pulse irregular at 90/min
- Respirations 20/min and unlabored
- Temperature 98.8°F (36°C)
- Lungs clear
- Skin warm and dry, with dry mucous membranes

   Laboratory values available are:
- Potassium 3.2 mEq/L
- Sodium 132 mEq/L
- Chloride 106 mEq/L
- BUN 30 mg/dL
- Creatinine 1.4 mg/dL
- Glucose 130 mg/dL
- Urinalysis 3–5 WBCs, 0–3 RBCs, positive bacteria, specific gravity 1.022

Discussion

1. What problems have you identified based on the resident's history and physical assessment?

2. What other laboratory tests would be helpful?

3. What nursing actions should you take immediately?

INTRODUCTION

Laboratory testing is a useful tool for nurses, who care for aging patients in a variety of health-care settings. There are many useful tests to assist the licensed practical nurse (LPN) in providing safe, quality care for older adults. Laboratory tests are often ordered on admission to a hospital or nursing home, or for elderly persons when visiting a primary care provider in an outpatient clinic. LPNs may also collect blood specimens in other settings, such as home health or hospice care, for evaluation in a laboratory at a later date. As an LPN, you have studied laboratory values and their meanings in your medical and surgical nursing classes. As a practicing LPN, you will use laboratory resources at the facility where you work to interpret laboratory values of older adults correctly. The purpose of this chapter is not to repeat that information, but rather provide you with a ready reference of common and significant tests for elderly people along with specific and pertinent information for aging patients. Rationale for testing is reviewed generally. In addition to this resource, advancing medical technology allows you easy access to Internet resources where general laboratory testing information and the meaning of those laboratory values are readily available. There are some Internet resources listed at the end of this chapter.

MEANING OF LABORATORY VALUES IN ELDERLY PATIENTS

Laboratory tests are a routine part of the health examination for all people. For many tests, the normal ranges are different for elderly people than for people younger than 65 years of age. For other tests, there is no change with age. In addition, elderly people may have greater deviations from normal laboratory indicators when under stress, and return to normal levels is often slower in elderly people than in younger people. Laboratory tests are useful because medical conditions are discovered and treatments can be monitored. The diagnosis and treatment of these conditions result in substantial improvement in health, even in elderly individuals with multiple health problems.

Relationship to Clinical Status

You, as the LPN, need to remember that all laboratory findings should never be considered in isolation, especially when dealing with often frail elderly persons seen in clinical settings. The elderly person's gender, dietary pattern, activity level, tobacco use, alcohol intake, current medications, and aggressive medical or nursing interventions may alter laboratory findings. It is essential that you consider all facets of the individual's health and habits when you review the laboratory results. For example, abnormal laboratory values may indicate a physiological stressor such as dehydration or a medication side effect rather than illness.

It is important to remember that behind every laboratory procedure there is a human being who might be anxious about the procedure itself or the results of the procedure.

HEALTHY PEOPLE 2020

Goals

Attain a longer high-quality life free of preventable disease, disability, injury, or premature death.

Promote quality of life and healthy behaviors across all life stages.

COMMON SCREENING TESTS

There are several relatively simple and common screening tests performed on elderly people. The physician or nurse practitioner may request other tests after these easy screening interventions are completed and the results reviewed. These screenings are often part of an outpatient well aging adult screening. It is important for you to know about them and what they screen for.

A routine laboratory evaluation generally consists of the following:

• Complete blood cell count (CBC)
• Serum glucose
• Serum creatinine level
• Serum electrolytes
• Thyroid function tests
• Urinalysis
• Stool guaiac test

This chapter discusses the most common laboratory tests ordered and their meanings for elderly people. The values shown under headings are normal reference values from Van Leeuwen (2015) *Davis's Comprehensive Handbook of Laboratory and Diagnostic Tests with Nursing Implications* (6th ed.) or Meiner (2011) *Gerontologic Nursing* (4th ed.). As an LPN, you must refer to the reference intervals used by the clinical laboratory where you work for the most precise reference ranges.

Tuberculin Skin Test

Negative result	<6 mm of induration
Borderline positive	6–10 mm of induration
Positive result	>10 mm of induration

General Information

The tuberculin skin test, using purified protein derivative (PPD), is the screening method of choice for the detection of tuberculosis. Up to 25% of older adults who are clinically ill with tuberculosis show no reaction (<10 mm of induration) to intradermal injections of 1 mL of tuberculin. Some older adults who show no initial reaction. Most people who react positively to the test have no clinical evidence of infection.

Nursing home residents, whose risk of infection is five times greater than that of nonresidents, should be screened with a tuberculin skin test on admission and annually thereafter. Although the incidence of infection is low, treatment with antituberculosis medication is effective, in congregate living situations reducing risk of epidemic infection.

Nursing Implications

Anergy (lack of reaction to specific antigens) is common in elderly people. Because of this decreased ability to elicit an inflammatory response to the intradermal tuberculin solution, a second intradermal PPD injection is recommended 1 to 2 weeks after the first one (two-step testing process). All PPDs should be placed with appropriate intradermal technique and should be done annually.

Urinalysis

Appearance	Clear yellow/straw
Specific gravity	1.005–1.035
pH	4.5–8.0

General Information

Normal urine in an elderly person should test negative for glucose, ketones, blood, bilirubin, lupus erythematosus, protein nitrates, and calculi, although traces of protein may be present. There may be zero to three red blood cells (RBCs), zero to four white blood cells (WBCs), a few epithelial cells, and a few crystals per high-power field on microscopic examination. Elderly people commonly have the presence of zero to three hyaline casts on low-power field. In addition, 10% to 50% of older people have asymptomatic bacteriuria. Refer to Table 22.1 for urinalysis specifics.

Nursing Implications

• As you care for older adults, you can encourage adequate and appropriate nutrition and fluid intake. LPNs can discuss bladder hygiene, including frequent hand washing, regular urine elimination, and proper use of toilet paper (front to back).
• Usually a midstream, clean-catch specimen is requested.
• All urine collected for culture or sensitivity studies must be in a sterile container and should be refrigerated within 10 minutes of collection. If left an hour or more at room temperature, pH changes occur. Normal occurring bacteria can split urea into ammonia and the urine becomes alkaline (higher pH).
• First-morning and fasting urine specimens are collected when the individual awakens. This morning specimen is the most concentrated urine of the day. Analysis of this fasting urine

Evidence-Based Practice

Donewerth, J.J. (2011). Laboratory and diagnostic tests. In Meiner, S. (ed.). Gerontologic nursing (4th ed., pp. 368–399). St. Louis, MO: Elsevier Mosby.

Donewerth (2011) reported on two evidenced-based studies related to urinalysis specimens and results. The first study, by Avorn and colleagues (1994), reported on 65 women who were incontinent for at least 2 weeks and who had an intimal random urine specimen with a clean-catch specimen collected each month for 6 months. The women were randomly selected to drink 10 oz. of cranberry juice or 10 oz. of a placebo drink during the study period. The findings suggested that drinking cranberry juice decreased urinary tract bacterial counts. In a second study, by Midthun and associates (2004), experienced CNAs collected 97 clean-catch urine specimens from residents able to provide that type of urine sample and who were also antibiotic free for 2 weeks. After urine collection, the CNAs were asked to identify strong, foul, or fruity urine odor on incontinence pads. It was believed that odor was a sign of urinary tract infection (UTI). No urine odors were identified as foul or fruity. In 28 of the 97 urines, a strong smell was detected. Culture of all urine specimens found that just over half of the strong-odor urines (15 of 28) had positive bacteria growth in the culture, whereas about one-fourth of the urines without odor (17 of 69 specimens) were positive for bacterial growth. This finding suggests that urine smell means looking for the source of the odor, such as diabetes or dehydration.

Questions

1. What other patient-care activities promote quality care for incontinent patients and reduce the risk for UTI?
2. How does this reported evidence change the way LPNs may care for patients from a quality care viewpoint?
3. What other types of laboratory studies or blood work could help provide evidence for urinary incontinence or urinalysis changes?

TABLE 22.1 URINALYSIS DIPSTICK SCREEN

Urinary Substance Tested	Reference Value	Significance of the Reference Value
Color	Yellow, amber	Some medications change urine color
Appearance	Clear	Pus, casts, blood, bilirubin can change color
Odor	Ammonia-based	or appearance of urine (less clear to cloudy)
	Foul or fruity	Dehydration or lower fluid intake concentrates urine (color or odor change noted)
		Bacteria and other excreted wastes affect urine odor sometimes
pH	4.0–8.0	Vegetarian diet (fruit and vegetables) elevate pH (alkaline)
		High-protein diet (meat and eggs) lower pH (acidic)
		Acidic: diarrhea; diabetes mellitus; respiratory acidosis; COPD or asthma; metabolic acidosis

Continued

TABLE 22.1   URINALYSIS DIPSTICK SCREEN—cont'd

Urinary Substance Tested	Reference Value	Significance of the Reference Value
		Alkaline: vomiting, gastric suction; diuretics; UTI; metabolic alkalosis; respiratory alkalosis
Specific gravity	Adult: 1.001–1.035	Low: renal failure; diuresis; hypothermia; over-hydration
	Elders: range lowers from decreased ability to concentrate urine	High: dehydration; water restriction; vomiting; diarrhea
Protein	Negative	Positive protein: diabetes mellitus; congestive heart failure; systemic lupus; malignant hypertension
Glucose	Negative	Positive glucose: diabetes mellitus; Cushing's syndrome; severe stress; drug interactions
Ketones	Should be negative	Positive ketones: uncontrolled diabetes mellitus; starvation; high-protein diet; excessive aspirin use; dehydration; diabetic ketoacidosis
Nitrites	Negative	Positive nitrites leukocyte esterase and bacteria:
Bacteria	Negative	Probable UTI
	Elders: May be positive without reported symptoms	Probable UTI
	Older female: More common bacteria >70 years	
Leukocyte esterase	Negative	Identifies enzyme activity of WBCs (bacterial presence)
Bilirubin	0.1–1.0 unit/dL	Positive bilirubin and urobilinogen: hepatic disease (liver; gallbladder; biliary tract)
Urobilinogen	Negative	Positive urobilinogen: Hemolytic process; UTIs
Blood	Adult: negative	Positive blood: Cystitis or prostatitis; renal trauma; kidney stones

COPD, chronic obstructive pulmonary disease; UTI, urinary tract infection; WBC, white blood cell.

for protein, nitrite, glucose, and urinary sediment is most accurate at this time.

- A screening urine containing bacteria, protein, leukocyte esterase, nitrites or blood should be cultured. A microscopic examination of the urine may also be done to assess for crystals or stones, casts, epithelial cells, or other urine sediment (solid matter) (see Box 22.1).

- For all urinary testing and specimen collection, you will need to instruct the patient on why each test is being ordered (screening or diagnostic).

BOX 22.1 24-HOUR URINE SPECIMENS

A 24-hour urine specimen is collected to study a variety of urinary sediments and substances. It is often ordered based on a routine urinalysis or a comprehensive metabolic profile (CMP) blood test.

The most common 24-hour urine tests are ordered to assess renal function. The urine collected is evaluated for creatinine, blood urea nitrogen (BUN), protein, and sometimes calcium, potassium, phosphate, or sodium (electrolytes). The glomerular filtration rate (GFR) and creatinine clearance values are determined using a specific formula. A serum creatinine level is needed to calculate the values, and it is drawn on the day the urine specimen is returned.

Nursing Implications

You will be responsible for providing the patient with a container to collect the urine in, along with instructions on how to collect the specific urine specimen requested. A 24-hour urine specimen measures the average excretion for substances eliminated in variable amounts during the day.

Proper collection of a 24-hour urine requires that the first void of the day be discarded and the time noted. Urine is collected until the next day's first morning void at or before the designated start time the day before. If one urine specimen during the 24 hours is discarded or spilled, the test will not be accurate. All urine needs to be refrigerated until it is returned to the laboratory.

It is important for you to remind those persons collecting the urine specimen to make sure they drink adequate fluids and do not exercise heavily or have excessive protein intake because that alters the test results.

• All random urine specimens need at least 10 mL of urine for analysis; sometimes you will need more volume.
• It is important for you to provide water to hydrate the patient if he or she is unable to void unless there is a reason that would alter the test results.

• LPNs should be aware of medications that can change urine color.

Urinary tract infection (UTI) is a specific health issue common in elderly people. The highest incidence of reported UTIs is in long-term care facilities. This is in part because urinary tract pathogens become resistant to antibiotics in nursing homes. Incontinence of urine and stool, poor hygiene, and an age-related decreased immune response are other contributing factors.

1. Typical UTI symptoms are:
   Frequency
   Burning
   Hematuria
2. UTI in an older person often presents differently:
   Nocturia
   Incontinence
   Confusion
   Anorexia
   Lethargy

Stool for Occult Blood (Stool Guaiac)

Negative result   Absence of test solutions (reagent) color

General Information

Assessment of a stool specimen for blood is a relatively easy and inexpensive laboratory test to identify the presence of blood in the stool or gastrointestinal (GI) tract. Bleeding is common in older people, especially in individuals taking aspirin-containing medications and nonsteroidal anti-inflammatory drugs (NSAIDs). It is estimated that about 2.5 mL of blood per day appears in the stool. Hemorrhoids and colorectal cancer are the most common causes of minor bleeding in elderly people.

Abnormal bleeding from the GI tract may be either occult (hidden) or obvious by observation. Minor bleeding can decrease hemoglobin and hematocrit and cause symptoms of fatigue and weakness. The fecal occult blood test is useful in screening for colorectal cancer.

Nursing Implications

• There are various tests for fecal occult blood, all requiring the contact of a reagent with a stool specimen.
• A single stool smear can be obtained with a gloved hand during a rectal examination as

These women are glad their mother performs routine screenings each year.

part of a digital rectal examination (DRE) to check the prostate gland in a male patient or during a female pelvic examination or Pap test.

- A positive test result, indicated by color (usually blue), occurs when there is more than the normal amount of GI blood present.
- The presence of hemorrhoids, common in elderly individuals, especially if there is chronic constipation, can result in a positive stool guaiac.
- It is recommended that at least three separate random stool specimens be collected and that the sample of stool applied to the test card be from at least two areas of each stool.
- You should instruct the person to avoid red meats, vitamin C intake, iron supplements, and aspirin for 2 to 3 days before testing to avoid invalidating the results.
- You should always check the manufacturer's directions and suggestions on how to perform the test.

 ## HEMATOLOGIC TESTING

Blood is the body fluid that transports nutrients, cells, electrolytes, and metabolic wastes. Most laboratory tests analyze specific components of the blood with particular reference values determined as a normal range based on random public samples. Reference values vary slightly depending on the laboratory used and its accepted reference range. LPNs use laboratory tests to aid in safe quality care because many elderly patients present with vague signs or symptoms that are seen in a variety of common chronic diseases.

One of the most common laboratory or hematologic tests to determine the cellular elements of the blood and overall health of an individual is the CBC. Plasma or serum refers to the fluid substance of the blood. Plasma actually contains fibrinogen, a clotting substance, whereas serum is the fluid without the fibrinogen.

Today a machine performs most routine CBC analysis. When this test is ordered, it is called a CBC with auto diff, meaning the cellular components are determined with technology rather than manually as was done in the past. There are times when the physician or nurse practitioner may order a blood smear or CBC with manual diff. The term 'diff' means differential and refers to the different types of cells in the blood count; erythrocytes, or RBCs, and leukocytes, or WBCs, are the main cellular components of the blood. Generally, there are no apparent age-related changes in reference values for a CBC laboratory test. It is important to remember that blood counts may vary with altitude.

The comprehensive metabolic profile (CMP) is used to assess blood values inclusive of common electrolytes, liver enzymes, renal function indicators, glucose, overall protein, and albumin. Additional common blood tests ordered for seniors include vitamin B_{12}, folic acid, thyroid-stimulating hormone (TSH), calcium and phosphorus, magnesium, coagulation studies (prothrombin time [PT], partrial thromboplastin time [PTT], and international normalized ratio [INR]), uric acid, immune globulins, and lipoproteins (lipid profile).

Complete Blood Count

The CBC includes RBC count, hemoglobin, hematocrit, RBC indices, WBC count, platelets, and frequently, but not always, a differential. Values for the CBC do not change with age.

Red Blood Cell Count

Male	4.7–6.1 million cells/mcL
Female	4.2–5.4 million cells/mcL

General Information

The RBC count is a usefulf hematological test to diagnose anemia, polycythemia, cardiac or renal disease, and other bone marrow abnormalities in combination with other blood or urine tests.

There are six differentiated RBC markers in a CBC:

1. Total number of RBCs
2. Hemoglobin (Hgb)

3. Hematocrit (HCT)
4. Mean corpuscle volume (MCV)
5. Mean corpuscle hemoglobin (MHC)
6. Mean corpuscle hemoglobin concentration (MCHV).

The last three markers are the characteristics of individual RBCs.

Decreased RBC Count
Anemia
Fluid overload
Kidney problems
Bone marrow invasion of other cells or tumors
Recent hemorrhage
Chronic illness
Autoimmune diseases

Increased RBC Count
Polycythemia (altitude related)
Dehydration
Hypoxia
Congestive heart failure
Impaired pulmonary ventilation
Abnormal hemoglobin
Significant physical training (i.e., marathon races; more elders are participating in them)

Hemoglobin

Male	13.8–17.2 g/dL
Female	12.1–15.1 g/dL

General Information
Normal Hgb levels are maintained throughout life in healthy individuals. Hemoglobin concentration in whole blood parallels the RBC count, meaning that if RBCs increase, so does Hgb, and vice versa. For elderly adults who already suffer with decreased energy levels associated with general aging and chronic disease, the lower Hgb level affects oxygen binding and overall cellular and physical energy.

Increased Hemoglobin
Polycythemia
Dehydration
High altitude
Chronic obstructive pulmonary disease (COPD) or other obstructive lung disease

Decreased Hemoglobin
Anemia
Dietary iron deficiency and/or poor iron absorption

Recent hemorrhage (GI bleeding is a common reason in elders)
Fluid retention causing hemodilution kidney disease

Hematocrit

Male	47.0 ± 5.0%
Female	42.0 ± 5.0%

General Information
Hematocrit measures the percentage by volume of packed RBCs in whole blood. It is determined by spinning the blood and the heavier RBCs settle to the bottom. The value is a percentage (ratio) of cells to serum.

Decreased Hematocrit
Anemia
Hemodilution
Bone marrow disease
Kidney disease
Rheumatoid arthritis
Liver disease (cirrhosis)
Relationship to aging and decrease in intrinsic factor 7th–9th decade of life

Increased Hematocrit
Polycythemia
Significant volume depletion occurs with associated increased blood urea nitrogen (BUN) and creatinine.

Red Blood Cell Indices

MCV (RBC size)	
Male	78–100 fL
Female	79–102 fL
MCH (RBC color/Hgb content)	25–35 pg/cell
MCHC (RBC color/Hgb content)	31%–37%

General Information
RBC indices aid in the diagnosis and classification of anemias by providing information about the size, hemoglobin concentration, and hemoglobin weight of an average RBC.

Nursing Implications
You will need to be aware of your patient's RBC count along with his or her Hgb and Hct levels to understand if the patient is at risk for venous thrombosis from elevated values. Clot formation and pain most commonly occur in the

lower leg (calf area). This is termed a deep vein thrombosis (DVT).

Compression of the calf or leg promotes better circulation, and you may be required to assist patients with TED hose use. If bedrest is ordered for a patient in your care, you will need to ensure the patient follows that recommendation along with elevation of the affected limb.

If the RBC, Hgb, and Hct are low, patients will have fatigue. The physician may order iron supplementation and you will want to educate the patient on ways to conserve energy.

If levels are extremely low, a blood or packed red blood cell (PBRC) transfusion may be ordered by the physician.

White Blood Cell Count

4,500–10,000 cells/mμL

General Information

The WBC count is used to identify infectious or inflammatory processes, to evaluate the need for further tests, and to monitor the older person's response to chemotherapy or radiation therapy. There is a decrease in the WBC count with age because of an overall reduction in lymphocyte cells. The major implication of fewer lymphocytes is a decreased ability to resist and fight infection.

Decreased WBC Count (Leukopenia)

Bone marrow depression from primary disease such as leukemia, myeloma, and other tumors
Reactions to antineoplastics or other toxins
Viral infections, such as influenza and infectious hepatitis, which are more common in older adults
Sepsis
Radiation treatments
Drug use, including phenytoin, NSAIDs, and metronidazole
General nutritional deficiency

Increased WBC Count (Leukocytosis)

Infection
Inflammation
Tissue necrosis
Leukemia
Excessive exercise
Stress (common in elderly individuals due to physiological as well as emotional stress, which can be related to finances, loneliness, and functional decreases, among other things)

BOX 22.2   WHITE BLOOD CELL CELLULAR FUNCTIONS

- Neutrophils: Reflect general phagocytosis of bacteria and foreign substances and control inflammation
- Eosinophils: Reflect allergic responses, parasitic infection, and autoimmune diseases
- Basophils: Reflect acute allergic response, stress reactions, and bone marrow disease
- Lymphocytes: Reflect infections, systemic lupus, response to chemotherapy or radiation, leukemia, and infectious hepatitis
- Monocytes: Reflect tuberculosis, chronic infections or inflammatory disease, and response to drug therapy

---

White Blood Cell Differential

There are five kinds of WBCs: neutrophils, lymphocytes, monocytes, eosinophils, and basophils. Each WBC cell type functions as part of the body's defense system against infectious or other foreign substances. WBC types are most often expressed as percentage (%) or the ratio the individual WBC type per 100 WBC cells.

In elderly persons, an infection may not be accompanied by an increase in the number of WBCs. The WBC differential is necessary to detect and diagnose disease. It often is collected along with other blood or urine tests.

Neutrophils	1.6–6.7 K/mcL or 55%–70%
Eosinophils	0.0–0.5 K/mcL or 1%–5%
Basophils	0.0–0.3 K/mcL or 0%–3%
Lymphocytes	1.2–3.4 K/mcL or 16%–46%
Monocytes	0.2–1.0 K/mcL or 4%–11%

General Information

The WBC differential helps determine the severity of an infection, detect allergic reactions and parasitic infections, identify various leukemias, and assess the individual's capacity to resist and overcome infection.

Neutrophils can be differentiated to include bands, which are immature neutrophils, and segmented neutrophils known as segs, which are mature neutrophils. These values are important for cancer patients, individuals undergoing treatments

This older couple goes to the hospital outpatient department monthly to have blood drawn to assist in their medication management. They understand the importance of monitoring their medication levels.

that suppress bone marrow, and for elderly patients who are prone to infection and who often do not manifest the same signs or symptoms of infection as younger adults. An increase in bands requires further investigation. Neutropenia is a significant syndrome with specific nursing considerations for the LPN.

Platelet Count

130,000–400,000/mcL

General Information

Thrombocytes, or platelets, are cellular fragments found in the blood and are necessary for clotting. A clot forms as the cells aggregate or join together to form a plug necessary for clot formation and hemostasis. Platelets contribute to phospholipid activity in the coagulation process.

Decreased Platelet Count (Thrombocytopenia)

Hemorrhage
Bone marrow disease
Chemotherapy or radiation
Prescribed anticoagulation therapy
Folic acid or vitamin B_{12} deficiency
Disseminated intravascular coagulation (DIC)
Idiopathic thrombocytopenia
Systemic lupus
Drugs (furosemide, indomethacin, penicillin, phenytoin, quinidine sulfate, salicylates, thiazides, tricyclic antidepressants, and others)
Destruction resulting from immune disorders, radiation, or mechanical injury

Increased Platelet Count (Thrombocytosis)

Iron-deficiency anemia
Hemorrhage: Splenectomy
Rheumatoid arthritis
Polycythemia vera
Malignancy or other tumor formation
High altitudes
Persistent cold temperature
Strenuous exercise

Erythrocyte Sedimentation Rate

A slight increase is noted for normal reference value in the fifth to sixth decades.

Male <50 years old	0–9 mm/hr
Male >60 years old	1–20 mm/hr
Female <50 years old	1–20 mm/hr
Female >60 years old	1–30 mm/hr

General Information

The erythrocyte sedimentation rate (ESR), also known as the sed rate, is a useful hematology test to measure how fast RBCs settle into the bottom of a laboratory tube with gravity over one hour. The faster the cells fall, the smaller the RBC size; the slower the fall, the larger the RBCs.

The value of the ESR is that it is an inexpensive lab screening easily obtained when a CBC is drawn. The ESR is not a specific test, meaning without other laboratory values it may be difficult to know the source of the inflammatory process. It does indicate changes in fibrin, reactive proteins, and autoimmune globulins leading to better quality of care as the reasons for the elevations are explored. Serial ESR evaluations monitor resolution of infection, inflammation, or vasculitis.

Increased ESR

Polymyalgia or fibromyalgia syndromes
Temporal arteritis (common in the elderly)
Rheumatoid versus osteoarthritis differential
Chronic inflammatory disease
Infection
Malignancy
Vascular collagen disease

Decreased ESR

Sickle cell anemia
Liver disease
Polycythemia
Elevated blood glucose

Folic Acid and Vitamin B$_{12}$

Folic acid	3.1–17.5 ng/mL
Vitamin B$_{12}$	> 250 pg/mL

General Information

Folic acid, a vitamin B complex element, is necessary for RBC and WBC function. Folic acid decrease indicates protein malnutrition, anemia, and liver or renal disease. Alcohol use and other prescribed drugs can decrease this vitamin as well.

Vitamin B$_{12}$ is necessary for full development of the RBC. A decrease in B$_{12}$ level is associated with gastric malabsorption and gastric disease. Aging is not believed to be a factor for vitamin B$_{12}$ decrease; however, there is more pernicious anemia as people age.

If anemia is present, an iron level and/or total iron binding capacity (TIBC) may be ordered to assess overall health status, especially in patients with chronic disease.

Increased Folic Acid

Overuse of dietary supplement(s)
Leukemia
Vegan/vegetarian diet
Vitamin B$_{12}$ deficiency

Decreased Folic Acid

Poor nutrition (common in elders)
Anorexia
Malabsorption
   Celiac disease
   Chrohn's disease
   Cholestasis
Lymphoma
Pancreatic cancer
Pernicious anemia
Bowel resection
Liver disease

Nursing Implications

A deficiency of these vitamins affects overall energy and is often associated with macrocytic anemia. Vitamin B$_{12}$ is required for optimum RBC development.

There are some studies showing that a deficit of these vitamins contributes to dementia and Alzheimer's disease.

Metformin, a common oral drug for diabetes, may decrease folic acid and vitamin B$_{12}$. It is important for you to understand that patients with diabetes need to have these serum levels checked at least every other year.

Homocysteine, an inflammatory substance associated with coronary artery disease and cardiac events, is reduced if there are adequate levels of vitamin B$_{12}$, folic acid, and vitamin B$_6$. When they are elevated, this plasma substance level should be checked.

Coagulation Tests

Coagulation: Prothrombin Time (PT)

Normal	11.2–13.2 seconds with INR of 1.0
Therapeutic	1.5–2.0 times normal control

Prothrombin, or factor II, aids in the clotting process. The PT test, however not only measures prothrombin; it is a determination of the overall coagulatory cycle The partial thromboplastin time (PTT) test verifies blood thinning for heparin products. The International Normalized Ratio (INR) blood test verifies the results of the PT.

The PT test identifies the action and effectiveness of Coumadin (warfarin) treatment for blood thinning (It does not evaluate the effectiveness of heparin, another drug used to thin blood and prevent clotting.) The PTT test verifies blood consistency and appropriate anticoagulation for heparin products. The International Normalized Ratio (INR) blood test verifies the results of the PT test; it is the "standard" value from one lab to another regardless of the lab location.

PT is determined before initiation of warfarin therapy and then daily until maintenance dosage is established. Thereafter, PT determinations are made at 1- to 4-week intervals, depending on the stability of the person's therapeutic level. It may be checked weekly if there is variability or difficulty maintaining the ideal reference values.

Abnormal values (high) usually are the result of liver disease, especially cirrhosis, Vitamin K deficiency, or changes in gastric absorption (lack of bile salts) or long-term antibiotic therapy, which changes normal GI bacteria.

There is no clinical diagnostic significance for a low PT other than diet or pharmacology considerations; there are very rare malignancies that alter the PT and promote thrombophlebitis. Most thrombophlebitis is associated with RBC or platelet change, not PT changes. As the LPN you should be aware of new anticoagulation medications often replacing heparin and warfarin therapy.

International Normalized Ratio

Normal	1.0–1.50 with the ideal value as close to 1 as possible.
Therapeutic target	2.0–3.0 (ideally 2.5)

This test uses international standards to assess the validity of PT results. Before the 1980s there was great variance in PT references, causing difficulty for anticoagulation therapy and increased variability and associated bleeding issues from medication dose changes to stabilize the PT. It has become a standard of care for coagulopathy treatments.

Partial Thromboplastin Time or Activated Partial Thromboplastin Time

PPT normal	22.1–43.1 sec
APPT normal	25–36 sec
Therapeutic target for both	1.5–2.5 times normal control

GENERAL INFORMATION

The PTT test is primarily for assessment of therapeutic heparin interventions. It can be useful in identifying bleeding disorders, which change plasma clotting factors and indicate deficits of the body's intrinsic system (i.e., hemophilia or systemic lupus).

- Risk of serious hemorrhage is high in anticoagulated persons older than age 70, especially individuals at risk for falls.
- Many drugs have a potentiating or inhibiting effect on warfarin, so all medications being taken by an individual taking warfarin such sulfonamides, digoxin, and cephalosporins. Patients should avoid aspirin or NSAIDS. All medications must be reviewed. Diets high in vitamin K should be encouraged.
- You need to educate patients about the increased possibility of bleeding while taking anticoagulants and suggest strategies such avoidance of razors and applying pressure when scratched or cut.

Think Like a Nurse

Mrs. J. was diagnosed with pancreatic cancer and goes to an outpatient clinic laboratory weekly for blood draws to assist in medication management and assessment of the cancer progress. She knows how important the results are to her overall health.

1. List tests that are important for you to assess and review to monitor a patient with pancreatic or other gastrointestinal cancer.
2. Explain why you, as the LPN, need to review these laboratory values and screening tests.

- When PT or PTT values are abnormal, risk of bleeding or signs of bleeding such as hematuria, black tarry stools, hematemesis, bruising and petechiae, epistaxis, hemoptysis, continuous abdominal or head pain, faintness, or dizziness should be reviewed with the patient and the anticoagulant dose withheld. Notify the physician immediately.
- Periodic urinalyses and stool guaiac and liver function tests are carried out to detect hemorrhage or liver dysfunction.

COMPREHENSIVE METABOLIC PROFILE INDICATORS

Blood Glucose: Plasma

Fasting:

Normal	70–99 mg/dL
Elder adult	Increase of 1–2 mg/dL per decade
Prediabetes	100–125 mg/dL

Note: 40% of adults 50 years or older have prediabetes

Diabetes mellitus	>125 mg/dL

(Verify by glycolated hemoglobin [HgA1c] or two fasting blood glucose values)

Glycolated Hemoglobin

There is no information to show that the HgA1c changes with age.

Normal	<5.7%
Prediabetes	5.7%–6.4%
Diabetes	>6.5%
Goal for diabetic patients	7% or less

General Information

In elderly people, the exact definition of abnormal glucose tolerance is unclear. The National Institute of Diabetes, Digestive, and Kidney Diseases recommend serum glucose and HgA1c testing to screen for diabetes. There are three diagnostic categories of diabetes: type 1 diabetes, type 2 diabetes, and prediabetes inclusive of gestational diabetes and chronic marginally elevated fasting blood glucose. In the past, two elevated fasting serum or finger-stick values were suggested. Using the two separate laboratory values, a diagnosis of diabetes or prediabetes is confirmed with the HgA1c when the blood glucose is high normal to slightly elevated over time.

The HgA1c test measures the mean results of plasma glucose over a period of about 3 months. It is a good indicator of serum glucose and is a reliable test to show the absence or presence of diabetes as well as the prediabetes risk. There are numerous reasons that glucose level can change because many drugs and health conditions affect the plasma glucose levels.

1. Signs and symptoms of decreased blood plasma glucose or hypoglycemia include:
   Plasma blood glucose values less than 100 mg/dL
   Weakness
   Restlessness
   Hunger
   Nervousness
   Sweating
   Rapidly decreasing mental alertness in an elderly person without the above-listed common symptoms
2. Hypoglycemia may be caused by:
   Beta-blockers
   Ethanol
   Clofibrate
   Monoamine oxidase inhibitors
   Strenuous exercise
   Failure to refrigerate the blood sample and analyze it within a few hours of collection
3. Signs and symptoms of increased blood plasma glucose or hyperglycemia include:
   Plasma glucose levels that exceed 600 mg/dL can be life-threatening.
   Plasma glucose greater than 160–180 mg/dL is the average renal threshold, but can result in glucose presence in the urine, glycosuria, in older adults.

With aging there is a lack of the following symptoms or they may be present with a less obvious appearance:
   Urinary frequency
   Dehydration
   Weakness
4. Hyperglycemia may be caused by:
   Medications causing increased glucose levels such as:
   Chlorthalidone
   Thiazide diuretics
   Furosemide
   Oral contraceptives
   Benzodiazepines
   Phenytoin
   Phenothiazines
   Lithium
   Epinephrine
   Nicotinic acid
   Corticosteroids
   Recent illness or infection

Undetected or worsening hyperglycemia causes a mental status decrease that progresses more quickly to hyperosmolar coma in an older person with non–insulin-dependent diabetes mellitus.

Electrolytes

Normal values for electrolytes are the same for young and old. Numerous conditions, medications, and dietary factors influence electrolyte values. Common electrolyte-related causes of weakness in elderly people are hypernatremia (high sodium), hyponatremia (low sodium), and hypokalemia (low potassium). In general, electrolyte values represent what is in the serum and not in the cells. Electrolytes are present in the cells and often determine cellular activity and health. The two main electrolytes are sodium and potassium.

Sodium is primarily present in extracellular fluid (outside cells), whereas potassium, magnesium, and phosphate are intracellular electrolytes. When a positive electrolyte moves from extracellular to intracellular areas, a negative electrolyte sodium, bicarbonate, or chloride follows. There is evidence to support that low magnesium level is a risk for diabetes or elevated glucose and increased lipoproteins (cholesterol and triglyceride).

Sodium, Serum

Normal   136–145 mEq/L

GENERAL INFORMATION

Elderly people are at increased risk of serum sodium imbalance. Decreased sodium levels promote water excretion, and increased levels promote retention, primarily through stimulation or depression of aldosterone secretion. Loss of body water causes concentration of serum sodium (hypernatremia), whereas an increase in body water causes dilution of serum sodium (hyponatremia). Sodium also influences the acid-base balance, chloride or potassium levels, and neuromuscular function.

HYPONATREMIA

A sodium concentration of less than 136 mEq/L occurs when there is an excess of water in relation to total sodium.

1. Symptoms may be absent, or there may be:
   Fatigue
   Headache
   Restlessness
   Decreased skin turgor
   Nausea
   Muscle cramps and tremors
   Disorientation
   Confusion
   Coma
   Seizures
   Death
2. Causes of hyponatremia include:
   Vomiting
   Diarrhea
   Renal disorders
   Diuretics
   Congestive heart failure
   Cirrhosis
   Overhydration
   Adrenal insufficiency
   Use of nutritional support formulas
     without additional sodium
   Syndrome of inappropriate antidiuretic
     hormone secretion associated with
     numerous drugs and diseases

HYPERNATREMIA

A sodium concentration greater than 146 mEq/L is a result of a deficit of body water relative to total sodium content and is usually caused by dehydration.

1. Symptoms include:
   Weakness
   Thirst
   Restlessness
   Dry, sticky mucous membranes

QSEN

COMPETENCY: Quality Improvement (Knowledge, Skills)

Goals for LPNs Related to Laboratory Testing in the Elderly

Generally, laboratory employees are responsible for obtaining blood specimens from the people in your care. "Providing care that is respectful of and responsive to individual patient preferences, needs, and values and ensuring that patient values guide all clinical decisions" are integral parts of caring for elders (Drenkard, 2013, p. 4).

Often you, or a certified nursing assistant (CNA) you supervise, will be responsible for obtaining any urine, stool, wound, or sputum specimen needed for laboratory testing. Your priority is to gather all specimens correctly according to standards and protocols. That may seem difficult at times, but there is no reason to send a specimen to the laboratory if it is not collected correctly because it will provide an inaccurate result.

When an older person is asked to give you a midstream urine specimen, the patients may not understand what that means. Not wanting to look "dumb," the patient may not ask for an explanation. You must determine whether the person understands the instructions by asking for responses about what you expect him or her to do and perhaps even give a reason for doing it a specific way. When asked to cleanse the urinary meatus before voiding for a clean-catch specimen, an older person may think that is not "proper" and simply not do it. You are the person responsible to see that this is done correctly so that the urine specimen gives accurate results (Corbett & Banks, 2012, p. 61).

When obtaining a sputum specimen, you are the person who must see that the specimen comes from a deep cough so that it is the best specimen possible. Most people do not like mucus, and it may even be painful for the older person to cough deeply. You need to plan ahead and be prepared with a strategy to obtain the specimen needed so that the proper treatment can be started. As in all things you do, be patient and caring, because these are the hallmark behaviors of professionals in nursing.

Flushed skin
Oliguria
Diminished reflexes
2. Causes of hypernatremia include:
Inadequate fluid intake
Diarrhea
Polyuria associated with diabetes mellitus
Diuretics
Increased insensible water loss from fever
and tachypnea
Hypertension
Dyspnea
Edema
Kidney disease owing to a lack of
response to antidiuretic hormone
3. Causes of excess sodium concentration
include:
Increased dietary intake
Aldosteronism
Intravenous infusion of normal saline for
treatment of fluid loss or shock

Potassium, Serum
Normal 3.5–5.0 mEq/L

GENERAL INFORMATION
Potassium maintains cellular osmotic equilibrium
and helps regulate muscle activity by maintaining
electrical conduction within the cardiac and skeletal
muscles. Potassium also helps regulate acid-base
balance, enzyme activity, and kidney function.
Potassium deficiency develops rapidly because the
body has no effective way to conserve potassium.

HYPOKALEMIA
1. Signs and symptoms of hypokalemia
include:
Mental confusion
Rapid, weak, irregular pulse
Hypotension
Anorexia
Decreased reflexes
Muscle weakness
Paresthesia

2. Causes of hypokalemia include:
Diuretics
Diarrhea
Vomiting
Renal tubular acidosis
Malnutrition
Urinary potassium losses associated
with glycosuria and ketonuria and
with hyperaldosteronism

HYPERKALEMIA
1. Signs and symptoms of hyperkalemia
include:
Weakness
Malaise
Nausea
Diarrhea
Muscle irritability
Oliguria
Bradycardia
2. Causes of hyperkalemia include:
Renal failure
Cell damage from burns
Injuries
Chemotherapy
Acidosis
Addison's disease
Diabetes mellitus
3. Medications affecting serum potassium
level include:
Spironolactone
Triamterene
NSAIDs
Beta-blockers
Angiotensin-converting enzyme inhibitors
Penicillin G
Amphotericin B
Methicillin
Tetracycline

Calcium, Plasma
Normal   9–10.5 mg/dL

GENERAL INFORMATION
Calcium absorption becomes less efficient with
age in men and women. Inadequate dietary calcium is associated with the loss of bone that begins
in the 40s. Calcium helps regulate and promote
neuromuscular and enzyme activity, skeletal development, and blood coagulation. Parathyroid
hormone, vitamin D, calcitonin, and adrenal
steroids control calcium blood levels. Almost all
of the body's calcium is stored in the bones and
teeth. Serum calcium varies inversely with the
body's phosphorus level. The body requires ingestion of about 1 g per day of dietary calcium because calcium is excreted in the urine and feces.

HYPOCALCEMIA
1. Signs and symptoms of hypocalcemia
include:
Circumoral and peripheral numbness and
tingling

Muscle twitching
Facial muscle spasm
Muscle cramping
Seizures
Dysrhythmias

2. Causes of hypocalcemia include:
Insufficient activity of the parathyroid glands
Hypomagnesemia
Hyperphosphatemia owing to renal failure
Laxatives
Chemotherapy
Corticosteroids
Malabsorption
Acute pancreatitis
Alkalosis osteomalacia
Diarrhea
Rickets (vitamin D deficiency)

HYPERCALCEMIA

1. Signs and symptoms of hypercalcemia include:
Hypertension
Bone pain
Muscle hypotonicity
Nausea
Vomiting
Dehydration
Mental confusion
Coma
Cardiac arrest

2. Causes of hypercalcemia include:
Hyperparathyroidism
Thiazide diuretics
Cancer
Addison's disease
Hyperthyroidism
Paget's disease
Immobilization
Excessive vitamin D intake
Calcium-containing antacids
Androgens
Progestins or estrogens
Lithium carbonate

Phosphate, Serum
Normal   3–4.5 mg/dL

GENERAL INFORMATION
Phosphate helps regulate calcium levels, carbohydrate and lipid metabolism, and acid-base balance. Adequate levels of vitamin D are necessary for absorption of phosphates from the intestine. About 85% of the body's phosphate is found in bone. Calcium and phosphate have a reciprocal relationship. The kidneys regulate phosphate excretion to maintain a balance with serum calcium.

Chloride, Serum
Normal   98–106 mEq/L

GENERAL INFORMATION
Chloride interacts with sodium to maintain the osmotic pressure of the blood. Chloride is important in maintaining the acid-base balance in the body and varies inversely with the bicarbonate level. It also is an important electrolyte for maintaining the body's osmotic pressure. Low chloride levels correspond to low sodium and potassium levels. Chloride is also an important electrolyte for maintaining the body's osmotic pressure. Renal disease can decrease chloride excretion and cause fluid accumulation.

End Products of Metabolism

Blood Urea Nitrogen (BUN), Serum
Normal   8–25 mg/dL
Elderly adults   Slight increase as renal function decreases with age. If it is greater than 28–30 mg/dL, additional laboratory tests should be ordered to discover the reason.

Family is this woman's greatest joy. She appreciates the monthly laboratory work that is done for her at the nursing home where she resides. She doesn't worry about the results because she knows the physician and nurses will manage the situation for her. That leaves her more time to be with her family.

GENERAL INFORMATION

BUN is the main end product of protein metabolism. BUN level reflects protein intake, liver function, and kidney excretory capacity. The normal BUN value remains unchanged with age. Because protein intake is often low in elderly persons, BUN values may be normal even with impaired renal function. Elevation of BUN levels without serum creatinine elevation suggests dehydration.

There are usually no signs or symptoms of an increased BUN level other than the signs and symptoms associated with dehydration or other underlying renal disease. Likewise, with decreased BUN levels, the signs and symptoms are those of the underlying condition.

1. Causes of increased BUN levels include:
    Renal disease
    Reduced renal blood flow
    Urinary tract obstruction
    GI bleed
    Increased protein catabolism (starvation, burns)
    Drugs such as aminoglycosides, amphotericin B, and methicillin
2. Causes of decreased BUN levels include:
    Severe liver failure
    Malnutrition
    Overhydration
    Chloramphenicol use

Creatinine, Serum

Normal male:	0.6–1.5 mg/dL
Normal female:	0.6–1.1 mg/dL
Older adult:	Values decrease as muscle mass decreases and renal function changes

Levels greater than 5.0 mg/dL indicate a more than 50% decrease in nephron function.

GENERAL INFORMATION

Creatinine values also are unchanged with age. Because lean body mass declines with age, however, the total daily production of creatinine also declines, remaining less than 1.2 mg/dL. This causes an overestimate of renal function in elderly persons based on static measurements of serum creatinine.

Creatinine clearance declines by almost 10% per decade after 40 years of age and is a more reliable indicator of kidney function than BUN and serum creatinine values. In elderly people, creatinine clearance is important for determining the dosage for drugs that are cleared by the kidney to avoid drug toxicity. Creatinine levels change more slowly than BUN levels do, so monitoring the creatinine level is a better measure of kidney function in the elderly.

Causes of increased serum creatinine include:

- Renal disease
- Diabetic acidosis
- Starvation
- Muscle disease
- Hyperthyroidism
- Use of ascorbic acid
- Barbiturates
- Diuretics

A high serum creatinine level with nonspecifc symptoms may not indicate renal failure but rather be the result of weight loss and reports of weakness. Because the kidneys easily excrete creatinine with minimal tubular reabsorption, serum creatinine levels are directly related to the glomerular filtration rate (GFR).

Bilirubin, Serum

Total	0.1–1.0 mg/dL
Direct	0.0–0.4 mg/dL
Indirect	0.1–1.0 mg/dL

GENERAL INFORMATION

Bilirubin is the major product of hemoglobin breakdown and is excreted as a pigment in bile. The excretion of bilirubin depends on the normal production and destruction of RBCs and a functional hepatobiliary system, where bilir-ubin is conjugated and excreted. The direct bilirubin value increases with the obstruction of the flow of bile through the biliary system because this causes uptake of direct bilirubin into the circulation. Levodopa may cause false increases in bilirubin. GI bleeding can contribute to an elevated bilirubin value.

Uric Acid, Serum

Men	3.6–8.0 mg/dL
Women	2.3–6.0 mg/dL
Older male	2.0–8.5 mg/dL
Older female	2.0–8.0 mg/dL

GENERAL INFORMATION

Uric acid, the major end metabolite of dietary and endogenous purines, is excreted through the kidneys. Cell breakdown and catabolism of nucleic acids, excessive production and destruction of cells, and inability to excrete uric acid are causes of hyperuricemia. An increase in serum uric acid is found in various conditions, including gout, impaired renal function, congestive heart failure, hemolytic anemia, polycythemia, neoplasms, and psoriasis. Uric acid level is influenced by foods high in purine, so dietary measures are part of the treatment for an elevated uric acid level. Gout is the most common symptom manifested when levels increase, and all joints can be affected; the joints of the foot are the most common site.

Serum uric acid levels greater than 8 mg/dL in men and greater than 6 mg/dL in women are often associated with symptoms of gout. Gout is an acute inflammation of a joint, commonly the metatarsophalangeal joint of the great toe, caused by uric acid crystal accumulation.

Causes of increased serum uric acid levels include:

- Loop diuretics
- Thiazides
- Starvation
- High-purine diet
- Stress
- Alcohol abuse
- Chemotherapy
- Menopause

Levodopa, acetaminophen, ascorbic acid, and phenacetin may cause false elevations in uric acid levels.

Liver Function Tests

Most liver function tests remain unchanged in elderly people. The alkaline phosphatase level is frequently elevated in older adults as bone degeneration and decreased bone remodeling occur. Total alkaline phosphatase may increase owing to Paget's disease, bone fracture, trauma, or osteoporosis. For people taking tacrine (Cognex) for Alzheimer's disease, liver function tests are very important.

Alanine Aminotransferase (ALT)
Normal 10–56 U/L

Slight increase is noted in the seventh to ninth decade of life.

GENERAL INFORMATION
ALT, an enzyme necessary for tissue energy production, is present predominantly in the liver. It also is present in the kidney, heart, and skeletal muscles and is a relatively specific indicator of acute liver cell damage.

Causes of elevated ALT include:

- Fatty liver disease
- Tuberculosis
- Liver disease (cirrhosis)
- Different medications
- Cholecystitis
- Intrahepatic cholestasis
- Pancreatitis
- Hepatic congestion owing to heart failure
- Acute myocardial infarction
- Trauma
- Lead ingestion
- Carbon tetrachloride exposure

Falsely elevated ALT levels may be caused by barbiturate or narcotic analgesic use.

Aspartate Aminotransferase (AST) or Serum Glutamic-Oxaloacetic Transaminase (SGOT)
Normal   5–41 U/L

GENERAL INFORMATION
AST is an enzyme found in cells of the liver, heart, muscles, kidneys, pancreas, and RBCs. Serum levels are highest during acute cellular damage and decrease during tissue repair. The AST level is useful in monitoring the progress of myocardial infarction and acute liver disease. Tuberculosis and its subsequent treatment are both reasons for a rise in AST.

Causes of AST elevation include:

- Myocardial infarction
- Liver disease
- Extensive surgery
- Hemolytic anemia
- Pulmonary emboli
- Delirium tremens
- Diseases of the brain, muscle, pancreas, spleen, and lungs

Alkaline Phosphatase Level
Adult male   45–115 U/L
Adult female   30–100 U/L

Increased values are seen with each decade after 50 years. There are no parameters identified; age considerations and provider judgment are based on presentation of patient.

GENERAL INFORMATION
Alkaline phosphatase is an enzyme that is active in bone calcification and in lipid and metabolite transport. Serum alkaline phosphatase levels are sensitive to biliary obstruction by space-occupying hepatic lesions, such as tumors or abscesses, and to metabolic bone disease. Alka-line phosphatase

isoenzymes may be identified to differentiate hepatic and skeletal diseases. This test is not specific for source of cellular or organ change, so it is not used as often today as it was in the past. Decreases in the level of ALP can indicate malnutrition or excessive vitamin D intake. Anticonvulsants increase levels of this enzyme.

Causes of increased alkaline phosphatase include:

- Gallbladder disease associated with obstruction
- Paget's disease
- Bone metastasis
- Hyperparathyroidism
- Liver disease
- Osteomalacia

Creatinine Kinase (CK) or Creatinine Phosphokinase (CPK)

Normal male total	60–400 U/L
Normal female total	40–150 U/L

Isoenzyme Values

CK-I (BB or brain)	0%–1%
CK-II (MB or heart)	3% or 0–7.5 ng/mL
CK-III (MM or muscle)	95%–100%

Creatinine kinase is important for energy and is integral for muscular tissue function and health. Values of this enzyme are elevated after any muscular injury or activity. Because of this the enzyme is a useful marker for acute myocardial infarction (MI) and to assess progressive muscular diseases or necrosis of muscle from trauma.

If CK-II is greater than 10 U/L, then a cardiac event has not occurred. If it is greater than 12 U/L, it is likely the patient had an MI or other ischemic event other than angina. CK-II is present in the serum between 3 and 6 hours after acute MI. It peaks in about 24 hours and remains elevated for 3 days or less.

Troponins

Troponin I	>1.5 ng/mL positive for MI
Troponin T	>0.1–0.2 ng/mL positive for MI

Troponins are proteins found in muscle and increase with an acute MI. They are often drawn along with CK levels because they are present as early as 2 hours after the event and peak within 24 hours, as does the CK level. They remain elevated for up to 1 week so can be useful for assessment and treatment of an elderly person. This test is especially important for aging women, who often have different or vague heart attack symptoms and may not seek medical care as readily.

B-Natriuretic Peptide (BNP)

Normal reference	<100 pg/mL
Positive congestive heart failure	>100 pg/mL

This is a peptide found in the ventricles of the heart and is useful for detecting early to late changes in cardiac function related to hypertrophy of the ventricles. It is useful for diagnosing congestive heart failure because it is a cardiac-specific peptide.

NUTRITIONAL INDICATORS

Elderly persons require and consume fewer total calories per day than younger adults. Carbohydrate intake may increase slightly whereas fat and protein intakes generally decline in older people. Lean body mass and total body protein decrease, whereas the percentage of body fat increases with age.

It is crucial that you, as an LPN, recognize that elderly persons are often at risk for malnutrition. This risk is due to decreased mobility; cognitive and sensory deficits; chewing and swallowing difficulties; and loss of appetite because of medications, illness, or the environment. The increased occurrence of wounds, infection, and dehydration creates additional nutritional demands on elderly persons; however, the most significant causes of poor nutrition in older people are poverty and chronic illness.

Because of these physiological and societal factors, it is important to have baseline laboratory values for the following indices of nutritional status and to understand their significance:

- Total serum proteins measure visceral protein stores.
- Serum albumin is the most widely used indicator of protein status.
- Serum transferrin is an indicator of protein stores.
- Serum cholesterol indicates lipid mass.
- Serum creatinine indicates lean body mass.

The hemoglobin, hematocrit, and lymphocyte count included in the CBC reflect the body's ability to transport nutrients and resist disease. Other common nutritional indicators are iron and micronutrients such as vitamins and minerals.

FOCUSED LEARNING CHART

Elderly persons often are at risk for malnutrition. Possible reasons are:

Physical	Psychological	Environmental
Chronic illness*	Depression	Poverty*
Decreased mobility	Cognitive deficits	Inability to travel to grocery store
Sensory deficits		
Loss of appetite due to medications		
Chewing and swallowing difficulties		

* The most significant causes of malnutrition in the elderly.

Nutritional deficiencies are often identified only when an associated problem, such as weight loss, poor wound healing, or weakness, occurs. Treating an underlying cause such as medication use or an illness may correct the deficiency. Otherwise, an increased dietary intake of the nutrient or vitamin and mineral supplements may be indicated.

Protein Indicators

Total Serum Protein
6.0–8.0 g/dL

GENERAL INFORMATION

The major blood proteins are serum albumin and the globulins, which together equal the total serum protein value. The measurement of total protein is performed by protein electrophoresis and aids in the diagnosis of protein deficiency; blood dyscrasias; and hepatic, GI, renal, and neoplastic diseases.

1. Low serum protein symptoms include:
   Dermatitis
   Hair thinning
   Muscle wasting
   Weakness
   Poor wound healing

2. Causes of increased total protein include:
   Dehydration
   Diabetic acidosis
   Infections
   Multiple myeloma
   Monocytic leukemia
   Chronic alcoholism
   Chronic inflammatory disease
   Edema
   Tissue breakdown
   Poor wound healing

3. Causes of decreased total protein include:
   Malnutrition
   Hepatic disease
   Renal disease
   GI disease
   Hodgkin's disease
   Trauma, such as burns, hemorrhage, and shock
   Hyperthyroidism
   Congestive heart failure

Albumin, Serum
Normal   3.1–4.3 g/dL

GENERAL INFORMATION

Albumin values of less than 3.0 g/dL indicate protein malnutrition and are accompanied by an increased incidence of morbidity and mortality. Albumin maintains oncotic pressure and transports substances such as bilirubin, fatty acids, hormones, and drugs that are insoluble in water.

1. Albumin is increased in multiple myeloma and with dehydration.
2. Causes of decreased albumin include:
   Malnutrition
   Liver and/or renal disease
   Collagen diseases
   Rheumatoid arthritis
   Metastatic carcinoma
   Hyperthyroidism
   Essential hypertension
   Use of cytotoxic agents

Globulins, Serum

Normal   2.6–4.1 g/dL

GENERAL INFORMATION

The four types of globulins identified by protein electrophoresis are found in differing quantities in various conditions. Alpha$_1$ globulin, alpha$_2$ globulin, and beta globulin are carrier proteins that transport lipids, hormones, and metals through the blood. Gamma globulin is an important component of the immune system.

Causes of increased globulins include:

• Tuberculosis
• Chronic syphilis
• Subacute bacterial endocarditis
• Myocardial infarction
• Multiple myeloma
• Collagen diseases
• Rheumatoid arthritis
• Diabetes mellitus
• Hodgkin's disease

NURSING IMPLICATIONS

Because a consistent relationship between protein intake and serum albumin levels has not been established, a high-protein diet is not advised except for individuals with evidence of protein calorie malnutrition. Protein allowance is the same for older people as for younger people: 0.8 g/kg body weight. Protein should provide at least 12% of total calories for the healthy older person. The proteins from animal sources such as beef, poultry, fish, and dairy products are the most complete, whereas complementary vegetable proteins have less biological value. Some older people may need nutritional supplementation through oral, enteral, or parenteral routes if malnutrition is severe.

Iron Indicators

Iron, Serum

Male	80–180 mg/dL
Female	60–160 mg/dL

GENERAL INFORMATION

Iron appears in the plasma bound to the glycoprotein transferrin. Iron is essential in the production and function of hemoglobin and other compounds. Dietary iron is absorbed by the intestine and distributed in the body for synthesis, storage, and transport. The body has no mechanism for eliminating excessive iron; total body and bone marrow iron stores increase with advancing age, although serum iron may be depleted. Serum iron values should be interpreted together with the total iron-binding capacity (TIBC) and serum ferritin. Bone marrow and liver biopsy and iron absorption or excretion studies may be necessary to obtain a definitive diagnosis in iron-related disease. A decrease in serum iron with an increased TIBC occurs in iron-deficiency anemia, which is most commonly caused in elderly persons by GI blood loss or malabsorption.

Ferritin, Serum

Normal   20–400 ng/mL

GENERAL INFORMATION

Ferritin is an iron-storage protein. Serum ferritin level indicates the amount of available iron stored in the body. It is measured to distinguish between iron deficiency (decreased ferritin level) and chronic infection or inflammation (increased or normal ferritin level).

1. Causes of increased serum ferritin include:
   Liver disease
   Iron overload
   Leukemia
   Hodgkin's disease
   Chronic renal failure
   Hemolytic anemias
   Acute or chronic infection and inflammation
2. Ferritin is decreased only with chronic iron deficiency

Total Iron-Binding Capacity (Transferrin), Serum

250–410 mg/dL

GENERAL INFORMATION

TIBC decreases with age and reflects the transferrin content of the serum. Transferrin, a beta globulin protein, transports circulating iron that is stored in various forms in the bone marrow, liver, and spleen. In protein-energy malnutrition, TIBC is less than 250 mg/dL (see previous discussion under serum iron).

Lipoproteins

Total Plasma Cholesterol

Desired	<200 mg/dL
Borderline	200–239 mg/dL
High	≥240 mg/dL

High-Density Lipoprotein (HDL) Cholesterol

Desired	>35 mg/dL

Low-Density Lipoprotein (LDL) Cholesterol

Desired	130 mg/dL
Borderline	130–159 mg/dL
High	160 mg/dL
Triglycerides	160 mg/dL

General Information

Blood lipid and lipoprotein cholesterol levels, which are influenced by heredity, diet, and obesity, are directly related to atherosclerotic heart disease in elderly people. Higher HDL cholesterol, lower LDL cholesterol, and a decreased level of plasma triglycerides all are associated with decreased incidence of coronary heart disease.

In women, the increase in plasma total cholesterol with age is due primarily to an increase in LDL cholesterol. HDL cholesterol increases slightly in men older than 65 years but decreases in women of the same age. Without intervening therapy, the risk for coronary heart disease in elderly people gradually increases.

Total cholesterol and HDL cholesterol should be measured in screening tests for the elderly population. The findings of a high initial cholesterol value should be followed by two subsequent evaluations because there may be significant daily variations in values. Older persons may have a total cholesterol of less than 200 to 240 mg/dL but have elevated LDL cholesterol and decreased HDL cholesterol and so have an increased risk of coronary heart disease. Conversely, if HDL cholesterol is high, accounting for a total cholesterol level greater than 200 mg/dL, there is a reduced risk for coronary heart disease. Total cholesterol and HDL cholesterol may be obtained from non-fasting blood samples. Triglyceride levels are accurate only after a 12-hour fast. LDL cholesterol levels may be calculated after total cholesterol, HDL cholesterol, and triglycerides are known.

Lipid abnormalities are often genetic. Causes of secondary lipid elevation include:

- Diets high in saturated fat or cholesterol
- Excessive alcohol intake
- Estrogen supplements
- Thiazide diuretics
- Beta blockers
- Smoking
- Uncontrolled diabetes
- Hypothyroidism
- Uremia
- Corticosteroid use
- Sedentary lifestyle
- Morbid obesity

Cholesterol levels less than 120 to 156 mg/dL have been associated with increased mortality in nursing home residents. Causes of decreased cholesterol include:

- Malnutrition
- Hyperthyroidism
- Chronic obstructive pulmonary disease

Nursing Implications for Lipid Abnormalities

- Weight control
- Increased physical activity
- Restriction of alcohol
- Cessation of smoking
- Restriction of dietary fat

Dietary restrictions should be cautiously initiated so that adequate calorie and protein intake is considered in the elderly. Drug therapy to control lipid levels may be beneficial in older persons with known coronary heart disease or high risk of disease.

DRUG MONITORING AND TOXICOLOGY

Drug monitoring is important when the margin of safety between therapeutic and toxic blood levels is narrow. Drug blood levels are useful guides in maintaining therapeutic levels and in identifying toxic levels of drugs. Not all drugs have a known therapeutic blood level even though toxic levels have been identified. Some drugs, such as amphetamines, are monitored through urine testing. Elderly persons metabolize and eliminate drugs more slowly than middle-aged adults, which heightens the importance of drug monitoring.

Three commonly monitored drugs—digoxin, theophylline, and phenytoin—are discussed because they require close observation by the LPN. Numerous classes of drugs are commonly checked for therapeutic or toxic levels. Review the list in Box 22.3. Refer to a basic laboratory manual for specific drug therapeutic and toxic values.

Digoxin (Lanoxin) Level, Serum

Therapeutic	0.5–20 ng/mL
Toxic	2.5 ng/mL

General Information

Digoxin, used in the treatment of congestive heart failure and cardiac arrhythmias, has a prolonged half-life in elderly patients because of its reduced renal clearance. Serum digoxin level has a narrow therapeutic range, and digitalis toxicity is relatively common in elderly persons despite the availability of tests for serum drug levels.

Common side effects of digitalis toxicity include:

- Visual changes
- Headache
- Nausea and vomiting
- Weakness and fatigue

Weakness and fatigue are sometimes the only indicators of digitalis toxicity in an elderly person.

Quinidine significantly increases the serum level of digoxin. Consequently, the digoxin dose must be reduced when both of these drugs are prescribed. Also, a change from tablet to elixir preparation of digoxin increases the absorption and serum level, so that the digoxin dose again needs to be reduced. Low serum potassium levels and high serum calcium levels increase the risk of serious arrhythmias in persons receiving digoxin therapy.

Nursing Implications

- Draw blood samples for determining serum digoxin levels at least 5 to 6 hours after the

BOX 22.3 COMMONLY MONITORED MEDICATION LEVELS

Alcohol

Ethanol
Isopropanol (rubbing alcohol)
Methanol (antifreeze)

Amphetamines (Urine Testing)

Amphetamine
Dextroamphetamine
Methamphetamine (Desoxyn)
Phenmetrazine (Preludin)

Antiarrhythmics

Disopyramide (Norpace)
Lidocaine (Xylocaine)
Procainamide (Pronestyl)
Propranolol (Inderal)
Quinidine (Quinaglute and others)
Verapamil (Calan, Isoptin)

Antibiotics

Amikacin (Amikin)
Gentamicin (Garamycin)
Kanamycin (Kantrex)
Netilmicin (Netromycin)
Tobramycin (Nebcin)

Anticonvulsants

Carbamazepine (Tegretol)
Ethosuximide (Zarontin)
Phenobarbital (Luminal)
Phenytoin (Dilantin)
Primidone (Mysoline)

Antidepressants

Amitriptyline
Nortriptyline (Pamelor, Aventyl)
Desipramine (Norpramin)
Doxepin (Sinequan and others)
Imipramine (Tofranil)
Lithium (Lithobid)

Barbiturates and Hypnotics

Amobarbital (Amytal)

Glutethimide (Doriden)

Pentobarbital (Nembutal)

Phenobarbital (Luminal)

Secobarbital (Seconal)

Bronchodilators

Aminophylline

Theophylline (Theo-Dur and others)

Cardiac Glycosides

Digitoxin (Crystodigin)

Digoxin (Lanoxin)

Hemoglobin Derivatives

Carboxyhemoglobin (Hg = CO)

Methemoglobin

Sulfhemoglobin

Non-narcotic Analgesics

Acetaminophen (Tylenol and others)

Salicylates (aspirin)

Phenothiazines

Chlorpromazine (Thorazine)

Prochlorperazine (Compazine)

Thioridazine (Mellaril)

Trifluoperazine (Stelazine)

General Information

Theophylline, a bronchodilator, may or may not be associated with improved respiratory effort on spirometry testing. Nevertheless, theophylline improves mucociliary clearance of the lungs and may improve myocardial contractility, stimulate respirations, and act as a mild diuretic. Even though this is a useful drug for chronic obstructive pulmonary disease (COPD), it is used less frequently today because of the side effect profile, multiple drug interactions, and development of other medications that are effective without the same side effect profile. Most of them have fewer drug interactions as well.

Wide variations in the rate and extent of absorption and rate of metabolism for theophylline result in peak-to-trough fluctuations in serum concentrations and subsequent subtherapeutic or toxic responses.

Possible theophylline toxicity symptoms
    include:
    Anorexia
    Abdominal discomfort
    Nausea
    Vomiting
    Dizziness
    Shakiness
    Restlessness
    Irritability
    Palpitations
    Tachycardia
    Hypotension
    Heart arrhythmias and seizures

daily dose and preferably just before the next scheduled daily dose.
- Check the apical pulse for 1 full minute.
- Suspect digitalis toxicity when there is a sudden change in heart rhythm or pulse (especially a decrease).
- Withhold the medication and report to the physician when there is a sudden change in pulse or rhythm.
- Monitor the serum potassium level, especially if the person is taking diuretics.

Theophylline, Serum

| Therapeutic | 10–20 µg/mL |
| Toxic | 20 µg/mL |

Nursing Implications

- Dizziness is a common side effect at the initiation of theophylline use in elderly people. Theophylline elimination is reduced in persons with heart failure, kidney or liver disease, and alcoholism.
- Fever also changes the metabolism and action of this drug. Smoking and phenytoin use increase the elimination of theophylline so that an increase in dosage is required. Macrolide antibiotics such as erythromycin may increase serum theophylline levels and cause toxicity.
- The serum level must be checked when signs or symptoms of toxicity develop or when medications affecting serum levels are added or discontinued.

• Regular monitoring of serum concentrations of theophylline is necessary to determine therapeutic dosage.

Phenytoin (Dilantin), Serum

Therapeutic	10–20 µg/mL
Toxic	30 µg/mL

General Information

Phenytoin, an anticonvulsant that also has antiar-rhythmic properties, is metabolized by the liver and excreted in the bile and partially by the kidneys. Phenytoin has many potentially serious adverse reactions and side effects that necessitate monitoring of several parameters, including liver, kidney, thyroid, and hemato-logical functioning.

1. Potential adverse reactions and side effects include:
   Drowsiness
   Mental confusion
   Tremors
   Bradycardia
   Hypotension
   Photophobia
   Blurred vision
   Nausea
   Vomiting
   Epigastric pain
   Abnormal blood counts
   Fever
   Skin eruptions
   Pneumonitis
2. Acute kidney or liver dysfunction results in toxic drug levels.
3. Causes for decreased serum levels include:
   Chronic alcohol abuse
   Antacids
   Antihistamines
   Antineoplastics
   Barbiturates
   Excess of folic acid
   Rifampin
4. Causes for increased serum levels include:
   Acute intake of alcohol
   Anticoagulants
   Aminosalicylic acid
   Benzodiazepines
   Cimetidine
   Dexamethasone
   Estrogens
   Isoniazid

Methylphenidate
Phenothiazines
Salicylates
Sulfonamides
Phenylbutazone

Nursing Implications

• Liver and thyroid function tests, blood counts, and urinalysis are recommended before the initiation of therapy, at monthly intervals during early therapy, and at regular intervals thereafter.
• Lower doses are given to older adults and individuals with liver or kidney impairment.
• When phenytoin is given intravenously, vital signs and cardiac function must be monitored closely.
• Serum concentrations of magnesium, folic acid, vitamin D, and vitamin K may be decreased with phenytoin therapy and should be monitored.
• Symptoms of low serum magnesium may mimic symptoms of phenytoin toxicity.

 CONCLUSION

The use and interpretation of laboratory results are extremely important to substantiate clinical judgment and provide comprehensive health assessments in elderly people. With changes in demographics and lifestyles of elderly adults along with meaningful and frequent advances in medical knowledge, common laboratory tests will continue to be used to support and achieve goals for the best personal health of each individual as well as the expanding community of elders nationally.

Physiological changes in older persons, presence of disease, use of medications, variance in diets, and exercise will affect some laboratory reference values. Chronic syndromes and physiological aging processes contribute to changes in several specific substances in routine urine and blood specimens, and these laboratory procedures guide LPNs in best interventions and practices for complex and co-morbid health conditions.

It is necessary to monitor changes in an individual's laboratory values periodically to compare changes of the individual's laboratory values and assess overall morbidity for the individual patient. Laboratory results can also be matched with test values of other older adults in similar situations for evaluation of disease or treatments.

Understanding laboratory values in the elderly population is a continuing and sometimes challenging endeavor for all health-care practitioners. It is important for you to refer consistently to comprehensive laboratory manuals and individual laboratory reference intervals used in a particular locality and to have specialized printed, digital, or Internet gerontological references available. You can always contact the laboratory analyzing the specimens or peers you work with for collaborative information and answers. As new information becomes available, the interpretation of laboratory data will become more precise and useful in determining care for older people.

CASE STUDY SOLUTIONS

1. Underweight with risk of malnutrition

   Heart arrhythmia with possible orthostatic hypotension

   Probable urinary tract infection with urinary incontinence

   Anorexia and nausea possibly related to medications or urinary tract infection

   Recurrent falls with several possible causes, including weakness owing to decreased food and fluid intake, hypokalemia and hyponatremia, difficulty ambulating because of degenerative arthritis, orthostatic hypotension because of dehydration, and infection

2. CBC to assess for anemia and infection

   Digoxin level to check for toxicity as a cause of anorexia and nausea

   Urine culture and sensitivity to identify and quantify urine bacteria and determine antibiotic sensitivity

   Total protein to evaluate nutritional status

3. Safety measures to prevent falls, such as having Mr. K. call for assistance before getting up to go to the restroom. Advise him to change positions slowly from lying to sitting and then from sitting to standing. Consider a bedside commode because he has urinary incontinence and difficulty ambulating.

   Provide fluids and simple, easily digested foods in frequent small amounts.

   If nausea occurs, notify the physician.

   Withhold digoxin until the level value is obtained. Report to the physician.

   Withhold the furosemide because Mr. K. is dehydrated and has hypokalemia and hyponatremia, probably as a result of the diuretic. Report to the physician.

   Check any stools for occult blood because ibuprofen (an NSAID) is often the cause of GI bleeding. If the CBC indicates iron-deficiency anemia, the physician will probably discontinue this medication. Acetaminophen (Tylenol) may be used on a regular schedule to control arthritic pain.

REVIEW QUESTIONS

1. All laboratory test results for older adults should be:
   1. Evaluated against younger clients
   2. Evaluated against the other older adults on the unit
   3. Evaluated against the client's total clinical situation
   4. Evaluated against the person's CBC results

2. With the incidence of tuberculosis (TB) increasing among elderly people, it is critical for the LPN to know that:
   1. TB skin tests are inaccurate on people older than age 65
   2. When there is no initial reaction to the TB skin test in elderly people, it should be given again 1 week later
   3. It is unnecessary and expensive to do TB screening on nursing home residents
   4. Isoniazid is not an effective TB drug of choice for the elderly

3. What two tests determine if an individual is on the right dose of warfarin (Coumadin)?
   1. PT and PTT.
   2. INR and PTT
   3. BNP and INR
   4. INR and PT

4. Potassium deficiency develops:
   1. Slowly in elderly persons
   2. In the kidneys
   3. Rapidly because there is no way to conserve potassium
   4. Only when using diuretics

5. Every elderly person with a low serum albumin level should be:
   1. Put on a high-protein diet
   2. Put on bedrest
   3. Put on a diet of 12% complete proteins
   4. Put on vitamin supplements

REFERENCES

Corbett J.V., & Banks, A. (2012) *Laboratory tests and diagnostic procedures with nursing diagnoses* (8th ed.). New York, NY: Prentice Hall.

Drenkard, K.N. (2013). Patient-centered care. American Association of Colleges of Nursing. www.aacn.nche.edu/qsen/workshop-details/orlando/KD-PCC.pdf

Meiner, S.E. (2011). *Gerontologic nursing* (4th ed.). St. Louis, MO: Elsevier Mosby.

Van Leeuwen, A. M. & Bladh, M. L. (2015). *Davis's comprehensive handbook of laboratory and diagnostic tests with nursing implications* (6th ed.). Philadelphia, PA: F.A. Davis Company

WEB RESOURCES

24-hour urine protein: www.nlm.nih.gov/medlineplus/ency/article/003622.htm

Therapeutic drug levels: www.nlm.nih.gov/medlineplus/ency/article/003430.htm

Appendix A

Sample Advance Directives: Living Will and Power of Attorney for Health Care

The following document is reproduced courtesy of Caring Connections, 1731 King Street, Suite 100, Alexandria, VA 22314. It is a sample for the state of California. To get a similar document for your state, please go to Caring Connection's Web site at www.caringinfo.org or call them at 800-658-8898.

INTRODUCTION TO YOUR CALIFORNIA ADVANCE HEALTH CARE DIRECTIVE

This packet contains a legal document, a **California Advance Health Care Directive,** that protects your right to refuse medical treatment you do not want, or to request treatment you do want, in the event you lose the ability to make decisions yourself. You may complete any or all of the first four parts, depending on your advance planning needs. You must complete part 5.

Part 1 is a **Power of Attorney for Health Care**. This part lets you name someone (an agent) to make decisions about your health care. Unless otherwise written in your advance directive, your power of attorney for health care becomes effective when your primary doctor determines that you lack the ability to understand the nature and consequences of your health care decisions or the ability to make and communicate your health care decisions. If you want your agent to make health care decisions for you now, even though you are still capable of making health care decisions, you can include this instruction in your power of attorney for health care designation.

Part 2 includes your **Individual Instructions**. This is your state's living will. It lets you state your wishes about health care in the event that you can no longer speak for yourself and you may limit the individual instructions to take effect only if a specified condition arises.

Part 3 allows you to express your wishes regarding organ donation.

Part 4 of this form lets you designate a physician to have primary responsibility for your health care.

Part 5 contains the signature and witnessing provisions so that your document will be effective.

This form does not expressly address mental illness. If you would like to make advance care plans regarding mental illness, you should talk to your physician and an attorney about an advance directive tailored to your needs.

Note: These documents will be legally binding only if the person completing them is a competent adult, who is 18 years of age or older, or an emancipated minor.

INSTRUCTIONS FOR YOUR CALIFORNIA ADVANCE HEALTH CARE DIRECTIVE

How do I make my advance health care directive legal?

You must sign and date your advance directive or direct an adult to do so for you if you are unable to sign it yourself.

Your signature must be witnessed by or you must acknowledge your signature before a notary public or two adult witnesses. Your two adult witnesses may not be
- your health care provider or an employee of your health care provider,
- the operator or an employee of a community care facility,
- the operator or an employee of a residential care facility for the elderly, or
- the person you have appointed as an agent, if you have appointed an agent.

In addition, one of your witnesses must be unrelated to you by blood, marriage, or adoption and not entitled to any portion of your estate.

If you are a patient in a skilled nursing facility when you execute your advance directive, one of your witnesses must be a patient advocate or ombudsman.

Whom should I appoint as my agent?

Your agent is the person you appoint to make decisions about your health care if you become unable to make those decisions yourself. Your agent may be a family member or a close friend whom you trust to make serious decisions. The person you name as your agent should clearly understand your wishes and be willing to accept the responsibility of making health care decisions for you.

Your agent cannot be
- your supervising health care provider,
- the operator of a community care facility or residential care facility where you are receiving care, or
- the employee of a health care institution where you are receiving care or employee of a community care facility or residential care facility where you are receiving care, unless:
  - the employee is related to you by blood, marriage, or adoption,
  - the employee is your registered domestic partner, or
  - the employee is your coworker at the facility or institution.

If you have a conservator appointed for you as part of involuntary commitment proceedings under the Lanterman-Petris-Short Act, that conservator cannot be appointed as your agent unless you are represented by a lawyer who signs a certificate stating that you have been advised of your rights. If this applies to you, you should talk with your lawyer about your rights, the applicable law, and the potential consequences involved.

On the other hand, you may include in your advance directive a nomination for the individual appointed as your conservator, if necessary. The court will consider your nomination in any protective proceeding.

You can appoint a second and third person as your alternate agents. An alternate agent will step in if the person(s) you name as agent is/are unable, unwilling or unavailable to act for you.

Should I add personal instructions to my advance directive?

One of the strongest reasons for naming an agent is to have someone who can respond flexibly as your medical situation changes and deal with situations that you did not foresee. If you add instructions to this document it may help your agent carry out your wishes, but be careful that you do not unintentionally restrict your agent's power to act in your best interest. In any event, be sure to talk with your agent about your future health care and describe what you consider to be an acceptable "quality of life."

What if I change my mind?

Except for the appointment of your agent, you may revoke any portion or this entire advance directive at any time and in any way that communicates your intent to revoke. This could be by telling your agent or physician that you revoke, by signing a revocation, or simply by tearing up your advance directive.

In order to revoke your agent's appointment, you must either tell your supervising health care provider of your intent to revoke or revoke your agent's appointment in a signed writing.

If you execute a new advance directive, it will revoke the old advance directive to the extent of any conflict between the two documents.

Unless you specify otherwise in Part 2, if you designate your spouse as your agent, that designation will automatically be revoked by divorce or annulment of your marriage.

What other important facts should I know?

Your agent, if you appoint one, does not have authority to authorize convulsive treatment, psychosurgery, sterilization, or abortion, or to have you committed or placed in a mental health treatment facility.

CALIFORNIA ADVANCE HEALTH CARE DIRECTIVE - PAGE 1 OF 13

Explanation

You have the right to give instructions about your own health care. You also have the right to name someone else to make health care decisions for you. This form lets you do either or both of these things. It also lets you express your wishes regarding donation of organs and the designation of your primary physician. If you use this form, you may complete or modify all or any part of it. You are free to use a different form.

Part 1 of this form is a **power of attorney for health care**. Part 1 lets you name another individual as agent to make health care decisions for you if you become incapable of making your own decisions or if you want someone else to make those decisions for you now even though you are still capable. You may name an alternate agent to act for you if your first choice is not willing, able, or reasonably available to make decisions for you. (Your agent may not be an operator or employee of a community care facility or a residential care facility where you are receiving care, or an employee of the health care institution where you are receiving care, unless your agent is related to you, is your registered domestic partner, or is a co-worker. Your supervising health care provider can never act as your agent.)

Unless the form you sign limits the authority of your agent, your agent may make all health care decisions for you. This form has a place for you to limit the authority of your agent. You need not limit the authority of your agent if you wish to rely on your agent for all health care decisions that may have to be made. If you choose not to limit the authority of your agent, your agent will have the right to:

(a)   Consent or refuse consent to any care, treatment, service, or procedure to maintain, diagnose, or otherwise affect a physical or mental condition;

(b)   Select or discharge health care providers and institutions;

(c)   Approve or disapprove diagnostic tests, surgical procedures and programs of medication;

(d)   Direct the provision, withholding, or withdrawal of artificial nutrition and hydration and all other forms of health care, including cardiopulmonary resuscitation; and

(e)   Make anatomical gifts, authorize an autopsy, and direct the disposition of your remains.

Explanation Continued

Part 2 of this form lets you give specific **instructions** about any aspect of your health care, whether or not you appoint an agent. Choices are provided for you to express your wishes regarding the provision, withholding, or withdrawal of treatment to keep you alive, as well as the provision of pain relief. Space is provided for you to add to the choices you have made or for you to write out any additional wishes. If you are satisfied to allow your agent to determine what is best for you in making end-of-life decisions, you need not fill out part 2 of this form.

Part 3 of this form lets you express an intention to donate your bodily organs and tissues following your death.

Part 4 of this form lets you designate a physician to have primary responsibility for your health care.

After completing this form, sign and date the form in **Part 5**. The form must be signed by two qualified witnesses or acknowledged before a notary public. Give a copy of the signed and completed form to your physician, to any other health care providers you may have, to any health care institution at which you are receiving care, and to any health care agents you have named. You should talk to the person you have named as agent and alternate agent(s) to make sure that he or she understands your wishes and is willing to take the responsibility.

You have the right to revoke this advance health care directive or replace this form at any time.

INSTRUCTIONS

PART 1: POWER OF ATTORNEY FOR HEALTH CARE

(1) DESIGNATION OF AGENT: I designate the following individual as my agent to make health care decisions for me:

PRINT THE NAME,
HOME ADDRESS
AND HOME AND
WORK TELEPHONE
NUMBERS OF YOUR
PRIMARY
AGENT

_____

(Name of individual you choose as agent)

_____

(address)   (city) (state)   (zip code)

_____

(home phone)   (work phone)

OPTIONAL: If I revoke my agent's authority or if my agent is not willing, able, or reasonably available to make a health care decision for me, I designate as my first alternate agent:

PRINT THE NAME,
HOME ADDRESS
AND HOME AND
WORK TELEPHONE
NUMBERS OF YOUR
FIRST ALTERNATE
AGENT
(OPTIONAL)

_____

(Name of individual you choose as first alternate agent)

_____

(address)

_____

(city)   (state)   (zip code)

_____

(home phone)   (work phone)

OPTIONAL: If I revoke the authority of my agent and first alternate agent or if neither is willing, able, or reasonably available to make a health care decision for me, I designate as my second alternate agent:

PRINT THE NAME,
HOME ADDRESS
AND HOME AND
WORK TELEPHONE
NUMBERS OF YOUR
SECOND
ALTERNATE
AGENT
(OPTIONAL)

_____

(Name of individual you choose as second alternate agent)

_____

(address)

_____

(city)   (state)   (zip code)

_____

(home phone)   (work phone)

CALIFORNIA ADVANCE HEALTH CARE DIRECTIVE — PAGE 4 OF 13

ADD INSTRUCTIONS HERE ONLY IF YOU WANT TO LIMIT THE POWER OF YOUR AGENT

(2) AGENT'S AUTHORITY: My agent is authorized to make all health care decisions for me, including decisions to provide, withhold, or withdraw artificial nutrition and hydration, and all other forms of health care to keep me alive, except as I state here:

_____
_____
_____
_____
_____

(Add additional sheets if needed.)

(3) WHEN AGENT'S AUTHORITY BECOMES EFFECTIVE: My agent's authority becomes effective when my primary physician determines that I am unable to make my own health care decisions unless I mark the following box. If I mark this box [   ], my agent's authority to make health care decisions for me takes effect immediately.

INITIAL THE BOX IF YOU WISH YOUR AGENT'S AUTHORITY TO BECOME EFFECTIVE IMMEDIATELY

(4) AGENT'S OBLIGATION: My agent shall make health care decisions for me in accordance with this power of attorney for health care, any instructions I give in Part 2 of this form, and my other wishes to the extent known to my agent. To the extent my wishes are unknown, my agent shall make health care decisions for me in accordance with what my agent determines to be in my best interest. In determining my best interest, my agent shall consider my personal values to the extent known to my agent.

CROSS OUT AND INITIAL ANY STATEMENTS IN PARAGRAPHS 4, 5, OR 6 THAT DO NOT REFLECT YOUR WISHES

(5) AGENT'S POSTDEATH AUTHORITY: My agent is authorized to make anatomical gifts, authorize an autopsy, and direct disposition of my remains, except as I state here, in paragraph (2) above, or in Part 3 of this form:

_____

_____

_____

(6) NOMINATION OF CONSERVATOR: If a conservator of my person needs to be appointed for me by a court, I nominate the agent designated in this form. If that agent is not willing, able, or reasonably available to act as conservator, I nominate the alternate agents whom I have named, in the order designated.

PART 2: INSTRUCTIONS FOR HEALTH CARE

If you fill out this part of the form, you may strike any wording you do not want.

(7) END-OF-LIFE DECISIONS: I direct that my health care providers and others involved in my care provide, withhold, or withdraw treatment in accordance with the choice I have marked below: (**Initial only one box**)

INITIAL THE PARAGRAPH THAT BEST REFLECTS YOUR WISHES REGARDING LIFE-SUPPORT MEASURES

[   ] (a) **Choice NOT To Prolong Life**
I do not want my life to be prolonged if (1) I have an incurable and irreversible condition that will result in my death within a relatively short time, (2) I become unconscious and, to a reasonable degree of medical certainty, I will not regain consciousness, or (3) the likely risks and burdens of treatment would outweigh the expected benefits,

OR

[   ] (b) **Choice To Prolong Life**
I want my life to be prolonged as long as possible within the limits of generally accepted health care standards.

(8) RELIEF FROM PAIN: Except as I state in the following space, I direct that treatment for alleviation of pain or discomfort should be provided at all times even if it hastens my death:

ADD INSTRUCTIONS HERE ONLY IF YOU WANT TO LIMIT PAIN RELIEF OR COMFORT CARE

_____

_____

_____

_____

_____

_____

_____

_____

CALIFORNIA ADVANCE HEALTH CARE DIRECTIVE — PAGE 6 OF 13

ADD OTHER INSTRUCTIONS, IF ANY, REGARDING YOUR ADVANCE CARE PLANS

THESE INSTRUCTIONS CAN FURTHER ADDRESS YOUR HEALTH CARE PLANS, SUCH AS YOUR WISHES REGARDING HOSPICE TREATMENT, BUT CAN ALSO ADDRESS OTHER ADVANCE PLANNING ISSUES, SUCH AS YOUR BURIAL WISHES

ATTACH ADDITIONAL PAGES IF NEEDED

© 2005 National Hospice and Palliative Care Organization 2014 Revised.

(9) OTHER WISHES: (If you do not agree with any of the optional choices above and wish to write your own, or if you wish to add to the instructions you have given above, you may do so here.) I direct that:

_____

_____

_____

_____

_____

_____

_____

_____

_____

_____

_____

_____

_____

_____

_____

_____

(Add additional sheets if needed.)

PART 3: DONATION OF ORGANS AT DEATH
(OPTIONAL)

ORGAN
DONATION
(OPTIONAL)

(10) Upon my death: (initial applicable box)

INITIAL THE BOX
THAT AGREES WITH
YOUR WISHES
ABOUT ORGAN
DONATION

[   ] (a) I do not give any of my organs, tissues, or parts and do
not want my agent, conservator, or family to make a
donation on my behalf,

[   ] (b) I give any needed organs, tissues, or parts,

OR

[   ] (c) I give the following organs, tissues, or parts only

_____
_____
_____

STRIKE THROUGH
ANY USES YOU DO
NOT AGREE TO

My gift is for the following purposes:
(strike any of the following you do not want)
    (1) Transplant
    (2) Therapy
    (3) Research
    (4) Education

CALIFORNIA ADVANCE HEALTH CARE DIRECTIVE — PAGE 8 OF 13

PART 4: PRIMARY PHYSICIAN
(OPTIONAL)

PRINT THE NAME, ADDRESS AND TELEPHONE NUMBER OF YOUR PRIMARY PHYSICIAN (OPTIONAL)

(11) I designate the following physician as my primary physician:

_____
(name of physician)

_____
(address)

_____
(city)   (state)   (zip code)

_____
(phone)

PRINT THE NAME, ADDRESS AND TELEPHONE NUMBER OF YOUR ALTERNATE PRIMARY PHYSICIAN (OPTIONAL)

OPTIONAL: If the physician I have designated above is not willing, able, or reasonably available to act as my primary physician, I designate the following physician as my primary physician:

_____
(name of physician)

_____
(address)

_____
(city)   (state)   (zip code)

_____
(phone)

(12) EFFECT OF COPY: A copy of this form has the same effect as the original.

PART 5: EXECUTION

This Health Care Directive will not be valid unless it is EITHER:

(A)   Signed by two (2) qualified adult witnesses who are personally known to you or to whom you have proven your identity by convincing evidence and who are present when you sign or acknowledge your signature. Your witnesses may not be

- your health care provider or an employee of your health care provider,
- the operator or an employee of a community care facility,
- the operator or an employee of a residential care facility for the elderly, or
- the person you have appointed as an agent, if you have appointed an agent.

In addition, one of your witnesses must be unrelated to you by blood, marriage, or adoption and not entitled to any portion of your estate. (Use Alternative 1, below, if you decide to have your signature witnessed.)

OR

(B)   Witnessed by a notary. (Use Alternative 2, below (page 12), if you decide to have your signature notarized.)

IF YOU CHOOSE TO SIGN WITH WITNESSES, USE ALTERNATIVE 1, BELOW

IF YOU CHOOSE TO HAVE YOUR SIGNATURE NOTARIZED, USE ALTERNATIVE 2, BELOW (PAGE 12)

THERE ARE SPECIAL WITNESSING REQUIREMENTS IF YOU LIVE IN A SKILLED NURSING FACILITY

If you are a patient in a skilled nursing facility when you execute your advance directive, one of your witnesses must be a patient advocate or ombudsman. This witness must sign the statement on page 13, even if you have had your advance directive notarized.

© 2005 National Hospice and Palliative Care Organization 2014 Revised.

CALIFORNIA ADVANCE HEALTH CARE DIRECTIVE - PAGE 10 OF 13

OPTION 1: Sign before a Witness

SIGN AND DATE THE DOCUMENT AND THEN PRINT YOUR NAME AND ADDRESS

_____   _____
(date)   (sign your name)

_____
(print your name)

_____
(address)

_____
(city)   (state)   (zip code)

STATEMENT OF WITNESSES

I declare under penalty of perjury under the laws of California (1) that the individual who signed or acknowledged this advance health care directive is personally known to me, or that the individual's identity was proven to me by convincing evidence, (2) that the individual signed or acknowledged this advance directive in my presence, (3) that the individual appears to be of sound mind and under no duress, fraud, or undue influence, (4) that I am not a person appointed as an agent by this advance directive, and (5) that I am not the individual's health care provider, an employee of the individual's health care provider, the operator of a community care facility, an employee of an operator of a community care facility, the operator of a residential care facility for the elderly, nor an employee of an operator of a residential care facility for the elderly.

WITNESSING PROCEDURE

BOTH OF YOUR WITNESSES MUST AGREE WITH THIS STATEMENT

First Witness:

_____   _____
(date)   (signature of witness)

_____
(printed name of witness)

_____
(address)

_____
(city)   (state)   (zip code)

ONE WITNESS MUST ALSO SIGN THE STATEMENT ON PAGE 11

Second Witness:

_____   _____
(date)   (signature of witness)

_____
(printed name of witness)

_____
(address)

_____
(city)   (state)   (zip code)

HAVE YOUR WITNESSES SIGN AND DATE THE DOCUMENT AND THEN PRINT THEIR NAME AND ADDRESS

© 2005 National Hospice and Palliative Care Organization 2014 Revised.

ONE OF YOUR WITNESSES MUST ALSO SIGN THIS STATEMENT

ADDITIONAL WITNESS STATEMENT

I further declare under penalty of perjury under the laws of California that I am not related to the individual executing this advance health care directive by blood, marriage, or adoption, and, to the best of my knowledge, I am not entitled to any part of the individual's estate upon his or her death under a will now existing or by operation of law.

_____   _____
          (date)   (signature of witness)

CALIFORNIA ADVANCE HEALTH CARE DIRECTIVE - PAGE 12 OF 13

ALTERNATIVE NO. 2: NOTARY PUBLIC

SIGN AND DATE THE DOCUMENT AND THEN PRINT YOUR NAME AND ADDRESS

_____ _____
(date)   (sign your name)

_____
(print your name)

_____
(address)

_____
(city)   (state)   (zip code)

A NOTARY PUBLIC MUST FILL OUT THIS PORTION OF THE FORM

State of California   )
) SS.
County of _____)

On _____ before me,_____
                                                        (insert name of notary public)
personally appeared _____,
                                        (insert the name of principal)

Who proved to me on the basis of satisfactory evidence to be the person(s) is/are subscribed to the within instrument and acknowledged to me that he/she/they executed the same in his/her/their authorized capacity(ies), and that by his/her their signature(s) on the instrument the person(s), or the entity upon behalf of which the person(s) acted, executed the instrument.

I certify under PENALTY OF PERJURY under the laws of the state of California that the foregoing paragraph is true and correct.

WITNESS my hand and official seal.

NOTARY SEAL

_____
(signature of notary)

THIS SECTION
MUST BE
COMPLETED
BY A PATIENT
ADVOCATE OR
OMBUDSMAN IF
YOU ARE A
RESIDENT IN A
SKILLED NURSING
FACILITY

STATEMENT OF PATIENT ADVOCATE OR OMBUDSMAN
I declare under penalty of perjury under the laws of California that I am
a patient advocate or ombudsman as designated by the State
Department of Aging and that I am serving as witness as required by
section 4675 of the Probate Code.

_____   _____
(date)   (signature)
_____
(printed name)

_____
(address)

_____
(city)   (state)   (zip code)

Courtesy of Caring Connections
1731 King St., Suite 100, Alexandria, VA 22314
www.caringinfo.org, 800/658-8898

Appendix B

Answers to Review Questions

Chapter 1
1. 3
2. 1
3. 2
4. 4
5. 1, 2, 3, and 4
6. 1

Chapter 2
1. 2
2. 1
3. 1
4. 4
5. 2

Chapter 3
1. 4
2. 3
3. 2
4. 2
5. 4
6. 3

Chapter 4
1. 2
2. 3
3. 3
4. 4
5. 1

Chapter 5
1. 1
2. 2
3. 2
4. 3
5. 1

Chapter 6
1. 3
2. 1
3. 1
4. 2
5. 2

Chapter 7
1. 1, 2, 4, 5, 6, 7
2. 1
3. 3
4. 4
5. 4

Chapter 8
1. 3
2. 3

3. 4
4. 4
5. 1

Chapter 9
1. 2
2. 4
3. 1, 5
4. 4
5. 4

Chapter 10
1. 3
2. 4
3. 4
4. 1
5. 4

Chapter 11
1. 1
2. 2
3. 1
4. 2
5. 4

Chapter 12
1. 4
2. 3
3. 2
4. 4
5. 4
6. 3

Chapter 13
1. 2
2. 2
3. 3
4. 3
5. 2
6. 2

Chapter 14
1. 2
2. 1
3. 2
4. 3
5. 4

Chapter 15
1. 3
2. 1
3. 2
4. 4
5. 2

Chapter 16
1. 2
2. 3
3. 3
4. 4
5. 4

Chapter 17
1. 2
2. 3
3. 4
4. 4
5. 2

Chapter 18
1. 4
2. 3
3. 4
4. 3
5. 4

Chapter 19
1. 2
2. 4
3. 1
4. 4
5. 4

Chapter 20
1. 4
2. 2
3. 3
4. 4
5. 4

Chapter 21
1. 1
2. 2
3. 2
4. 3
5. 4
6. 3
7. 4

Chapter 22
1. 3
2. 2
3. 4
4. 3
5. 3

Index

Note: Page numbers followed by f refer to figures; page numbers followed by t refer to tables.

Abdomen, assessment of, 300–301
Absorption, of medications, 395–396
ACA. *See* Affordable Care Act.
Acceptance stage of grief, 201
Accessory muscles, 29
Accommodation to dysfunction, 383–384
Acting out, sexual, 357
Active exercise, in rehabilitative and restorative care, 379. *See also* Exercise.
Active listening, 234–235
Activities, 182–185. *See also* Exercise.
 benefits of, 182, 183–184, 186
 in environmental management, 214–215
Activities of daily living (ADLs), 28–29
 assessment of, 307
 definition and examples of, 307
 instrumental, 28, 29, 308–309, 308f
 in rehabilitative and restorative care, 386
 and self-care, 119
Acute care facilities, 222
Acute illness. *See also specific types*.
 vs. chronic conditions, 271–273
 and mobility problems, 317
 as transition, 48–49
AD. *See* Alzheimer's disease.
ADLs. *See* Activities of daily living.
Admission, case study of, 58–61
ADRs. *See* Adverse drug reactions.
Adult day services (ADS), 217–218
Advanced beginner CNAs, 238–239
Advance directives, 97–98, 205–206
Adverse drug reactions (ADRs), 391, 397, 398t
Advocates, nurses as, 375
Aerobic exercises, 115
Affordable Care Act (ACA), 101–102
Age groups, new definitions of, 7
Ageism, 6, 23–24
Age-related changes. *See also specific types*.
 case study of, 20, 34
 normal, description of, 28–33
 pharmacotherapeutics affected by, 391–393
 restorative care affected by, 376–377
Aggressive behavior, 233–235
Aging, 19–35
 attitudes toward, 22–24
 demographics of, 6–8, 20–21

impact on nursing, 21–22
 normal process of, 27–33
 theories of, 24–27
Agitated delirium, as sign of imminent death, 206
Agitation, 356–357
AHA. *See* American Hospital Association.
AIDS, 134, 263–264
Alanine aminotransferase (ALT), 427
Albumin, 429–430
Alcohol abuse, 117–119, 365, 399
Alkaline phosphatase, 427–428
ALT. *See* Alanine aminotransferase.
Alzheimer's disease (AD), 363–364
American Association of Poison Control Centers, 136
American Hospital Association (AHA), Patient's Bill of Rights, 91
Amino acids, 151–152
Anemia, sickle cell, 165–166
Anger
 progressively lowered stress threshold and, 44
 as stage of grief, 200
Antacid abuse, 398–399
Antibiotics, organisms resistant to, 265
Antidepressants, 359
Anxiety, indicators of, 132
Apnea, sleep, 190, 329
Arthritis, 284
Asian Americans, 169–171
Aspartate aminotransferase (AST), 427
Assertive communication, 233–234
Assessment
 of environments of care, 212–214
 functional, 306–309, 377
 holistic, 292
 in management and leadership, 236
 of medication therapy, 401–402
 in nursing process, 63–64, 68
 of nutrition, 147, 149, 327
 of pain, 186–187
 physiological. *See* Physiological assessment.
 psychological. *See* Psychological assessment.
 of spiritual needs, 49–50, 380
Assignments, care, 238–240
Assisted-living communities, 61, 62, 219–220
AST. *See* Aspartate aminotransferase.
Attitudes, toward aging, 22–24

Attorney, power of, 97, 205
Authoritarian leadership style, 227–228

Baby boomers, 7
Bags, safety, 136–137
Balance, 318
Bargaining stage of grief, 200–201
Basophils, 418
Bathrooms
 fall prevention in, 129
 as source of infection, 262
Bedrest, 317
Bedside caregivers, nurses as, 374
Beers criteria, 399–400
Behavioral interventions, for chronic incontinence, 322–323
Behavior problems
 assertive behavior in response to, 233–235
 violent, 357
Benner, Patricia, 238–239
Bilirubin, 426
Black Americans, 164–167
Bladder. *See also* Urinary incontinence.
 normal age-related changes in, 31
 in rehabilitative and restorative care, 379, 386
 retraining of, 322, 386
Blood
 normal age-related changes in, 28
 in stool, test for, 415–416
Blood glucose test, 421–422
Blood tests, 416–421
Blood urea nitrogen (BUN), 425–426
Blood vessels, normal age-related changes in, 28
B-natriuretic peptide (BNP), 428
Body image, 49
Bones, normal age-related changes in, 29–30, 315
Bowel continence, in rehabilitative and restorative care, 379–381, 386
Braden scale, 301, 302f–303f
Breast self-examination, 305–306, 305f
Breath sounds, adventitious, 300
BUN. *See* Blood urea nitrogen.
Butler, Robert, 23

CAAs. *See* Care Area Assessments.
CAD. *See* Coronary artery disease.
Calcium
 need for, 155
 testing of, 424–425

Calculating skills, definition and
    assessment of, 338–339
CAM. *See* Confusion Assessment
    Method.
Canada, medications from, 394
Carbohydrates, 149
Carbon monoxide poisoning, 136
Cardiovascular system
    assessment of, 274, 298
    common chronic conditions in,
        275–279
    and falls, 127
    in mobility problems, 316
    normal age-related changes in,
        28–29, 316
Care Area Assessments (CAAs), 63–64
Care Area Triggers (CATs), 64
Care/caring, 3–17. *See also specific
    settings and types of care.*
    climate of, 213
    environments of. *See* Environments.
    human, 11–14, 92
    philosophies of, 4, 8–11
    quality of, management of, 246–247
    reasons to study, 12–13
Case managers, nurses as, 375
Cataracts, 282
    case study of, 270, 288
Catheters, urinary (UCs), 261
CATs. *See* Care Area Triggers.
CBC. *See* Complete blood count.
Central nervous system. *See* Nervous
    system.
Cerebrovascular accident (CVA). *See*
    Stroke.
Certified nursing assistants (CNAs)
    delegation to, 240–241
    education of, 245–246
    five points of clinical expertise of,
        238–240
    in planning process, 69–70
Charting, 70–71
CHF. *See* Congestive heart failure.
Chloride
    need for, 155–156
    testing of, 425
Choices
    guided, 352
    in transitional outcomes, 42–43
Cholesterol tests, 431
Chronic illness and diseases. *See also
    specific types.*
    vs. acute conditions, 271–273
    common types of, 7, 110, 184,
        275–287
    and infections, 258
    management of, 110–111
    and mobility problems, 316–317
    wellness promotion with, 110–111
Chronic obstructive pulmonary disease
    (COPD), 190–191, 283–284
Chronopharmacology, 401

Circadian rhythms, 189, 401
CK. *See* Creatinine kinase.
Clear-liquid diets, 157
Climate of caring, 213
Clinical expertise, five points of,
    238–240
Clinical status, relationship of
    laboratory values to, 411
Closed questions, 352
Clothing, and falls, 127–128
CNAs. *See* Certified nursing assistants.
Coagulation tests, 420–421
Cognition
    changes in, and pharmacotherapeutics,
        392–393
    definition of, 336
Cognitive disorders
    as barriers to sleep, 191
    safety concerns with, 131–132
Cognitive functions, 336–339
Cold, risks associated with, 130–131
Comfort measures, 384
Communication
    assertive, 233–234
    assessment of, 338
    in end-of-life care, 202
    with families, 231–232
    general guidelines for, 350–356
    with interdisciplinary teams, 232–233
    in management and leadership,
        229–235
    nonverbal, 230, 231, 354–355
    with patients and residents,
        230–231
    with people with dementia, 358,
        362–363
    with people with psychological
        problems, 350–356, 358
    verbal, 230, 352
Community-based care, 219
Competent CNAs, 239
Complete blood count (CBC), 416
Complete proteins, 152
Comprehensive metabolic profile
    indicators, 421–428
Computers, in nursing process, 72
Condoms, 262–263
Confidentiality
    in end-of-life care, 202
    as legal and ethical issue, 100
Confusion Assessment Method (CAM),
    341, 342
Congestive heart failure (CHF),
    190–191, 276–277
Consent, informed, 96–97
Constipation, 323
Continence training, 386
Continuing care retirement
    communities, 62, 220
Continuity theory of aging, 26
COPD. *See* Chronic obstructive
    pulmonary disease.

Coronary artery disease (CAD),
    275–276
Counselors, nurses as, 374–375
CPK. *See* Creatinine phosphokinase.
Creatinine, 426
Creatinine kinase (CK), 428
Creatinine phosphokinase (CPK), 428
Crisis management, 237
Crutch walking, 385
Cruzan, Nancy, 97
Culturally specific care, 161–179
    of Asian Americans, 169–171
    of black Americans, 164–167
    case study of, 162, 177
    communication in, 353
    end-of-life, 203
    of European Americans, 171–172
    of Hispanic Americans, 172–175
    of Jewish Americans, 175–176
    of Native Americans, 167–169
Culture, 162–164
    definition of, 162
    vs. ethnicity, 163
    ethnocentrism based on, 162–163
Custodial care, 24, 372
Customer focus, 246–247
CVA (cerebrovascular accident).
    See Stroke.

Daily living activities. *See* Activities of
    daily living.
Day services, adult (ADS), 217–218
Death. *See also* End-of-life care.
    imminent signs of, 206–207
    mystery of, 198–199
    of spouse, 48
    stages of grief and, 199–201
Decision-making
    in end-of-life care, 203–206
    in management and leadership,
        235–237
Degenerative joint disease, 284, 315–316
Delegation, 240–241
Delirium, 361–362
    agitated, as sign of imminent
        death, 206
    assessment of, 340–342
    causes of, 361
    definition of, 361
    vs. depression, 360, 360t, 361
    incontinence caused by, 321
    safety concerns with, 131–132
Dementia, 362–364
    in Alzheimer's disease, 363–364
    as barrier to sleep, 191
    characteristics of, 362
    communicating with people with,
        358, 362–363
    vs. depression, 360, 360t, 361
    safety concerns with, 131–132
    stages of disorientation in,
        362–363, 364

Democratic leadership style, 228–229
Demographics of aging, 6–8, 20–21
Denial stage of grief, 200
Dependability, in end-of-life care, 202
Depression, 358–361
    assessment of, 341–342, 360
    case study of, 182, 193
    vs. dementia and delirium, 360,
        360t, 361
    indicators of, 132
    risk factors for, 359, 359t
    as stage of grief, 201, 359
    and suicide, 360–361
    treatment of, 359–360
Despair, vs. integrity, 14–15, 26
Deterioration, delay of, 383
Developmental disabilities, 365
Developmental tasks, 14–15, 26
Dexterity, changes in, 392
Diabetes, type 2, 285–286
    culture and, 168
    risk factors for, 285–286
    symptoms of, 286
Diagnoses. See Medical diagnoses;
        Nursing diagnoses.
Diet. See Nutrition.
Digoxin, 432–433
Dilantin, 434
Directives, advance, 97–98, 205–206
Disabilities
    developmental, 365
    as transitions, 48
Disasters, safety in, 136–137
Diseases. See Illness and diseases.
Disorientation, stages of, 362–364
Distress, 116, 188
Distribution, drug, 396
Disuse osteoporosis, 315
DME. See Durable medical equipment.
Documentation
    computerized, 72
    of implementation of plans, 70–71
    of physiological assessment, 309
    of plans of care, 68–70
Down's syndrome, 365
Drug abuse, 117–119, 365. See also
        Medications.
Drug-resistant organisms, 265
Durable medical equipment (DME), and
        falls, 128
Dysfunction, accommodation to,
        383–384

Ears, assessment of, 295–296. See also
        Hearing.
Eclectic leadership style, 229
Education
    of employees, 245–246
    of patients. See Patient education.
Educators, nurses as, 374
Elder abuse, 98, 135, 139
Eldercare Locator, 135

Elder self-neglect, 362
Electrolytes
    need for, 155–157
    testing of, 422–425
Elimination, changes in, 31–32,
        320–323. See also Incontinence.
Elite-old population, 7
Emergency situations, safety in,
        136–140
Emerson, Ralph Waldo, 40
Emotional maturity, in end-of-life
        care, 202
Empathy
    in end-of-life care, 202–203
    with people with psychological
        problems, 352–353
Employees, management of, 242–246
Endocrine system
    assessment of, 275
    common chronic conditions in,
        285–287
End-of-life (EOL) care, 197–209
    advance directives on, 205–206
    case study of, 198, 208
    cultural differences in, 203
    hospice in, 204
    imminent signs of death in, 206–207
    palliative care in, 204
    qualities needed for, 201–203
    stages of grief in, 199–201
Endurance-building exercises, 115
Enmeshment, 335
Environments of care, 211–224. See
        also specific types.
    assessment of, 212–214
    case study of, 212, 223
    in fall prevention, 128–129
    improving characteristics of, 44
    and infection, 261–262
    management of, 13, 212–215
    relocation trauma and, 215, 216
    types of, 61, 62, 215–222
    visual inspections of, 139–140
Envy, 173
EOL. See End-of-life.
Eosinophils, 418
Erectile dysfunction drugs, 134
Erikson, Eric, 14–15, 26
Errors
    in employee evaluation, 244
    medical, legal liability for, 93
Erythrocyte sedimentation rate (ESR),
        419–420
Esophagus, normal age-related changes
        in, 31
ESR. See Erythrocyte sedimentation rate.
Essential amino acids, 151–152
Ethics, 90–93. See also Legal and
        ethical issues.
    case study of, 90, 103
    definition of, 90–91
    vs. law, 91–93

Ethnicity, 163–164
    vs. culture, 163
Ethnocentrism, 162–163
Etiquette, 232
European Americans, 171–172
Eustress, 116
Evaluation
    of employees, 243–245
    in management and leadership, 237
    of medication therapy, 403–404
    in nursing process, 71–72
Examinations. See Physical
        examinations.
Excretion, of medications, 396–397
Exercise, 182–185
    amount of, 114, 187
    benefits of, 182–184, 186
    in rehabilitative and restorative
        care, 379
    types of, 114–115, 185
    in wellness, 113–116
Expert CNAs, 239
Expertise, clinical, five points of,
        238–240
Extremes, questions about, 358
Extreme temperatures, 130–131,
        138–139
Extrinsic factors, in falls, 318–319
Eyes, assessment of, 295. See also
        Vision.

Face, assessment of, 294–295
Failure to thrive, 361
Fall risks, 126–129, 318–320
    contributing factors in, 127, 318–319
    in home visits, listening and watching
        for, 138–139
    prevention measures for, 127–129,
        319–320
Families
    changes in roles and relationships
        in, 48
    communication with, 231–232
Fats, dietary, 149, 152
Feeding tubes, 158, 386
Feil, Naomi, 362
Ferritin, 430
Fiber, dietary, 323
Financial considerations
    cost of medications, 395
    and health insurance, 100–102
Fire safety, 136
Fitness, in wellness, 113–116
Flexibility, in end-of-life care, 202
Flexibility exercises, 114
Flooding, 136
Fluoride, 156
Flu vaccines, 260
Folate, 153–154
Folic acid test, 420
Food. See Nutrition.
Food-borne diseases, 261

Food journals, 149
Food poisoning, 136, 261
Friction, in pressure ulcers, 324, 326
Full-liquid diets, 157
Function
    assessment of, 306–309, 377
    definition of, 28, 29, 382
    normal age-related changes in, 28–33
    in rehabilitative and restorative care,
        377, 382–383
Functional assessment, 306–309, 377
Functional incontinence, 322

Gait
    in crutch walking, 385
    and falls, 319
Gastroesophageal reflex disease
        (GERD), 190–191
Gastrointestinal (GI) system
    assessment of, 274, 300–301
    and falls, 127
    normal age-related changes in, 31
Gender ratios, 7–8
Genetics, theory of aging based on,
        24–25
Genitourinary system
    assessment of, 274
    and falls, 127
    normal age-related changes in, 31–32
Genuineness, 352–353
GERD. See Gastroesophageal reflex
    disease.
Geriatric Depression Scale, Short
    Form, 342
Geriatrics, definition of, 5, 22
Gerontological nursing, 4–6
Gerontology, 4–6
    definition of, 4–5, 22
    need for nurses in, 5–6
Gerotranscendence, 14–15, 287
Glaucoma, 282
Globulins, 430
Goals, definition of, 376
Goal setting
    in management and leadership,
        236–237
    in nursing process, 67–69
    in rehabilitative and restorative care,
        378–379
Grief
    coping with, 117, 359
    stages of, 199–201, 359
Group therapy, for psychological
    problems, 365–366
Guided choices, 352

Habit training, 322
Hair, normal age-related changes in, 30
Half-life of drugs, 391
Hallucinations, 357
Halo error, 244
Hand hygiene, 258

HDL. See High-density lipoprotein.
Head, assessment of, 294–295
Health
    changes in, as transition, 48–49
    as continuum, 108–110
    definitions of, 106
    well-being and safety in, 292, 292f
Health-care proxy, 97, 205
Health emergencies, 137–138
Health insurance, 100–102
Health Insurance Portability and
        Accountability Act (HIPPA), 100
Health promotion. See Wellness.
Healthy People 2020, 114, 126, 129,
        185, 273, 411
Hearing changes
    common types of, 282–283
    normal age-related, 33
    and pharmacotherapeutics, 392
Heart, normal age-related changes in, 28
Heart failure
    case study of, 292, 311
    congestive, 190–191, 276–277
Heat, risks associated with, 130
Hematocrit tests, 417
Hematologic tests, 416–421
Hemoglobin tests, 417
Herpes Zoster vaccine, 260
Hierarchy of needs, 67
High-density lipoprotein (HDL)
    cholesterol, 431
HIPPA. See Health Insurance Portability
    and Accountability Act.
Hiring process, 242–243
Hispanic Americans, 172–175
History
    physiological, 292–306
    sexual, 263
HIV/AIDS, 134, 263–264
Holism, 9
Holistic assessment, 292
Holistic caring, 3–17
    basic concepts of, 9–10
    definition of, 9
    teamwork in, 10–11
Holistic wellness, 106. See also Wellness.
Home care
    environment of, 61, 218–219
    safety concerns to check on during
        visits, 138–140
Home remedies, 397–398
Homonymous hemianopsia, 280, 281f
Hospice care, 204, 219
Hospital care, 61, 222
HTN. See Hypertension.
Human caring, 11–14, 92
Humor, in end-of-life care, 202
Hygiene, hand, 258
Hypercalcemia, 425
Hyperkalemia, 424
Hypernatremia, 423–424
Hypertension (HTN), 277–278

Hyperthermia, 130, 131
Hypocalcemia, 424–425
Hypokalemia, 424
Hyponatremia, 423
Hypothermia, 130–131
Hypothyroidism, 286–287

IADLs. See Instrumental activities of
    daily living.
Iatrogenic disorders, 330
    case study of, 314, 331
Identification, of key processes for
    improvement, 246–247
IDTs. See Interdisciplinary teams.
Illness and diseases. See also specific
        types.
    acute. See Acute illness.
    case study of, 314, 331
    chronic. See Chronic illness.
    common types of, 313–332
    as continuum, 108–110
    medical diagnoses of, 66–67
    and mobility problems, 314–317
    as transition, 48
Imminent death, signs of, 206–207
Immobility. See Mobility changes.
Immune system, maintaining healthy,
    257–259
Immunizations, 257, 259–261
Implementation
    in management and leadership, 237
    of medication therapy, 403
    in nursing process, 70–71
    in rehabilitative and restorative care,
        379–382
Incentives, 108–109
Incomplete proteins, 152
Incontinence, 320–323
    acute, 321–322
    case study of, 182, 193–194
    chronic, 322–323
    normal age-related changes and,
        31–32, 320
    in rehabilitative and restorative care,
        379–381, 386
    training to prevent, 386
Infection(s), 255–268. See also
        specific types.
    case study of, 256, 267
    environmental cleanliness and,
        261–262
    immune system and, 257–259
    immunizations and, 259–261
Influenza vaccines, 260
Informed consent, 96–97
Injuries, from falls, 318–320
Insomnia, 190–191
Instructions, giving, 352
Instrumental activities of daily living
        (IADLs), 28, 29
    assessment of, 308–309, 308f
    definition and examples of, 308

Insurance
  health, 100–102
  long-term care, 101
Integrity, vs. despair, 14–15, 26
Integumentary system. *See also* Skin.
  assessment of, 301
  infections in, 258–259
  normal age-related changes in, 30–31
Interdisciplinary teams (IDTs),
  communication in, 232–233
International normalized ratio, 421
Interviews, in hiring process, 242–243
Intestines, normal age-related changes
  in, 31
Intimacy needs, 98–100. *See also*
  Sexuality.
Intrapulmonary changes, 29
Intrinsic factors, in falls, 318–319
Involvement, in environmental
  management, 214–215
Iodine, 156
Iron
  need for, 156
  testing of, 430–431
Isolation, and mental health
  disorders, 132

Jewish Americans, 38, 175–176
Job changes, 47–48
Joints
  degenerative joint disease in, 284,
    315–316
  maintenance of, in rehabilitative and
    restorative care, 379
  normal age-related changes in,
    29–30, 315
Journals, food, 149

Katz ADL scale, 307
Kitchens, as source of infection, 262
Krysl, Marilyn, 46–47
Kübler-Ross, Elisabeth, 199–200

Laboratory tests, 409–437
  case study of, 410, 436
  drug monitoring, 431–434
  hematologic, 416–421
  meaning of values, 411
  metabolic, 421–428
  screening, 412–416, 434
Laissez faire leadership style, 228
Latino Americans, 172–175
Lawton's IADL scale, 308, 308f
Laxative abuse, 399
LDL. *See* Low-density lipoprotein.
Leadership. *See* Management and
  leadership.
Legal and ethical issues, 89–104
  advance directives, 97–98
  case study of, 90, 103
  confidentiality, 100
  elder abuse, 98

financial considerations, 100–102
informed consent, 96–97
intimacy needs, 98–100
law vs. ethics, 91–93
liability, 93–94
negligence, malpractice, and
  omission, 94–95
patient rights, 91, 367
restraints, 90, 95–96, 103, 367
Leniency error, 244
Lesbian, gay, bisexual, and transgender
  (LGBT) population, 132–134
Liability, legal, 93–94
Life expectancies, 7
Life review, 52–53
Life story, writing, 52
Lifestyles
  and immune system, 257
  and wellness, 117–119
Life support, advance directives on,
  97–98
Lipoproteins, 431
Liquid diets, 157
Listening
  active, 234–235
  in end-of-life care, 202–203
  in holistic care, 10
  to people with psychological
    problems, 353
  for safety concerns, in home visits,
    138–139
Liver function tests, 427–428
Living wills, 97–98, 205
Long-term care facilities, 61–62,
  220–221
Long-term care insurance, 101
Long-term memory (LTM), 336–337
Low-density lipoprotein (LDL)
  cholesterol, 431
LTM. *See* Long-term memory.
Lungs, normal age-related changes
  in, 29
Lymphocytes, 418

MA-C. *See* Medication Aide – Certified.
Macular degeneration, 282
Magnesium, 155
Malnutrition, 326–328
  assessment of, 327
  and pressure ulcers, 325
  risk factors for, 147, 327, 429
Malorientation, in dementia, 363, 364
Malpractice, 94–95
Management
  of chronic diseases, 110–111
  of environments of care, 13, 212–215
  of quality of care, 246–247
  of stress, 116, 188
Management and leadership, 225–252
  care planning hoop in, 235–237, 236f
  case study of, 226, 249–250
  communication in, 229–235

definition and use of terms, 227
of personnel, 242–246
priority setting in, 238–242
quality of care in, 246–247
roles in, 227
styles of, 227–229
Marginalized people, 14
Maslow, Abraham, 67
Masturbation, 99–100
Matching technique, 354
MDROs. *See* Multidrug-resistant
  organisms.
MDS. *See* Minimum data set.
Medicaid, 8, 101
Medical diagnoses, 269–290. *See also*
  specific diagnoses.
  acute vs. chronic, 271–273
  case study of, 270, 288
  vs. nursing diagnoses, 66–67
Medicare, 8, 101
Medication Aide–Certified (MA-C),
  241–242
Medications, 389–407. *See also specific*
  types.
  abuse of, 117–119, 365, 398–399
  age-related changes affecting impact
    of, 391–393
  Beers criteria for, 399–400
  challenges of taking correctly, 393
  chronopharmacology of, 401
  common forms of misuse of, 393,
    397–399
  cost of, 395
  definitions related to, 391
  disposal of, 400
  drug-resistant organisms and, 265
  and falls, 128
  incontinence caused by, 321
  laboratory tests monitoring, 431–434
  nursing process with, 401–404
  pharmacokinetics of, 395–397
  polypharmacy and, 393–395
  promoting safe use of, 400–401
  for psychological problems, 366–367
  side effects of, 397, 398t
Memory
  assessment of, 336, 340
  depression and, 341–342
  impairments in, 336
  types of, 336–337
Mental health, 334–339
  characteristics of wellness in, 335
  cognitive functions in, 336–339
  definition of, 334
  disorders of. *See* Psychological
    problems.
  tools for assessment of, 339–342
Mental status examinations,
  339–340, 340t
Metabolic diseases, 285–287
Metabolic tests, 421–428
Metabolism, of medications, 396

Methicillin-resistant *Staphylococcus aureus* (MRSA), 265
Mexico, medications from, 394
Micturition, normal age-related changes in, 31
Middle-old population, 7
Minerals, 154–156, 157
Mini-Cog, 339, 340t, 341
Mini-Mental Status Exam (MMSE), 339, 340t, 341
Minimum data set (MDS)
    definition of, 64
    establishment of, 63
    problem areas identified by, 65–66
    sample, 60, 76f–87f
Mirroring technique, 354
MMSE. *See* Mini-Mental Status Exam.
Mobility changes, 314–317
    causes of, 315–317
    constipation caused by, 323
    incontinence caused by, 321
    and pressure ulcers, 324
Modified diets, 157
Monocytes, 418
Mosquitoes, 266
Motivation, 108–109
Mouth, assessment of, 296
Movement. *See also* Mobility changes.
    normal age-related changes in, 32
    repetitive, in dementia, 363–364
MRSA. *See* Methicillin-resistant *Staphylococcus aureus*.
Multicratic leadership style, 229
Multidrug-resistant organisms (MDROs), 265
Muscle strength
    exercises for, 114
    normal age-related changes in, 29–30, 315
Musculoskeletal system
    assessment of, 274, 304–305
    common chronic conditions in, 284–285
    and falls, 127
    in mobility problems, 315–316
    normal age-related changes in, 29–30, 315
Muslim Americans, 50, 165
MyPlate food guide, 149–150

Nails, normal age-related changes in, 30
NANDA. *See* North American Nursing Diagnosis Association.
Napping, 188
Narcotic drugs, 186
National Council of State Boards of Nursing (NCSBN), 240
Native Americans, 167–169
Natural disasters, safety in, 136–137
NCSBN. *See* National Council of State Boards of Nursing.
Neck, assessment of, 294–295

Needs, hierarchy of, 67
Negligence, 94–95
Nervous system
    assessment of, 274–275, 296–297
    common chronic conditions in, 279–283
    and falls, 127
    normal age-related changes in, 32–33
Neurons, normal age-related changes in, 32
Neutrophils, 418–419
Nightingale, Florence, 9, 212, 246
Nitrogen balance, 152
Nocturnal myoclonus, 191
Noncompliant patients, 108–109
Nonessential amino acids, 151–152
Nonverbal communication, 230–231, 354–355
Normal aging process, 27–33
North American Nursing Diagnosis Association (NANDA), 64–65
Nose, assessment of, 295
Novice CNAs, 238
Nurse practice acts (state laws), 93, 240
Nurses
    as end-of-life care providers, 201–203
    roles in rehabilitative and restorative care, 374–376
Nursing
    gerontological, 4–6
    holistic, 9–11
    philosophy of, 8–11
    transcultural, 163
Nursing diagnoses, 64–66
    case study of, 60–61
    vs. medical diagnoses, 66–67
    with medication therapy, 402
Nursing facilities (intermediate care), 220
Nursing homes, 220–221
    patient education on, 221
    stereotypes of, 24
    types of, 220
Nursing process, 62–72, 63f
    assessment in, 63–64, 68
    case study of, 58–61
    computers in, 72
    definition of, 62
    diagnosis in, 64–66
    evaluation in, 71–72
    implementation in, 70–71
    with medications, 401–404
    planning in, 67–70
Nutrient theory of aging, 26
Nutrition, 145–160
    altered status, 326–328
    assessment of, 147, 149, 327
    case study of, 146, 159
    and falls, 127, 128
    and immune system, 257
    needs of older adults, 149–157

    in rehabilitative and restorative care, 386
    theory of aging based on, 26
    tracking intake of, 148–149
    types of diet plans, 157–158
    and weight changes, 147–148
    in wellness, 112

OBRA. *See* Omnibus Budget Reconciliation Act.
O'Grady, Tim Porter, 21
Old-old population, 7
Omission, acts of, 94–95
Omnibus Budget Reconciliation Act (OBRA), 63, 95, 372
Open questions, 352
Oral cavity, normal age-related changes in, 31
Organizational involvement, total, 246
Orientation
    assessment of, 337, 340
    definition of, 337
    disorientation, 362–364
    malorientation, 363–364
Osteoarthritis, 284, 315–316
Osteoporosis, 30, 285, 315
OTC. *See* Over-the-counter.
Outcomes
    of care, identifying, 67–69
    of transitions, influencing, 41–44
Overflow incontinence, 322
Over-the-counter (OTC) medications, 397–398

Pain
    assessment of, 186–187
    as barrier to rest, 185–188
Palliative care
    in end-of-life care, 204
    in rehabilitative and restorative care, 384
Paranoia, 364–365
Parenteral nutrition (PN), 158
Parkinson's disease (PD), 281–282
Partial thromboplastin time (PTT) test, 420–421
Participative leadership style, 228–229
Passive behavior, 233–234
Paternalism, 14
Patient Care Partnership, 91
Patient education
    on assessment tools, 342
    on delirium, 362
    on immunizations, 257
    on incontinence, 321
    on medications, 403
    on nursing homes, 221
    on peripheral vascular disease, 279
    on pressure ulcers, 326
    in rehabilitative and restorative care, 374

on screening tests, 434
on self-care, 378
on skin lesions, 301
Patient Protection and Affordable Care Act (ACA), 101–102
Patient's Bill of Rights, 91
Patient Self-Determination Act, 97
PD. *See* Parkinson's disease.
PDCA (Plan, Do, Check, and Act) cycle, 247
Pelvic muscle exercises, 322–323
Perception, definition and assessment of, 336–337
Peripheral vascular disease, 278–279
Peripheral vascular system, assessment of, 297–298
Permissive leadership style, 228
Personalization, in environmental management, 13, 214
Personal space, in environmental management, 13, 214
Personnel management, 242–246
Pets, as source of infection, 261–262
Pharmacodynamics, definition of, 391
Pharmacokinetics
age-related changes in, 395–397
definition of, 391
Pharmacology, 389–407. *See also* Medications.
case study of, 390, 405
common problems in, 397–401
definition of, 391
Pharmacotherapeutics
age-related changes affecting, 391–395
definition of, 391
Phenytoin, 434
Philosophies of care, 8–11
case study of, 4, 16
characteristics of, 8–9
holistic, 9–11
Phosphate tests, 425
Phosphorus, 155
Photographs, collecting and organizing, 52–53
Physical examinations. *See also* Physiological assessment.
need for regular, 110
techniques for, 292, 294–306
Physical therapy, and falls, 128
Physiological assessment, 291–312
case studies of, 59–60, 292, 311
documentation of, 309
functional assessment in, 306–309
history in, 292–293
review of systems in, 294–306
Physiological changes, normal age-related, 28–33. *See also specific types.*
Physiological problems. *See* Illness and diseases.
Physiological theories of aging, 24–26, 27

PIM. *See* Potentially inappropriate medications.
Place orientation, 340
Plan, Do, Check, and Act (PDCA) cycle, 247
Planning, in nursing process. *See* Plans of care.
Planning hoop, 235–237, 236f
Plans of care, 67–70
design of, 67–70
documentation of, 68–70
evaluation of, 71–72
implementation of, 70–71
with medication therapy, 402–403
sample, 72, 73f
Plasma proteins, 157
Plasma tests, 421–422
Platelet count, 419
PLST. *See* Progressively lowered stress threshold.
PN. *See* Parenteral nutrition.
Pneumococcal vaccine, 260–261
Pneumonia, 258
Poisoning
carbon monoxide, 136
food, 136, 261
Polypharmacy, 393–395
Posture
and falls, 318
transitional, 128
Potassium
need for, 156
testing of, 424
Potentially inappropriate medications (PIM), 399–400
Poverty, definition and impacts of, 166
Power of attorney, 97, 205
Prayer, 51
Prediabetes, 285
Presbycusis, 282–283
Presbyopia, 282
Pressure ulcers, 324–326
assessment of risk, 301, 325
Braden scale of risk, 301, 302f–303f
definition of, 324
prevention of, 325–326
risk factors for, 324–325
staging of, 325
treatment of, 326
Priority setting
in management and leadership, 238–242, 248
in nursing process, 67
Privacy
in environmental management, 13, 214
in psychological assessment, 343
Problem-solving skills, definition and assessment of, 339
Proficient CNAs, 239
Progressively lowered stress threshold (PLST), 44–47

Prompted voiding, 322
Pronouns, vague, 358
Protein binding, 391
Proteins
need for, 149–152, 157
testing of, 429–430
Prothrombin time (PT) test, 420–421
Proxy, health-care, 97, 205
Psychological assessment, 333–348
case study of, 334, 346
cognitive functions in, 336–339
techniques for, 343–344
timing and frequency of, 342–343
tools for, 339–342, 340t
use of results of, 344–345
validity and reliability of scales, 342–343
Psychological health
developmental tasks in, 14–15, 26
in rehabilitative and restorative care, 377–378
Psychological problems, 349–369. *See also specific types.*
agitation caused by, 356–357
as barriers to sleep, 191
case study of, 350, 368
definition of, 350
group therapy for, 365–366
guidelines for communicating with people with, 350–356, 358
indicators of, 132
patient rights and, 367
psychotropic medications for, 366–367
safety concerns with, 131–132, 138–139, 351
somatization of, 367
stress-related, 356–357
terminology of, 351
Psychological theories of aging, 26–27
Psychological well-being, health and safety in, 292, 292f
Psychosocial well-being, in rehabilitative and restorative care, 381
Psychotropic medications, 366–367
PT. *See* Prothrombin time.
PTSD, indicators of, 132
PTT. *See* Partial thromboplastin time.
Pulmonary disease, chronic obstructive (COPD), 190–191, 283–284
Pulmonary system
assessment of, 274
common chronic conditions in, 283–284

Quality of care, management of, 246–247
Questions
about extremes, 358
open vs. closed, 352
Quinlan, Karen Ann, 97

RAI. *See* Resident Assessment
    Instrument.
RAPs. *See* Resident assessment
    protocols.
RBC. *See* Red blood cell.
Reality orientation, 366
Recency error, 244
Red blood cell (RBC) count, 416–417
Red blood cell (RBC) indices, 417–418
Rehabilitative and restorative care,
    371–388
    assessment of goals of, 382–384
    case study of, 372, 387
    changes affecting goals of, 376–378
    clinical implications of, 384–386
    vs. custodial care, 24, 372
    definitions of, 372–374
    development of goals for, 378–379
    implementation of goals in, 379–382
    nursing roles in, 374–376
Relationships
    definition of, 117
    in families, changes in, 48
    loss of, 117
    with people with psychological
        problems, 350–352
Relaxers, quick, 116
Religious belief
    case study of, 38, 54
    significance of, 39–40, 49–51
    vs. spirituality, 49
Relocation trauma, 215, 216
Reminiscence, 365
Remotivation, 365–366
Renal function, normal age-related
    changes in, 31
Repetitive motion, in dementia,
    363–364
Reproductive system
    assessment of, 305–306, 305f
    normal age-related changes in, 32
Researchers, nurses as, 375–376
Resident(s)
    communication with, 230–231
    definition and use of term, 62, 67
Resident Assessment Instrument
    (RAI), 63–65
Resident assessment protocols
    (RAPs), 63
Resocialization, 366
Resources, for addressing safety
    concerns, 140
Respiratory system
    assessment of, 298–300
    infections in, 258
    in mobility problems, 316
    normal age-related changes in,
        29, 316
Rest, 185–189
    benefits of, 182
    pain as barrier to, 185–188
    stress as barrier to, 188

Restless leg syndrome (RLS), 191
Restlessness, terminal (TR), 206
Restorative care. *See* Rehabilitative and
    restorative care.
Restraints, use of, 95–96, 367
    case study of, 90, 103
Retirement, as transition, 47–48
Retirement communities, continuing
    care, 62, 220
Review of systems, 273–275, 294–306
Rights, patient, 91, 367
RLS. *See* Restless leg syndrome.

Safety, well-being and health in,
    292, 292f
Safety concerns, 13, 125–143
    case study of, 126, 141
    elder abuse, 135, 139
    in emergency situations, 136–138,
        139, 140
    in environmental management,
        213–214
    extreme temperatures, 130–131,
        138–139
    falls, 126–129, 138–139
    in home visits, evaluating, 138–140
    mental health, 131–132,
        138–139, 351
    sexuality, 132–134, 139
    skin integrity, 129–130, 138–139
Sandwich generation, 48
Screening tests, 412–416, 434
Self-care, 119–120, 378, 386
Self-feeding, 386
Self-neglect, elder, 362
Self-responsibility, 119–120
Sense words, preferred, 358, 358t
Sensory changes
    common types of, 282–283
    and falls, 127
    normal age-related, 33
    and pharmacotherapeutics, 391–392
Serum glutamic-oxaloacetic
    transaminase (SGOT), 427
Sexual history, 263
Sexuality
    acting out, 357
    providing for intimacy needs, 98–100
    in rehabilitative and restorative
        care, 381
    safety measures regarding,
        132–134, 139
Sexually transmitted infections (STIs)
    and diseases (STDs), 134, 262–264
Sexual orientation, 132–134
SGOT. *See* Serum glutamic-oxaloacetic
    transaminase.
Shearing, in pressure ulcers, 324, 326
Shingles vaccine, 260
Short Portable Mental Status
    Questionnaire (SPMSQ), 339,
    340t, 341

Short-term memory (STM), 336–337
Sickle cell anemia, 165–166
Side effects of medications, 397, 398t
Sinuses, assessment of, 295
Skeleton, normal age-related changes
    in, 29
Skilled nursing facilities (SNF), 61, 220
Skin
    assessment of, 301
    common problems with, 324–326
    infections in, 259
    normal age-related changes in, 30
    normal vs. abnormal lesions on,
        301, 304t
    pressure ulcers on, 301, 302f–303f,
        324–326
    protecting integrity of, 129–130,
        138–139
Sleep, 189–192, 328–329
    case study of, 182, 194
    disorders of, 190–192, 329
    importance of, 182–183, 189
    during naps, 188
    normal age-related changes in,
        32–33, 189, 328–329
    normal patterns of, 189, 328
    strategies for promoting, 189, 329
Sleep apnea, 190, 329
Sleeping medications, 329
SNF. *See* Skilled nursing facilities.
Social function
    assessment of, 309
    definition of, 307, 309
Social Security, definition of, 8
Sodium
    need for, 155
    testing of, 422–424
Soft diets, 157
Somatization, 367
Speaking slowly, 358
Spirituality
    assessment of, 49–50, 380
    case study of, 38, 54
    in rehabilitative and restorative care,
        380–381
    vs. religion, 49
    significance of, 39–40, 49–51
SPMSQ. *See* Short Portable Mental
    Status Questionnaire.
Spouse, death of, 48
Standard precautions, 259
Staphylococcus aureus, methicillin-
    resistant (MRSA), 265
Statistics, high-quality, in total quality
    management, 246–247
STDs. *See* Sexually transmitted
    infections.
Stereotypes, 22–24
Stimulation, in environmental
    management, 13, 214
STIs. *See* Sexually transmitted
    infections.

STM. *See* Short-term memory.
Stomach, normal age-related changes in, 31
Stool, test for occult blood in, 415–416
Strengthening
  case study of, 182, 193
  exercises for, 114–115
Stress, 115–116
  as barrier to rest, 188
  common causes of, 45, 116
  management of, 116, 188
  progressively lowered threshold for, 44–47
  psychological problems caused by, 356–357
  of relocation, 215
Stress incontinence, 322
Stroke, 279–281
  case study of, 314, 331
  effects of, 280–281, 281f
  types of, 279–280
Subculture theory of aging, 26
Substance abuse, 117–119, 132, 365
Suicide risk, 360–361
Sundown syndrome, 329
Supplemental Social Security, definition of, 8
Supreme Court, U.S., 97
Sweat glands, normal age-related changes in, 30
Symbols, universal, 354–355, 355t

Tai chi, 284
Taste, changes in
  normal age-related, 33
  and pharmacotherapeutics, 392
TB. *See* Tuberculosis.
Tdap. *See* Tetanus, diphtheria, and pertussis.
Teams
  holistic, 10–11
  interdisciplinary, communication in, 232–233
Temperatures, extreme, 130–131, 138–139
Terminal restlessness (TR), 206
Territoriality, in environmental management, 214
Tests. *See* Laboratory tests.
Tetanus, diphtheria, and pertussis (Tdap) vaccine, 259–260
Theophylline, 433–434
Therapeutic diets, 157–158
Thinking, definition and assessment of, 338
Throat, assessment of, 296
TIBC. *See* Total iron-binding capacity.
Time confusion, in dementia, 363–364
Time orientation, 340
Tolerance, in end-of-life care, 202–203

Tools
  high-quality, in total quality management, 246–247
  for psychological assessment, 339–342, 340t
Total iron-binding capacity (TIBC), 431
Total quality management (TQM), 246–247
Total serum protein, 429
Touch
  nonverbal communication through, 354, 354t, 355
  normal age-related changes in, 33
  and pharmacotherapeutics, 392
Toxicology, 431–434
TQM. *See* Total quality management.
TR. *See* Terminal restlessness.
Transcultural nursing, 163
Transferrin, 431
Transitions, 37–56
  case study of, 38, 54
  common characteristics of, 41
  common types of, 40–41, 47–49
  definition of, 38–39
  influencing outcomes of, 41–44
  perception of, 43–44
  preparation for, 43
  progressively lowered stress threshold and, 44–47
  resolving problems with, 51–53
  significance of, 38–40
  spirituality in, 39–40, 49–51
Transpersonal caring, 213
Trauma, relocation, 215–216
Treatment strategies, for chronic conditions, 111
Troponins, 428
Tube feedings, 158, 386
Tuberculin skin test, 412
Tuberculosis (TB), 264–266
  case study of, 256, 267
  test for, 412

UCs. *See* Urinary catheters.
Ulcers. *See* Pressure ulcers.
Universal precautions, 259
Universal symbols, 354–355, 355t
Urge incontinence, 322
Uric acid, 426–427
Urinalysis, 412–415, 413t–414t
Urinary catheters (UCs), 261
Urinary incontinence, 320–323
  acute, 321–322
  chronic, 322–323
  costs of, 320
  definition of, 320
  in rehabilitative and restorative care, 379
Urinary system, assessment of, 306
Urinary tract infections (UTIs), 258, 321, 415

Urination, frequent, in insomnia, 190–191
Urine specimens, 24-hour, 415
UTIs. *See* Urinary tract infections.

Vague pronouns, 358
Validation groups, 366
Validation Method, 358, 362–363
Values, in communication, 353
Vegetation stage of dementia, 363–364
Verbal communication, 230, 352
Violent behavior, 357
Vision changes
  common types of, 282–283
  and falls, 319
  normal age-related, 33
  and pharmacotherapeutics, 391–392
Visual inspections, for safety concerns, 139–140
Vitamin B_{12} test, 420
Vitamins, 152–154

Walking programs, in rehabilitative and restorative care, 384–386
Water
  functions of, 156–157
  need for, 156–157
Water-borne diseases, 261
Watson, Jean, 11–14, 92, 213
WBC. *See* White blood cell.
Wear and tear theory of aging, 25
Weight
  and nutrition, 147–148
  reasons for changes in, 147–148
Well-being
  health and safety in, 292, 292f
  psychosocial and spiritual, in rehabilitative and restorative care, 381
Wellness, 105–123
  case study of, 106, 121
  with chronic diseases, 110–111
  as continuum, 108–110
  exercise and fitness in, 113–116
  health-promotion activities in, 107–108, 109–110
  lifestyles and, 117–119
  in mental health, 335
  nutrition in, 112
  objective of, 107
  regular physical exams in, 110
  self-care in, 119–120
West Nile virus, 266
White blood cell (WBC) count, 418
White blood cell (WBC) differential, 418–419
White blood cells, functions of, 418
Writing, of life story, 52
Yoga, 315
Young-old population, 7

Zinc, 156